Priorities in
CRITICAL CARE
NURSING

Priorities in CRITICAL CARE NURSING

FOURTH EDITION

LINDA D. URDEN, RN, DNSc, CNA, FAAN
Director, Outcomes Research
Clarian Health Partners
Indianapolis, Indiana;
Adjunct Associate Professor
Adult Health Department
Indiana University
Indianapolis, Indiana

KATHLEEN M. STACY, RN, MS, CNS, CCRN
Nurse Manager/Clinical Nurse Specialist
Intermediate Care Unit
Palomar Medical Center Escondido, California;
Adjunct Faculty Member
School of Nursing, College of Health and Human Services
San Diego State University
San Diego, California

MARY E. LOUGH, RN, MS, CNS, CCRN
Clinical Nurse Specialist
Medical/Surgical/Trauma ICU
Stanford Hospital and Clinics
Stanford, California;
Associate Clinical Professor
Department of Physiological Nursing
University of California, San Francisco
San Francisco, California

With 200 illustrations

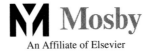
Mosby
An Affiliate of Elsevier

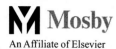

An Affiliate of Elsevier

11830 Westline Industrial Drive
St. Louis, Missouri 63146

NOTICE

Nursing is an ever-changing field. Standard safety precautions must be followed, but as new research and clinical experience broaden our knowledge, changes in treatment and drug therapy may become necessary or appropriate. Readers are advised to check the most current product information provided by the manufacturer of each drug to be administered to verify the recommended dose, the method and duration of administration, and contraindications. It is the responsibility of the licensed health care provided, relying on experience and knowledge of the patient, to determine dosages and the best treatment for each individual patient. Neither the Publisher nor the editors assume any liability for any injury and/or damage to persons or property arising from this publication.

The Publisher

Library of Congress Cataloging-in-Publication Data

Priorities in critical care nursing / [edited by] Linda D. Urden, Kathleen M. Stacy, Mary
     E. Lough.—4th ed.
          p.; cm.
     Includes bibliographical references and index.
     ISBN 0-323-02481-5 (alk. paper)
          1. Intensive care nursing. I. Urden, Linda Diann. II. Stacy, Kathleen M. III. Lough,
Mary E.
          [DNLM: 1. Critical Care. 2. Nursing Care. WY 154 P958 2003]
     RT120.I5E83 2003
     610.73′6–dc22

                                                                                        2003061506

Executive Publisher: Barbara Nelson Cullen
Developmental Editor: Adrienne Simon
Publishing Services Manager: John Rogers
Project Manager: Doug Turner
Designer: Amy Buxton

Printed in the United States of America

Last digit is the print number: 9   8   7   6   5   4   3   2

Contributors

Kim Blount, RN, MSN, CCRN
Cardiovascular Clinical Nurse Specialist
Carolinas Medical Center
Charlotte, North Carolina

Beverly Carlson, MS, RN, CNS
Cardiac Research Project Director
Sharp Healthcare;
San Diego, California

JoAnn M. Clark, RN, MSN, CGNP, CFNP
Gerontological and Family Nurse Practitioner
Assistant Clinical Professor
Internal Medicine/Medicine for Seniors
University of California, San Diego
La Jolla, California

Joni Dirks, RN, MS, CCRN
Clinical Nurse Specialist
Department of Veterans Affairs Medical Center
Palo Alto, California

Barbara J. Draude, RN, MSN
Assistant Professor
Middle Tennessee State University
School of Nursing
Mufreesboro, Tennessee

Lorraine Fitzsimmons, DNS, FNP, BC
Graduate Program Chair
Advanced Practice Nursing of Adults and the Elderly
San Diego State University School of Nursing
San Diego, California

Ruth N. Grendell, RN, DNSc
Professor of Nursing (Emerita)
Point Loma Nazarene University
San Diego, California;
Adjunct Professor University of Phoenix
San Diego, California

Lynne Jett, RN, C, MSN
Instructor, BSN Program
California State University, Dominguez Hills
Dominguez Hills, California

Karen L. Johnson, PhD, RN, CCRN
Assistant Professor
University of Maryland School of Nursing
Baltimore, Maryland

Mary E. Lough, RN, MS, CNS, CCRN
Clinical Nurse Specialist
Medical/Surgical/Trauma ICU
Stanford Hospital and Clinics
Stanford, California;
Associate Clinical Professor
Department of Physiological Nursing
University of California, San Francisco
San Francisco, California

Jeanne M. Maiden, RN, MS, CNS, CCRN
Critical Care Clinical Nurse Specialist
University of California at San Diego Medical Center
San Diego, California

Kathleen A. Mendez, RN, MS, CNS, CCRN
Nurse Manager/Clinical Nurse Specialist
Cardia Care Unit
Palomar Medical Center
Escondido, California

Judith K. Glann Mitchell, RN, MSN, CCRN, CNS/Rx, ACNP
Cardiovascular/Critical Care Clinical Nurse Specialist/Rx
New Mexico VA Healthcare System
Albuquerque, New Mexico

Mary Courtney Moore, RN, RD, PhD
Research Assistant Professor
Vanderbilt University School of Medicine
Nashville, Tennessee

Kathy C. Richards, PhD, RNP
Research Health Scientist
Central Arkansas Veterans Healthcare System;
Associate Professor
University of Arkansas for Medical Sciences College of
  Nursing
Little Rock, Arkansas

Mary Schira, PhD, RN, APRN, BC, ACNP
Associate Clinical Professor
Director, Acute Care and Emergency
Nurse Practitioner Programs
University of Texas at Arlington
School of Nursing
Arlington, Texas

Kathleen M. Stacy, RN, MS, CNS, CCRN
Nurse Manager/Clinical Nurse Specialist
Intermediate Care Unit
Palomar Medical Center
Escondido, California;
Adjunct Faculty Member
School of Nursing, College of Health and Human Services
San Diego State University
San Diego, California

Sheila Cox Sullivan, PhD, RN
Associate Professor and Associate Dean
College of Nursing
Harding University
Searcy, Arkansas

Linda D. Urden, RN, DNSc, CNA, FAAN
Director, Outcomes Research
Clarian Health Partners
Indianapolis, Indiana;
Adjunct Associate Professor
Adult Health Department
Indiana University
Indianapolis, Indiana

Reviewers

Joyce Oppenheimer, MSN, RN
Assistant Professor
Nursing Department
Endicott College
Beverly, Massachusetts

Sandra O'Sullivan, MS, RN, CCRN
Clinical Academic Instructor
Pennsylvania State University
School of Nursing
University Park, Pennsylvania

Marilyn Pase, RN, MSN
Associate Professor
Department of Nursing
New Mexico State University
Las Cruces, New Mexico

Michaelynn Paul, RN, BSN, CCRN
Instructor
Walla Walla College
School of Nursing
Portland, Oregon

To critical care nurses who strive for excellence in care
LDU

For my wonderful family -
James, Sherrie-Anne, and Meniko
Thank you for all your loving support!

For my wonderful staff in the Intermediate Care Unit
Thank you for all your positive affirmations!
KMS

Dedicated to my mother,
Margaret Agnes Greally Lough
MEL

Preface

We are grateful to the many students, nurses, and educators who made the first three editions of *Priorities in Critical Care Nursing* successful. We actively solicited input from users of the third edition and incorporated their comments and suggestions regarding format, content, and organization for this book. The emphasis continues to be on priorities for the critical care nurse. We believe that prioritizing conditions and issues will assist critical care nurses in quickly assessing and intervening in the most efficient and effective manner.

ORGANIZATION

The book is again organized around alterations in dimensions of human functioning that span the biopsychosocial realms.

Organizationally, the book comprises ten major units. The chapter content of Unit One, *Foundations of Critical Care Nursing Practice*, forms the basis of practice regardless of the physiologic alterations of the critically ill patient. Although chapters in this book may be studied in any sequence, we recommend that Chapter 1, *Caring for the Critically Ill Patient*, be studied first because it clarifies the major assumptions on which the book is based.

Unit Two, *Common Problems in Critical Care*, examines potential critical care practice problems and is divided into six chapters: *Psychosocial Alterations*, *Sleep Alterations*, *Nutritional Alterations*, *Gerontologic Alterations*, *Pain Management*, and *Sedation Assessment and Management*.

Unit Three, *Cardiovascular Alterations*, Unit Four, *Pulmonary Alterations*, and Unit Five, *Neurologic Alterations*, are each organized according to the following three-chapter format:

Assessment and Diagnosis
Disorders
Therapeutic Management

This organization permits easy retrieval of information for students and clinicians and provides flexibility for the educator to individualize teaching methods by assigning chapters that best suit student needs.

Unit Six, *Renal Alterations*, Unit Seven, *Gastrointestinal Alterations*, and Unit Eight, *Endocrine Alterations*, are each organized according to the following two-chapter format:

Assessment and Diagnostic Procedures
Disorders and Therapeutic Management

Unit Nine, *Multisystem Alterations*, addresses disorders that affect multiple body systems and necessitate discussion as a separate category. Unit Nine is organized in a two-chapter format:

Trauma
Shock and Multiple Organ Dysfunction Syndrome

Unit Ten, *Nursing Management Plans of Care*, contains the core of critical care nursing practice in a nursing process format: signs and symptoms, nursing diagnosis, outcome criteria, and nursing interventions. The nursing management plans of care are referenced throughout the book within the *Nursing Diagnosis Priorities* boxes.

Finally, the Appendix, *Physiologic Formulas for Critical Care*, features commonly encountered hemodynamic and oxygenation formulas and other calculations presented in easily understood terms.

NURSING DIAGNOSIS AND MANAGEMENT

The power of research-based critical care practice has been incorporated into nursing interventions. To foster critical thinking and decision making, a boxed menu of nursing diagnoses complete with specific etiologic or related factors accompanies each medical disorder and major medical treatment discussion and directs the learner to the section of the book where appropriate nursing management is detailed.

In keeping with the emphasis on priorities in critical care, *Nursing Diagnosis Priorities* boxes list the most urgent potential nursing diagnoses to be addressed. To facilitate student learning, the nursing management plans of care incorporate nursing diagnoses, etiologic or related factors, clinical manifestations, and interventions with rationales. The nursing management plans of care are liberally cross-referenced throughout the book for easy retrieval by the reader.

NEW TO THIS EDITION

New to this edition are the following chapters:

Chapter 1, *Caring for the Critically Ill Patient*
Chapter 9, *Sedation Assessment and Management*

Chapter 1 content includes an overview of critical care and contemporary critical care practice, including nursing roles, professional organizations, standards of practice, and evidence-based practice. Holistic critical care nursing methodologies are discussed, as well as nursing's unique contribution to health care. Interdisciplinary planning for care of the critically ill patient is described in the areas of care models, care management tools, and managing variances. Chapter 9 focuses on sedation and oversedation in the critical care setting. The content comprises the different levels of sedation, the role of assessment tools to determine sedation requirements, and both pharmacologic and non-pharmacologic interventions.

A feature new to this edition is the *Collaborative Management Priorities* boxes in the nursing management sections. These boxes focus on the aspects of multidisciplinary care in the management of patients in the critical care setting. Another new feature is the *Patient Safety Priorities* boxes accompanying each therapeutic management chapter, as appropriate. The purpose of these boxes is to highlight for the learner any safety issue that is specific and related to the chapter discussion.

LEARNER ENHANCEMENTS

To accompany the *Priorities in Critical Care Nursing* textbook, the teaching and learning package has been revised for this edition. The *Instructor's Resource* provides a variety of aids to help enhance the course instruction. It is available both on-line on the Evolve Web site and on CD. Included are sample course outlines with teaching strategies, a test-bank of over 500 questions with answers and rationales, and PowerPoint lecture slides of key text, tables, and boxes. In addition, an electronic image collection of 125 images from the book is included.

The Evolve Web site also includes WebLinks, which allow you to directly access hundreds of active Web sites keyed to each chapter of the book. These WebLinks are constantly updated so that you will have access to the most cutting-edge information in the field.

This edition of *Priorities in Critical Care Nursing* has become Web-active with open-book quizzes available on the *Student Resource* portion of the Evolve Web site. Students can test their knowledge and review key issues using this helpful study tool.

Priorities in Critical Care Nursing, fourth edition, represents our continued commitment to bringing you the best in all things a textbook can offer: the best and brightest in contributing and consulting authors; the latest in scientific research befitting the current state of health care and nursing; an organizational format that exercises diagnostic reasoning skills and is logical and consistent; and outstanding artwork and illustrations that enhance student learning. We pledge our continued commitment to excellence in critical care education.

ACKNOWLEDGMENTS

The talent, hard work, and inspiration of many people have produced the fourth edition of *Priorities in Critical Care Nursing*. We appreciate the assistance of our acquisition editor, Barbara Nelson Cullen, and our developmental editor, Adrienne Simon. We are also grateful to our project manager, Doug Turner, for his scrupulous attention to detail.

Linda D. Urden
Kathleen M. Stacy
Mary E. Lough

Contents

UNIT ONE

FOUNDATIONS OF CRITICAL CARE NURSING PRACTICE

LINDA D. URDEN

Caring for the Critically Ill Patient

Objectives

- Describe critical care nursing roles.
- Discuss the importance of holistic care for the critically ill patient and family.
- Articulate nursing's unique role in health care.
- List and discuss the six phases of the nursing process in critical care.
- Compare and contrast interdisciplinary critical care management models and tools.
- Explain the safety issues in the critical care environment.

evolve Be sure to check out the free exercises on-line at *http://evolve.elsevier.com/Urden/priorities/*

CONTEMPORARY CRITICAL CARE

Critical care today is provided to patients by a multidisciplinary team of health care professionals who have in-depth education in the specialty field of critical care. The team consists of physician intensivists, specialty physicians, nurses, advanced-practice nurses and other specialty nurse clinicians, pharmacists, respiratory therapy practitioners, other specialized therapists and clinicians, social workers, and clergy. Critical care is provided in specialized units or departments, with a focus on the continuum of care and efficient transition of care from one setting to another.

CRITICAL CARE NURSING ROLES

Nurses provide and contribute to the care of critically ill patients in a variety of roles. The most prominent role for the professional registered nurse (RN) is that of direct care provider. Other nurse clinicians also contribute to patient care, including patient educators, cardiac rehabilitation specialists, physician's office nurses, and infection control specialists. The specific types of expanded-role nursing positions are determined by individual organizational resources and needs.

Advanced-practice nurses (APNs) have met educational and clinical requirements beyond the basic nursing educational requirements for all nurses. The APNs in critical care areas are predominantly the clinical nurse specialist (CNS) and the nurse practitioner (NP) or acute care nurse practitioner (ACNP). APNs have a broad depth of knowledge and expertise in their specialty area and manage complex clinical and systems issues. The organizational system and existing resources of an institution determine what roles may be needed and how these roles function.

CNSs serve in specialty roles that require their clinical, teaching, research, leadership, and consultative abilities. They work in direct clinical roles and systems or administrative roles and in various other settings in the health care system. They may be organized by specialty, such as cardiovascular, or function, such as cardiac rehabilitation. CNSs also may be designated as case managers for specific patient populations.

NPs and ACNPs manages clinical care of a group of patients and have various levels of prescriptive authority, depending on the state and practice area in which they work. They also provide care consistency, interact with families, plan for patient discharge, and provide teaching to patients, families, and other members of the heath care team.[1]

CRITICAL CARE NURSING STANDARDS

The American Association of Critical-Care Nurses (AACN) has established nursing standards to provide a framework for critical care nurses. The standards are authoritative statements that describe the level of care and performance by which the quality of nursing care can be judged. Standards serve as descriptions of expected nursing roles and responsibilities.[2] The six AACN *Standards of Care for Acute and Critical Care Nursing* are prescriptive of a competent level of nursing practice (Box 1-1). The AACN also provides eight standards of professional practice (Box 1-2).

EVIDENCE-BASED PRACTICE

Much of early medical and nursing practice was based on nonscientific traditions that resulted in variable and haphazard patient outcomes.[3] These traditions and rituals, which were based on folklore, "gut instinct," trial and error, and personal preference, were often passed down from one generation of practitioners to another.[3-5]

The dramatic and multiple changes in health care and the ever-increasing presence of managed care in all geographic regions have resulted in greater emphasis on demonstrating the effectiveness of treatments and practices on outcomes.[6] In addition, increased emphasis is placed on efficiency, cost-effectiveness, quality of life, and patient satisfaction ratings.[7] It has become essential for nurses to use the best data available to make patient care decisions and carry out the appropriate nursing interventions. Through a scientific basis, with its ability to explain and predict, nurses are able to provide research-based interventions with consistent, positive outcomes.

Box 1-1 **AACN Standards of Care for Acute and Critical Care Nursing**

STANDARD OF CARE I: ASSESSMENT

The nurse caring for acute and critically ill patients collects relevant patient health care data.

STANDARD OF CARE II: DIAGNOSIS

The nurse caring for acute and critically ill patients analyzes the assessment data in determining diagnoses.

STANDARD OF CARE III: OUTCOME IDENTIFICATION

The nurse caring for acute and critically ill patients identifies individualized, expected outcomes for the patient.

STANDARD OF CARE IV: PLANNING

The nurse caring for acute and critically ill patients develops a plan of care that prescribes interventions to attain expected outcomes.

STANDARD OF CARE V: IMPLEMENTATION

The nurse caring for acute and critically ill patients implements interventions identified in the plan of care.

STANDARD OF CARE VI: EVALUATION

The nurse caring for acute and critically ill patients evaluates the patient's progress toward attaining expected outcomes.

From American Association of Critical-Care Nurses: *Standards of care for acute and critical care nursing*, Aliso Viejo, Calif, 1998, The Association.

Box **1-2**   AACN Standards of Professional Practice for Acute and Critical Care Nursing

STANDARD OF PROFESSIONAL PRACTICE I: QUALITY OF CARE

The nurse caring for acute and critically ill patients systematically evaluates the quality and effectiveness of nursing practice.

STANDARD OF PROFESSIONAL PRACTICE II: INDIVIDUAL PRACTICE EVALUATION

The nurse caring for acute and critically ill patients reflects knowledge of current professional practice standards, laws, and regulations.

STANDARD OF PROFESSIONAL PRACTICE III: EDUCATION

The nurse caring for acute and critically ill patients maintains current knowledge and competency in the care of acute and critically ill patients.

STANDARD OF PROFESSIONAL PRACTICE IV: COLLEGIALITY

The nurse caring for acute and critically ill patients interacts with and contributes to the professional development of peers and other health care providers as colleagues.

STANDARD OF PROFESSIONAL PRACTICE V: ETHICS

The nurse's decision and actions on behalf of acute and critically ill patients are determined in an ethical manner.

STANDARD OF PROFESSIONAL PRACTICE VI: COLLABORATION

The nurse caring for acute and critically ill patients collaborates with the team, consisting of patient, family, and health care providers, in providing patient care in a healing, humane, and caring environment.

STANDARD OF PROFESSIONAL PRACTICE VII: RESEARCH

The nurse caring for acute and critically ill patients uses clinical inquiry in practice.

STANDARD OF PROFESSIONAL PRACTICE VIII: RESOURCE UTILIZATION

The nurse caring for acute and critically ill patients considers factors related to safety, effectiveness, and cost in planning and delivering patient care.

From American Association of Critical-Care Nurses: *Standards of care for acute and critical care nursing*, Aliso Viejo, Calif, 1998, The Association.

HOLISTIC CARE

The high-technology–driven critical care environment is fast paced and directed toward monitoring and treating life-threatening changes in patient conditions. For this reason, attention is often focused on the technology and treatments necessary for maintaining stability in the physiologic functioning of the patient. Great emphasis is placed on technical skills and professional competence and responsiveness to critical emergencies. Concern has been voiced about the lesser emphasis on the caring component of nursing in this fast-paced, highly technologic health care environment.[8,9] Nowhere is this more evident than in areas where critical care nursing is practiced. Keeping the *care* in nursing care is one of our greatest challenges.[9] The critical care nurse must be able to deliver high-quality care skillfully, using all appropriate technologies, while incorporating psychosocial and other holistic approaches as appropriate to the time and the patient's condition.

The caring aspect between nurses and patients is fundamental to the nurse-patient relationship and to the health care experience. Holistic care focuses on human integrity and stresses that the body, mind, and spirit are interdependent and inseparable. Thus, all aspects need to be considered in planning and delivering care.[10]

Health care providers clearly understand that a patient's physical condition progresses in fairly predictable stages, depending on the presence or absence of comorbid conditions. Less clearly understood is the effect of psychosocial issues on the healing process. For this reason, special consideration must be given to determining the unique interventions that will positively impact each individual patient and help the patient progress toward desired outcomes.

An important aspect in the care delivery to and recovery of critically ill patients is the personal support of family members and significant others. The value of both patient-centered and family-centered care should not be underestimated.[11] It is important for families to be included in care decisions and to be encouraged to participate in the care of the patient as appropriate for the patient's level of needs and the family's level of ability.

Cultural diversity in health care is not a new topic but is gaining emphasis and importance as the world becomes more accessible to all as the result of increasing technologies and interfaces with places and peoples. Diversity includes not only ethnic sensitivity but also sensitivity and openness to differences in lifestyles, opinions, values, and beliefs. Unless cultural differences are taken into account, optimal health care cannot be provided. More attention has been directed recently at determining the physiologic and disease development and progression differences among various ethnic groups. Mortality rates from cardiovascular disease are significantly higher for both black men and black women than for white men and white women. The prevalence of coronary heart disease is highest in black women, followed by Mexican American men.[12] An increased sensitivity to the health care needs and vulnerabilities of all groups must be developed by care providers.

Cultural competence is one way to ensure that individual differences related to culture are incorporated into the plan of care.[13,14] Nurses must possess knowledge about biocultural, psychosocial, and linguistic differences in diverse populations to make accurate assessments. Interventions must then be tailored to address the uniqueness of each patient and family.

NURSING'S UNIQUE ROLE IN HEALTH CARE

Nursing is dynamic and responds to the changing nature of societal needs.[15] Four key features of contemporary nursing practice are described as follows[15]:

1. Attention to the full range of human experiences and responses to health and illness without restriction to a problem-focused orientation
2. Integration of objective data with knowledge gained from an understanding of the patient's or group's subjective experience
3. Application of scientific knowledge to the processes of diagnosis and treatment
4. Provision of a caring relationship that facilitates health and healing

The phenomena of concern to nurses are human experiences and responses to birth, illness, and death. Specifically, nursing care focuses on the following areas[15]:

- Physiologic and pathophysiologic processes
- Care and self-care processes
- Physical and emotional comfort, discomfort, and pain
- Emotions related to experiences of birth, health, illness, and death
- Meanings ascribed to health and illness
- Decision-making and choice-making abilities
- Perceptual orientations
- Relationships, role performance, and change processes within relationships

THE NURSING PROCESS

The nursing process is a method for making clinical decisions. It is a way of thinking and acting in relation to the clinical phenomena of concern to nurses. The nursing process is a systematic decision-making model that is cyclic, not linear. By virtue of its evaluation phase, the nursing process incorporates a feedback loop that maintains quality control of its decision-making outputs. Similar to a problem-solving method, the nursing process begins with an assessment phase and offers an organized, systematic approach to clinical problems. Unlike a problem-solving method, however, the nursing process is continuous, not episodic (Figure 1-1).

Nursing Diagnosis

The North American Nursing Diagnosis Association (NANDA) has supported the continued development and evolution of research-based nursing diagnoses.[16] With nursing diagnosis as a component of their decision-making methods, nurses necessarily become more systematic in the collection and interpretation of data and accomplish a

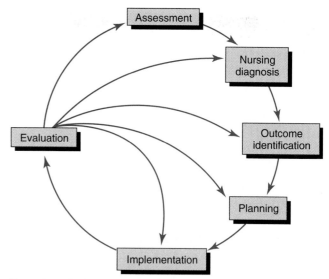

Figure 1-1   Cyclic nature of the nursing process. (Modified from Fortinash K, Holoday-Worret P: *Psychiatric nursing care plans,* ed 4, St Louis, 2002, Mosby.)

change in the substance of clinical nursing operations, from symptom management to problem solving. The most essential and distinguishing feature of any nursing diagnosis is that it describes a health condition *primarily resolved by nursing interventions or therapies.*

Some nursing diagnoses need accompanying qualifiers or specifiers based on the characteristics of the health problem as it manifests itself in a particular patient (Box 1-3). For example, the diagnosis *Fear* needs specification as to the object of the patient's particular fear, such as death, pain, disfigurement, or malignancy.

Outcome Identification

The emphasis on patient outcomes has become increasingly important in the provision of quality care and services. It is important that nurse-sensitive outcomes are delineated so that nursing care and services can be described and understood by all health care professionals, consumers, and payers.[17,18] Outcome statements consist of highly specific indicators that will be used by the nurse in the evaluation phase as criteria that either (1) the actual diagnosis has been resolved or reduced or (2) the risk diagnosis has not occurred. An outcome statement is a projection of the expected influence that the nursing intervention will have on the patient in relation to the identified diagnosis.

Outcome criteria should be measurable, desirable, and attainable, with full consideration given to patient/nurse resources. Measurable outcome criteria consist of recognizable patient behaviors, statements, and physiologic parameters. Many of the phenomena that critical care nurses diagnose and treat are readily measurable, such as adequacy of spontaneous ventilation, cardiac output, and tissue perfusion. Outcome statements are made further measurable by

Box **1-3** Format for Nursing Diagnoses

ACTUAL PROBLEM (THREE-PART STATEMENT)

Part 1: Nursing diagnosis

Altered Tissue Perfusion: Myocardial

Part 2: Etiologic factors (related to:)

Acute myocardial ischemia secondary to CAD

Part 3: Defining characteristics

Angina >30 min but <6 hr
ST-segment elevation on 12-lead ECG
Elevation of CK and CK-MB enzymes
Apprehension

RISK PROBLEM (TWO-PART STATEMENT)

Part 1: Nursing diagnosis

Risk for Aspiration

Part 2: Etiologic factors (related to:)

Impaired laryngeal sensation or reflex
Impaired laryngeal peristalsis or tongue function
Impaired laryngeal closure or elevation
Increased gastric volume
Increased intragastric pressure
Decreased lower esophageal sphincter pressure
Decreased antegrade esophageal propulsion

CAD, Coronary artery disease; ECG, electrocardiogram; CK, creatine kinase; CK-MB, MB isoenzyme of creatine kinase.

indicating the date and time of anticipated attainment. The individual patient's baseline and patterns and the available nurse/patient resources are the dominant considerations in a projection of desired outcome versus normative values.

Planning

During the planning phase, comprehensive planning of all care and services for the patient is done. The process consists of collaboration by the nurse with all appropriate health care providers, the patient, and family members as well as significant others.

Implementation

Implementation is the action component of planning. The nursing treatment plan is carried out in this phase of the nursing process. Assessment and evaluation are continuous throughout the implementation phase.

Nursing Interventions

Also known as *nursing orders* or *nursing prescriptions*, nursing interventions constitute the treatment approach to an identified health alteration. Interventions are selected to satisfy the outcome criteria and prevent or resolve the nursing diagnosis. Interventions have the greatest impact when they are directed at the etiologic/related factors of the diagnosis

or, in the case of a risk diagnosis, the risk factors. This approach stipulates that the etiologic factors of a problem can be modified by nursing management.

Evaluation

Evaluation of attainment of the expected patient outcomes occurs formally at intervals designated in the outcome criteria. Informal evaluation occurs continuously. The evaluation phase and the associated activities may be the most important dimensions of the nursing process.

INTERDISCIPLINARY CRITICAL CARE MANAGEMENT

The managed care environment has placed emphasis on examining methods of care delivery and processes of care by all health care professionals. Partnerships have been formed or strengthened, with a focus on increasing quality of care and services while containing or decreasing costs. Coordination of care in critical care units has been demonstrated to influence patient outcomes significantly.[19]

Case Management

Case management is the process of overseeing the care of patients and organizing services in collaboration with the patient's physician or primary health care provider. The case manager may be a nurse, allied health care provider, or the patient's primary care provider. Case managers are usually assigned to a specific population group, and they facilitate effective coordination of care services as patients move in and out of different settings. Ideally, the case manager oversees the care of the patient across the continuum of care.

Outcomes Management

Outcomes management refers to a model aimed at managing the outcomes of care by the use of various tools, quality improvement processes, and interdisciplinary team involvement and action. Specifically, emphasis is placed on consistent standards of care, measurement of disease-specific clinical outcomes as well as patient functioning and well-being, and assessment of clinical and outcome data for the specific conditions.[20] Outcomes management also takes place in multiple settings across the continuum of care. Professional nurse outcomes managers ensure that variances from the plan of care are addressed in a timely manner. They also examine aggregate information with the team for quality improvement in the interdisciplinary plan of care.

Care Management Tools

Many quality improvement tools are available to providers for care management.

Clinical Pathway

The clinical pathway presents an overview of the entire multidisciplinary plan of care for routine patients. It focuses on the critical elements in the care of certain patient populations and may track variances from the pathway. Pathways are developed by a multidisciplinary team based on a specific diagnosis or condition and integrated with the most recent research and best practices from the literature. Pathways are ideal for high-volume diagnosis groups that are amenable to standardization. Many pathways are incorporated into the medical record or computerized, making them a permanent part of the clinical record.

Algorithm

An algorithm is a stepwise decision-making flowchart for a specific care process or processes. Algorithms are more focused than clinical pathways and guide the clinician through the "if, then" decision-making process, addressing patient responses to particular treatments. Well-known examples of algorithms are the advanced cardiac life support (ACLS) algorithms published by the American Heart Association.

Practice Guideline

A practice guideline is usually developed by a professional organization (e.g., AACN, Society of Critical Care Medicine, American College of Cardiology) or a government agency (e.g., Agency for Health Care Research and Quality). Practice guidelines are generally written in text prose style rather than in the flowchart format of pathways and algorithms. Practice guidelines are used as resources in formulating the pathway or algorithm.

Protocol

A protocol is a common tool in research studies. Protocols are more directive and rigid than pathways or guidelines, and providers should not vary from a protocol. Patients are screened carefully for specific entry criteria before being started on a protocol. The many national research protocols include those for cancer and chemotherapy studies. Protocols are helpful when built-in "alerts" signal the provider to potentially serious problems. Computerization of protocols assists providers in being more proactive to dangerous drug interactions, abnormal laboratory values, and other untoward effects that are preprogrammed into the computer.

Order Set

An order set consists of preprinted provider orders that are used to expedite the order process once a standard has been validated through analytic review of practice and research. Order sets complement and increase compliance with existing practice standards. Sets can also be used to represent the algorithm or protocol in order format.

SAFETY ISSUES IN CRITICAL CARE

Patient safety has become a major focus of health care consumers as well as providers of care and administrators of health care institutions. The U.S. Institute of Medicine publication *Crossing the Quality Chasm: a New Health System for the 21st Century* (2001) has been the impetus for debate and actions to improve the safety of health care environments. The information indicates that health care too often results in harm to patients and routinely fails to deliver its potential benefits.[21]

Patient safety has been described as an ethical imperative implied in health care professionals' actions and interpersonal processes.[22] "Critical care units are busy, complex environments where the margins of error are narrow and the demands for safety are crucial."[23] In this environment, patients are particularly vulnerable because of compromised physiologic status, multiple technologic and pharmacologic interventions, and multiple care providers often working rapidly. It is essential that care delivery processes that minimize the opportunity for errors are designed and that a *safety culture* rather than a "blame culture" is created.[24] When an injury or inappropriate care occurs, it is crucial that health care professionals promptly explain to the patient and family how the injury or mistake occurred and the short-term and long-term effects. The patient and family should be informed that the factors involved in the injury will be investigated so that steps can be taken to reduce or avoid the likelihood of similar injury to other patients.

The *Safe Medical Device Act* (SMDA) of 1990 requires that hospitals report serious or potentially serious device-related injuries or illness of patients and employees to the manufacturer of the device and, if death is involved, to the U.S. Food and Drug Administration (FDA). In addition, implantable devices must be documented and tracked.[25] The SMDA serves as an "early warning" system so that the FDA can obtain information on device problems. Failure to comply with this act will result in civil action.

REFERENCES

1. Kleinpell R: Reports of role descriptions of acute care nurse practitioners, *AACN Clin Issues* 9(2):290-295, 1998.
2. American Association of Critical-Care Nurses: Practice resources, www.aacn.org.
3. Omery A, Williams RP: An appraisal of research utilization across the United States, *J Nurs Adm* 29(12):50-56, 1999.
4. Wojner AW: Why do we do the things we do? Stop the carnage of nursing research, *AACN News* 17(4):2, 12, 2000.
5. Mick D: Folklore, personal preference, or research-based practice, *Am J Crit Care* 9(1):6-7, 2000.
6. Rosswurm MA, Larrabee JH: A model for change to evidence-based practice, *Image J Nurs Sch* 31(4):317-322, 1999.
7. McPheeters M, Lohr KN: Evidence-based practice and nursing: commentary, *Outcomes Manag Nurs Pract* 3(3):99-101, 1999.
8. Panting K: Intensive care/intensive cure: the future of critical care? *Crit Care Nurse* 15(12):100, 1995.
9. Miller KL: Keeping the care in nursing care: our biggest challenge, *J Nurs Adm* 25(11):29-32, 1995.
10. Marlano C: Holistic ethics, *Am J Nurs* 101(1):24A-24C, 2001.
11. Powers PH et al: The value of patient- and family-centered care, *Am J Nurs* 100(5):84-88, 2000.
12. Alspach G: Time for sensitivity training: cultural diversity in cardiovascular disease, *Crit Care Nurse* 20(3):14-24, 2000.

13. Gonzales R, Gooden M, Porter C: Eliminating racial and ethnic disparities in health care, *Am J Nurs* 100(3):56-58, 2000.
14. Leonard B, Plotnikoff GA: Awareness: the heart of cultural competence, *AACN Clin Issues* 11(1):51-59, 2000.
15. American Nurses' Association: *Nursing's social policy statement,* Washington, DC, 1995, The Association.
16. North American Nursing Diagnosis Association: *Nursing diagnosis: definitions and classification,* Philadelphia, 1999, The Association.
17. Brooten D, Naylor M: Nurses' effect on changing patient outcomes, *Image J Nurs Sch* 27(2):95-99, 1995.
18. Himali U: A unified nursing language: the missing link in establishing nursing-sensitive patient outcomes, *Am Nurs* 27(2):23, 1995.
19. Knaus W et al: An evaluation of outcome from intensive care in major medical centers, *Ann Intern Med* 104:410-418, 1986.
20. Wojner A: Outcomes management: an interdisciplinary search for best practice, *AACN Clin Issues* 7(1):133-145, 1996.
21. Institute of Medicine: *Crossing the quality chasm: a new health system for the 21st century,* Washington, DC, 2001, National Academy Press.
22. White GB: Patient safety: an ethical imperative, *Nurs Econ* 20(4):195-197, 2002.
23. Benner P: Creating a culture of safety and improvement: a key to reducing medical error, *Am J Crit Care* 10(4):281-284, 2001.
24. Smith AP: In search of safety: an interview with Gina Pugliese, *Nurs Econ* 20(1):6-12, 2002.
25. Jensen JR: FDA's Safe Medical Device Act, *Risk Manag Rep* 1(2):1-4, 1997.

LINDA D. URDEN

2

Ethical and Legal Issues

Objectives

- Discuss ethical principles as they relate to critical care patients.
- Discuss the concept of medical futility.
- Describe what constitutes an ethical dilemma.
- List steps for making ethical decisions.
- Identify legal and professional obligations of critical care nurses.
- Describe the elements of certain torts that may result from critical care nursing practice.
- Identify and discuss specific legal issues in critical care nursing practice.

evolve Be sure to check out the free exercises on-line at *http://evolve.elsevier.com/Urden/priorities/*

MORALS AND ETHICS

Morals are the "shoulds," "should nots," "oughts," and "ought nots" of actions and behaviors and have been related closely to sexual mores and behaviors in Western society. Religious and cultural values and beliefs largely mold a person's moral thoughts and actions. Morals form the basis for action and provide a framework for evaluation of behavior.

Ethics are concerned with the "why" of the action rather than with whether the action is right or wrong, good or bad. Ethics implies that an evaluation is being made and is theoretically based on or derived from a set of standards.

ETHICAL PRINCIPLES

Certain ethical principles were derived from classic ethical theories that are used in health care decision making. *Principles* are general guidelines that govern conduct, provide a basis for reasoning, and direct actions. The six ethical principles discussed here are autonomy, beneficence, nonmaleficence, veracity, fidelity, and justice (Box 2-1).

Autonomy

The concept of autonomy appears in all ancient writings and early Greek philosophy. In health care, autonomy can be viewed as the freedom to make decisions about one's own body without the coercion or interference of others. Autonomy is a freedom of choice or a self-determination that is a basic human right. It can be experienced in all human life events.

The critical care nurse is often "caught in the middle" in ethical situations, and promoting autonomous decision making is one of those situations. As the nurse works closely with patients and families to promote autonomous decision making, another crucial element becomes clear. Patients and families must have all the information about a particular situation before they can make a decision that is best for them. They not only should be given all the pertinent information and facts but also must have a clear understanding of what was presented.[1] In this situation the nurse assumes one of the most important roles of the health care team, that is, as *patient advocate*, providing more information as needed, clarifying points, reinforcing information, and providing support during the decision-making process.

| Box **2-1** | Ethical Principles in Critical Care |

- Autonomy
- Beneficence
- Nonmaleficence
- Veracity
- Fidelity
  - Confidentiality
  - Privacy
- Justice/allocation of resources

Beneficence

The concept of doing good and preventing harm to patients is a sine qua non for the nursing profession. However, the ethical principle of beneficence, which requires that one *promote* the well-being of patients, indicates the importance of this duty for the health care professional. The principle of beneficence presupposes that harms and benefits are balanced, leading to positive or beneficial outcomes.

In approaching issues related to beneficence, conflict with the principle of autonomy is common. *Paternalism* exists when the nurse or physician makes a decision for the patient without consulting the patient.

Traditional health care has been based on a paternalistic approach to patients. Many patients are still more comfortable in deferring all decisions about care and treatment to their health care provider. Active involvement by various organizations and agencies in regard to health care has demonstrated a trend toward the public's need and desire for more information about health care in general, as well as more about alternative treatments and providers. Paternalism, or *maternalism* in the case of female providers, may always be a possibility in the health care setting, but enlightened consumers are causing a change in this practice of health care professionals.

Nonmaleficence

The ethical principle of nonmaleficence, which dictates that one *prevent* harm and correct harmful situations, is a prima facie duty for the nurse. Thoughtfulness and care are necessary, as is balancing risks and benefits. Beneficence and nonmaleficence are on two ends of a continuum and are often adhered to differently, depending on the views of the practitioner.

Veracity

Veracity, or truth telling, is an important ethical principle that underlies the nurse-patient relationship.

Veracity is important when soliciting informed consent because the patient needs to be aware of all potential risks of and benefits to be derived from specific treatments or alternative therapies.[2-4] Again, the critical care nurse may be in the middle of a situation where all the facts and information about a particular treatment option are not disclosed. Sometimes information has been given accurately to the patient and family but has been delivered with bias or in a misleading way. Veracity must guide all areas of practice for the nurse, that is, in colleague relationships and employee relationships, as well as in the nurse-patient relationship.

Fidelity

Fidelity, or faithfulness and promise keeping to patients, is also a sine qua non for nursing. It forms a bond between individuals and is the basis of all relationships, both professional and personal. Regardless of the amount of autonomy that patients have in the critical care areas, they still depend on the nurse for many types of physical care and emotional support. A trusting relationship that establishes and maintains an open atmosphere is positive for all involved.[5] Making a promise to a patient is voluntary for the nurse, whereas having respect for a patient's decision making is a moral obligation.[6]

Fidelity extends to the family of the critical care patient. When a promise is made to the family that they will be called if an emergency arises or that they will be informed of any other special events concerning the patient, the nurse must make every effort to follow through on the promise. Fidelity not only will uphold the nurse-family relationship but also will reflect positively on the nursing profession as a whole and on the institution where the nurse is employed.

Confidentiality is one element of fidelity that is based on traditional health care professional ethics. Confidentiality is described as a right whereby patient information can be shared only with those involved in the care of the patient. An exception to this guideline might be when the welfare of others will be put at risk by keeping patient information confidential. Again in this situation, the nurse must balance ethical principles and weigh risks with benefits. Special circumstances, such as the existence of mandatory reporting laws, will guide the nurse in certain situations.

Privacy also has been described as being inherent in the principle of fidelity. Privacy may be closely aligned with confidentiality of patient information and a patient's right to privacy of his or her person, such as maintaining privacy for the patient by pulling the curtains around the bed or making sure that the patient is adequately covered.

Justice

The principle of justice is often used synonymously with the concept of *allocation of scarce resources*. With escalating health care costs, expanded technologies, an aging population with their own special health care needs, and in some cases a scarcity of health care personnel, the question of how to allocate health care becomes even more complex.

The application of the justice principle in health care is concerned primarily with divided or portioned allocation of goods and services, which is termed *distributive justice*. As health care resources become increasingly scarcer, allocation of resources to certain programs and rationing of resources within certain programs will become more evident.

MEDICAL FUTILITY

The concept of medical futility has resulted in various discussions and proposed criteria and formulas to predict outcomes of care.[7] Medical futility has both a qualitative and a quantitative basis and can be defined as "any effort to achieve a result that is possible but that reasoning or experience suggests is highly improbable and that cannot be systematically reproduced."[8]

Therapy or treatment that achieves its predictable outcome and desired effect is, by definition, effective. Effect must be distinguished from benefit, however; although predictable and desired, the effect is nonetheless futile if it is of no benefit to the patient.

END-OF-LIFE CARE

Despite the advances of technologies and lifesaving treatments performed in critical care units, many people die there. Depending on available and accessible subacute care or hospice units, patients may receive care in critical care units for several days before their death. During this time, most if not all "traditional" critical care technologies, treatments, and interventions are withdrawn or not used, with limited end-of-life decision making and care management for these patients.[9] The person's identity is closely linked with a dignified death, and health care providers must facilitate the environment and care so that death can occur in a dignified manner. When it is acknowledged, death can be seen as a "passage" instead of failure to save the life.[10]

End-of-life (EOL) care is especially challenging for critical care nurses because their practice is focused on those with critical conditions, monitoring for emergent physiologic changes, and performing interventions to alleviate adverse outcomes.[9,11,12] EOL care refers to the final days or weeks of life when death is imminent.[13] During this time, palliative care is given, as collaboratively planned by the patient, family, and health care team members. *Palliative care* focuses on symptom relief and promotes favorable outcomes by assisting patients and families to reach their personal goals during the EOL experience. It is essential that critical care nurses confront the "care and comfort" for patients who will not live, and understand strategies to address EOL issues and care for their patients and families. Numerous resources exist to facilitate their understanding of EOL issues,[14,15] including chaplains, social workers, hospice staff, and other spiritual advisors.

ETHICAL FOUNDATION FOR NURSING PRACTICE

Traditional theories of professions include a code of ethics upon which the practice of the profession is based. It is by adherence to a code of ethics that the professional fulfills an obligation to provide quality practice to society.

A professional ethic is based on three elements: (1) the professional code of ethics, (2) the purpose of the profession, and (3) the standards of practice of the professional. The code of ethics developed by the professionals is the delineation of its values and relationships with and among members of the profession and society. The need for the profession and its inherent promise to provide certain duties form a contract between nursing and society. The professional standards describe specifics of practice in a variety of settings and subspecialties. Each element is dynamic, and ongoing evaluations are necessary as societal expectations change, technologies increase, and the profession evolves.

Nursing Code of Ethics

The American Nurses' Association (ANA) provides the major source of ethical guidance for the nursing profession. The *Code of Ethics for Nurses* serves as the basis for nurses in analyzing ethical issues and decision making (Box 2-2).[16]

What Is an Ethical Dilemma?

In general, ethical cases are not always clear-cut or "black and white." The most common ethical dilemmas encountered in critical care are forgoing treatment and allocating the scarce resources of critical care. Before the application of any decision model is made, it must be determined whether a true ethical dilemma exists. Thompson and Thompson[17] delineate the following three criteria for defining moral and ethical dilemmas in clinical practice:

1. An awareness of the different options
2. An issue that has different options
3. Two or more options with true or "good" aspects, with the choice of one option over the other compromising the option not chosen

Steps in Ethical Decision Making

To facilitate the ethical decision-making process, a model or framework must be used so that all parties involved will consistently and clearly examine the multiple ethical issues that arise in critical care (Box 2-3).

Step One

First, the major aspects of the medical and health problems must be identified. In other words, the scientific basis of the problem, potential sequelae, prognosis, and all data relevant to the health status must be examined.

Step Two

The ethical problem must be clearly delineated from other types of problems. *Systems problems* result from failures and inadequacies in the health care facility's organization and operation or in the health care system as a whole and are often misinterpreted as ethical issues. *Social problems* arising from conditions in the community, state, or country as a whole also are occasionally confused with ethical issues. Social problems can lead to *systemic problems*, which can constrain responses to ethical problems.

Step Three

Although categories of necessary additional information will vary, whatever is missing in the initial problem presentation should be obtained. If not already known, the health prognosis and potential sequelae should be clarified. Usual demographic data (e.g., age, ethnicity, religious preferences, educational/economic status) may be considered in the decision-making process. The role of the family or extended family and other support systems needs to be examined. Any desires that the patient may have expressed about the treatment decision, either in writing or in conversation, must be obtained.

Step Four

The patient is the primary decision maker and autonomously makes these decisions after receiving information about the alternatives and sequelae of treatments or lack of treatment. In many ethical dilemmas the patient is not competent to make a decision, however, as when the patient is comatose or otherwise physically or mentally unable to make a decision. In these cases, surrogates are designated or court

---

Box 2-2   Code of Ethics for Nurses

1. The nurse, in all professional relationships, practices with compassion and respect for the inherent dignity, worth, and uniqueness of every individual, unrestricted by considerations of social or economic status, personal attributes, or the nature of health problems.
2. The nurse's primary commitment is to the patient, whether an individual, family group, or community.
3. The nurse promotes, advocates for, and strives to protect the health, safety, and rights of the patient.
4. The nurse is responsible and accountable for individual nursing practice and determines the appropriate delegation of tasks consistent with the nurse's obligation to provide optimum patient care.
5. The nurse owes the same duties to self as to others, including the responsibility to preserve integrity and safety, to maintain competence, and to continue personal and professional growth.
6. The nurse participates in establishing, maintaining, and improving health care environments and conditions of employment conducive to the provision of quality health care and consistent with the values of the profession through individual and collective action.
7. The nurse participates in the advancement of the profession through contributions to practice, education, administration, and knowledge development.
8. The nurse collaborates with other health care professionals and the public in promoting community, national, and international efforts to meet health needs.
9. The profession of nursing, as represented by associations and their members, is responsible for articulating nursing values, for maintaining the integrity of the profession and its practice, and for shaping social policy.

From American Nurses' Association: *Code of ethics for nurses with interpretive statements*, Washington, DC, 2002, The Association.

Box **2-3**   Steps in Ethical Decision Making
1. Identify the health problem. 2. Define the ethical issue. 3. Gather additional information. 4. Delineate the decision maker. 5. Examine ethical and moral principles. 6. Explore alternative options. 7. Implement decisions. 8. Evaluate and modify actions.

appointed because the urgency of the situation requires a quick decision.

Others who are involved in the decision also need to be identified at this time, such as family, nurse, physician, social worker, clergy, and members of other disciplines in close contact with the patient. The role of the nurse must be examined. It may not be necessary for the nurse to make a decision at all; rather, the nurse's role may be simply to provide additional information and support to the decision maker.

Step Five

Personal values, beliefs, and moral convictions of all persons involved in the decision process need to be known. Whether actually achieved through a group meeting or through personal introspection, values clarification facilitates the decision-making process.

General ethical principles also need to be examined in regard to the case at hand. For example, are veracity, informed consent, and autonomy being promoted? Beneficence and nonmaleficence will be analyzed as they relate to a patient's condition and desires. Close examination of these principles will reveal any compromise of ethical or moral principles for either the patient or the health care provider and will assist in decision making.

Step Six

After the identification of alternative options, the outcome of each action must be predicted. This analysis helps the person select the option with the best "fit" for the specific situation or problem. Both short-range and long-range consequences of each action must be examined, and new or creative actions must be encouraged. Consideration also must be given to the "no action" option, which is another choice.

Step Seven

When a decision has been reached, it is usually after much thought and consideration.

Step Eight

Evaluation of an ethical decision serves both to assess the decision at hand and to provide a basis for future ethical decisions. If outcomes are not as predicted, it may be possible to modify the plan or to use an alternative that was not originally chosen.

LEGAL RELATIONSHIPS

When a professional nurse commences employment in a critical care facility, three legal relationships are formed. First, on accepting employment, the relationship between the nurse and the *employer* is formed. Second, on assuming the care of a patient, a relationship is created between the *patient* and nurse. Third, every state has a law that mandates the entry-level educational requirements that must be met for a person to become licensed to practice nursing. The act of licensing creates a legal relationship between the nurse and the *state*.

These relationships impose legal obligations. The nurse owes a patient the duty of reasonable and prudent care under the circumstances. The nurse owes the employer the duty of competency and the ability to follow policies and procedures; other contractual duties may exist as well. The nurse owes the state and public the duty of safe, competent practice as legally defined by practice standards.

The critical care nurse's legal duties are enforceable, and the nurse can be held legally accountable for breach or violation through a variety of laws and legal processes. Nurses, hospitals, patients, and other health care providers can be involved in a variety of legal disputes, including negligence and professional malpractice, incompetence, unauthorized practice, unprofessional or illegal conduct, workers' compensation, and contract and labor disputes.

Tort Liability

The area of civil law is divided into many categories, two of which are contracts and torts. The law of *contracts* contains a set of rules governing the creation and enforcement of an agreement between two or more parties (entities or individuals). For example, contract law may apply to a dispute between the nurse, as employee, and an institution, as employer. In contrast, a *tort* is a type of civil wrong or injury that results from a breach of a legal duty. Tort law is generally divided into intentional and unintentional torts, strict liability, and specific torts (Box 2-4).

Intentional torts involve (1) a mind-set indicative of purpose and (2) an act. Intent exists when the person forms a mental design to achieve a particular outcome and consequence. Assault, battery, false imprisonment, trespass, and intentional infliction of emotional distress are all examples of intentional torts. In each of these torts, a specific act is required, and there is purposeful interference with a person or property.

In *assault* the act is a behavior that places the *plaintiff* (person being wronged who later sues) in fear or apprehension of offensive physical contact; in civil law the *defendant* is the person being sued for wronging another. *Battery* is the unlawful or offensive touching of or contact with the plaintiff or something attached to the plaintiff. *False imprisonment*

Box **2-4**	Classification of Torts

INTENTIONAL TORTS
Assault
Battery
False imprisonment
Trespass
Infliction of mental or emotional distress

SPECIFIC TORTS
Defamation
  Slander
  Libel
Invasion of privacy

UNINTENTIONAL TORTS
Negligence
Medical/nursing treatment torts
  Professional malpractice
Abandonment

STRICT LIABILITY
Products liability

is detaining, confining, or restraining another against the person's will. The two types of *trespass* involve (1) a person's land and (2) an individual's personal property. These acts are defined as "unauthorized entry onto land of another" or "unauthorized handling of another's personal property." In addition, the law protects a person's interest in peace of mind through the tort claim of "infliction of mental or emotional distress." The act in this case, however, must involve extreme misconduct or outrageous behavior.

Unintentional torts involve failures or breach of nursing duties that lead to harm, including negligence, malpractice, and abandonment. *Negligence* is the failure to meet an ordinary standard of care, resulting in injury to the patient or plaintiff. *Malpractice* is a type of professional liability based on negligence and includes professional misconduct, breach of a duty or standard of care, illegal or immoral conduct, or failure to exercise reasonable skill, all of which lead to harm (see later discussion). *Abandonment* is a type of negligence in which a duty to give care exists, is ignored, and results in harm to a patient. It is the absence of care and the failure to respond to a patient that may give rise to an allegation of abandonment.

Specific torts involve privacy and reputation interests and include invasion of privacy and defamation. *Defamation* is composed of two torts: *slander* (oral defamation) and *libel* (written defamation). Defamation is not the mere statement or writing of words that injures a person's reputation or good name; the words also must be communicated to another. If the words are true, this may provide a defense against a defamation claim. *Invasion of privacy* involves the violation of a person's right to privacy. Nurses can invade another's

privacy by revealing confidential information without authorization or by failing to follow the patient's health care decisions.

Nurses can avoid allegations of these specific claims by (1) making statements about another's reputation only when necessary and substantiated by fact and (2) respecting another's privacy and autonomy and maintaining a confidential relationship with the patient.

Administrative Law and Licensing Statutes

A second type of law and legal process in which nurses are involved is administrative law and the regulatory process. This area of law governs the nurse's relationship with the *government*, either state or federal. Administrative law involves the rules of the government's activities in regulating health care delivery and practice; the rules of investigation, procedure, and evidence differ from those of civil and criminal law. Several government health care agencies are involved in such regulation.

A state has the power to regulate nursing because the state is responsible for the health, safety, and welfare of its citizens. Therefore, establishing minimal entry-level requirements, standards of nursing practice, and educational requirements are acceptable state actions. State legislatures create laws governing nursing practice, generally termed *nurse practice acts*, and a unit of the state government within the executive branch is responsible for the enforcement of nursing laws. This unit is often called the *State Board of Nursing* or *Board of Nurse Examiners*; however, the name varies by state. Standards also vary by state, which is another important reason that nurses should seek advice from counsel licensed to practice law in their own state.

Negligence and Malpractice

As defined earlier, negligence is an unintentional tort involving a breach of duty or failure (through an act or an omission) to meet a standard of care, causing personal harm. Malpractice is a type of professional liability based on negligence in which the defendant is held accountable for breach of a duty of care involving special knowledge and skill. These torts have several elements, all of which the plaintiff has the burden of proving.

The law recognizes four elements of negligence and malpractice. The first element, a *duty*, or legal obligation, requires the person ("actor") to conform to a certain standard of conduct for the protection of others against unreasonable risks. The critical care nurse's legal duty is to act in a reasonable and prudent manner, as any other critical care nurse would act under similar circumstances. The standard is that of a critical care nurse, a professional with special knowledge and skill in critical care. The standard is that owed at the time the incident or injury occurred, not at the time of litigation. In most jurisdictions the standard of care is a *national* standard, as opposed to a local or community standard. General critical care nursing duties are implied by statute and administrative rules and regulations and are stated explicitly in judicial decisions (Box 2-5).

The second element, *breach of duty*, involves a failure on the actor's part to conform to the standard required. *Causation*, the third element, involves proving that the actor's breach was reasonably close or causally connected to the resulting injury. This is also referred to as *proximate cause*. The fourth element, *injury* or damages, must involve an actual loss or damage to the plaintiff or his or her interest. A plaintiff may claim different types of damages, such as compensatory and punitive. Patient injury can range in value, depending on what happened to the patient. The plaintiff must produce evidence of the damages and their value. If the nurse breaches a standard of care that leads to injury, the plaintiff must show what amount of money will compensate for his or her injuries. The goal of the compensation is to provide the amount of money that will return the plaintiff to the position that existed before the injury occurred.

Res ipsa loquitur, "the thing speaks for itself," is a rule of evidence used by plaintiffs in negligence or malpractice litigation. It is a rebuttable presumption or inference of negligence by the defendant, which arises on the plaintiff's proof that (1) the injury is one that ordinarily does not happen in the absence of negligence and (2) the instrumentality causing the injury was in the defendant's exclusive management and control. The burden then shifts to the defendant to prove absence of negligence. For example, negligence can be inferred when muscle ischemia and necrosis occur as a result of improper body positioning and the application of splints or restraints. Negligence can also be inferred from a foreign object left in a patient's body cavity after surgery.

Because critical care nurses deal with life-threatening situations, any patient injury is potentially severe or may result in death. Should the injury occur as a result of alleged negligence, the nurse may be held liable for the patient's death and also for the resulting loss to surviving family members. All states have "wrongful death" acts, and a number of states have both "death" acts and "survival" acts, which are prosecuted concurrently. With the two causes of action, the expenses, pain and suffering, and loss of earnings of the decedent up to the time of death are allocated to the survival action, and loss of benefits to the survivors is allocated to the wrongful death action.

Specific critical care nursing actions have resulted in litigation (Box 2-6). In such cases the nurse's action is central to the lawsuit. However, nurses are named as sole defendant or codefendant in a comparatively small percentage of cases. Although this pattern is changing, physicians and hospitals are generally named as defendants.

Typically, nursing negligence cases involve breach or failure in six general categories (Box 2-7). The first category includes the use of defective equipment or the failure to perform safety and maintenance assessments. Nurses have made errors in drug identification, administration, and dosages. Nurses have failed to report changes in patient status to physicians in a timely manner. Nurses have not communicated to supervisors a physician's failure to respond to the nurse's communication. Failure to supervise and assist patients who subsequently fall is also a source of nursing negligence. Improper wound care with resulting infection and incorrect instrument and sponge counts in the surgical setting have also led to patient injury and lawsuits.

Legal Doctrines and Theories of Liability

In tort law the nurse's action may be examined and legal duties defined according to the following theories of liability:

Box 2-5 Legal Duties of Critical Care Nurses

- Observe.
- Assess.
- Conduct ongoing observations and assessments.
- Recognize significance of information.
- Report.
- Plan, implement, and evaluate care.
- Respond to changes.
- Interpret and carry out orders.
- Take reasonable measures to ensure patient safety.
- Exercise professional judgment.
- Properly perform procedures.
- Follow hospital policies and procedures.
- Record and document.

Box 2-6 Select Critical Care Nursing Actions in Negligence Lawsuits

GENERAL

Failure to advise physician/supervisor of change in patient's health status
Failure to monitor patients at requisite intervals
Failure to adhere to established institutional protocols
Failure to assess patients' clinical status adequately
Failure to respond to alarms
Failure to maintain accurate, timely, and complete medical records
Failure to carry out treatment and evaluate treatment results properly
Failure to use safe, functional equipment

SPECIFIC

Failure to provide supplemental oxygen when the ventilator cannot be promptly reattached
Failure to use intravenous (IV) infusion equipment properly, causing extensive fluid extravasation
Failure to monitor IV infusions, recognize infiltration, and discontinue IV therapy
Failure to recognize signs of intracranial bleeding
Failure to investigate patient's complaint of pain and discover hematoma under blood pressure cuff

Box **2-7**	Six General Categories of Nursing Negligence

1. Improper administration of treatments
2. Improper administration of medications
3. Inadequate or false written and verbal communication
4. Insufficient supervision of patients
5. Improper postoperative treatment and wound care
6. Incorrect perioperative instrument and sponge counts

- Personal liability
- Vicarious liability: respondeat superior
- Corporate liability
- Other liability doctrines (e.g., temporary or borrowed servant, captain of the ship)

Under the theory of *personal liability*, each individual is responsible for his or her own actions, including the critical care nurse, supervisor, physician, hospital, and patient. Each has responsibilities that are uniquely his or her own. In contrast to personal liability, the individual may be afforded the protection of personal immunity.

Vicarious liability is indirect responsibility, such as the liability of an employer for the acts of the employee. Under the doctrine of *respondeat superior*, a "master" is liable for certain wrongful acts of a "servant," as is a principal for those of an agent. An employer may be liable for an employee's acts that are performed within the legitimate scope of employment. In critical care the nurse typically is an employee of a hospital. However, nurses may be independent contractors with the hospital through critical care nursing agencies or businesses. If the latter is the case, the nurse is not an employee of the hospital, and the hospital is not vicariously liable for the nurse's action.

Corporate liability is the liability attached to the corporate entity (e.g., the hospital) for its own corporate activities and decisions.

Other doctrines, such as *temporary servant* or *borrowed servant* and *captain of the ship*, may apply to the critical care nurse and the critical care unit. These doctrines are used when the plaintiff argues that the physician is responsible for the nurse's actions, even though the nurse is an employee of the hospital, not of the physician. If it can be shown that the nurse acted under the direction and control of the physician, the physician may be accountable for the nurse's actions. However, these doctrines are becoming increasingly uncommon. What viability remains is typically found in cases involving nurse anesthetists and operating room nurses.

NURSE PRACTICE ACTS

The practice of nursing is regulated by the state. As a general rule, the state's police power to regulate prevails, as long as the state's actions are not arbitrary or capricious. All nurses must be licensed to practice under their individual state's licensure statutes. *Licensure* authorizes (1) the right to practice and (2) access to employment. Therefore licensure is a property right that is constitutionally protected. Every state has legislation that defines the legal scope of nursing practice and defines unprofessional and illegal conduct that may lead to investigation and disciplinary action by the state and sanctions on the right to practice. The state nurse practice act establishes entry requirements, definitions of practice, and criteria for discipline. Although licensure is mandatory for registered nurses (RNs), statutory content varies among the states.

Generally, state law contains two definitions of nursing: one for the RN (or professional nurse) and one for the licensed practical (or vocational or technical) nurse. These definitions determine titles that may be used by nurses, the scope of nursing practice, and requirements for entering the nursing profession. In some states, advanced RN practice, prescriptive authority for certain nurses, and third-party reimbursement are also defined by statute.

Mandatory continuing education requirements are also defined by statute in most states. The state authorizes its board of nursing to monitor practice, implement standards of care, enforce rules and regulations, and issue sanctions. *Sanctions* include additional education, restricted practice, supervised practice, license suspension, and license revocation. Some form of disciplinary action generally occurs as a result of unauthorized practice, negligence or malpractice, incompetence, chemical or other impairment, criminal acts, or violations of specific nurse practice act provisions.

The scope of medical practice is also statutorily defined, and in most states a physician is given broad discretion to delegate tasks to others. Physicians may delegate to critical care nurses through written protocols or standing orders, which must be written, dated, and signed by the physician; standing orders and protocols must be updated regularly. The nurse must be adequately prepared to follow the protocol and perform with a reasonable degree of skill, care, and diligence as performed by similar nurses under similar circumstances. Protocol and standing orders should identify unambiguously the corresponding roles of hospital administrators, nurses, and physicians. Within a state's jurisdiction, however, the scope of medical practice and the scope of nursing practice often overlap because each practice may authorize the same functions. Such overlapping creates problems at the regulatory level and will expand as the role of nursing continues to evolve.

Chemical impairment is a common reason for disciplinary action. In some states the impaired nurse may avoid serious sanctions by voluntarily suspending practice and entering a rehabilitation program. This must be done with the advice of counsel (the nurse's own lawyer). Generally, this option is available as long as no patient has been harmed because of the nurse's impairment.

SPECIFIC PATIENT CARE ISSUES

Myriad legal issues and controversies exist in the field of critical care. Concerns often arise in the areas of (1) informed consent and authorization for treatment and (2) the patient's right to accept or refuse medical treatment.

Informed Consent and Authorization for Treatment

There are two types of consent: express and implied. *Express consent* may be written or verbal and is the consent given specifically for nonroutine procedures. *Implied consent* may be implied in fact, an assumption based on patient behavior (e.g., patient extending arm for venipuncture or nodding approval), or may be implied in law (e.g., unconscious, hemorrhaging patient in emergency department). This discussion summarizes the elements of valid informed consent, the adequacy of consent and negligent nondisclosure, and exceptions to consent requirements and the duty to disclose.

Valid consent must be (1) voluntary, (2) obtained, and (3) informed. Although consent can be verbal or written, most hospital policies require that informed, voluntary consent to nonroutine procedures be obtained and confirmed in writing, as signed and dated by the patient, physician, and witness (if required). Most informed consent statutes provide that a consent in writing to a medical or surgical procedure that meets the consent and disclosure requirements of the statute creates a legal presumption that informed consent was given.

In the vast majority of jurisdictions the decision maker (person giving consent) must be a legally competent adult (i.e., having reached age of majority, or age 18 years in most states). Competence is a legal judgment, and as a general rule, there is a legal presumption of patient competence.[18] A person is mentally incompetent (thereby rendering a consent invalid) if adjudicated incompetent. A person must likewise have the capacity (a medical and nursing judgment) to give consent. The patient must be oriented and understand what he or she has been told, and current medications must be documented. For adults legally adjudicated incompetent, the guardian may give consent if the guardian has been given this authority.

Minors are legally incompetent, and consent is obtained from the parent or guardian. In many jurisdictions, however, there are two important exceptions to this rule: (1) mature minors may consent to treatment for substance abuse, sexually transmitted disease, and matters involving contraception and reproduction; and (2) emancipated minors may consent to treatment in general. Minors are considered "emancipated" if married or divorced before the age of majority, if in the military service, or if living independently with parental consent.

Consent must also be informed and timely. The physician has a duty to disclose the diagnosis, condition, prognosis, material risks/benefits associated with the treatment or procedure, explanation of the treatment, providers of the treatment (who is performing, supervising, and assisting in procedure), material risks and benefits of alternative therapy, and the probable outcome (including material risks/benefits) if the patient refuses the treatment or procedure. Failure to disclose such information or inadequate disclosure with resultant injury may constitute negligence and give rise to tort claims of malpractice, battery, negligent nondisclosure, and abandonment. Consent is generally valid for 7 to 30 days. However, the time at which consent expires must be explicitly stated in the institutional policy and procedure manual.

There are many exceptions to consent requirements and the duty to disclose, and clearly the exceptions vary according to jurisdiction. Emergencies constitute one exception, unless the patient refuses treatment or has previously made a competent and informed refusal. States vary significantly in the following treatment situations: endangered fetal viability, alcohol or other drug detoxification, emergency blood transfusion, cesarean birth, and substance abuse during pregnancy. Jurisdictions also vary on the issue of sources of consent (informal directives) for the incompetent patient or the patient in an emergency who has no legal guardian. Alternatives include consensus from as many next of kin as possible, with evidence that (1) the treatment is reasonable and necessary, and (2) the family's decision would not be contrary to the patient's wishes, known as *substituted judgment* (made by a surrogate decision maker). Another alternative is a court order for treatment. In the absence of substituted judgment, many courts use the "best interests" standard.

Right to Accept or Refuse Medical Treatment

The right to consent and informed consent includes the right to refuse treatment. In most cases a competent adult's decision to refuse even life-sustaining treatment is honored.[19-23] The underlying rationale is that the patient's right to withdraw or withhold treatment is not outweighed by the state's interest in preserving life. The right to refuse treatment is *not* honored in some situations, including (but not limited to) the following:

1. The treatment relates to a contagious illness that threatens the health of the public.
2. Innocent third parties will suffer (e.g., parent's wish to refuse blood transfusion to child most likely would be overruled to save child's life).
3. The refusal violates ethical standards.
4. Treatment must be instituted to prevent suicide and to preserve life.

When patients refuse treatment, complex ethical, legal, and practical problems arise. Hospitals should have specific policies to guide nurses in these areas, and nurses' participation in hospital or institutional ethics committees is strongly advised.

Withholding and Withdrawing Treatment

As stated, an adult has the right to refuse treatment, even treatment that sustains life. This right means that the critical care nurse may participate in the withholding or withdrawing of treatment. Historically, the distinction between withholding and withdrawing treatments was considered the issue of importance, but this is no longer the case. Health care decisions become most complex when patients lose competency and capacity to make their own decisions personally.

Advance Directives

The U.S. Congress passed landmark legislation known as the *Patient Self-Determination Act/Omnibus Budget Reconciliation Act (OBRA) of 1990.*[24-33] The statute requires that all adults must be provided written information on an individual's rights under state law to make medical decisions, including the right to refuse treatment and the right to formulate advance directives.

The law mandates that providers of health care services under Medicare and Medicaid must comply with requirements relating to patient advance directives, which are written instructions recognized under state law for provisions of care when persons are incapacitated. Providers may not be reimbursed for the care they provide unless the requirements of this provision are met.

Providers must have written policies and procedures (1) to inform all adult patients at initiation of treatment of their right to execute an advance directive and of the provider's policies on the implementation of that right, (2) to document in the medical record whether an individual has executed an advance directive, (3) *not* to condition care and treatment or otherwise discriminate on the basis of whether a patient has executed an advance directive, (4) to comply with state laws on advance directives, and (5) to provide information and education to staff and the community on advance directives.

Patients themselves can provide clear direction by preparing in advance written documents that specify their wishes.[34] These documents are termed *advance directives* and include the living will and durable power of attorney for health care. To be effective in a jurisdiction, both these directives must be statutorily or judicially recognized. The *living will* specifies that if certain circumstances occur, such as terminal illness, the patient will decline specific treatment, such as cardiopulmonary resuscitation and mechanical ventilation. The living will does not cover all treatment; in some states, for example, nutritional support may not be declined through a living will. The *durable power of attorney for health care* is a directive through which a patient designates an "agent," someone who will make decisions for the patient if the patient becomes unable to do so. Critical care nurses whose patients have executed advance directives must follow state law provisions and the hospital's policies and require education regarding advance directives and their important role in patient advocacy.[35]

Orders Not to Resuscitate

Hospital policies that address orders to withhold or withdraw treatment should exist in all critical care units. For example, orders not to resuscitate, typically referred to as *do-*

not-resuscitate (DNR) orders, should be governed by written policies, including (but not limited to) the following:

1. DNR orders should be entered in the patient's record with full documentation by the responsible physician about the patient's prognosis and the patient's agreement (if he or she is capable) or, alternatively, the family's consensus.
2. DNR orders should have the concurrence of another physician designated in the policy.
3. Policies should specify that orders are reviewed periodically (some policies require daily review).
4. Patients with capacity must give their informed consent.
5. For patients without capacity, that incapacity must be thoroughly documented, along with the diagnosis, prognosis, and family consensus.
6. Judicial intervention before writing a DNR order is usually indicated when the patient's family does not agree or there is uncertainty or disagreement about the patient's prognosis or mental status. As a general rule, however, in the absence of conflict or disagreement, DNR orders are legal in a majority of jurisdictions if executed clearly and properly.
7. Policies should specify who is to be contacted and notified within the hospital administration.

Other orders to withhold or withdraw treatment may involve mechanical ventilation, dialysis, nutritional support, hydration, and medications such as antibiotics. The legal and ethical implications of these orders for each patient must be carefully considered. Hospitals should have written policies on all orders to withhold and withdraw treatment. Policies must cover how decisions will be made, who will decide, and what roles the patient, family, health care providers, and the institution will play. Policies must be developed that consider state laws and judicial opinions.

REFERENCES

1. Correll N: Identifying patient's needs helps with ethical dilemmas, *AACN News* 17(6):4, 2000.
2. Dennis BP: The origin and nature of informed consent: experiences among vulnerable groups, *J Prof Nurs* 15(5):285, 1999.
3. Crow KG, Matheson L, Steed A: Informed consent and truth telling: cultural direction of healthcare providers, *J Nurs Adm* 30(3):148, 2000.
4. Michael JE: Stay in-the-know regarding informed consent, *Nurs Manag* 33(5):22-23, 2002.
5. Washington G: Trust: a critical element in critical care nursing, *Focus Crit Care* 17(5):418, 1990.
6. Aroskar M: *Fidelity and veracity: questions of promise keeping, truth telling and loyalty.* In Foweler M, Levine-Ariff J, editors: *Ethics at the bedside*, Philadelphia, 1987, Lippincott.
7. Ewer MS: The definition of medical futility: are we trying to define the wrong term? *Heart Lung* 30(1):3-4, 2001.
8. Schneiderman LJ, Jecker NS, Jonsen AR: Medical futility: its meaning and ethical implications, *Ann Intern Med* 112(12):949, 1990.
9. Miller PA, Forbes, Boyle DK: End-of-life care in the intensive care unit: a challenge for nurses, *Am J Crit Care* 10(4):230-237, 2001.

10. Benner P: Death as a human passage: compassionate care for persons dying in critical care units, *Am J Crit Care* 10(5):355-359, 2001.
11. White KR, Coyne PJ, Patel UB: Are nurses adequately prepared for end-of-life care? *J Nurs Scholarsh* 33(2):147-151, 2001.
12. Puntillo KA et al: End-of-life issues in intensive care units: a national random survey of nurses' knowledge and beliefs, *Am J Crit Care* 10(4):216-229, 2001.
13. Ferrell BR, Coyle N: A review of palliative care nursing, *Am J Nurs* 102(5):26-31, 2002.
14. http://www.aacn.nche.edu/ELNEC/ajn.htm
15. http://www.palliativecarenursing.net
16. American Nurses' Association: *Code of ethics for nurses with interpretive statements*, Washington, DC, 2002, The Association.
17. Thompson J, Thompson H: *Bioethical decision-making for nurses*, Norwalk, Conn, 1985, Appleton-Century-Crofts.
18. Northrop CE, Kelly ME: *Legal issues in nursing*, St Louis, 1987, Mosby.
19. *Bouvia v Superior Court*, 225 Cal Rptr 297; 179 C.A.3d 1127, *review denied* (Cal App 1986).
20. *In re Farrell*, 529 A.2d 404 (NJ 1987).
21. *McKay v Bergstedt*, 801 P.2d 617 (Nev 1990).
22. *State v McAfee*, 385 S.E.2d 651 (Ga 1989).
23. Wilson-Clayton ML, Clayton MA: Two steps forward, one step back: *McKay v Bergstedt*, *Whittier Law Rev* 12:439, 1991.
24. *Advance directives for health care: deciding today about your care in the future*, Des Moines, 1991, Iowa Hospital Association, Iowa Medical Society, Iowa State Bar Association.
25. *Put it in writing: a guide to promoting advance directives*, Chicago, 1991, American Hospital Association (800-242-2626).
26. Cate FH, Gill BA: *The Patient Self-Determination Act: implementation issues and opportunities*, Washington, DC, 1991, Annenberg Washington Program.
27. *Advance directive protocols and the Patient Self-Determination Act: a resource manual for the development of institutional protocols*, New York, 1991, Choice in Dying (212-366-5540; formerly Society for the Right to Die/Concern for Dying).
28. Emanuel L, Emanuel E: The medical directive: a new comprehensive advance care document, *JAMA* 261(22):3, 288, 1989.
29. *The Patient Self-Determination Act of 1990: implementation in Iowa hospitals*, Des Moines, 1991, Iowa Hospital Association (515-288-1955).
30. *Advance medical directives*, Arlington, Va, 1991, National Hospice Organization (703-243-5900).
31. *The patient self-determination directory and resources guide*, Washington, DC, 1991, National Health Lawyers Association (202-833-1100).
32. *Patient Self-Determination Act/Omnibus Budget Reconciliation Act of 1990*, Pub No 101-508, Sec 4206, 42 USC Sec 1395cc(a)(1) (1990).
33. *Advance directives*, Des Moines, Iowa, 1991, Unisys (800-776-6045).
34. Douglas R, Brown HN: Patients' attitudes toward advance directives, *J Nurs Scholarsh* 34(1):61-65, 2002.
35. Ryan CJ et al: Perceptions about advance directives by nurses in a community hospital, *Clin Nurse Spec* 15(6):246-252, 2001.

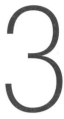

KIM BLOUNT

Patient and Family Education

Objectives

- Adapt and apply teaching-learning theory to the critical care setting.
- Perform a learning needs assessment.
- Construct a teaching plan for patients in the critical care unit.
- Discuss four methods of instruction and the appropriateness of each to the critical care setting.
- Describe informational needs of families of critically ill patients.

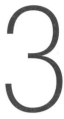 Be sure to check out the free exercises on-line at *http://evolve.elsevier.com/Urden/priorities/*

EDUCATIONAL CHALLENGES

Providing education is a fundamental part of the overall plan for any patient's care. According to the Joint Commission on Accreditation of Healthcare Organizations (JCAHO), the goal of patient/family education is to improve health outcomes by promoting healthy behavior and involvement in care and care decisions.[1] Because admission to a critical care unit is generally an unexpected event, it presents special challenges to providing effective patient/family education.

The critical care nurse must set priorities that place maintenance of immediate physical and psychologic safety above health promotion and educational needs. When the patient's clinical condition allows, however, the education plan can be initiated with continuation throughout the hospital stay into discharge. All patients and families must receive specific information (Box 3-1). Time constraints and the necessity to set priorities of care may limit the actual amount of time available for educating patients and families.

Along with a belief in the patient's right to know, the patient's right *not* to know must be respected when patients prefer not to learn about their illnesses. Simple basic information about monitors and unit policy, for example, usually suffices in these cases. Indeed, more information than can be processed and integrated can greatly increase anxiety and may result in slower recovery. Individuals have the right to accept, adopt, or reject the information provided in educational encounters.

ADULT LEARNING PRINCIPLES

Central to successful implementation of an educational plan in the critical care and telemetry environment is the incorporation of the principles of adult learning theory.[2] Adults must be ready to learn, having moved from one developmental or educational task to the next. They need to know *why* it is important to learn something before they can actually learn it. Inherent in their attitudes is a responsibility for their own decisions. Consequently, they may resent when others try to force different beliefs on them. Adults bring a wealth of experience to the learning environment that must be recognized and promoted in educational techniques. Because their orientation to learning is *life centered*, the tasks being taught should focus on current problem resolution. Finally, motivation for the adult learner arises out of internal pressures such as self-esteem and quality of life.

TEACHING-LEARNING PROCESS

The teaching-learning process is a dynamic, continuous activity (Box 3-2). Teaching is not just the passing of facts and information from one person to another. Learning is both growth and development. It is an active process that occurs internally over time and cannot be forced. Learning involves altering behavior to produce changes in one or more of the three learning domains: knowledge, attitudes, and skills.[3]

Assessment

Assessment is the gathering of information for the purposes of identifying actual or potential learning needs. It identifies gaps in the knowledge, attitudes, and skills the patient or family has regarding the illness, environment, or lifestyle (Box 3-3). Knowing this information will allow the nurse to develop a collaborative, individualized, need-targeted education plan of care. The assessment process does not stop after the completion of the admission assessment; it is continuous and ongoing.

Patients and families may be so overwhelmed by what they see or have already been told that they may be unable to identify their own learning needs. The bedside nurse is responsible for involving both the patient and the family in the assessment process and discovering what they want and need to know. Involving patients and families in this process gives value to their needs and assists them in gaining some

---

Box 3-1 Essential Critical Care Information for the Patient/Family

- Orientation to the various care providers and the services they deliver
- Orientation to the unit environment (e.g., call light, bed controls)
- Orientation to unit routines and plan of care: visiting hours, frequency of monitoring and nurse assessments, venipunctures to obtain blood specimens, daily weights, special shift routines
- Explanations regarding reasons for equipment, monitors, and associated alarms (e.g., cardiac monitor, ventilator, intravenous [IV] lines, IV pumps, pacemaker, pulse oximetry)
- Explanation of all procedures and expected sensations/discomforts both in and off the unit
- Medications given: drug name, reason for receiving, side effects to report to nurse/others
- Immediate plan of care
- Transition to next level of care: reason for transfer, environment, staffing, availability of care providers
- Discharge plan: medications, diet, activity, pathophysiology of disease, symptom management, special procedures and associated equipment, when to call health care provider, available community resources

---

Box 3-2 Steps in the Patient/Family Education Process

- Assess learning needs and readiness to learn.
- Develop an educational plan of care.
- Implement the plan of care.
- Evaluate outcomes.
- Document the process.

Box **3-3**   **Assessment Questions for the Critically Ill Patient and Family**

- What brings you to the hospital? Can you tell me what happened? Can you tell me more?
- What have you been told so far about your (your family member's) condition and plan of care?
- What is the most important thing for you to know right now?
- What would you like to know? What information can I give you right now?
- Who are your main support people?
- Has anything like this ever happened to you (your family) before?
- Have you (your family) ever been in an intensive care unit or hospital before?
- Do you have any special concerns that we need to address right now?

Modified from Reeder J: *AACN Clin Issues* 2:188-194, 1991.

control over a situation in which they may feel powerless. Active participation and control stimulate the motivation to receive information, as well as make the overall education process more satisfying; in essence, the patient/family will learn more.

Assessing ability, willingness, and readiness to learn is an essential part of developing and implementing an education plan of care. Readiness to learn is the motivation to try out new concepts and behaviors.[4] The *ability* to learn is the capacity of the learner to understand, pay attention, and comprehend the material being taught. *Willingness* to learn describes the learner's openness to new ideas and concepts. Several factors affect ability, willingness, and readiness to learn as well as the ability to cope and adapt to the current situation. These factors include physiologic, psychologic, sociocultural, financial, and environmental aspects.[3-5]

Development of Education Plan

The education plan must be ongoing, interactive, and consistent with the patient's plan of care and education level (see Box 3-1). Information gathered from the assessment must be analyzed and used to prioritize education needs, formulate a nursing diagnosis, and develop an education plan of care. The nurse also must consider the patient's clinical and emotional status when setting education priorities. The education plan should include (1) expected outcomes, (2) objectives, (3) content to be taught, (4) interventions, (5) available education materials, and (6) appropriate teaching strategies. Box 3-4 provides a sample education plan for patients undergoing coronary artery bypass surgery. Refer to the Nursing Management Plan for Deficient Knowledge (p. 482).

Implementation of Education Plan

Patients in the critical care environment are educated in many informal interactions with the nurse, and the knowl-

edge gained fosters patient understanding and well-being. Educational opportunities can be present during various nursing care activities, such as bathing and administration of medication. Each encounter with the patient/family must be viewed as a teaching opportunity. At times during the hospitalization, however, more formal or structured educational experiences may be required.

Learning Environment

As discussed, patient barriers to learning are related to physiologic, emotional, and motivational factors. To structure a successful teaching-learning experience in a critical care area, the nurse must also carefully assess the environmental and iatrogenic barriers that affect the interaction. Bright lights, unpleasant odors, unfamiliar noises, and untidy surroundings can distract patients and add to cognitive impairment. Control of these factors can facilitate the learning process. Factors that cannot be controlled must be explained to the patient to alleviate anxiety and facilitate a trusting relationship between patient and nurse.

Teaching Methods

There are three basic methods of teaching: lecture, discussion, and demonstration. The selection of the methods will be determined by various factors, including patient clinical status, readiness to learn, cognitive abilities, learning style, instructional time, and availability of teaching materials and resources. In addition, innovative methods of teaching and presentation of educational materials must be developed and used efficiently to maximize existing resources.[6]

Lecture. Lecture is the presentation of information in a highly structured format to a group. In this method the teacher provides a great deal of material but may not provide ample opportunities for teacher-learner interaction. This style of teaching is inappropriate for acutely ill patients in the critical care unit, although it may be useful in the telemetry unit. Optimally, the group size should be arranged to enable the learners to ask questions and receive appropriate feedback on content presented.

Discussion. Discussion is less structured than lecturing and allows an exchange and feedback between the teacher and learner. The teacher can adapt the material to meet the needs of the individual or group. Discussion groups can be effective with hospitalized patients when a group with similar problems and at similar stages of adaptation can be gathered. Individual discussion with patients/families is appropriate and valuable during the acute phase of illness because it allows them to express their feelings and interpretations.

Demonstration. Demonstration involves acting out a procedure while giving appropriate explanations to provide the learner with a clear idea of how to perform a task. Patients can then practice the skill and can be given feedback about their performance. This method is often used in the acute care setting, as when coughing/deep breathing or taking one's own pulse is taught.

Box 3-4   **Teaching Plan for Patient Undergoing Coronary Artery Bypass Surgery**

PREOPERATIVE PHASE

During preoperative educational interactions the nurse should assess the patient/family's level of anxiety and the effect on the ability or desire to learn. Preoperative education should be individualized to prepare the patient appropriately for the surgery, to provide education about postoperative care, and to minimize anxiety. Before the teaching-learning experience, the nurse should do the following:

- Assess the patient's level of anxiety and desire to learn about the upcoming surgery.
- Individualize the preoperative teaching plan based on assessment findings.

Areas to Consider in Teaching Session

- Review of coronary artery bypass graft (CABG) procedure
- Time leaving room for surgery, length of surgery, location of family waiting area
- Surgical preparation and shave
- Nothing by mouth (NPO) after midnight
- What to expect when awakening from anesthesia
- Sights and sounds of recovery room/critical care unit
- Tubes and drains: chest tubes, hemodynamic monitoring lines, Foley catheter, intravenous lines, pacemaker wires (if appropriate), endotracheal tube (inability to speak with tube in place)
- Discomfort to expect from incisions; availability of pain medication
- Coughing/deep breathing practice
- Use of incentive spirometer
- When, how long, and how often family can visit
- Usual length of critical care unit stay

Other Nursing Actions

- Reassure patient/family that many staff members and much activity around bedside are normal and do not indicate complications.
- Elicit and answer any specific questions that patient/family may have at this time.
- Determine specific needs and desires for day of surgery (e.g., patient needs hearing aid or glasses as soon as possible).
- Meet with family alone to offer support and address concerns that they may not want to express to the patient.

CRITICAL CARE UNIT PHASE

Patient/family education is designed to meet immediate needs and reduce anxiety in the critical care unit phase. Appropriate content to address at this time includes the following:

- Basic explanation of bedside equipment
- Review of tubes and drains
- Turning, coughing, deep breathing
- Use of incentive spirometry
- Use of oxygen equipment
- Orientation to time, place, and situation
- Explanation of procedures

- Basic purpose of medications
- Explanation of normal progression in early postoperative period
- Basic range-of-motion (ROM) exercises (e.g., ankle circles, point and flex)

Other Nursing Actions

- Reassure patient/family of normal progression.
- Repeat and reinforce information as necessary.
- Answer questions as they arise.
- Begin early to prepare patient for transfer to prevent transfer anxiety.
- Determine family learning needs and address these needs with patient or in separate teaching sessions as appropriate

STEP-DOWN UNIT PHASE

After transfer from the critical care unit, patient/family educational needs increase. Short daily educational sessions should be planned to cover the following content:

- Basic pathophysiology of coronary artery disease (CAD)
- Review of CABG procedure
- Risk factors for CAD
- Upper extremity ROM exercises
- Dietary recommendations (salt-modified diet, fat/cholesterol-modified diet)
- Taking of own pulse
- Recognition and treatment of angina (use of nitroglycerin)

Other Nursing Actions

- Use audiovisual materials in teaching sessions or as reinforcement of content.
- Provide printed take-home materials outlining important content.
- Answer questions as they arise.

DISCHARGE TEACHING

Before discharge the following content should be covered with the patient and family:

- Activity guidelines
- Lifting restrictions
- Incision care
- Possibility of patient being extremely fatigued or depressed after discharge
- Guidelines for return to work, driving, and sexual activity
- Medication safety and administration

Other Nursing Actions

- Reassure patient that "ups and downs" are normal.
- If necessary, reassure patient/family that likelihood of cardiac emergencies at home is minimal.
- Provide printed material for further study by patient/family.
- Answer questions as they arise.
- Provide phone number for patient/family to call when further questions arise.

Other Methods of Instruction

In addition to the three basic methods, several other approaches are available to deliver or augment information in a patient teaching program. These methods include commercially prepared or custom-designed printed materials, bedside videotape programs, and computer-assisted patient education programs.

Written Materials. Written materials can be very useful tools in patient/family education. These materials allow repetition and reinforcement of content and provide basic information in printed form for reference later. To be useful, however, the content must be accurate and current, and the patient/family must be able to read and understand it.

Low literacy levels are considered to be a barrier to successful patient/family education and the teaching-learning process.[7] Typical patient education materials are written at or above the eighth-grade or ninth-grade reading level and may be out of reach for many people.[4,8] Almost 20% of the U.S. adult population have low literacy skills and read at or below the fifth-grade reading level.[9] To help overcome the problem of low literacy, it is recommended that patient education materials be printed at or below the fifth-grade reading level[8,10] (Box 3-5).

Audiovisual Media. Using media devices can be an excellent method of instruction. Use of overhead projectors, slides, pictures, videos, and closed-circuit patient education TV channels are the most frequently used audiovisual media strategies. These methods entertain the learners as much as "tell" them important information they should know. This type of media can provide "nice to know" information as well as "need to know" information. Viewing a video alone does not ensure retention of material or knowledge acquisition. Patient education channels and videos should not replace nurse interaction and should be used jointly. The nurse must review with the learner the content presented to reiterate key points and evaluate the outcome.

Closed-circuit television (CCTV) is a common service in many health care settings. CCTV is best used as one component of a comprehensive educational program and is not intended to be used alone. CCTV allows for viewing of the session at a time that best suits the patient/family and can be stopped, restarted, or repeated as necessary.

Computer-assisted Instruction. Computer-assisted instruction (CAI) is new in the patient/family education arena. Although personal computers are now commonplace, this learning medium may not be suitable for some individuals because comfort levels with technical aspects of the computer vary. The learner must pay attention to the material being presented and must not be preoccupied with learning how to use the "mouse." Many computer systems available to the general public for learning purposes have "touch screens" that are easy to use and do not depend on the learner being familiar with computers. These CAI programs are generally easy to use, self-directed, and presented in a pleasurable, colorful format.

Internet Websites. Patients and families often use Internet websites to research information regarding the illness or condition of concern. Websites contain a wealth of information, but not all the information is accurate. The nurse must advise the patient/family of this fact and ask them to print out and bring in such material so that it can be discussed.

Evaluation
What to Evaluate

The evaluation process helps the nurse determine the effectiveness of patient/family education interventions. The nurse must decide how well the learner has met the expected outcomes and objectives. Evaluation should be done as each intervention is carried out to allow the nurse to give feedback to the patient/family and revise the education plan of care to accommodate continued learning needs. It is also important to assess the patient/family's response to the process. The response to the teaching-learning interaction includes the level of interest, willingness to learn, and level of participation.

How to Evaluate

There are several ways to determine the effectiveness of the teaching-learning process. Evaluating knowledge can be done through verbal questioning or written testing on the topic. Questioning provides an interactive avenue for the nurse to assess whether the learner has retained the information taught. Verbal questioning should occur not only immediately after the teaching event but also later to

---

Box **3-5**	Example of Different Reading Levels in Critical Care Education

COLLEGE READING LEVEL

Consult your physician immediately with the onset of chest discomfort, shortness of breath, or increased perspiration.

TWELFTH-GRADE READING LEVEL

Call your physician immediately if you experience chest discomfort, shortness of breath, or increased sweatness.

EIGHTH-GRADE READING LEVEL

Call your doctor immediately if you start having chest pain or shortness of breath or feel sweaty.

FOURTH-GRADE READING LEVEL

Call your doctor right away if you start having chest pain, can't breathe, or feel sweaty.

assess knowledge retention. Some CAI programs include a posttest that provides participants with immediate feedback on their learning. Written tests may also be administered to assess knowledge retention but are infrequently used in the critical care setting.

Observation and return demonstration represent the evaluation of choice for the skills-learning domain. For the patient/family to be "checked off" on a particular skill, they should be able to perform it independently, using the nurse only as a resource for questions. Endotracheal suctioning, placing condom catheters, and performing dressing changes are common tasks that patients and families may be asked to learn. Because of the increasingly complex care patients now require at home after discharge, these skills may be the entire focus of teaching before discharge.

It is important to remember that not every teaching moment is a success, and the nurse should not have feelings of guilt or failure when the learner has not achieved the desired objective. Revisiting and revising the goals and objectives during the teaching-learning session may be necessary to meet the ever-changing needs of the patient or family (Box 3-6).

Documentation

Documentation of the teaching-learning process is multifaceted and should reflect each component in the education plan of care. Whenever a teaching-learning encounter has been completed, the interaction, material taught, and learner response must be recorded.[11] The assessment documentation should include assessment of patient/family learning needs, abilities, preferences, and readiness to learn as well as potential barriers to learning. The remainder of the documentation should include the expected outcome/goals, objectives, interventions, who was taught, what was taught, materials used, patient/family response to teaching, and any follow-up education or materials needed.

Informational Needs of Families in Critical Care

Family members and significant others of critically ill patients are integral to the recovery of their loved ones. When planning for the overall care of patients, nurses and other caregivers need to consider the informational and emotional support needs of this group.[12] Families of critically ill patients report their greatest need is for information.[13] Flexible visiting hours and informational booklets regarding the critical care experience are recommended to meet this need (Box 3-7).[14]

PREPARATION OF PATIENT/FAMILY FOR TRANSFER FROM CRITICAL CARE

Transferring a patient from the critical care unit to a step-down unit may result in anxiety and stress. At this time, patients and families have become dependent on the monitors, equipment, constant nursing attention, and abundant information received while in the critical care unit. The patient has become secure knowing that immediate physiologic and emotional needs are being met. A strong bond has often developed between the staff and the family. Many patients and families are reluctant to give up that bond and believe that their needs will not be met as well on a step-down unit. To avoid anxiety and provide the patient and family with some control over the event, nurses need to prepare them for the transfer process.

Preparation for transfer should start after the patient has been stabilized and the life-threatening event that resulted in hospitalization has subsided. The stressor at this point is not the now-familiar critical care environment but the unfamiliar step-down environment. Explanations as to where the patient will be transferred, the reason for transfer, and the name of the nurse who will be providing care should be provided as soon as known. Before transfer, information about changes in care, expectations for self-care, and visiting hours should be provided to the patient/family. Family members should also be contacted concerning exactly when the patient will be transferred so they can be present during the transfer or made aware of the patient's new location.

Box 3-6 **Teaching Strategies for Critical Care Nurses**

- Assess patient/family learning needs.
- Assess patient/family readiness to learn.
- Set realistic and measurable goals.
- "Clump" information together in the most simple and understandable manner.
- Provide opportunity for demonstration and practice of new skills.
- Provide simple, clear, written instructions; consider videotape or alternative format as appropriate to patient/family learning style and teaching material.
- Provide feedback and opportunity for review of information.
- Individualize regimen to patient lifestyle and preferences.
- Reinforce new knowledge and behaviors.
- Ensure appropriate follow-up (e.g., community resources, support groups, home health care).

Box 3-7 **Informational Requirements of Families with a Critically Ill Patient**

- Have questions answered honestly.
- Know the facts about the patient's prognosis.
- Know the results of procedures as soon as possible.
- Have staff inform family members of the patient's status.
- Know why things are being done.
- Know about possible complications.
- Receive explanations that can be understood.
- Know exactly what is being done.
- Know about the staff providing care.
- Receive directions about what to do during a procedure.

Modified from Miracle VA, Hovenkamp G: *Am J Crit Care* 3(3):155, 1994.

The education plan of care and tips learned by the critical care staff about that particular patient and family should be communicated to the step-down unit staff. Most of the patient transfers made from the critical care unit to a step-down unit are planned events. At times, however, unplanned or unexpected transfers occur, usually when the critical care unit requires bed space for a more seriously ill patient. In this situation the transfer occurs quickly, either during the day or often at night. Families may be present in the hospital or may have gone home for the evening. This sudden need to transfer the patient can produce as much anxiety as the initial event, primarily because the patient/family may not feel ready for the transfer or may think they have lost control of the situation. Providing the patient/family with concrete evidence of improvement, such as more favorable vital signs or the need for fewer medications or tubes, can assure them of improvement in the patient's condition before unplanned transfers occur.

REFERENCES

1. Joint Commission on Accreditation of Healthcare Organizations: *Comprehensive accreditation manual for hospitals*, Oakbrook Terrace, Ill, 2000, The Commission.
2. Hansen M, Fisher JC: Patient-centered teaching from theory to practice, *Am J Nurs* 98(1):56, 1998.
3. Phillips LD: Patient education: understanding the process to maximize time and outcomes, *J Intraven Nurs* 22(1):19-35, 1999.
4. Rankin S, Stallings K: *Patient education: issues, principles, practices*, ed 3, Philadelphia, 1996, Lippincott.
5. Ruzicki D: Realistically meeting the educational needs of hospitalized acute and short-stay patients, *Nurs Clin North Am* 24(3):629-637, 1989.
6. Barnes LP: The illiterate client: strategies in patient teaching, *MCN Am J Matern Child Nurs* 17(3):127, 1992.
7. Quirk P: Screening for literacy and readability: implications for the advanced practice nurse, *Clin Nurse Spec* 14(1):26-32, 2000.
8. Doak C, Doak L, Root J: *Teaching patients with low literacy skills*, ed 2, Philadelphia, 1996, Lippincott.
9. Doak C et al: Improving comprehension for cancer patients with low literacy skills: strategies for clinicians, *CA Cancer J Clin* 48(3):151-162, 1998.
10. Klingbeil C, Speece M, Schubiner H: Readability of pediatric patient education materials, *Clin Pediatr (Phila)* 34(2):96-102, 1995.
11. Casey F: Documenting patient education: a literature review, *J Contin Educ Nurs* 26(6):257-260, 1995.
12. Doering LV, McGuire AW, Rourke D: Recovering from cardiac surgery: what patients want to know, *Am J Crit Care* 11(4):333-343, 2002.
13. Henneman EA, McKenzie JB, Dewa CS: An evaluation of interventions for meeting the information needs of families of critically ill patients, *Am J Crit Care* 1(3):85, 1993.
14. Miracle VA, Hovenkamp G: Needs of families of patients undergoing invasive cardiac procedures, *Am J Crit Care* 3(3):155, 1994.

UNIT TWO

COMMON PROBLEMS IN CRITICAL CARE

RUTH N. GRENDELL

4

Psychosocial Alterations

Objectives

- Explain the following coping strategies as they relate to critically ill patients: regression, suppression, denial, trust, religious beliefs, and family support.
- Describe the needs and coping mechanisms of families of critically ill patients.
- Explain interventions and nursing management for patients with coping alterations.
- Identify situations that increase the risk of disturbances of self-concept.

evolve Be sure to check out the free exercises on-line at *http://evolve.elsevier.com/Urden/priorities/*

33

Patients requiring critical care must cope with a variety of stressors. A patient's response to these stressors depends on individual differences, such as age, gender, social support, cultural background, medical diagnosis, current hospital course, and prognosis. A person's perceptions of self and relationships with others, of spiritual values, and of self-competency in social roles also play a major role in how he or she will respond to stress and illness. This chapter provides a theoretic basis for understanding these various issues and provides the nurse with additional insight into implementing holistic nursing care.

SELF-CONCEPT

The human self-concept is a major concern for nurses because nursing interventions that do not consider the individual in his or her wholeness, including the self-concept, will probably not be effective. The self-concept comprises attitudes about oneself; perceptions of personal abilities, body image, and identity; and a general sense of worth. The stressors imposed by physical illness, trauma, and surgical procedures can cause disturbances in the self-concept. A person's response to these stressors depends on a variety of individual differences (Box 4-1).

Box 4-1 Stressors in the Critical Care Setting

Patients' experience of critical illness and care will vary. However, each patient must cope with at least some of the following stressors:
- Threat of death
- Threat of survival, with significant residual problems related to the illness/injury
- Pain or discomfort
- Lack of sleep
- Loss of autonomy over most aspects of life and daily functioning
- Loss of control over environment, such as loss of privacy and exposure to light, noise, and general activity of the critical care unit, including the care of other patients
- Daily hassles or common frustrations
- Loss of usual role, and with that, loss of the arena in which usual coping mechanisms serve the patient
- Separation from family and friends
- Loss of dignity
- Boredom, broken only by brief visits, threatening stimuli, and frightening thoughts
- Loss of ability to express self verbally when intubated

Effects and response to the stressors depend on the individual's perception of the intensity of the stress and the following factors:
- Acute/chronic duration of stressors
- Cumulative effect of simultaneous stressors
- Sequence of stressors
- Individual's previous experience with stressors and coping effectiveness
- Amount of social support

The terms "self-concept" and "self-esteem" have often been used synonymously, with no clear-cut definitions made. However, theoretic models used in the development of measurements refer to the *self-concept* as the "self-schema," or knowledge, of abilities, beliefs, and values that influence behavior during interactions with others in the social and cultural environments. *Self-esteem* is most closely linked to one's sense of self-worth.[1-3] Although relatively stable, the self-concept can be modified by the developmental phases and social roles a person experiences over a lifetime.[3,4] Any event with unpredictable body changes and functions requires adjustments in the self-concept as well as a realistic readjustment to the role limitations that are imposed. These adjustment stages are complex and highly individualized.

A person faced with an intolerable situation may panic, may display behavior that distorts reality, and may exhibit excessive demands or may be suspicious of motives and methods of the caregivers. Depression and anxiety are common reactions as the person experiences a loss of control and worries over outcomes.[5,6] The illness experience may have different meanings for individuals from different cultures and ethnic groups. Assessment of their needs can be elicited through use of tools that include questions that are sensitive to cultural values.[2,6-8] Patients in critical care units usually do not have time to adjust to the illness conditions and may exhibit signs of shock, numbness, and avoidance of reality and may be unable to understand clearly the implications of the situation.[9,10] The patient is usually transferred to an intermediate care unit before a true acknowledgment phase occurs.

Body Image Disturbance

Body image is the mental picture an individual has of his or her body and its physical functioning at any given time. It includes one's attitudes and feelings about one's body in reference to appearance, build, health, performance ability, and gender-related concepts.[5] The body image develops over time from internal sensations of postural changes, contact with people and objects in the environment, emotional experiences, and fantasies. The ability to project possible images of one's self in the future that are highly desirable or feared may play a powerful role in motivating and regulating goal-directed behavior.[1]

Disturbances in body image arise when the person fails to perceive or adapt to the changes that are imposed by age, disease, trauma, or surgery. In some cases the person may feel betrayed by the body, which no longer seems "normal." Body image may also be altered by the need to incorporate a prosthetic device or a donated body part.[9,11] The disease or problem may be corrected by surgery and treatments, but when the result is visible to the patient and others, the change in body image can arouse intense feelings of anger, frustration, depression, and powerlessness.[9,12] The critical care nurse often begins the process of helping the patient live with this permanent alteration. Interventions by the nurse and other health team members focus on helping the person manage the physical changes and the psychosocial alterations.

Disturbances in Self-Esteem

Self-esteem, or self-measurement of one's worth, develops as a part of self-concept through the perceived appraisals of significant others.[1] The need for self-esteem is a part of the hierarchy of human needs postulated by Maslow.[13] Having high self-esteem helps a person deal with the environment and face the maturational and situational crises of life more easily. Persons with a well-developed self-esteem are at less risk for disturbances of self-esteem than those with poorly developed self-esteem.[4,11]

Self-esteem has been studied in a variety of contexts and is an important concept for nurses, who have a significant impact on ill patients' understanding.[5,11,14] Illness can rob the person of perspective and shrinks both the familiar world and the one of possibility, often leading to low self-esteem, powerlessness, helplessness, and depression.[5,6,15] A low self-regard impairs one's ability to adapt. The person may refuse to participate in self-care, may exhibit self-destructive behavior, or may be too compliant, asking no questions and permitting others to make all decisions.[16] Refer to the Nursing Management Plan for Situational Low Self-Esteem (p. 504).

POWERLESSNESS

Powerlessness, as a nursing diagnosis, is defined as the perception of the individual that one's own action will not significantly affect an outcome.[6,17,18] Unrelieved powerlessness may result in hopelessness (see Coping Mechanisms).

The causes of powerlessness include factors in the health care environment, interpersonal interactions, one's culture and religious beliefs, illness-related regimen, and a lifestyle of helplessness. The range in levels of powerlessness varies and depends on the person's perceived sense of control, the amount of losses experienced, and the availability of social support. Powerlessness can be manifested by delayed decision making or refusal to make decisions and by expressions of self-doubt in role performance. Frustration, anger, and resentment over being dependent on others often manifest as verbal expressions of dissatisfaction with care.[8]

Individuals vary in the amount of control they prefer.[16,19] The critical care unit routines may oppose or preclude any control by the patient. The person for whom control is important should be helped to continue to control as many areas of life as possible. On the other hand, a patient must be given the opportunity to choose not to control.

Rotter's early research on human behavior and perception of control has helped explain the variability of responses from persons in similar situations.[20] He proposed two major concepts of internal versus external locus of control. Individuals who have *internal* locus of control perceive themselves to be responsible for the outcome of events.

Individuals with *external* locus of control believe their actions will have no effect on outcomes of a situation. The scale to measure internal/external locus of control developed by Rotter is useful in assessing this personality trait, which is a relatively stable tendency.

Another aspect of powerlessness is *learned helplessness*, or *excessive dependence*.[21] A person who repeatedly experiences uncontrollable situations loses the motivation for making decisions about life events. Some people assume a "martyr" role and accept the illness state as their fate, thus doing nothing to improve their status. Others may find the sick role a gratifying means for gaining control over others by using their symptoms to gain attention.[22] Setting limits on these behaviors, encouraging independence and participation in self-care, providing counseling, and involving family members in establishing realistic goals are helpful strategies to assist the person to abandon this manipulative behavior.

Critically ill patients generally have experienced a rapid onset of illness without time to acquire the illness role. If "control" is defined as the ability to determine the use of time, space, and resources, admission to a critical care unit strips away this power. On admission, persons lose their independent status and become patients. Choice of clothing and use of other personal belongings are usually restricted in a critical care unit. Patients cannot decide who enters the room, who provides personal care, or who intrudes with painful treatments. Hospital rules usually are not open to modification. Patients may feel anxious because they are separated from a familiar environment and have restrictions on who may visit them.[23]

Poor interactions with the health care providers may make the situation worse. Patients may react aggressively, may try bargaining, or may refuse to comply with diagnostic and treatment regimens. They may resent the close scrutiny of the nurses and physicians and the invasion of their privacy. By virtue of their experiences with critical illness and care, people may lose sight of areas of influence they still do retain over themselves because so much control has been taken from them. Nursing emphasizes the patient's influence on control and thus helps to preserve it.[10,14] Refer to the Nursing Management Plan for Powerlessness (p. 498).

SPIRITUAL DISTRESS

Spiritual distress has been defined as the disruption in the life principle that pervades one's being and that integrates and transcends one's biologic and psychosocial nature.[17,18] Adherence to a particular philosophic, psychologic, sociologic, or political belief may bring a sense of one's value and of life's meaning. Threats imposed by any physiologic or psychologic illness and prolonged pain and suffering can challenge a person's spirituality.[24] Life-threatening illness causes a person to face his or her mortality. The provision of holistic nursing care is not limited to meeting a person's religious needs; it also encompasses all that provides meaning to life.

A person in spiritual distress may question the meaning of suffering and death in relation to a personal belief system. The person may express anger toward God or other supreme being, feelings of self-blame, or regret over inability to practice belief rituals. Individuals may even question the necessity for the therapeutic regimen. *Spiritual care* is described as health-promoting interventions that relieve the responses to stress affecting spiritual perspectives of individuals or groups.[25]

ACUTE CONFUSION AND DELIRIUM

Acute confusion, which encompasses *global cognitive impairment*, has not been clearly or consistently defined.[26] Synonyms include delirium (the medical term), intensive care unit (ICU) psychosis, postcardiotomy delirium, and acute brain failure. Additional terms are acute mental status change, acute organic reaction, metabolic encephalopathy, and reversible cognitive dysfunction. Orientation to person, time, and place and the ability to reason, follow directions, process incoming stimuli, and maintain concentration are lost. Confused persons may be aware of these disturbances and fear that they are "losing their minds." The confused state is a secondary response to *organic* causes (e.g., hypoxia, drugs, fluid-electrolyte imbalance) or *inorganic* causes (e.g., stress, sleep deprivation).

Onset is abrupt, and duration can be shortened if early diagnosis and treatment are initiated. Confusion develops in an estimated 50% of hospitalized elderly patients but is often misdiagnosed because of inaccurate assessment and assumptions that the mental deterioration is a result of aging.[27,28] More than 80% of reports of confused status in elderly patients are attributed to organic causes; dehydration and recent falls, hip fractures, and polypharmacy are additional risk factors for confusion. Behavioral symptoms may be subtle and varied. Prodromal symptoms include insomnia, distractibility, drowsiness, anxiety, and nightmares. Symptoms of acute confusion resemble those of dementia, which makes differentiation between the two conditions more difficult. However, dementia, which cannot be reversed, has a gradual onset and is of long duration (Table 4-1.)

Approximately 10% to 15% of all hospitalized medical-surgical patients experience symptoms of delirium. This percentage is increased by 30% to 40% in the critical care setting. Hospital stays are prolonged for this population.[19,26] An increased level of confusion may be the first indicator of a biologic problem or may be the result of environmental stressors.

Etiology

Understanding the causes and symptoms of delirium, knowing those at risk for developing delirium, and using appropriate measures to minimize causal factors are primary aspects of the critical care nurse role. Many causes of or contributors to delirium can occur for anyone at any given time. Three predisposing contributors to the development of delirium

are (1) age 60 years or older, (2) brain damage, and (3) a chronic brain disorder, such as Alzheimer's disease.

Drugs typically used in the ICU are contributing factors to delirium, including digitalis, antibiotics, steroids, β-adrenergic blockers, and respiratory stimulants. Additional causes of delirium include sleep deprivation, sensory deprivation/overload, and immobilization, which are common events in the ICU.[29]

The patient in the ICU is deprived of the restorative benefits of deep sleep and the rapid eye movement (REM) phase of sleep because of frequent interruptions by equipment noises, voices, and procedures. Bright overhead lights, absence of day-night cycles, immobility, pain, and medications contribute to the patient's disorientation to time and place. Daytime napping, complaints of fatigue, and slurred speech can result, as well as depression, cognitive impairment, and hallucinations. Delayed recovery, increased length of hospital stay, and seriousness of the sleep deprivation are closely related.

The literature reports more than 30 terms for describing the confusion syndrome.[26] Many of the terms are misleading, are narrow in scope, and give cause for overlooking some of the possible reasons for the behaviors. The *Diagnostic and Statistical Manual of Mental Disorders*[30] (currently the revised fourth edition, DSM-IV-R) uses the term *delirium* as the only official designation for this syndrome and has established specific criteria to use in making this diagnosis.

Assessment

Three forms of delirium have been identified: hyperactive, hypoactive, and a mixture of both forms.[26,31] Patients with *hyperactive delirium* may become violent; may remove intravenous lines, dressings, and catheters; may be extremely restless and try to get out of bed; may pick at things in the air; and may call out to persons who are not there. Sympathetic nervous system responses of tachycardia, dilation of pupils, diaphoresis, and facial flushing are evident. Patients with *hypoactive delirium* complain of extreme fatigue, are slow to respond, and have hypersomnolence that can progress to loss of consciousness. At times these individuals are absorbed in a dreamlike state, mumble to themselves, experience vivid hallucinations, and make inappropriate gestures. The third form of delirium is a mixture of agitation and hypoactive behaviors that may vary throughout the day. Symptoms and hallucinations seem to worsen during the night, often referred to as the *sundowner's syndrome*, with more lucid intervals during the day.

Mental Status Examination

The mental status examination is a full, criteria-based assessment of the patient's cognitive function and thought processes. Although the examination is rarely conducted in its entirety in the critical care setting, knowledge of its main components will enhance the nurse's effectiveness in

Table 4-1   Comparison of Delirium and Dementia: Course and Symptoms

Area of Interest	Delirium	Dementia
Onset	Sudden; global cognitive impairment. Symptoms may fluctuate throughout day; may be more severe at night, in the dark, or on awakening.	Gradual; global cognitive impairment that is slowly progressive over time.
Duration	Most often *reversible* when treated appropriately. Symptoms may remain indefinitely if cause is not determined.	Generally *irreversible*. Alzheimer's disease is the most common form.
Etiology	Infection, medications, ICU stressors (see Box 4-1), hospitalization, fluid-electrolyte imbalance, disease (e.g., myocardial infarction, CVA). *Delirium often occurs when severe infection/illness is superimposed in patients with Alzheimer's disease.*	Several theories: infection, neurotoxic agents (aluminum), angiopathy and blood-brain barrier incompetence, multiple small CVAs or cardiovascular problems, neurotransmitter/receptor deficiencies, abnormal proteins and by-products, genetic defects. *Elderly persons are most vulnerable.*
Orientation	Loss of orientation to person, place, and time and ability to reason or follow instructions; hallucinations and illusions, mind wandering, incoherent speech, sudden speech outbursts, swearing, poor judgment.	Difficulty with abstract thinking; impaired judgment; difficulty in finding words; loss of communication with others; loss of "personhood," passive behaviors, eventually requires dependent care.
Memory	Impaired, especially involving recent events.	Recent and remote memory impaired; degree of impairment varies; slow recall; frequent short-term deficit.
Psychomotor actions	Continual, aimless activity common, or variable with hypokinetic/hyperkinetic or mixed activity; easily agitated, startled, or distracted.	Normal or may have apraxia.
Sleep	Disturbed sleep-wake cycle; may be reversed (nighttime wakefulness/daytime napping). Symptoms of depression may be present (withdrawal/isolation).	Sleep may be fragmented. Symptoms of depression may be present (withdrawal/isolation, nighttime wakefulness/daytime napping, somatic complaints); affects 20%-30% of patients with dementia.

Data from Henry M: *Am J Nurs* 102(3):49-55, 2002; Colling KA: *J Nurs Scholarsh* 32(3):239-244, 2000; Pace-Murphy K, Dyer C, Gleason M: In Fortinash K, Holoday-Worret P, editors: *Psychiatric mental health nursing,* St Louis, 2000, Mosby; and Graham I: *J Clin Nurs* 8(6):675-683, 1999.
ICU, Intensive care unit; *CVA,* cerbrovascular accident (stroke).

collecting data to document findings by using accepted terminology and identifying issues that need further assessment (Box 4-2).

Management

Sedation is prescribed for patients with hyperactive delirium. *Risperidone* (Risperdal) is now preferred over haloperidol in treatment of delirium because it produces less sedation and fewer extrapyramidal (pseudoparkinsonian) symptoms. It also has fewer anticholinergic effects (e.g., dry mouth, constipation, urinary retention). Risperidone has been effective in treating aggression, agitation, and other psychotic symptoms of dementia. It is classified as an atypical (serotonin/dopamine antagonist) antipsychotic because of its effectiveness in treating both positive and negative symptoms of schizophrenia. A regular dosing schedule is preferred rather than waiting until symptoms recur before giving another dose. A combination of risperidone and *lorazepam* (Ativan), a benzodiazepine drug with a short half-life, allows lower doses of each drug to be given. This combination is most useful in treating delirium related to alcohol or benzodiazepine withdrawal.[26,32]

When delirium is considered to be secondary to pain, narcotics can be administered. However, the paradoxical effects of depressed respirations and cardiac output can exacerbate the delirium. The elderly patient in particular benefits from smaller doses given on a regular basis.[26]

Finally, neuromuscular blocking agents are sometimes used for severely agitated patients who are on mechanical ventilation to effect a decrease in oxygen consumption, to promote synchrony with the ventilator, and to increase tissue oxygenation. These complex drugs can be dangerous but do not affect consciousness, cognition, or pain levels, which

---

| Box **4-2** | **The Mental Status Examination** |

GENERAL OBSERVATIONS
- Appearance
- Reaction to interviewer
- Behavior and psychomotor activity

SENSORIUM AND INTELLIGENCE
- Level of consciousness
- Orientation
- Memory
- Intellectual function
- Judgment
- Comprehension

THOUGHT PROCESSES
- Form of thought
- Content of thought
- Mood
- Affect
- Insight

---

would require the addition of sedatives or analgesics.[32] Refer to the Nursing Management Plan for Acute Confusion (p. 469) for specific nursing interventions.

COPING MECHANISMS

When a patient copes effectively, what he or she is doing to cope often goes unnoticed. Emotionally the patient seems relatively comfortable, is a cooperative recipient of care, and exhibits nonproblematic behavior. The patient may be using multiple appropriate coping mechanisms that help to manage a problem or stressful situation. Refer to the Nursing Management Plan for Powerlessness (p. 498) for specific nursing interventions.

Regression

Regression is an unconscious defense mechanism that involves a retreat, in the face of stress, to behavior characteristic of an earlier developmental level.[33] Regression allows the patient to give up his or her usual role, autonomy, and privacy to become the passive recipient of medical and nursing care. In fact, the patient who does *not* regress jeopardizes his or her care. Conversely, the patient who becomes *too* regressed presents another problem. Regression is a normal reaction to severe burns, and the person may become childlike in interactions with staff, whining, clinging to staff, and attempting to keep the nurse at the bedside. In both cases the patient must know the limits set on behavior if he or she is to receive essential care. The patient is best served when limits are set in a supportive manner.

Although the behavior of these patients can provoke confrontations or reprimands, such responses should be avoided. These responses from staff may only worsen a situation in which a patient is already struggling with issues of dependence and autonomy.

Suppression

Suppression is a conscious, intentional process in which patients push ideas, problems, or desires out of their conscious thoughts.[33] Patients often use suppression when their problems are overwhelming and they are in no position to resolve them. Before becoming ill, for example, an individual may have been struggling to meet financial obligations but now uses suppression to postpone dealing with this concern until later in the recovery phase.

Denial

According to the North American Nursing Diagnosis Association (NANDA), denial includes both conscious and unconscious attempts to disavow knowledge or the meaning of an event. This text uses the psychoanalytic definition of denial, "an unconscious defense mechanism that reduces anxiety by eliminating or reducing the seriousness of the perceived threat," to allow for the distinction between denial and suppression. When used by a critically ill patient, denial reduces the anxiety and the threat of the illness.[17]

The degree to which denial is used varies among patients and may vary in the same patient at different times. Patients also may deny different aspects of the illness.

Trust

Trust manifests in the critical care patient as the belief that the staff will see the patient through the illness, managing any untoward event that might occur. Trust is an unconscious process in which the patient transfers the trust learned in early significant relationships onto caregivers in the present.[23,34]

Hope

Although hope has long been recognized as a significant factor in patient recovery and survival, the phenomenon receives little attention until the patient becomes hopeless. Hope is the expectation that a desire will be fulfilled. It can exist even in the face of a realistic appraisal of a grim situation.[34] Hope supports the patient and helps the patient endure the physical and psychologic insults of the daily experience. Hope is central to resilience and spiritual strength.[6,15,35,36]

Spiritual Beliefs and Practices

Spiritual beliefs and practices may provide the patient with some measure of acceptance of an illness, a sense of mastery and control, a source of hope and trust beyond the limits the staff can provide, and the strength to endure the current stress. A patient may discuss personal beliefs and concerns openly or view the subject as a private and personal matter.[6,24,37]

Use of Family Support

The patient may use the presence of a supportive family to cope with critical illness. The patient with a supportive family knows that family members share a past and hope for a future with the patient. They love the patient as a person and member of the family. The patient also realizes that family members know him or her in ways the staff cannot. With family the patient may know that his or her experience is truly understood, even when little is said. Family members also may be involved in the patient's personal care and may attend to the practical problems the patient cannot, such as managing finances.[38]

Sharing Concerns

Sharing concerns with a caring and understanding listener can relieve some of the patient's spiritual and emotional distress. The patient is consoled knowing that he or she is not alone and that someone knows and cares about what the patient is experiencing.[14,34] The patient may share concerns with family members. However, the patient may be reluctant to upset loved ones further or may have a family for whom such communication is not the norm. A patient who relies on this coping mechanism will benefit from a nurse who recognizes when a patient needs to talk and who knows how to listen.

COPING ASSESSMENT

Ineffective coping may be suggested in patient behaviors. Overt hostility, severe regression, and noncompliance with treatment may suggest ineffective coping. The patient may also report such problems as severe anxiety, despondence, and despair. The nurse who suspects that coping is ineffective should consider a number of factors before questioning the patient directly.

It is not always clear whether the patient's coping is truly ineffective and intervention by the nurse is indicated. Witnessing problematic behavior can be very uncomfortable, especially when that behavior is directed at the caregiver. Careful evaluation of one's reaction to the behavior is needed to discover whether patient care can continue to be provided objectively by the nurse alone, or whether consultation with other team members is needed to alleviate the problem.[8,9,23,24]

COPING ENHANCEMENT

Some patients remember well their time in the ICU, whereas others have few memories of the experience. A recent study revealed that the overall psychosocial need of ICU patients was a feeling of safety. Nurses providing emotional support and encouragement, supplying information about patients' progress, helping them regain some control and independence, instilling a sense of hope, and building a close trusting relationship with family members made the patients feel safe. The patients felt reassured by the nurses' professional skill performance and sensitivity to their emotional and spiritual needs.[10,14,38] Essential techniques for effective interventions include an attitude of caring; openness and warmth; and withholding judgment until the nurse "knows" the patient (has an understanding of the individual's perception about self), the current illness or problem, and the type of social support available. Assessment skills are essential, as is a willingness to become involved when the potential for, or use of, ineffective coping mechanisms exists.

Teaching the patient new coping skills may be impossible, because individuals have a repertoire of defense and coping mechanisms, both conscious and unconscious, that they automatically bring into play when facing stressful situations. A person who is experiencing extreme psychologic stress cannot learn new methods to manage these defense mechanisms. However, the nurse may help to reduce the level of anxiety by employing active listening, encouraging support from family members and other caregivers, and introducing changes in the environment as appropriate. In this way the nurse can facilitate the changes the patient must make. It is extremely important that the patient express an interest in learning and recognize a personal need for help.[6,36]

A patient's trust in the nurse's competence in the physical and technical aspects of care aids in the patient's participation. Hope is instilled when the nurse and other caregivers display a sense of realistic optimism regarding the patient's progress. Patients must receive honest feedback because they are keen observers of their caregivers and read them well. Trust and hope are easily lessened when inappropriate information is given.[38] Refer to the Nursing Management Plan for Anxiety (p. 475) and Ineffective Coping (p. 495) for specific nursing interventions.

Supporting Family Members

Patient-centered care is also family-centered care. Consideration of nonbiologic or nonlegal partners of the patient as members of the patient's support system is also necessary in providing holistic care. The nurse's support of family members at the bedside can enhance the value of the visits for the patient,[36-38] and other supportive interventions should be considered (Box 4-3).[39] Patients often look to the family for love, understanding, support, and care in matters they cannot attend to themselves.

Supporting Spiritual Care

There is a certain amount of uncertainty in all illness experiences, and it affects a person's adaptation and outcomes. *Uncertainty* has been defined as a multidimensional concept related to the inability to determine the meaning of illness-related events.[12,33] Self-reflection, with a focus on examining issues that attack the self, is a component of the search for meaning.[25] Separation from religious rituals/ties and intense suffering can induce spiritual distress for patients and their families. Using a spiritual assessment tool to identify a person/family's perception of their current situation, inner strengths, self-concept, and beliefs helps the nurse in supporting spiritual care.[6,24,25]

Box **4-3**	Interventions to Support Family Members

1. Identify a family spokesperson and support persons.
2. Identify a primary nursing contact for the family.
3. Establish a mechanism for family access to the patient.
4. Promote access to the patient, and ensure consistency in adhering to unit routines.
5. Establish a mechanism to contact the family and to update on changes in patient status.
6. Provide information based on family needs.
7. Ensure support services are available, and refer to specialized services as needed.
8. Explain all procedures using understandable terms.
9. Include family in providing care.
10. Provide a comfortable environment for the family.
11. Include family in end-of-life planning, and provide palliative care and support for terminally ill patients and families.

Modified from Twibell RS: *Dimens Crit Care Nurs* 17(2):100-112, 1998.

REFERENCES

1. Stein K, Rose R, Markus H: Self-schemas and possible selves as predictors and outcomes of risky behaviors in adolescents, *Nurs Res* 47(2):96-106, 1998.
2. Mendyka B: Exploring culture in nursing: a theory-driven practice, *Holistic Nurs Pract* 15(1):32-41, 2000.
3. Coopersmith S: *The antecedents of self-esteem*, San Francisco, 1967, Freeman.
4. Judge T, Erez A, Bono J, Thoresen C: Are measures of self-esteem, neuroticism, locus of control and generalized self-efficacy indicators for a common core construct? *J Pers Soc Psychol* 83(3):693-710, 2002.
5. Polusky S: Street music or the blues? The lived experience and social environment of depression, *Public Health Nurs* 17(4):292-299, 2000.
6. Bay E et al: Chronic stress, sense of belonging, and depression among survivors of traumatic brain injury, *J Nurs Scholarsh* 34(3):221-226, 2002.
7. Beck AT et al: The measurement of pessimism: the hopelessness scale, *J Couns Clin Psychol* 42(6):861, 1974.
8. National Institute of Mental Health: Depression, www.nimh.nih.gov, 2002.
9. Kaba E, Thompson D, Burnard P: Coping after heart transplantation: A descriptive study of heart transplant recipients' methods of coping, *J Adv Nurs* 32(4):930-936, 2000.
10. Hupcey J: Feeling safe: The psychosocial needs of ICU patients, *J Nurs Scholarsh* 32(4):361-367, 2000.
11. Shaffer R, Corish C: Cardiac surgery and women: cardiac surgery. Part 2. Recovery, *J Cardiovasc Nurs* 12(4):14-31, 1998.
12. McCormick K: A concept analysis of uncertainty in illness, *J Nurs Scholarsh* 34(2):127-131, 2002.
13. Maslow H: *Motivation and personality*, New York, 1954, Harper & Row.
14. Whittemore R: Consequences of not "knowing the patient," *Clin Nurs Spec* 14(2):75-81, 2000.
15. Gibson J, Kenrick M: Pain and powerlessness: the experience of living with peripheral vascular disease, *J Adv Nurs* 24(4):737-745, 1998.
16. Colling K: A taxonomy of passive behaviors in people with Alzheimer's, *J Nurs Scholarsh* 32(3):239-244, 2000.
17. North American Nursing Diagnosis Association: *Nursing diagnosis: definitions and classifications*, St Louis, 2001-2002, The Association.
18. Ackley B, Ladwig G: *Nursing diagnosis handbook: a guide to planning care*, St Louis, 2001, Mosby.
19. Hustey F, Meldon S: The prevalence and documentation of impaired mental status in elderly emergency department patients, *Ann Emerg Med* 39(3):248-253, 2002.
20. Rotter JB: Generalized expectancies for internal versus external control of reinforcement, *Psychol Monogr* 80(609):1, 1966.
21. Janis IL, Rodin J: Attribution, control, and decision-making: social psychology and health care. In Stone GC, Adler NC, editors: *Health psychology—a handbook*, San Francisco, 1979, Jossey-Bass.
22. Seligman ME: *Helplessness: on depression, development and death*, San Francisco, 1975, Freeman.
23. Grendell R: Psychologic aspects of physiologic illness. In Fortinash K, Holoday-Worret P, editors: *Psychiatric mental health nursing*, ed 2, St Louis, 2000, Mosby.
24. Dossey B, Dossey L: Holistic modalities and healing moments, *Am J Nurs* 98(6):44-47, 1998.
25. Carson V, Green H: Spiritual well-being: a predictor of hardiness in patients with acquired immunodeficiency syndrome, *J Prof Nurs* 8(4):209-220, 1992.

26. Henry M: Descending into delirium, *Am J Nurs* 102(3):49-56, 2002.

27. Graham I: Reflective narrative and dementia care, *J Clin Nurs* 8(6):675-683, 1999.

28. McDougall G, Balyer J: Decreasing mental frailty in at-risk elders, *Geriatr Nurs* 19(4):220-224, 1998.

29. Redeker N: Sleep in acute care settings: an integrative review, *J Nurs Scholarsh* 32(1):31-38, 2000.

30. American Psychiatric Association: *Diagnostic and statistical manual of mental disorders*, rev ed 4 (DSM-IV-R), Washington, DC, 2000, The Association.

31. Pace-Murphy K, Dyer C, Gleason M: Delirium, dementia, and amnestic and other cognitive disorders. In Fortinash K, Holoday-Worret P, editors: *Psychiatric mental health nursing*, ed 2, St Louis, 2000, Mosby.

32. Key J, Hayes E: *Pharmacology: a nursing process approach*, Philadelphia, 2000, Saunders.

33. Holoday-Worret P: Foundations of psychiatric mental health nursing. In Fortinash K, Holoday-Worret P, editors: *Psychiatric mental health nursing*, ed 2, St Louis, 2000, Mosby.

34. Gelling L: The role of hope for relatives of critically ill patients: a review of the literature, *Nurs Stand* 4(1):33-38, 1999.

35. Roberts S, Johnson L, Kelly B: Fostering hope in the elderly congestive heart patient in critical care, *Geriatr Nurs* 20(4):195-199, 1999.

36. Morse J, Penrod J: Linking concepts of enduring, uncertainty, suffering, and hope, *Image J Nurs Sch* 31(2):145-150, 1999.

37. Taylor K: Standards of holistic nursing practice, *AORTN* 72 (6):1080, 2000.

38. Hupcey JE: Establishing the nurse-family relationship in the intensive care unit, *West J Nurs Res* 20(2):180-194, 1998.

39. Twibell RS: Family coping during critical illness, *Dimens Crit Care Nurs* 17(2):100-112, 1998.

SHEILA COX SULLIVAN
KATHY C. RICHARDS

5

Sleep Alterations

Objectives

- Define the stages of sleep.
- Explain the three physiologic effects that occur during rapid eye movement (REM) sleep.
- Describe changes in sleep resulting from the aging process.
- Define dysfunctional sleep.
- Name three commonly prescribed critical care medications that decrease REM sleep.
- Describe evidence-based practice methods for promoting sleep in critical care.

evolve Be sure to check out the free exercises on-line at *http://evolve.elsevier.com/Urden/priorities/*

SLEEP PHYSIOLOGY

Humans spend about one third of their lives engaged in a process known as *sleep*. Although little is known at present about the physiologic process or the degree to which sleep affects us, researchers are learning more about sleep every day. The behavioral definition of sleep is a reversible behavioral state of perceptual disengagement from and unresponsiveness to the environment.[1] Research involving simultaneous monitoring using the electroencephalogram (EEG), electrooculogram (EOG), and electromyogram (EMG) has shown that there are two distinct stages of sleep: *nonrapid eye movement* (NREM) and *rapid eye movement* (REM).

SLEEP STAGES
Nonrapid Eye Movement Sleep

Humans experience three states of being. They are either awake (Figure 5-1), in REM sleep, or in NREM sleep, which can be further divided into stages 1 through 4, with each stage a progressively deeper sleep state. Adults usually enter sleep through NREM *stage 1* sleep (Figure 5-2), which is a transitional, lighter sleep state from which the patient can be easily aroused by light touch or softly calling his or her name. Stage 1 is demonstrated by an EEG pattern of low-voltage, mixed-frequency waveforms with vertex sharp waves. A patient with severely disrupted sleep may experience an increase in the amount of stage 1 sleep throughout the sleep cycle. As a patient makes the transition from awake to asleep, a brief memory impairment may result.[1] Patients may experience muscle jerks and recall vivid images on awakening. These reactions, called *hypnic myoclonia*, are not pathologic but can cause the patient to awaken feeling frightened.

In NREM *stage 2*, sleep deepens, and the patient is more difficult to arouse. As stage 2 continues, high-voltage, slow-wave activity begins to appear. When these slow waves represent 20% of the EEG activity per page, they meet the criteria for NREM *stage 3* sleep. Stage 3 slow waves continue

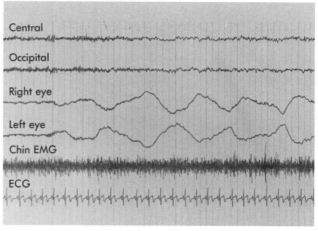

Figure 5-2   NREM stage 1 sleep.

to develop until 50% of the EEG waveforms are slow wave, which meets the criteria for *stage 4* sleep. Stages 3 and 4 often are combined and referred to as *slow-wave sleep*, or *delta sleep* (Figure 5-3). Delta sleep has the highest arousal threshold.

NREM sleep is dominated by the parasympathetic nervous system. The body tries to maintain a homeostatic regulation, resulting in a decreased level of energy expenditure. Blood pressure, heart and respiratory rates, and metabolic rate return to basal levels. EMG activity is lower in NREM versus wake states but not as low as that in REM sleep. A patient may experience sweating or shivering with temperature extremes in NREM sleep, but this ceases during REM sleep.[1]

During slow-wave sleep, 80% of growth-stimulating hormone is released, stimulating protein synthesis while sparing catabolic breakdown. The release of other hormones, such as prolactin and testosterone, suggests that anabolism is occurring during slow-wave sleep. Cortisol release peaks during early-morning hours, whereas melatonin is released only during darkness, and thyroid-stimulating hormone is

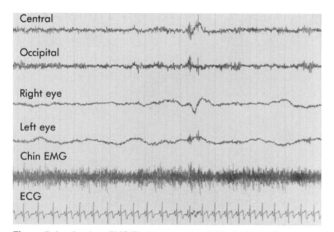

Figure 5-1   Awake. *EMG*, Electromyogram; *ECG*, electrocardiogram; upper tracings are EEG and EOG measurements.

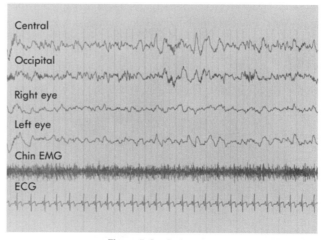

Figure 5-3   Delta sleep.

inhibited during sleep. Activities associated with NREM stage 4 sleep include protein synthesis and tissue repair, such as the repair of epithelial and specialized cells of the brain, skin, bone marrow, and gastric mucosa.[2] Some propose that NREM sleep is a restorative period that relieves the stresses of waking activities, whereas REM sleep serves to refuel creative brain stores. Table 5-1 lists the time spent in sleep stages for normal adults.

Rapid Eye Movement Sleep

Although REM sleep is also called the "dream stage," dreaming is not the exclusive property of any one stage. REM can be viewed as a highly active brain in a paralyzed body. REM sleep is frequently referred to as *paradoxical sleep* because some areas of the brain remain very active while others are suppressed. EMG waveforms are relatively slow low voltage with sawtooth waves present. Increased cortical activity occurs, with the EEG pattern resembling that of the awake state (Figure 5-4).

The sympathetic nervous system predominates during REM sleep.[3] Oxygen consumption increases, and blood pressure, cardiac output, and respiratory/heart rates become variable. The body's response to decreased oxygen levels and increased carbon dioxide levels is lowest during REM sleep. Cardiac efferent vagus nerve tone is generally suppressed during REM sleep, and irregular breathing patterns can lead to oxygen reduction, particularly in patients with pulmonary and cardiac disease. An increase in premature ventricular contractions and tachydysrhythmias may be associated with respiratory pauses during REM sleep.[3] Arterial pressure surges and increases in heart rate, coronary arterial tone, and blood viscosity may cause the combination of plaque rupture and hypercoagulability in patients with cardiac disease.[4]

SLEEP CYCLES

NREM and REM sleep cycles alternate throughout the night. Sleep onset usually occurs in stage 1 sleep, progressing through stages 2 to 4 and then going back to stage 2, at which time the person usually enters REM. This first cycle usually takes about 70 to 100 minutes, with later cycles lasting 90 to 120 minutes. Four to five cycles are completed during normal adult sleep. NREM sleep predominates during the first third of the night, whereas REM is more prominent during the last third. Brief episodes of wakefulness (usually

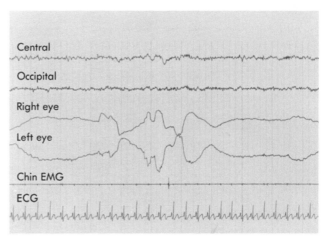

Figure 5-4   REM sleep.

less than 5%) tend to intrude later into the night and are usually not remembered the next morning.

The amount of sleep required is still debated. No set number of hours has been established, and sleep length may be determined by many factors, including genetic predisposition. A sufficient amount of sleep has been achieved when the person awakens without the alarm and proceeds through the day without feeling sleepy.

SLEEP CHANGES WITH AGE

Elderly persons most often complain about either excessive sleepiness or insomnia, and current research offers justification for both these complaints.[5] Sleep pattern changes in older adults include fewer episodes of stages 3 and 4 NREM and REM sleep.[6] Elderly persons also report that they do not sleep as soundly or feel as rested after awakening,[7] possibly because they do not consolidate their sleep into one session. They may go to bed, awake 4 hours later, stay awake for an extended period, then go back to sleep, resulting in fragmented sleep patterns.[8] Many of the diseases associated with aging may contribute to these nocturnal arousals, including diabetes, nocturia, cardiovascular symptoms, chronic pain, and depression.[8-10] In addition, sleep-related respiratory disorders and increased incidence of periodic leg movements in elders may further disrupt their sleep.[11] Increasing age brings many physical and social changes with which the elder must cope. Assessment of elderly clients must always include sleep history as an indicator of mental health because depression is a common struggle for this population.[12]

PHARMACOLOGY AND SLEEP

Many drugs essential to treatment of critically ill patients impact sleep quality (Table 5-2).[13-16] It is important to understand the relationship between various medications and the sleep of patients in the critical care unit. Pathophysiology and age may profoundly affect not only medication absorption and elimination but also how patients cope with their illness and their ability to maintain health.

Table 5-1	Time Spent in Sleep Stages for Normal Adults

Stage	Percent of Nocturnal Sleep
1	2-5
2	45-55
3	3-8
4	10-15
REM	20-25

Table 5-2 Pharmacologic Management: Select Drugs That Affect Sleep and Wakefulness

Class	Drug	Effect	Comments
HYPNOTICS[13]			
Benzodiazepines		↓ SWS, ↑ TST, ↓ WASO, ↓ stage 1, mild REM suppression	↑ Apnea, ↑ daytime residual sedation, mild respiratory depression, ↓ psychomotor function
Immediate acting	Quazepam	Half-life 20-120 hr	
	Temazepam	Half-life 8-20 hr	
Long acting	Flurazepam	Half-life 40-250 hr	
Rapid acting	Triazolam	Half-life 2-6 hr	
	Estazolam	Half-life 8-24 hr	Rebound insomnia
Nonbenzodiazepines		No effect on REM or SWS	No cognitive or performance impairment; ↓ abuse potential; can be taken in middle of night
Rapid acting	Zolpidem	Half-life 1 hr	
	Zaleplon	Half-life 1 hr	
STIMULANTS[14]			
Nonsympathomimetics	Nicotine	↑ SL, ↓ TST, ↓ REM	
	Amphetamines	↓ REM, ↓ SWS, ↓ TST, ↑ WASO	
	Xanthine derivatives: coffee, chocolate, tea; scopolamine; strychnine; pentylenetetrazol; modafinil	↓ TST, ↑ REM, ↓ SWS, ↑ SL, ↑ WASO	Less daytime fatigue
Direct sympathomimetics	Isoproterenol, epinephrine, norepinephrine, phenylephrine, phenylpropanolamine, apomorphine	↑ Wake, ↑ REM onset, ↓ fatigue, ↓ sleepiness	↑ Blood pressure, ↓ heart rate
Indirect sympathomimetics	Amphetamine, methamphetamine, cocaine, pipradol, methylphenidate, tyramine	↑ WASO, ↑ daytime SL, ↓ sleepiness	Narcolepsy treatment, ↑ cognitive tasks
	Pemoline		Possible liver damage
ANTIHYPERTENSIVES[14]			
β-Antagonists	Propranolol, metoprolol	↑ Wake, TWT, SL, ↓ REM	Insomnia, nightmares
α-2 Agonists	Atenolol, clonidine	↓ REM, ↓ TST in hypertensive patients, ↑ TST in normal subjects	Nightmares, sedation, ↓ concentration, mental slowing
	Methyldopa	↑ REM, ↑ TST	Sedation, insomnia, nightmares

Drug class	Examples	Sleep effects	Other effects
Diuretics	Hydrochlorothiazide, chlorthalidone, indapamide	No data	Central nervous system effects unlikely
Vasodilators	Hydralazine	No data	Depression, insomnia, anxiety
Catecholamine depletors	Reserpine	↑REM and stage shifts	
Calcium antagonists	Verapamil, nifedipine, diltiazem, amlodipine, felodipine, nisoldipine	No data	Insomnia, nightmares, depression, sedation, difficulty concentrating
ANTIHISTAMINES[14-16]			
Histamine H_1-receptor antagonists	H_1 antihistamines (*chem. class:* selective histamine H_1-receptor antagonist) (e.g., diphenhydramine, hydroxyzine, triprolidine)	↑Drowsiness, ↓SL	Impaired daytime performance
	H_1 antihistamines (*chem. class:* ethanolamine derivative H_1-receptor antagonist) (e.g., loratadine, terfenadine)	No sedation effects	
Histamine H_2-receptor antagonists	Histamine$_2$ antagonists (e.g., cimetidine, ranitidine)	May cause insomnia or somnolence	Drowsiness in patients; renal impairment
Antidepressants[14]			
Tricyclic antidepressants	Amitriptyline, doxepin, imipramine, trimipramine, clomipramine, desipramine, nortriptyline, protriptyline	↑TST, ↓wake	↓Psychomotor and cognitive performance and daytime drowsiness
Selective serotonin reuptake inhibitors	Fluoxetine	↑TST, ↑wake, ↑stage 1, ↑SEM	Mildly ↑psychomotor performance
	Paroxetine	↑Wake, ↓TST, ↑stage 1, ↑SL	
	Sertraline	No data	Insomnia: 7%-16% of patients
	Fluvoxamine	↓TST, ↑wake, ↑stage 1, ↑SL	Insomnia, no impairment in performance
	Citralopram	No change	↓Cognitive performance in elderly patients
	Trazodone	Variable, ↑TST possible, ↓SL	Some improved psychomotor performance
Monoamine oxidase inhibitors	Phenelzine, tranylcypromine, moclobemide, brofaromine	Daytime sleepiness because of ↓TST, ↑wake	

↓, Decreased; ↑, increased; SWS, slow-wave sleep; TST, total sleep time; WASO, wake after sleep onset; REM, rapid eye movement; SL, sleep latency; TWT, total wake time; SEM, slow eye movement.

SLEEP APNEA SYNDROMES

Sleep apnea syndrome, sometimes called *sleep-disordered breathing*, occurs when airflow is absent or reduced. Apneas during sleep can be divided into three types: obstructive, central, and mixed. In obstructive apnea the absence of airflow is caused by an obstruction in the upper airway. Complete obstruction lasting 10 seconds or longer is referred to as *obstructive apnea*, whereas a partial obstruction is known as *hypopnea*. In *central apnea*, airflow is absent because of lack of ventilatory muscle effort. The third type of sleep apnea syndrome, *mixed*, occurs when a combination of both obstructive and central patterns occurs in one apneic event. An apnea-hypopnea index (number of apneic and hypopneic episodes per hour divided by hours of sleep) of 5 or greater is diagnostic of sleep apnea syndrome.[17]

All types of sleep apnea syndrome are accompanied by arterial desaturation and potentially by hypoxemia, which may cause pulmonary vasoconstriction and increased systemic vascular resistance. However, desaturation and hypoxemia are most severe in the obstructive type.

Obstructive Sleep Apnea-Hypopnea Syndrome

Obstructive sleep apnea-hypopnea syndrome (OSAHS) occurs when obstruction in the upper airway causes at least five apneic or hypopneic events per hour of sleep. The incidence of OSAHS is believed to increase with age. Consequences include chronic hypoventilation syndrome, arousals that fragment sleep, cardiovascular changes such as hypertension,[18,19] cerebrovascular accident (stroke), ischemic heart disease, insulin resistance, ventricular hypertrophy,[20] and nocturnal angina.[21] Because of the cardiovascular complications and accidents caused by sleepiness, OSAHS is a significant condition that should be thoroughly evaluated.

The cause of OSAHS is not entirely understood, although upper airway structure, hormonal balance, and neural control are implicated. Factors that contribute to OSAHS are (1) anatomic narrowing of the upper airway, (2) increased compliance of the upper airway tissue, (3) reflexes affecting upper airway caliber, and (4) pharyngeal inspiratory muscle function.[22] Computed tomography scans of awake subjects have shown that patients with OSAHS have narrower airways than normal subjects. The narrower the airway, the more easily it becomes obstructed.

Unstable control of the respiratory nerves of the diaphragmatic, intercostal, and upper airway muscles can cause sleep apnea.[22] Hypothyroidism can alter respiratory controls and therefore contribute to OSAHS. Other contributing disorders are exogenous obesity, kyphoscoliosis, and autonomic dysfunction.

The patient with OSAHS develops cycles of hypoxemia, hypercapnia, and acidosis with each episode of apnea until the patient is aroused and airflow resumes. Alveolar hypoventilation accompanies each apneic episode and results in hypercapnia. Between episodes, alveolar ventilation improves, so there is no net retention of carbon dioxide.

With obstruction, inspiratory subatmospheric intrathoracic pressures are abnormally elevated. This increased pressure promotes a tendency for airways to collapse, resulting in both hemodynamic and electrocardiographic changes. The extremely elevated pressures in OSAHS patients who have apneic episodes in both REM and NREM stages cause systemic and pulmonary hypertension. Systemic pressures of 200/120 mm Hg (awake control: 130/80 mm Hg) and pulmonary artery pressures of 80/54 mm Hg (awake control: 30/20 mm Hg) have been reported.[21] Cardiac dysrhythmias associated with obstructive apnea include bradycardias, sinus arrest, and occasionally, second-degree heart blocks. After resumption of airflow, tachycardias typically occur. Thus bradycardia-tachycardia syndrome is associated with OSAHS.[21]

Assessment and Diagnosis

Careful monitoring of oxygen saturation and breathing patterns can help the critical care nurse identify OSAHS and assist in its diagnosis and treatment. Patients at risk for OSAHS may have the following: snoring, obesity, short, thick neck circumference, cardiovascular disease, systemic hypertension, pulmonary hypertension, sleep fragmentation, gastroesophogeal reflux, and an impaired quality of life.

OSAHSs frequently end in brief EEG arousals. Patients may experience hundreds of arousals and not even realize they awaken hundreds of times during the night. These arousals cause the patient to experience sleep fragmentation causing excessive daytime sleepiness. This cardinal symptom of OSAHS may lead to irritability, poor job performance, troubled relationships, depression, and impaired quality of life. Further, OSAHS is highly correlated to cardiovascular disease[20] and hypertension.[18,19]

Diagnosis of OSAHS is made with *polysomnography*, an overnight sleep study. Polysomnography is used to determine the number and length of apnea episodes and sleep stages, number of arousals, airflow, respiratory effort, and oxygen desaturation.

Medical Management

For patients with mild OSAHS (apnea-hypopnea index of 5 to 10), weight loss, sleeping on the side if apneas are associated with sleeping on the back, avoidance of sedative medications and alcohol before bedtime, and avoidance of sleep deprivation may be sufficient. Patients with moderate to severe levels of apnea may be treated with mechanical, surgical, or pharmacologic therapy. Treatment may vary depending on the type and severity of illness.

Continuous positive airway pressure (CPAP) via nasal mask is the treatment of choice. When a patient cannot tolerate CPAP, *bimodal* positive airway pressure (BiPAP), which provides separate pressures for inspiration and expiration, may be used.

Various surgical treatments are available for treatment of apnea and snoring. Patients with mild OSAHS or snoring alone may undergo an outpatient procedure called *laser uvulopalatopharyngoplasty* (LAUP), which uses lasers to remove excess tissue at the soft palate level. For patients who snore but do not have apnea, somnoplasty may provide relief. *Somnoplasty* involves inserting a small electrode into the soft palate and heating the tissue, causing the area to shrink and tighten.[23]

Uvulopalatopharyngoplasty (UPPP) was one of the first surgical procedures used to treat OSAHS. Essentially a large tonsillectomy is performed with all redundant tissue removed. Only about 50% of patients experience sleep apnea improvement.[23] Complications include speech impairment, inability to eat, hemorrhage, and infection. Although tracheostomy was the original procedure used to treat OSAHS, it is now used only in patients with the most severe forms of apnea who do not respond to other treatments.

Treatment of OSAHS with medication is usually a last resort and has proved to be very disappointing. *Protriptyline* has been shown to decrease apnea and reduce excessive daytime sleepiness by decreasing REM sleep apnea frequency that increases during REM sleep. Oxygen may be used to lower hypoxemia and nocturnal desaturations.

Nursing Management

The nurse's role in the management of OSAHS includes educating the patient and family about the syndrome and the consequences of noncompliance with treatment regimens. This education may also include preoperative teaching for surgical procedures such as UPPP. Monitoring of patients with OSAHS while in critical care should include assessment of the breathing patterns, hours of sleep, and pulse oximetry. Refer to the Nursing Management Plan for Disturbed Sleep Pattern (p. 484).

If patients are admitted to the critical care unit with a history of OSAHS, they need to use their home CPAP mask and equipment as part of their regular sleep routine. The nurse can promote compliance with the CPAP system through specific interventions for these patients (Box 5-1).

Postoperative monitoring after UPPP includes risk of aspiration, pain management, anxiety relief, patient education, and monitoring for respiratory complications, hemor-

rhage, infection, impaired speech, nutritional concerns, and sleep disturbances.

Central Sleep Apnea

Central sleep apnea can be seen on polysomnography as an absence of airflow and respiratory effort for at least 10 seconds. Complete loss of EMG activity in respiratory muscles would be expected because central sleep apnea is defined as a pause in respiration without ventilatory effort.[24]

Central sleep apnea is not a single disease but rather a group of disorders in which breathing ceases momentarily during sleep because of the transient withdrawal of central nervous system drive to the muscles of respiration.[25] A patient with central sleep apnea may also experience obstructive events.

Central sleep apnea may result from many physiologic and pathophysiologic events.[24] Possible causes of *nonhypercapnic* central sleep apnea include periodic breathing at high altitude, renal/metabolic disturbances, Cheyne-Stokes breathing, and idiopathic central apnea seen at sea level. *Hypercapnic* central sleep apnea may occur in many neuromuscular conditions, including spinal cord or brain injury, encephalitis, brain stem neoplasm or infarcts, muscular dystrophy, myasthenia gravis, bulbar poliomyelitis, and postpolio syndrome.

Assessment and Diagnosis

Clinical characteristics of hypercapnic central sleep apnea include respiratory failure, cor pulmonale, peripheral edema, polycythemia, daytime sleepiness, and snoring. Patients with nonhypercapnic central sleep apnea have clinical features very similar to those of OSAHS. Nonhypercapnic central sleep apnea characteristics include daytime sleepiness, insomnia or poor sleep, mild or intermittent snoring, and awakenings accompanied by choking or feeling short of breath. Frequently the patients are of normal body weight. Diagnosis is made by overnight polysomnography or sleep study, which will determine the respiratory and sleep patterns of the patient.

Medical Management

Because there are two types of central sleep apnea, two therapeutic approaches are available depending on the cause of the apnea. The hypercapnic patient who has worsening hypoventilation during sleep is best served by nocturnal ventilation. Most of these patients experience some respiratory muscle failure. One treatment for patients with nonhypercapnic apnea or heart failure is nasal CPAP, which also may provide a beneficial cardiovascular effect. Nocturnal oxygen supplementation may be effective as well. If CPAP is not tolerated, pharmacologic management may be used. *Medroxyprogesterone*, a respiratory stimulant, may improve ventilation in selected patients.[24] *Acetazolamide*, a carbonic anhydrase inhibitor that can result in metabolic acidosis, also may decrease frequency of apneic episodes.

Box **5-1** **Nursing Care for Patients Using CPAP**

- Make sure that the mask fits snugly.
- Maintain the prescribed airway pressure.
- Ensure that air is not leaking, especially to the eye area.
- Monitor skin integrity under the mask.
- Make sure that the patient does not experience gastric insufflation.
- Encourage compliance at home.

Nursing Management

For the nurse caring for a patient with central sleep apnea, patient and family education about the patient's condition and treatment regimen can help ensure patient compliance. The nurse needs to address any fear or anxiety about going to sleep. Nurses should caution patients to avoid alcohol or sedative medications. Weight loss is recommended if the patient is obese. The nurse must carefully monitor and assess the patient's respiratory status.

SLEEP PROMOTION IN CRITICAL CARE

Critical care nurses may promote sleep by determining potential causes of sleep disruption and addressing these causes directly. For example, patients with anxiety or pain may be soothed by nursing interventions that promote relaxation or comfort, such as massage.[26] Relaxing sounds[27] or music therapy, open visitation policies, and controlling noise and light in the unit environment may also promote rest. Finally, nurses should control the flow of interventions to allow times of consolidated nocturnal sleep.[28]

REFERENCES

1. Carskadon MA, Dement WC: Normal human sleep: an overview. In Kryger MH, Roth T, Dement WC, editors: *Principles and practice of sleep medicine*, ed 3, Philadelphia, 2000, Saunders.
2. Davidhizar RE, Poole VL, Giger JN: What nurses need to know about sleep, *J Nurs Sci* 1:61-67, 1995.
3. Douglas NJ: Respiratory physiology: control of ventilation. In Kryger MH, Roth T, Dement WC, editors: *Principles and practice of sleep medicine*, ed 3, Philadelphia, 2000, Saunders.
4. Krachman SL, D'Alonzo GE, Criner GJ: Sleep in the intensive care unit, *Chest* 107(6):1713-1720, 1995.
5. Ancoli-Israel S et al: Identification and treatment of sleep problems in the elderly, *Sleep Med Rev* 1:3-17, 1997.
6. Ancoli-Israel S: Sleep problems in older adults: putting myths to bed, *Geriatrics* 52(1):20-30, 1997.
7. Buysse DJ et al: Napping and 24-hour sleep/wake patterns in healthy elderly and young adults, *J Am Geriatr Soc* 40(8):779-786, 1992.
8. Vitiello MV: Normal versus pathologic sleep changes in aging humans. In Kuna ST, editor: *Sleep and respiration in aging*, New York, 1991, Elsevier Science.
9. Bliwise DL: Normal aging. In Kryger MH, Roth T, Dement WC, editors: *Principles and practice of sleep medicine*, ed 3, Philadelphia, 2000, Saunders.
10. Bliwise DL, King AC, Harris RB: Habitual sleep durations and health in a 50-65 year old population, *J Clin Epidemiol* 47(1):35-41, 1994.
11. Sloan E, Flint A: Circadian rhythms and psychiatric disorders in the elderly, *J Geriatr Psychiatry Neurol* 9(4):164-170, 1996.
12. Zarit S, Zarit J: *Mental disorders in older adults*, New York, 1998, Guilford Press.
13. Henderson WB: Hypnotics: basic mechanisms and pharmacology. In Kryger M, Roth T, Dement WC, editors: *Principles and practice of sleep medicine*, ed 3, Philadelphia, 2000, Saunders.
14. Schweitzer PK: Drugs that disturb sleep and wakefulness. In Kryger M, Roth T, Dement WC, editors: *Principles and practice of sleep medicine*, ed 3, Philadelphia, 2000, Saunders.
15. Obermeyer WH, Benca RM: Effects of drugs on sleep, *Neurol Clin* 14:827-840, 1996.
16. Nolen TM: Sedative effects of antihistamines: safety, performance, learning, and quality of life, *Clin Ther* 19:39-55, 1997.
17. Kryger MH: Management of obstructive sleep apnea-hypopnea syndrome: overview. In Kryger MH, Roth T, Dement WC, editors: *Principles and practice of sleep medicine*, ed 3, Philadelphia, 2000, Saunders.
18. Peppard P, Young T, Palta M, Skatrud J: Prospective study of the associate between sleep-disordered breathing and hypertension, *N Engl J Med* 342:1378-1384, 2000.
19. Nieto F et al: Sleep disordered breathing and neuropsychological deficits, *Am J Respir Crit Care Med* 156:1813-1819, 1997.
20. Moore T et al: Sleep-disordered breathing in men with coronary artery disease, *Chest* 109:659-663, 1996.
21. Weiss JW, Launois SH, Anand A: Cardiorespiratory changes in sleep-disordered breathing. In Kryger MH, Roth T, Dement WC, editors: *Principles and practice of sleep medicine*, ed 3, Philadelphia, 2000, Saunders.
22. Hudgel DW: Mechanisms of obstructive sleep apnea, *Chest* 101(2):541-549, 1992.
23. Krug P: Snoring and obstructive sleep apnea, *AORN J* 69:792-797, 1999.
24. White DP: Central sleep apnea. In Kryger MH, Roth T, Dement WC, editors: *Principles and practice of sleep medicine*, ed 3, Philadelphia, 2000, Saunders.
25. Bradley T, Phillipson E: Central sleep apnea, *Clin Chest Med* 13(3):493-505, 1992.
26. Richards KC, Gibson R, Overton-McCoy AL: Effects of massage in acute and critical care, *AACN Clin Issues* 11(1):77-96, 2000.
27. Williamson JW: The effects of ocean sounds on sleep after coronary artery bypass graft surgery, *Am J Crit Care* 1(1):91-97, 1992.
28. Olsen DM et al: Quiet time: a nursing intervention to promote sleep in neurocritical care units, *Am J Crit Care* 10(2):74-78, 2001.

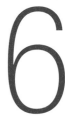

Nutritional Alterations

Objectives

- Describe the adverse effects of nutritional impairments on critically ill patients.
- Assess the nutritional status of critically ill patients with cardiovascular, pulmonary, neurologic, renal, gastrointestinal, and endocrine alterations.
- Recognize nutritional alterations associated with cardiovascular, pulmonary, neurologic, renal, gastrointestinal, and endocrine alterations.
- Collaborate with a multidisciplinary team in designing a nutrition program for critically ill patients.
- Identify complications of nutrition support and nursing interventions for prevention and management of these complications.

evolve Be sure to check out the free exercises on-line at *http://evolve.elsevier.com/Urden/priorities/*

METABOLIC RESPONSE TO STARVATION AND STRESS

Critically ill patients are at risk for a combination of starvation and the physiologic stress resulting from injury, trauma, major surgery, and sepsis. Starvation occurs because the person must have nothing by mouth (NPO) for surgical procedures, may be unable to eat because of disease-related factors, and may be hemodynamically too unstable to be fed. The physiologic stress causes an increased metabolic rate (hypermetabolism) that results in a rise in oxygen consumption and energy expenditure.

The hypermetabolic process results from hormonal changes caused by the stressful event. The sympathetic nervous system is stimulated, causing the adrenal medulla to release catecholamines (epinephrine and norepinephrine). Other hormones released in response to stress include glucagon, adrenocorticotropic hormone (ACTH), and antidiuretic hormone (ADH), as well as glucocorticoids and mineralocorticoids (e.g., cortisol, aldosterone). All these hormonal changes cause nutrient substrates, primarily amino acids, to move from peripheral tissues (e.g., skeletal muscle) to the liver for gluconeogenesis.

Unfortunately, this mobilization of substrates occurs at the expense of body tissue and function at a time when the needs for protein synthesis (e.g., for wound healing and acute-phase proteins) also are high. Hyperglycemia results from the effects of increased catecholamines, glucocorticoids, and glucagon. Loss of protein results in a negative nitrogen balance and weight loss.

UNDERNUTRITION: IMPLICATIONS FOR THE SICK OR STRESSED PATIENT

As many as 30% to 55% of hospitalized patients are believed to be at risk for malnutrition.[1] Although illness or injury is the major factor contributing to development of malnutrition, other possible contributing factors are (1) lack of communication among the nurses, physicians, and dietitians responsible for the care of these patients; (2) frequent diagnostic testing, which causes patients to miss meals or to be too exhausted for meals; (3) medications and other therapies that cause anorexia, nausea, or vomiting and thus interfere with food intake; (4) insufficient monitoring of nutrient intake; and (5) inadequate use of supplements, tube feedings, or total parenteral nutrition (TPN) to maintain the nutritional status of these patients.[2]

Critically ill patients receiving enteral tube feedings may have a daily intake of only approximately half the calories they require.[3] Nutritional status tends to deteriorate during hospitalization unless appropriate nutrition support is started early and continually reassessed.

Malnutrition is an ominous finding in seriously ill patients. Wound dehiscence, decubitus ulcers, sepsis, pulmonary infections, respiratory failure requiring ventilation, longer hospital stays, and death are more common among undernourished patients.[1,4-6]

ASSESSING NUTRITIONAL STATUS

A nutrition screening should be conducted on every patient. A brief questionnaire to be completed by the patient or significant other, the nursing admission form, or the physician's admission note usually provides enough information to determine whether the patient is at nutritional risk (Box 6-1). Any patient judged to be nutritionally at risk needs a more thorough nutrition assessment.

Biochemical Data

A wide range of laboratory tests can provide information about nutritional status, including blood and urine tests often used in the clinical setting (Table 6-1). No diagnostic tests for evaluation of nutrition are "perfect," and care must be taken in interpreting the results of the tests.

Clinical and Physical Manifestations

A thorough physical examination is an essential part of nutrition assessment. In assessing the patient for altered nutritional state, the nurse especially checks for signs of muscle wasting, loss of subcutaneous fat, skin or hair changes, and impaired wound healing (Box 6-2).

Diet and Health History

Information about dietary intake and significant variations in weight is a vital part of the history (Box 6-3). Dietary intake can be evaluated in several ways, including a diet record, a 24-hour recall, and a diet history.

Evaluating Assessment Findings

A patient rarely exhibits a lack of only one nutrient. Nutritional deficiencies usually are combined, with the patient lacking adequate amounts of protein, calories, and possibly vitamins and minerals. A common form of combined nutritional deficit among hospitalized patients is *protein-calorie malnutrition* (PCM). Two types of PCM are kwashiorkor and marasmus.

Box **6-1**	Patients at Risk for Malnutrition

- Involuntary loss or gain of a significant amount of weight (>10% of usual body weight in 6 months, >5% in 1 month), even if the weight achieved by loss or gain is appropriate for height
- Weight 20% more or less than ideal body weight, or body mass index <18.5 or >25
- Chronic disease
- Chronic use of a modified diet
- Increased metabolic requirements
- Illness or surgery that may interfere with nutritional intake
- Inadequate nutrient intake for >7 days
- Regular use of three or more medications
- Poverty

Table **6-1**   Common Blood and Urine Tests Used in Nutrition Assessment

Test	Comments
SERUM PROTEINS	
Albumin or prealbumin	Levels decrease with protein deficiency but also in liver failure; albumin levels are slow to change in response to malnutrition and repletion; prealbumin levels fall in response to trauma and infection.
HEMATOLOGIC VALUES	
Anemia	
Normocytic (normal MCV, MCHC)	Common with protein deficiency
Microcytic (decreased MCV, MCH, MCHC)	Indicative of iron deficiency (possibly from blood loss)
Macrocytic (increased MCV)	Common in folate and vitamin B_{12} deficiency
Decreased lymphocyte count	Common in protein deficiency

MCV, Mean corpuscular volume; MCHC, mean corpuscular hemoglobin concentration; MCH, mean corpuscular hemoglobin.

Kwashiorkor results in low levels of the serum proteins albumin, transferrin, and prealbumin; low total lymphocyte count; impaired immunity; loss of hair or hair pigment; edema resulting from low plasma oncotic pressure caused by a loss of plasma proteins; and an enlarged, fatty liver. *Marasmus* is recognizable by weight loss, loss of subcutaneous fat, and muscle wasting. In the

Box **6-2**   Clinical Manifestations of Nutritional Alterations

PROTEIN-CALORIE MALNUTRITION
Hair loss, dull dry brittle hair, loss of hair pigment
Loss of subcutaneous tissue, muscle wasting
Poor wound healing, decubitus ulcer
Hepatomegaly
Edema

VITAMIN DEFICIENCIES
Conjunctival and corneal dryness (vitamin A)
Dry scaly skin, follicular hyperkeratosis (papules result in "gooseflesh" appearance to skin) (vitamin A)
Gingivitis, poor wound healing (vitamin C)
Petechiae, ecchymoses (vitamin C or K)
Inflamed tongue, cracking at corners of mouth (riboflavin [vitamin B_2], niacin, folic acid, vitamin B_{12}, other B vitamins)
Edema, heart failure (thiamine [vitamin B_1])
Confusion, confabulation (vitamin B_1)

MINERAL DEFICIENCIES
Blue sclerae, pale mucous membranes, spoon-shaped nails (iron)
Hypogeusia (poor sense of taste), dysgeusia (bad taste), eczema, poor wound healing (zinc)

EXCESSIVE VITAMIN INTAKE
Hair loss, dry skin, hepatomegaly (vitamin A)

Box **6-3**   Nutrition History Information

INTAKE OF NUTRIENTS
Alcohol abuse
Anorexia, severe or prolonged nausea/vomiting
Confusion, coma
Poor dentition
Poverty

DIGESTION OR ABSORPTION OF NUTRIENTS
Previous gastrointestinal surgeries, especially gastrectomy, obesity surgery, and ileal resection
Certain medications, especially antacids and histamine H_2-receptor antagonists (reduce upper small bowel acidity), cholestyramine (binds fat-soluble nutrients), and anticonvulsants

NUTRIENT LOSSES
Blood loss
Severe diarrhea
Fistulas, draining abscesses, wounds, decubitus ulcers
Peritoneal dialysis or hemodialysis
Corticosteroid therapy (increased tissue catabolism)

NUTRIENT REQUIREMENTS
Fever
Surgery, trauma, burns, infection
Cancer (some types)
Physiologic demands (pregnancy, lactation, growth)

marasmic person, creatinine excretion in the urine is low, an indication of loss of muscle mass. Because PCM weakens muscles, increases vulnerability to infection, and can prolong hospital stays, the health care team should diagnose this serious disorder as quickly as possible so that appropriate nutritional intervention can be implemented.

NUTRITION AND CARDIOVASCULAR ALTERATIONS

Diet and cardiovascular disease may interact in a variety of ways. On the one hand, excessive nutrient intake, manifested by overweight or obesity and a diet rich in cholesterol and saturated fat, is a risk factor for development of arteriosclerotic heart disease. On the other hand, the consequences of chronic myocardial insufficiency may include malnutrition.

Nutrition Assessment

A nutrition assessment provides the nurse and other health care team members with the information necessary to plan the cardiovascular patient's nutrition care and education (Box 6-4). The major nutritional concerns relate to appropriateness of body weight and the levels of serum lipids and blood pressure.

Nutrition Intervention

Myocardial Infarction

The following guidelines will assist the nurse in providing appropriate nutritional care for the patient in the immediate post–myocardial infarction period:

- Limit meal size for the patient with severe myocardial compromise or postprandial angina.
- Monitor the effect of caffeine on the patient, if caffeine is included in the diet.
- Use caution in serving foods at temperature extremes.

Hypertension

A substantial number of individuals with hypertension are "salt sensitive," with their disorder improving when sodium intake is limited. Therefore restriction of sodium intake, usually to 2.5 g or less/day, is often advised to help control hypertension.[7] One teaspoon of salt provides about 2.3 g of sodium. Most salt substitutes contain potassium chloride

---

| Box **6-4** | Common Findings in Patients with Cardiovascular Disease |

- Overweight/obesity, underweight (cardiac cachexia)
- Abdominal fat: increased risk of cardiovascular disease with waist measurement >102 cm (>40 inches) for men and >88 cm (>35 inches) for women
- Elevated total serum cholesterol, LDL cholesterol, and triglycerides
- Wasting of muscle and subcutaneous fat (cardiac cachexia)
- Sedentary lifestyle
- Excessive intake of saturated fat, cholesterol, salt, and alcohol
- Angina, respiratory difficulty, fatigue during eating
- Medications that impair appetite (e.g., digitalis preparations, quinidine)

LDL, Low-density lipoprotein.

---

and may be used with the physician's approval by the patient who has no renal impairment. A diet rich in fruits, vegetables, and low-fat dairy products (the DASH, or Dietary Approaches to Stopping Hypertension, diet) combined with a sodium restriction is often more effective than sodium restriction alone.[8]

Heart Failure

Nutrition intervention for the patient with heart failure is designed to reduce fluid retained within the body and thus reduce the preload. Because fluid accompanies sodium, limitation of sodium is necessary to reduce fluid retention. Specific interventions include limiting salt intake, usually to 5 g/day or less, and limiting fluid intake as appropriate. If fluid is restricted, the daily fluid allowance is usually 1.5 to 2 L/day, to include both fluids in the diet and those given with medications and for other purposes.

Cardiac Cachexia

The severely malnourished cardiac patient often develops heart failure. Therefore sodium and fluid restriction, as previously described, is appropriate. It is important to concentrate nutrients into as small a volume as possible and to serve small amounts frequently, rather than three large meals daily. The individual should be encouraged to consume calorie-dense foods and supplements. Good choices include meats and poultry, cheeses, yogurt, frozen yogurt, and ice cream.

Because the patient is likely to tire quickly and to suffer from anorexia, enteral tube feeding may be necessary. Typical tube feeding formulas provide 1 calorie per milliliter (cal/ml), but more-concentrated products are available to provide adequate nutrients in a smaller volume. The nurse must monitor the fluid status of these patients carefully when they are receiving nutrition support. Assessing breath sounds and observing for presence and severity of peripheral edema and changes in body weight are performed daily or more frequently. A consistent weight gain of more than 0.11 to 0.22 kg (0.25 to 0.5 lb) per day usually indicates fluid retention rather than gain of fat and muscle mass.

NUTRITION AND PULMONARY ALTERATIONS

Malnutrition has extremely adverse effects on respiratory function, decreasing surfactant production, diaphragmatic mass, vital capacity, and immunocompetence. Patients with acute respiratory disorders find it difficult to consume adequate oral nutrients and can rapidly become malnourished. Individuals who have an acute illness superimposed on chronic respiratory problems are also at high risk. Almost three fourths of patients with chronic obstructive pulmonary disease (COPD) have had weight loss. Patients with undernutrition and end-stage COPD, however, often cannot tolerate the increase in metabolic demand that occurs during refeeding. In addition, they are at significant risk for development of cor pulmonale and may fail to tolerate the fluid required for delivery of enteral or parenteral nutrition support. Prevention of severe nutritional deficits, rather than correction of deficits once they have occurred, is important in nutritional management of these patients.

Nutrition Assessment

Common findings in nutrition assessment related to pulmonary alterations are summarized in Box 6-5. The patient with respiratory compromise is especially vulnerable to the effects of fluid volume excess and must be assessed continually for this complication, particularly during enteral and parenteral feeding.

Nutrition Intervention
Prevent or Correct Undernutrition/Underweight

The nurse and dietitian work together to encourage oral intake in the undernourished or potentially undernourished patient who is capable of eating. Small, frequent feedings are especially important because a very full stomach can interfere with diaphragmatic movement. Mouth care should be provided before meals and snacks to clear the palate of the taste of sputum and medications. Administering bronchodilators with food can help to reduce the gastric irritation caused by these medications.

Because of anorexia, dyspnea, debilitation, or need for ventilatory support, however, many patients will require enteral tube feeding or TPN. It is especially important for the nurse to be alert to the risk of pulmonary aspiration in the patient with an artificial airway. To reduce the risk of pulmonary aspiration during enteral tube feeding, the nurse should (1) keep the patient's head elevated at least 45 degrees during feedings, unless contraindicated; (2) discontinue feedings 30 to 60 minutes before any procedures that require lowering the head; (3) keep the cuff of the artificial airway inflated during feeding, if possible; (4) monitor the patient for increasing abdominal distention; and (5) check tube placement before each feeding (if intermittent) or at least every 4 to 8 hours if feedings are continuous.

Avoid Overfeeding

Overfeeding increases the production of carbon dioxide (CO_2). This is unlikely to be significant in the patient who is eating foods. Instead, it is an iatrogenic complication of TPN or enteral feeding. Arterial CO_2 tension ($PaCO_2$) may rise sufficiently to make it difficult to wean a patient from the ventilator. A balanced regimen with both lipids and carbohydrates providing the nonprotein calories is optimal for the patient with respiratory compromise, and the patient needs to be reassessed continually to ensure that caloric intake is not excessive.

Prevent Fluid Volume Excess

Pulmonary edema and failure of the right side of the heart, which may be precipitated by fluid volume excess, further worsen the status of the patient with respiratory compromise. Maintaining careful intake and output records allows for accurate assessment of fluid balance. Usually the patient requires no more than 35 to 40 ml/kg/day of fluid. For the patient receiving nutrition support, fluid intake can be reduced by (1) using 20% or 30% lipid emulsions as a source of calories, (2) using tube feeding formulas providing at least 2 cal/ml (the dietitian can recommend appropriate formulas), and (3) choosing oral supplements that are low in fluid.

NUTRITION AND NEUROLOGIC ALTERATIONS

Because neurologic disorders such as stroke and closed head injury tend to be long-term problems, these patients require good nutritional care to prevent nutritional deficits and promote well-being.

Nutrition Assessment

Nutrition-related assessment findings vary widely in the patient with neurologic alterations, depending on the type of disorder present (Box 6-6).

Box 6-5 Common Findings in Patients with Pulmonary Disease

- Underweight
- Elevated carbon dioxide partial pressure related to overfeeding
- Edema, dyspnea, signs of pulmonary edema related to fluid volume excess
- Poor food intake related to dyspnea
- Unpleasant taste in mouth from sputum production or bronchodilator therapy
- Endotracheal intubation preventing oral intake

Box 6-6 Common Findings in Patients with Neurologic Alterations

- Hyperglycemia (with corticosteroid use)
- Wasting of muscle and subcutaneous fat related to disuse or to poor food intake
- Poor food intake related to altered state of consciousness
- Dysphagia or other chewing/swallowing difficulties
- Ileus resulting from spinal cord injury or use of pentobarbital
- Hypermetabolism resulting from head injury
- Decubitus ulcers

Nutrition Intervention: Prevent or Correct Nutrition Deficits

Oral Feedings

Patients with dysphagia or weakness of the swallowing musculature often experience the greatest difficulty in swallowing dry foods and thin liquids (e.g., water) that are difficult to control.

Tube Feedings and Total Parenteral Nutrition

Patients who are unconscious or unable to eat because of severe dysphagia, weakness, ileus, or other reasons require tube feedings or TPN. Prompt initiation of nutrition support must be a priority in the patient with neurologic impairment. Needs for protein and calories are increased by infection and fever, as in the patient with encephalitis or meningitis. Needs for protein, calories, zinc, and vitamin C are increased during wound healing, as in trauma patients and those with decubitus ulcers.

Patients with neurologic deficits have an increased risk of certain complications (particularly pulmonary aspiration) during tube feeding and therefore require especially careful nursing management. Patients of most concern are (1) those with an impaired gag reflex, such as some patients with cerebrovascular accident (stroke); (2) those with delayed gastric emptying, such as patients in the early period after spinal cord injury and patients with head injury treated with barbiturate coma; and (3) those likely to experience seizures. To help prevent pulmonary aspiration, the patient's head is kept elevated, if not contraindicated; when elevation of the head is not possible, administering feedings with the patient in the prone or lateral position will allow free drainage of emesis from the mouth and decrease the risk of aspiration.

Administering *phenytoin* with enteral formulas decreases the absorption of the drug and the peak serum level achieved. The phenytoin dosage must be adjusted appropriately. Phenytoin levels should be monitored carefully in patients receiving enteral feedings.

Hyperglycemia is a common complication in patients receiving corticosteroids. Regular monitoring of blood glucose is an important part of their care. They may require insulin to control the hyperglycemia.

Prompt use of nutrition support is especially important for patients with head injuries because head injury causes marked catabolism, even in patients who receive barbiturates, which should decrease metabolic demands. Head-injured patients rapidly exhaust glycogen stores and begin to use body proteins to meet energy needs, a process that can quickly lead to PCM. The catabolic response is partly a result of corticosteroid therapy in head-injured patients. However, the hypermetabolism and hypercatabolism are also caused by dramatic hormonal responses to this type of injury.[9] Levels of cortisol, epinephrine, and norepinephrine increase as much as seven times normal. These hormones increase the metabolic rate and caloric demands, causing mobilization of body fat and proteins to meet the increased

energy needs. Furthermore, head-injured patients undergo an inflammatory response and may be febrile, creating increased needs for protein and calories. Improvement in outcome and reduction in complications have been observed in head-injured patients who receive adequate nutrition support early in the hospital course.[10]

NUTRITION AND RENAL ALTERATIONS

Providing adequate nutrition care for the patient with renal disease can be extremely challenging. Although renal disturbances and their treatments can greatly increase needs for nutrients, necessary restrictions in intake of fluid, protein, phosphorus, and potassium make delivery of adequate calories, vitamins, and minerals difficult. Thorough nutrition assessment provides the basis for successful nutrition management in patients with renal disease.

Nutrition Assessment

Some common assessment findings in individuals with renal disease are listed in Box 6-7.

Nutrition Intervention

The goal of nutrition interventions is to administer adequate nutrients, including calories, protein, vitamins, and minerals, while avoiding excesses of protein, fluid, electrolytes, and other nutrients with potential toxicity.

Protein

The kidney is responsible for excreting nitrogen from amino acids or proteins in the form of *urea*. Thus, when urinary excretion of urea is impaired in renal failure, blood levels of urea rise. Excessive protein intake may worsen uremia. However, the patient with renal failure often has (1) other physiologic stresses that actually increase protein/amino acid needs; (2) losses from dialysis, wounds, and fistulae; use of corticosteroid drugs that exert a catabolic effect; (3) increased endogenous secretion of catecholamines, corticosteroids, and glucagon, all of which can cause or

---

Box **6-7**	Common Findings in the Patient with Renal Failure

- Underweight (may be masked by edema)
- Electrolyte imbalances
- Hypoalbuminemia related to protein restriction and amino acid losses in dialysis
- Anemia related to inadequate erythropoietin production and blood loss with hemodialysis
- Hypertriglyceridemia related to use of glucose as osmotic agent in dialysis and use of carbohydrates to supply needed calories
- Wasting of muscle and subcutaneous tissue (may be masked by edema)
- Poor dietary intake related to protein and electrolyte restrictions

aggravate catabolism; (4) metabolic acidosis, which stimulates protein breakdown; and (5) catabolic conditions (e.g., trauma, surgery, sepsis). Therefore patients with acute renal failure need adequate amounts of protein to avoid catabolism of body tissues. Approximately 1.5 to 1.7 g of protein/kg/day has successfully maintained adequate protein nutrition in these patients.[11,12]

During hemodialysis and arteriovenous hemofiltration, amino acids are freely filtered and lost, but proteins such as albumin and immunoglobulin are not lost. Both proteins and amino acids are removed during peritoneal dialysis, creating a greater nutritional requirement for protein. Protein needs are estimated at approximately 1.0 to 1.2 g/kg/day for stable patients receiving hemodialysis or hemofiltration and 1.2 to 1.3 g/kg/day for those receiving peritoneal dialysis.[13,14] Patients in the process of wound healing and those with ongoing protein losses have greater needs.

Fluids

The patient with renal insufficiency usually does not require a fluid restriction until urine output begins to diminish. Patients receiving hemodialysis are limited to a fluid intake resulting in a gain of no more than 0.45 kg (1 lb) per day on the days between dialysis. This generally means a daily intake of 500 to 750 ml plus the volume lost in urine. With the use of continuous peritoneal dialysis, hemofiltration, or hemodialysis, the fluid intake can be liberalized.[15] This more liberal fluid allowance permits more adequate nutrient delivery, whether by oral, tube, or parenteral feedings. Enteral formulas containing 1.5 to 2.0 cal/ml or more provide a concentrated source of calories for tube-fed patients who require fluid restriction. Intravenous lipids, particularly 20% emulsions, can be used to supply concentrated calories for the TPN patient. Intradialytic TPN can be used to supply an additional source of nutrients at a time when the fluid can be rapidly removed in dialysis.[16,17]

Energy (Calories)

Energy needs are not increased by renal failure, but adequate calories must be provided to avoid catabolism.[11] It is essential that the renal patient receive an adequate number of calories to prevent catabolism of body tissues to meet energy needs. Catabolism not only reduces the mass of muscle and other functional body tissues but also releases nitrogen that must be excreted by the kidney. Adults with renal insufficiency need about 30 to 35 cal/kg/day, compared with the 25 to 30 cal/kg/day needed by healthy adults, to prevent catabolism and ensure that all protein consumed is used for anabolism rather than to meet energy needs.[11] After renal transplantation, when the patient initially receives large doses of corticosteroids, it is especially important to ensure that caloric intake is adequate (usually 25 to 35 cal/kg/day) to prevent undue catabolism.

Hypertriglyceridemia is found in a substantial number of patients with renal disorders. This condition is worsened by excessive intake of simple refined sugars, such as sucrose (table sugar) or glucose. Glucose in the peritoneal dialysate may be a significant calorie source and a contributing factor in hypertriglyceridemia. Approximately 70% of the glucose instilled during peritoneal dialysis to serve as an osmotic agent may be absorbed, and this must be considered part of the patient's carbohydrate intake. The glucose monohydrate used in intravenous and dialysate solutions supplies 3.4 cal/g. Thus, if a patient receives 4.25% glucose (4.25 g glucose/100 ml solution) in the dialysate, the patient receives the following:

$$42.5 \text{ g/L} \times 70\% \times 3.4 \text{ cal/g} = 101 \text{ cal/L of dialysate}$$

To help control hypertriglyceridemia, only about 30% to 35% of the patient's calories should come from carbohydrates, including glucose from the dialysate, with the major portion of dietary carbohydrate coming from complex carbohydrates (starches and fibers).

NUTRITION AND GASTROINTESTINAL ALTERATIONS

Because the gastrointestinal (GI) tract is so inherently related to nutrition, it is not surprising that impairment of the GI tract and its accessory organs has a major impact on nutrition. Two of the most serious GI-related illnesses seen among critical care patients are hepatic failure and pancreatitis.

Nutrition Assessment

Common assessment findings in patients with GI disease are listed in Box 6-8.

Nutrition Intervention
Hepatic Failure

Because the diseased liver has impaired ability to deactivate hormones, levels of circulating glucagon, epinephrine, and cortisol are elevated. These hormones promote catabolism of body tissues and cause glycogen stores to be exhausted.

Box 6-8   Common Findings in Patients with Gastrointestinal Disease

- Underweight related to malabsorption (from inadequate production of bile salts and pancreatic enzymes), anorexia, or poor intake (from pain caused by eating)
- Hypoalbuminemia (may result primarily from liver damage, not malnutrition)
- Hypocalcemia related to steatorrhea
- Hypomagnesemia related to alcohol abuse
- Anemia related to blood loss from bleeding varices
- Wasting of muscle and subcutaneous fat
- Confusion, confabulation, nystagmus, and peripheral neuropathy related to thiamine deficiency caused by alcohol abuse (Wernicke-Korsakoff syndrome)
- Steatorrhea

Release of lipids from their storage depots is accelerated, but the liver has decreased ability to metabolize them for energy. Furthermore, inadequate production of bile salts by the liver results in malabsorption of fat from the diet. Therefore body proteins are used for energy sources, producing tissue wasting.

The *branched-chain amino acids* (BCAAs)—leucine, isoleucine, and valine—are especially well used for energy, and their levels in the blood decline. Conversely, levels of the *aromatic amino acids* (AAAs)—phenylalanine, tyrosine, and tryptophan—rise as a result of tissue catabolism and impaired ability of the liver to clear them from the blood. The AAAs are precursors for neurotransmitters in the central nervous system (serotonin and dopamine). Rising levels of AAAs may alter nerve activity within the brain, leading to symptoms of encephalopathy. In addition, the damaged liver cannot clear ammonia from the circulation adequately, and ammonia accumulates in the brain. The ammonia may contribute to the encephalopathic symptoms and also to brain edema.[18,19]

Fluid and Electrolyte Status. Ascites and edema result from a combination of factors. There is decreased colloid osmotic pressure in the plasma because of the reduction of production of albumin and other plasma proteins by the diseased liver, increased portal pressure caused by obstruction, and renal sodium retention from secondary hyperaldosteronism. To control the fluid retention, restriction of sodium (usually 500 to 1500 mg [20 to 65 mEq] daily) and fluid (1500 ml or less daily) is generally necessary, in conjunction with administration of diuretics. Patients are weighed daily to evaluate the success of treatment. Also, laboratory data and physical status must be closely observed for potassium deficits caused by diuretic therapy and hyperaldosteronism.

Nutritious Diet. A diet with adequate protein helps to suppress catabolism and promote liver regeneration. Stable patients with cirrhosis usually tolerate 0.8 to 1.0 g of protein/kg/day. Patients with severe stress or nutritional deficits have increased needs, as much as 1.0 to 1.5 g/kg/day. If encephalopathy occurs or appears to be impending, however, tolerance of protein is impaired, and protein intake is reduced to 0.5 g/kg/day or less.

A diet adequate in calories (at least 30 cal/kg daily) is provided to help prevent catabolism and to prevent the use of dietary protein for energy needs. Moderate amounts of fat are given unless the patient has steatorrhea, in which case it is necessary to rely heavily on carbohydrates and medium-chain triglycerides (MCTs) to meet caloric needs. Soft foods are preferred because the patient may have esophageal varices that might be irritated by hard or dry foods. Because alcoholism is often the cause of hepatic failure and the diets of alcoholic patients are low in zinc, vitamin B complex, folate, and magnesium, supplements of these nutrients are usually provided daily.

Anorexia, malaise, and confusion may interfere with oral intake, and the nurse may need to provide much encouragement to the patient to ensure intake of an adequate diet.

Small, frequent feedings are usually accepted better by the anorexic patient than are three large meals daily. The nurse must assess the patient's neurologic status daily to evaluate tolerance of dietary protein. Increasing lethargy, confusion, or asterixis may signal a need for decreased protein intake. Anorexia, coupled with the unpalatable nature of the very-low-sodium, very-low-protein diet required in impending coma, may result in a need for tube feedings.

BCAA-enriched products have been developed for enteral and parenteral nutrition of patients with hepatic disease. In patients with encephalopathy who do not tolerate standard diets or nutrition support products, BCAA-enriched products may improve electroencephalogram (EEG) results and arousal, as well as nutritional status.[20] Patients with liver failure often receive lactulose, which causes diarrhea. If oral or tube feedings are also administered, diarrhea from concurrent administration of lactulose is not to be confused with intolerance of the feedings.

The patient who undergoes successful liver transplantation is usually able to tolerate a regular diet with few restrictions. Intake during the postoperative period must be adequate to support nutritional repletion and healing; 1.0 to 1.2 g of protein/kg/day and approximately 30 cal/kg/day are usually sufficient. Immunosuppressant therapy (corticosteroids and tacrolimus) contributes to glucose intolerance. Dietary measures to control glucose intolerance include (1) obtaining approximately 30% of dietary calories from fat, (2) emphasizing complex sources of carbohydrates, and (3) eating several small meals daily, with some of the day's carbohydrates in each meal. Moderate exercise often helps to improve glucose tolerance.

Pancreatitis

Food intake stimulates pancreatic secretion and thus increases the damage to the pancreas and the associated pain. Pancreatic insufficiency, with inadequate release of trypsin, chymotrypsin, and pancreatic lipase and amylase, results in impaired digestion and subsequent loss of nutrients in the stool. Fat malabsorption is the most marked effect of pancreatic insufficiency. Fat lost in the stools is accompanied by loss of calcium, zinc, and other minerals, along with the fat-soluble vitamins. Digestion and absorption of protein may also be impaired. In chronic pancreatitis, impaired glucose tolerance or frank diabetes is common because of destruction of the insulin-secreting beta cells of the pancreas.

Prevent Nutrition Deficits. An important goal of nutrition therapy in patients with acute pancreatitis or in exacerbations of chronic pancreatitis is to avoid further damage to the pancreas by providing little stimulus for enzyme secretion. Until recently, the common practice was to give TPN to patients with acute bouts of pancreatitis to reduce stimulation of the pancreas. However, evidence suggests that enteral feedings delivered below the level of the pancreatic duct provide little stimulation for pancreatic secretion.[21]

The results of randomized studies comparing TPN with *total enteral nutrition* (TEN, or enteral tube feeding) indicate that TEN is preferable to TPN in patients with severe acute pancreatitis, reducing the costs of care and risk of sepsis and improving clinical outcome.[22,23] Low-fat formulas and those with fat provided by MCTs are more readily absorbed than formulas that are high in long-chain triglycerides (e.g., corn or sunflower oil).

Levels of antioxidant nutrients (e.g., fat-soluble vitamins A and E, selenium) are low in patients with pancreatitis, probably because of poor absorption (related to pancreatic insufficiency) and increases in oxidative stress.[24] Water-miscible forms of the fat-soluble vitamins are available and may be better absorbed than the usual formulations.

When oral intake is possible, small, frequent feedings of low-fat foods are least likely to cause discomfort. Alcohol intake should be avoided because it worsens the tissue damage and the pain associated with pancreatitis. Guidelines for treatment of diabetes are appropriate for the care of the patient with glucose intolerance or diabetes related to pancreatitis (see following discussion).

NUTRITION AND ENDOCRINE ALTERATIONS

Endocrine alterations have far-reaching effects on all body systems and thus affect nutritional status in a variety of ways. One of the most common endocrine problems, both in the general population and among critically ill patients, is diabetes mellitus.

Nutrition Assessment

Common assessment findings in individuals with endocrine alterations are listed in Box 6-9. Because of the prevalence of patients with non–insulin-dependent (*type 2*) diabetes mellitus among the hospitalized population, the acute nutritional problems most often noted in patients with endocrine alterations are related to glycemic control.

Nutrition Intervention
Nutrition Support and Blood Glucose Control

Patients with insulin-dependent (*type 1*) diabetes mellitus or endocrine dysfunction caused by pancreatitis often have weight loss and malnutrition as a result of tissue catabolism because they cannot use dietary carbohydrates to meet energy needs. Although patients with type 2 diabetes are more likely to be overweight than underweight, they too may become malnourished as a result of chronic or acute infections, trauma, major surgery, or other illnesses. Nutrition support should not be neglected simply because a patient is obese, since PCM develops even in these patients. When a patient is not expected to be able to eat for at least 5 to 7 days or when inadequate intake persists for that period, initiation of tube feedings or TPN is indicated. No disease process benefits from starvation, and development or progression of nutritional deficits may contribute to complications such as decubitus ulcers, pulmonary or urinary tract infections, and sepsis, which prolong hospitalization, increase the costs of care, and may even result in death.

Blood glucose control is especially important in the care of surgical patients. Hyperglycemia in the early postoperative period is associated with increased rates of nosocomial infection. To maintain tight control of blood glucose, glucose levels are monitored regularly, usually several times a day until the patient is stable. Regular insulin added to the solution is the most common method of managing hyperglycemia in the patient receiving TPN. Multiple injections of regular insulin may be used to maintain tight control of blood glucose in the enterally fed patient.

In patients receiving enteral tube feedings, the transpyloric route (via nasoduodenal, nasojejunal, or jejunostomy tube) may be the most effective because gastroparesis may make intragastric tube feedings impossible or inadequate. Transpyloric feedings are given continuously or by slow intermittent infusion, since dumping syndrome and poor absorption often occur if feedings are given rapidly into the small bowel. For the continuously tube-fed patient with diabetes, control of blood glucose may be improved either with continuous insulin infusion or by use of a formula containing fiber, if such a formula is not contraindicated. Fiber may slow the absorption of the carbohydrate in the formula, producing a more delayed and sustained glycemic response.

Severe Vomiting or Diarrhea

When insulin-dependent patients experience vomiting and diarrhea severe enough to interfere significantly with oral intake or to result in excessive fluid and electrolyte losses, adequate carbohydrates and fluids must be supplied. If patients are receiving oral feedings, they may not be able to adhere to their usual diet but generally need to consume 10 to 15 g of carbohydrates every 1 to 2 hours.[25] Small amounts of food or liquids taken every 15 to 20 minutes are generally tolerated best by the patient with nausea and vomiting. Foods and beverages containing approximately 15 g of carbohydrate include ½ cup of regular gelatin, ½ cup of custard, ¾ cup of regular ginger ale, ½ cup of regular soft drink, and ½ cup of orange or apple juice. Blood glucose levels should be monitored at least every 2 to 4 hours, and the urine should be tested for ketones if blood glucose levels are greater than 250 mg/dl or the patient seems especially ill.[25]

Box **6-9**	Common Findings in Patients with Endocrine Disease

- Hyperglycemia related to poor diabetic control, infection, trauma/burns, or glucocorticoid use
- Elevated hemoglobin A_{1c} related to chronic poor diabetic control
- Hypoglycemia related to vomiting or poor food intake without adjustment of the dosage of insulin or oral hypoglycemic agents

ADMINISTERING NUTRITION SUPPORT
Enteral Nutrition

Whenever possible, the enteral route is the preferred method of feeding. Patients with abdominal trauma in particular have lower morbidity and mortality rates if fed enterally rather than parenterally.

There are a variety of commercial enteral feeding products, some of which are designed to meet the specialized needs of the critically ill. Products designed for the stressed patient with trauma or sepsis are usually rich in glutamine, arginine, and antioxidant nutrients (e.g., vitamins C, E, and A; selenium). The antioxidants help to reduce oxidative injury to the tissues (e.g., from reperfusion injury). Some products can be consumed orally, but it can be difficult for the critically ill patient to consume enough orally to meet the increased needs associated with stress.

Oral Supplementation

Oral supplementation may be necessary for patients who can eat and have normal digestion and absorption but simply cannot consume enough regular foods to meet caloric and protein needs. Patients with mild to moderate anorexia, burns, or trauma may be included in this category.

Tube Feeding

Tube feedings are used for patients who have at least some digestive and absorptive capability but are unwilling or unable to consume enough by mouth. Patients with profound anorexia and those experiencing severe stress (e.g., major burns, trauma) that greatly increases their nutritional needs often benefit from tube feedings. Individuals who require elemental formulas because of impaired digestion or absorption or specialized formulas for altered metabolic conditions such as renal or hepatic failure usually require tube feeding because the unpleasant flavors of the free amino acids, peptides, or protein hydrolysates used in these formulas are very difficult to mask.

Location and Type of Feeding Tube. Nasal intubation is the simplest and most common route for gaining access to the GI tract; this method allows access to the stomach, duodenum, or jejunum. *Tube enterostomy*—a gastrostomy or jejunostomy—is used primarily for long-term feedings (6 to 12 weeks or more) and when obstruction makes the nasoenteral route inaccessible. Tube enterostomies may also be used for the patient who is at risk for tube dislodgment because of severe agitation or confusion. A conventional gastrostomy or jejunostomy is often performed at the time of other abdominal surgery. The *percutaneous endoscopic gastrostomy* (PEG) tube has become extremely popular because it can be inserted without the use of general anesthetics. Percutaneous endoscopic jejunostomy (PEJ) tubes are also used.

Transpyloric feedings via nasoduodenal, nasojejunal, or jejunostomy tubes are typically used when there is a risk of pulmonary aspiration, because theoretically the pyloric sphincter provides a barrier that lessens the risk of regurgitation and aspiration. If nasogastric tubes are used, choosing the smallest possible tube diameter reduces the risk of gastroesophageal reflux and pulmonary aspiration. Transpyloric feedings have an advantage over intragastric feedings for patients with delayed gastric emptying, such as those with head injury, gastroparesis associated with uremia or diabetes, or postoperative ileus. Small bowel motility returns more quickly than gastric motility after surgery, and thus it is often possible to deliver transpyloric feedings within a few hours of injury or surgery.[26,27] Promotility agents such as metoclopramide may improve feeding tolerance.[28]

Nursing Management. The nurse's role in delivery of tube feedings usually includes (1) insertion of the tube, if a temporary tube is used; (2) maintenance of the tube; (3) administration of the feedings; (4) prevention and detection of complications associated with this form of therapy; and (5) participation in assessment of the patient's response to tube feedings.

Tube Placement. Critical care nurses are usually familiar with tube insertion, and therefore this topic is not discussed here. However, it is well to remember that if transpyloric positioning is desirable, administration of metoclopramide or erythromycin before tube insertion increases the likelihood of tube passage through the pylorus.[29]

Correct tube placement must be confirmed before initiation of feedings and regularly throughout the course of enteral feedings. Radiographs are the most accurate way of assessing tube placement, but repeated radiographs are costly and can expose the patient to excessive radiation. An inexpensive and relatively accurate alternative method involves assessing the pH of fluid removed from the feeding tube; some tubes are equipped with pH monitoring systems.

If the pH is less than 4.0 in patients not receiving gastric acid inhibitors, or less than 5.5 in patients who are receiving acid inhibitors, the tube tip is likely to be in the stomach.[30] Intestinal secretions usually have a pH greater than 6.0, and respiratory tract fluids usually have a pH greater than 5.5. The esophagus may have an acid pH, which may cause confusion between esophageal and gastric placement. However, other clues can help in identifying a tube that has its distal tip in the esophagus: it may be especially difficult to aspirate fluid out of the tube; a large portion of the tube may extend out of the body (although a tube inserted to the proper length could be coiled in the esophagus); and belching often occurs immediately after air is injected into the tube.[30]

Assessing both the pH and the *bilirubin* concentration of fluid aspirated from the feeding tube is a promising new method for confirming tube placement.[31] The bilirubin concentration in tracheobronchial and pleural fluid and in the stomach is approximately 90% less than in the intestine. Therefore the nurse who obtains fluid with a pH greater than 5.0 and a low bilirubin concentration from a feeding tube can be relatively sure that the distal tip of the tube is in the pulmonary system.[31] Measurement of end-tidal CO_2 also shows promise for confirming tube placement in ventilated patients.[32]

Formula Delivery. Careful attention to administration of tube feedings can prevent many complications. Very clean or aseptic technique in the handling and administration of the formula can help prevent bacterial contamination and a resultant infection. The optimal schedule for delivery of feedings also is important. Tube feedings may be administered intermittently or continuously.

Bolus feedings, which are intermittent feedings delivered rapidly into the stomach or small bowel, are likely to cause distention, vomiting, and dumping syndrome with diarrhea. Instead of using bolus feedings, nurses can gradually drip intermittent feedings, with each feeding lasting 20 to 30 minutes or longer, to promote optimal assimilation. The question of which feeding schedule—continuous or intermittent—is superior in critically ill patients remains unanswered.

Prevent or Correct Complications. Some of the more common complications of tube feeding are pulmonary aspiration, diarrhea, constipation, tube occlusion, and delayed gastric emptying (Table 6-2).

Total Parenteral Nutrition

Total parenteral nutrition refers to the delivery of all nutrients by the intravenous (IV) route. TPN is used when the GI tract is not functional or when nutritional needs cannot be met solely via the GI tract. Likely candidates for TPN include patients who have a severely impaired absorption (as in short bowel syndrome, collagen-vascular diseases, and radiation enteritis), intestinal obstruction, peritonitis, and prolonged ileus. In addition, some postoperative, trauma, and burn patients may need TPN to supplement the nutrient intake they are able to tolerate via the enteral route.

Routes for Delivery

TPN may be delivered through either central or peripheral veins. Because it requires an indwelling catheter, central vein TPN carries an increased risk of sepsis as well as potential insertion-related complications such as pneumothorax and hemothorax. Air embolism is also more likely with central vein TPN. However, central venous catheters provide very secure IV access and allow delivery of more hyperosmolar solutions than does peripheral TPN. TPN solutions containing 25% to 35% dextrose are often delivered through central veins, which provides an inexpensive source of calories.

Patients requiring multiple IV therapies and frequent blood sampling usually have multilumen central venous catheters, and TPN is often infused through these catheters. Clearly, patients requiring multilumen catheters are likely to be seriously ill and immunocompromised, and scrupulous aseptic technique is essential in maintaining multilumen catheters. The manipulation involved in frequent changes of IV fluid and obtaining blood specimens through these catheters increases the risk of catheter contamination.

TPN via peripheral vein rarely is associated with serious infectious or mechanical complications but does require good peripheral venous access. Therefore it may not be appropriate for patients receiving multiple IV therapies. Peripherally inserted central catheters (PICCs) allow central venous access through long catheters inserted in peripheral sites. This reduces the risk of complications associated with percutaneous cannulation of the subclavian vein (e.g., subclavian vein laceration, pneumothorax, chylothorax) and provides an alternative to peripheral TPN, but the PICC approach carries an increased risk of phlebitis and catheter malfunction.[33]

Nursing Management

Nursing management of the patient receiving TPN includes catheter care, administration of solutions, prevention or correction of complications, and evaluation of patient responses to IV feedings.

The indwelling central venous catheter provides an excellent nidus for infection. Catheter-related infections arise from endogenous skin flora, contamination of the catheter hub, seeding of the catheter by organisms carried in the bloodstream from another site, or contamination of the infusate. Good handwashing and scrupulous aseptic technique in all aspects of catheter care and TPN delivery are the primary steps for prevention of catheter-related infections. Other measures to reduce the incidence of catheter-related infections include (1) using maximal barrier precautions (cap, mask, sterile gloves, sterile drape) at the time of insertion, (2) tunneling the catheter underneath the skin, (3) cleaning the insertion site with antiseptics at regular intervals, and (4) maintaining cleanliness of the catheter hub (decontamination with antiseptics and reducing the number of tubing changes and other manipulations at the hub).[34] Newer approaches for reducing catheter-related infections include use of catheters impregnated with an antiseptic agent, including chlorhexidine, chlorhexidine and silver sulfadiazine, silver ions, and antibiotics (e.g., rifampin, minocycline); antibiotic locks in the catheter when infusions are stopped; a catheter hub that includes an antiseptic chamber; and dressing materials that release silver ions or chlorhexidine during use to reduce catheter site colonization.[34-36]

TPN solutions usually consist of amino acids, dextrose, electrolytes, vitamins, minerals, and trace elements. Although dextrose–amino acid solutions are usually considered good growth media for microorganisms, these solutions actually suppress the growth of most organisms usually associated with catheter-related sepsis, except yeasts. Because the many manipulations required to prepare solutions increase the possibility of contamination, however, TPN solutions are best used with caution. Solutions should be

Table 6-2   Nursing Management of Enteral Tube Feeding Complications

Complication	Contributing Factor(s)	Prevention/Correction
Pulmonary aspiration	Feeding tube positioned in esophagus or respiratory tract Regurgitation of formula	Check tube placement before intermittent feeding and every 4-6 hr during continuous feedings by checking pH of fluid aspirated from tube. Consult with physician regarding use of transpyloric tube; elevate head to 45 degrees during feedings unless contraindicated; if head cannot be raised, position patient in lateral (especially right lateral, which facilitates gastric emptying) or prone position to improve drainage of vomitus from mouth; if head must be in dependent position, discontinue feedings 30-60 min earlier and restart them only when head can be raised. Keep cuff of endotracheal or tracheostomy tube inflated during feedings, if possible. Metoclopramide may improve gastric emptying and decrease risk of regurgitation. Check tracheobronchial secretions with glucose oxidase strips to facilitate diagnosis of aspiration.
Diarrhea	Medications with GI side effects (antibiotics, digitalis, laxatives, magnesium-containing antacids, quinidine, caffeine, others) Hypertonic formula or medications (e.g., oral suspensions of antibiotics, potassium, or other electrolytes), which cause dumping syndrome Bacterial contamination of formula Fecal impaction with seepage of liquid stool around impaction	Evaluate feeding tolerance every 2 hr initially, then less frequently as condition becomes stable; intolerance may be manifested by bloating, abdominal distention/pain, lack of stool/flatus, diminished/absent bowel sounds, tense abdomen, increased tympany, and nausea/vomiting; if intolerance is suspected, abdominal radiographs may be done to check for distended gastric bubble, distended loops of bowel, or air-fluid levels. Evaluate patient's medications to determine potential for causing diarrhea; consult pharmacist when necessary. Evaluate formula administration procedures to ensure feedings are not being given by bolus infusion; administer formula continuously or by slow intermittent infusion. Dilute enteral medications well. Use scrupulously clean technique in administering tube feedings; prepare formula with sterile water if concerns about safety of the water supply or if patient is seriously immunocompromised; keep opened containers of formula refrigerated and discard in 24 hr; discard enteral feeding containers and administration sets every 24 hr; hang formula no more than 4-8 hr unless prepackaged in sterile administration sets; be especially careful with feedings given to patients being fed transpylorically or those receiving cimetidine or antacids because they lack normal antibacterial barrier of stomach acid. Perform digital rectal examination to rule out impaction; see Constipation.
Constipation	Low-residue formula, creating little fecal bulk	Consult with physician regarding use of fiber-containing formula.
Tube occlusion	Medications administered via tube that either physically plug tube or coagulate formula, causing it to clog tube Sedimentation of formula Aspirating gastric contents to measure residual volumes (acidified protein from formula clots in tube)	If medications must be given by tube, avoid use of crushed tablets; consult with pharmacist to determine whether medications can be dispensed as elixirs or suspensions; irrigate tube with water before and after administering any medication; never add any medication to formula unless the two are known to be compatible. Irrigate tube every 4-8 hr during continuous feedings and after every intermittent feeding. It has been suggested that aspiration of gastric residuals be avoided with small-bore feeding tubes (8 Fr) and that patient tolerance be assessed by physical examination; if residuals are measured, flush tube thoroughly after returning the formula to stomach.
Gastric retention	Delayed gastric emptying related to head trauma, sepsis, diabetic or uremic gastroparesis, electrolyte balance, or other illness	Cause must be corrected, if possible; consult with physician about use of transpyloric feedings or metoclopramide to stimulate gastric emptying; encourage patient to lie in right lateral position frequently, unless contraindicated.

Modified from Moore MC: *Pocket guide to nutritional care*, ed 4, St Louis, 2000, Mosby.

Table 6-3   Nursing Management of Total Parenteral Nutrition (TPN) Complications

Complication	Clinical Manifestations	Prevention/Correction
Catheter-related sepsis	Fever, chills, glucose intolerance, positive blood culture	Use aseptic technique when handling catheter, IV tubing, and TPN solutions; hang solution bottle no longer than 24 hr and lipid emulsion no longer than 12-24 hr; use in-line 0.22-µm filter with TPN to remove microorganisms; avoid drawing blood, infusing blood or blood products, piggybacking other IV solutions into TPN IV tubing, or attaching manometers or transducers via TPN infusion line, if possible. If catheter-related sepsis suspected, remove catheter or assist in changing catheter over guidewire, and administer antibiotics as ordered.
Air embolism	Dyspnea, cyanosis, apnea, tachycardia, hypotension, "millwheel" heart murmur; mortality estimated at 50% (depends on quantity of air entering)	Use Luer-Lok connections; use in-line air-eliminating filter; have patient perform Valsalva maneuver during tubing changes; if patient is on ventilator, change tubing quickly at end expiration; maintain occlusive dressing over catheter site for at least 24 hr after removing catheter to prevent air entry through catheter tract. If air embolism suspected, place patient in left lateral decubitus and Trendelenburg positions (to trap air in apex of right ventricle, away from outflow tract), and administer oxygen and CPR as needed; immediately notify physician, who may attempt to aspirate air from the heart.
Pneumothorax	Chest pain, dyspnea, hypoxemia, hypotension, radiographic evidence, needle aspiration of air from pleural space	Thoroughly explain catheter insertion procedure to patient (patient who moves or breathes erratically is more likely to sustain pleural damage); perform x-ray examination after insertion or insertion attempt. If pneumothorax is suspected, assist with needle aspiration or chest tube insertion, if necessary.
Central venous thrombosis	Edema of neck/shoulder/arm on same side as catheter; development of collateral circulation in chest; pain in insertion site; drainage of TPN from insertion site; positive findings on venogram	Follow measures to prevent sepsis; repeat or traumatic catheterization is most likely to result in thrombosis. If thrombosis confirmed, remove catheter and administer anticoagulants and antibiotics as ordered.
Catheter occlusion or semiocclusion	No flow or sluggish flow through catheter	If infusion is stopped temporarily, flush catheter with saline or heparinized saline. If catheter appears to be occluded, attempt to aspirate the clot; if this is ineffective, physician may order thrombolytic agent such as streptokinase or urokinase instilled in catheter.
Hypoglycemia	Diaphoresis, shakiness, confusion, loss of consciousness	Infuse TPN within 10% of ordered rate; monitor blood glucose level until stable after discontinuance of TPN. If hypoglycemia present, administer oral carbohydrate; if patient is unconscious or oral intake is contraindicated, physician may order bolus of IV dextrose.
Hyperglycemia	Thirst, headache, lethargy, increased urine output	Administer TPN within 10% of ordered rate; monitor blood glucose level at least daily until stable; patient may require insulin added to TPN if hyperglycemia is persistent; sudden appearance of hyperglycemia in a patient who previously tolerated same glucose load may indicate onset of sepsis.

Modified from Moore MC: *Pocket guide to nutritional care*, ed 4, St Louis, 2000, Mosby.
IV, Intravenous; *CPR*, cardiopulmonary resuscitation.

prepared under laminar flow conditions in the pharmacy, with avoidance of additions on the nursing unit. Solution containers need to be inspected for cracks or leaks before hanging, and solutions must be discarded within 24 hours of hanging. An in-line 0.22-µm filter, which eliminates all microorganisms but not endotoxins, may be used in administration of solutions. Use of the filter, however, cannot be substituted for good aseptic technique.

In contrast to dextrose–amino acid solutions, IV lipid emulsions support the proliferation of many microorganisms. Furthermore, lipid emulsions cannot be filtered through an in-line 0.22-µm filter because some particles in the emulsions have larger diameters than this. Lipid emulsions are handled with strict asepsis and must be discarded within 12 to 24 hours of hanging. Mixing lipid emulsions with dextrose–amino acid TPN solutions saves nursing time, but the nurse must be extremely careful in administering these solutions. TPN solutions containing lipids cannot be filtered through an in-line 0.22-µm filter, and they support the growth of most bacteria and *Candida albicans* to a greater degree than do dextrose–amino acid TPN solutions.

Prevent or Correct Complications. Some of the more common and serious complications of TPN include catheter-related sepsis, air embolism, pneumothorax, central venous thrombosis, catheter occlusion, and metabolic imbalances such as hypoglycemia and hyperglycemia (Table 6-3).

REFERENCES

1. Middleton MH, Nazarenko G, Nivison-Smith I, Smederly P: Prevalence of malnutrition and 12-month incidence of mortality in two Sydney teaching hospitals, *Intern Med J* 31:455, 2001.
2. Kinn S, Scott J: Nutritional awareness of critically ill surgical high-dependency patients, *Br J Nurs* 10:704, 2001.
3. Kelly IE et al: Still hungry in hospital: identifying malnutrition in acute hospital admissions, *Q J Med* 93:93, 2000.
4. Sullivan DH, Sun S, Walls RC: Protein-energy undernutrition among elderly hospitalized patients: a prospective study, *JAMA* 281:2013, 1999.
5. McWhirter JP, Pennington CR: Incidence and recognition of malnutrition in hospital, *BMJ* 308:945, 1994.
6. Covinsky KE et al: The relationship between clinical assessments of nutritional status and adverse outcomes in older hopitalized medical patients, *J Am Geriatr Soc* 47:532, 1999.
7. National Education Programs Working Group: Report on the management of patients with hypertension and high blood cholesterol, *Ann Intern Med* 114:224, 1991.
8. Vollmer WM et al: Effects of diet and sodium intake on blood pressure: subgroup analysis of the DASH-sodium trial, *Ann Intern Med* 135:1019, 2001.
9. Wilson RF, Tyburski JG: Metabolic responses and nutritional therapy in patients with severe head injuries, *J Head Trauma Rehabil* 13:11, 1998.
10. Taylor SJ et al: Prospective, randomized, controlled trial to determine the effect of early enhanced enteral nutrition on clinical outcome in mechanically ventilated patients suffering head injury, *Crit Care Med* 27:2525, 1999.
11. Kierdorf HP: The nutritional management of acute renal failure in the intensive care unit, *New Horiz* 3:699, 1995.
12. Bellomo R et al: A prospective comparative study of moderate versus high protein intake for critically ill patients with acute renal failure, *Ren Fail* 19:111, 1997.
13. Mitch WE, Maroni BJ: Factors causing malnutrition in patients with chronic uremia, *Am J Kidney Dis* 33:176, 1999.
14. Kopple J: Therapeutic approaches to malnutrition in chronic dialysis patients: the different modalities of nutritional support, *Am J Kidney Dis* 33:180, 1999.
15. Riella MC: Nutrition in acute renal failure, *Ren Fail* 19:237, 1997.
16. Brewer ED: Pediatric experience with intradialytic parenteral nutrition and supplemental tube feeding, *Am J Kidney Dis* 33:205, 1999.
17. Cato Y: Intradialytic parenteral nutrition therapy for the malnourished hemodialysis patient, *J Intraven Nurs* 20:130, 1997.
18. Hazell AS, Butterworth RF: Hepatic encephalopathy: an update of pathophysiologic mechanisms, *Proc Soc Exp Biol Med* 222:99, 1999.
19. Albrecht J, Jones EA: Hepatic encephalopathy: molecular mechanisms underlying the clinical syndrome, *J Neurol Sci* 170:138, 1999.
20. Russell MK, Charney P: Is there a role for specialized enteral nutrition in the intensive care unit? *Nutr Clin Pract* 17:156, 2002.
21. McClave SA, Spain DA, Snider HL: Nutritional management in acute and chronic pancreatitis, *Gastroenterol Clin North Am* 27:421, 1998.
22. Kalfarentzos F et al: Enteral nutrition is superior to parenteral nutrition in severe acute pancreatitis: results of a randomized prospective trial, *Br J Surg* 84:1665, 1997.
23. Windsor AC et al: Compared with parenteral nutrition, enteral feeding attenuates the acute phase response and improves disease severity in acute pancreatitis, *Gut* 42:431, 1998.
24. Van Gossum A et al: Deficiency in antioxidant factors in patients with alcohol-related chronic pancreatitis, *Dig Dis Sci* 41:1225, 1996.
25. American Diabetes Association: *Medical management of type 1 diabetes*, ed 3, Alexandria, Va, 1998, The Association.
26. Singh G, Ram RP, Kahna SK: Early postoperative enteral feeding in patients with nontraumatic intestinal perforation and peritonitis, *J Am Coll Surg* 187:142, 1998.
27. Braga M et al: Artificial nutrition after major abdominal surgery: impact of route of administration and composition of the diet, *Crit Care Med* 26:24, 1998.
28. Booth CM, Heyland DK, Paterson WG: Gastrointestinal promotility drugs in the critical care setting: a systematic review of the evidence, *Crit Care Med* 30:1429, 2002.
29. Lord LM et al: Comparison of weighted vs. unweighted enteral feeding tubes for efficacy of transpyloric intubation, *JPEN J Parenter Enteral Nutr* 17:71, 1993.
30. Metheny NA et al: pH testing of feeding-tube aspirates to determine placement, *Nutr Clin Pract* 9:185, 1994.
31. Metheny NA et al: pH and concentration of bilirubin in feeding tube aspirates as predictors of tube placement, *Nurs Res* 48:189, 1999.
32. Burns SM, Carpenter R, Truwit JD: Report on the development of a procedure to prevent placement of feeding tubes into the lungs using end-tidal CO_2 measurements, *Crit Care Med* 29:936-939, 2001.
33. Vanek VW: The ins and outs of venous access. Part II, *Nutr Clin Pract* 17:142, 2002.
34. Krzywda EA, Andris DA, Edmiston CE: Catheter infections: diagnosis, etiology, treatment, and prevention, *Nutr Clin Pract* 14:178, 1999.
35. Spencer RC: Novel methods for the prevention of infection of intravascular devices, *J Hosp Infect* 43:S127, 1999.
36. Veenstra DL, Saint S, Sullivan SD: Cost-effectiveness of antiseptic-impregnated central venous catheters for the prevention of catheter-related bloodstream infection, *JAMA* 282:554, 1999.

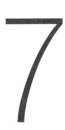

Gerontologic Alterations

BARBARA J. DRAUDE

Objectives

- Describe the age-associated physiologic changes that occur in the cardiovascular, respiratory, renal, gastrointestinal, hepatic, integumentary, and central nervous systems.
- State the clinical significance of age-related physiologic changes and the expected nursing considerations or interventions used in caring for older critical care patients.
- Relate the age-related changes in hepatic function and the accompanying pharmacokinetic changes to the administration of various cardiovascular medications.

evolve Be sure to check out the free exercises on-line at *http://evolve.elsevier.com/Urden/priorities/*

The process of senescence (growing old) is characterized by tissue and organ changes. These changes, along with the prevalence of chronic conditions in elderly patients, contribute to increased morbidity and mortality in the critical care unit. Aging is accompanied by physiologic changes in the cardiovascular, respiratory, renal, gastrointestinal, hepatic, integumentary, immune, and central nervous systems. With advancing age the incidence of disease increases, with cardiovascular and neoplastic diseases being the most common causes of death.[1] Although physiologic decline and disease processes influence each other, physiologic decline occurs independently of disease. Therefore changes in physiologic function are important to consider when caring for the elderly patient.

CARDIOVASCULAR SYSTEM

Advancing age has many effects on the cardiovascular system. Both the myocardium and the vascular system undergo a multitude of anatomic, cellular, and genetic changes that alter myocardial and peripheral vascular system function.[2]

Morphologic Changes in Myocardium

Myocardial collagen content increases with age.[3,4] *Collagen* is the principal noncontractile protein occupying the cardiac interstitium.[5] There are two types of collagen: type I and type III. The increase in myocardial stiffness in the aging heart probably results from an increase in *type I* collagen, which is associated with scar tissue formation and has a higher tensile strength.[5] *Type III* collagen is different from type I in that it is a "softer" type and is associated with the reparative process of wound healing.

Increased myocardial collagen content renders the myocardium less compliant. The decrease in myocardial compliance can adversely affect diastolic filling (through decreased distensibility and dilation) and myocardial relaxation. Consequently, the left ventricle must develop a higher filling pressure for a given increase in ventricular volume. The functional consequence could be an increase in myocardial oxygen consumption. Under normal physiologic conditions, an increase in myocardial oxygen demand is met with a corresponding increase in coronary artery blood flow. In the presence of coronary artery disease, however, coronary artery blood flow can be limited because of atherosclerotic-mediated narrowing of the coronary arteries. Thus the patient is at risk for developing myocardial ischemia and infarction. Clinical manifestations of myocardial ischemia include electrocardiographic (ECG) changes and chest pain. However, the sensation of chest pain is altered in the elderly person.

The aging heart undergoes a modest degree of hypertrophy that is similar to pressure overload–induced hypertrophy. Such hypertrophy entails a thickening of the left ventricular wall without appreciable changes in left ventricular cavity size.[6] The increase in left ventricular wall thickness is a result primarily of myocyte hypertrophy (increase in muscle cell size). In elderly individuals the myocardial hypertrophy may be caused by corresponding increases in aortic impedance and systemic vascular resistance.[7]

Myocardial Contraction and Relaxation

Myocardial contractility depends on numerous factors. However, the most important determinants of myocardial contraction are the intracellular level of free calcium (Ca^{++}) and the sensitivity of the contractile proteins for calcium.[8] Peak contractile force in the senescent myocardium is unaltered, suggesting that neither the amount of Ca^{++} during systole nor the sensitivity of the contractile proteins for calcium is altered. The prolonged duration of contraction (systole) is caused in part by a slowed or delayed rate of myocardial relaxation.[2,9]

Myocardial relaxation depends on removal of calcium from the cell by uptake into the sarcoplasmic reticulum (SR) and extrusion of calcium across the plasma membrane (sarcolemma) by the action of the sarcolemmal sodium-calcium exchanger and sarcolemmal Ca^{++}–adenosine triphosphatase (ATPase) pump.[8] In heart cells the decrease in Ca^{++} concentration at the start of diastole results primarily from uptake into the SR and to a lesser extent from efflux from the cell via the sarcolemmal sodium-calcium exchanger and Ca^{++}-ATPase pump. The age-associated decrease in the rate of relaxation may partly result from a reduced rate of calcium uptake (sequestration) by the SR.[10,11] Calcium uptake by the SR occurs through a Ca^{++}-ATPase pump embedded in the SR membrane.

Hemodynamics and Electrocardiogram

Resting (supine) heart rate (HR) decreases with age.[12,13] HR is an important determinant of cardiac output (CO), and the normal resting heart beats approximately 70 times a minute. At rest or with minimal activity, the elderly person probably will not experience any untoward cardiovascular effect (e.g., decrease in CO) with a HR of 62 beats/min. However, if the HR response is attenuated during exercise, the elderly person's capacity for exercise may be limited.

Resting CO and stroke volume (SV) are not changed with advancing age. At rest, left ventricular end-diastolic volume (LVEDV, preload), end-systolic volume (volume of blood remaining in ventricle after systole), and ejection fraction are not affected by age.[14] In the elderly human myocardium the early-diastolic filling period and isovolumic phase of myocardial relaxation are prolonged.[15,16] Although suggestive of diastolic dysfunction, these changes do not translate into decreases in LVEDV or SV.[15,16] Aging also is associated with a moderate increase in pulmonary artery pressure.[17]

Advancing age produces changes in the ECG. R-wave and S-wave amplitude decrease significantly in persons older than 49 years, whereas QT-interval duration increases, reflecting the prolonged rate of relaxation (Table 7-1).[18]

Table **7-1**   Age-Related Changes in Electrocardiographic Variables

ECG Variable	Age (years)			
	<30	30-39	40-49	>49
R-wave amplitude (mm)	10.43	10.53	9.01	9.25
S-wave amplitude (mm)	15.21	14.21	12.22	12.42
Frontal plane axis (degrees)	48.93	48.13	36.50	38.83
PR-segment duration (ms)	15.89	16.23	16.04	16.25
QRS-complex duration (ms)	7.64	7.51	7.36	8.00
QT-interval duration (ms)	37.83	37.50	37.99	39.58
T-wave amplitude (ms)	5.21	4.57	4.31	4.42

Data from Bachman S, Sparrow D, Smith LK: *Am J Cardiol* 48:513, 1981.
ms, Milliseconds.

The most common dysrhythmia occurring in elderly individuals is *premature ventricular contraction*. Other common types of dysrhythmias are sinus node dysfunction (atrial fibrillation, atrial flutter, paroxysmal supraventricular tachycardia) and atrioventricular conduction disturbances.[18,19] Because the majority of patients are asymptomatic, the use of antidysrhythmics is not generally recommended. The side effects and toxic effects of antidysrhythmics impose greater risk than the mortality or morbidity related to the dysrhythmia. In contrast, in symptomatic patients with malignant ventricular dysrhythmias (sustained ventricular tachycardia/fibrillation), pharmacologic therapy is warranted.[19]

Baroreceptor Function

Baroreceptor reflex function is altered with aging.[20] Baroreceptors, located at the bifurcation of the common carotid artery and aortic arch, are mechanoreceptors that respond to stretch and other changes in the blood vessel wall.[8] Impulses arising in the baroreceptor region project to the vasomotor center (nucleus of tractus solitarius) in the medulla. Abrupt changes in blood pressure caused by increases in peripheral resistance, CO, or blood volume are sensed by the baroreceptors, resulting in an increase in the impulse frequency to the vasomotor center within the medulla. This increase inhibits vasoconstrictor impulses arising from the vasoconstrictor region within the medulla.[8] The result is a decrease in HR and peripheral vasodilation; both these effects return the blood pressure to within normal limits.

Postural hypotension was once thought to occur more frequently in elderly persons and to be related to age. However, recent studies have shown that the prevalence of postural hypotension is quite low in elderly persons.[21,22] The prevalence of *orthostatic* hypotension is greater in institutionalized elderly patients who are receiving antihypertensive medications.[23]

Left Ventricular Function

In most individuals, aging is associated with a decline in exercise performance. The thickening of the left ventricular wall along with stiffening of the aortic and mitral valves makes the aging heart less able to provide adequate contractile strength.[24] With advancing age the maximal HR achieved during exercise is attenuated; however, the decreased HR response is accompanied by an increase in LVEDV and SV. This augmentation in LVEDV and SV offsets the attenuated HR response and maintains CO in exercise.

Healthy older persons have no age-associated decline in CO during exercise, but other factors (e.g., neural functioning, skeletal/joint functioning, pulmonary function) may limit an older individual's ability to exercise.

Peripheral Vascular System

The effects of aging on the peripheral vascular system are reflected in the gradual but linear rise in systolic blood pressure.[25,26] Diastolic blood pressure is less affected by age and generally remains the same or decreases.[26]

Important determinants of systolic blood pressure include the compliance of the vasculature and the blood volume within the vascular system. Similar to the heart, the compliance of the vasculature is determined by its cell type and tissue composition. With advancing age the intimal layer thickens, principally because of an increase in smooth muscle cells that have migrated from the medial layer, and the amount of connective tissue (collagen, elastic tissue) increases.[25] These changes occur in the intima of the large and distal arteries. This gradual decrease in arterial compliance, or "stiffening of the arteries," is known as *arteriosclerosis*. Arteriosclerotic and atherosclerotic processes cause the arteries to become progressively less distensible, altering the vascular pressure-volume relationship. These changes are clinically significant because small changes in intravascular volume are accompanied by disproportionate increases in systolic blood pressure. The decrease in arterial compliance and disproportionate increase in systolic blood pressure may lead to an increase in afterload and the development of concentric (pressure-induced) ventricular hypertrophy in the elderly patient.[27]

Arterial pressure is also governed by the amount of blood volume, which in turn is regulated by plasma levels of sodium and water and the activity of the renin-angiotensin system.[28] Plasma renin activity declines with age, and aging per se has no appreciable effect on sodium and water home-ostasis.[29,30] As noted later, however, age-related changes occur in renal tubular function, and the glomerular filtration rate (GFR) decreases, both of which can affect overall sodium and water homeostasis. Circulating levels of sodium-regulating hormones, such as natriuretic hormone, aldos-terone, and antidiuretic hormone (ADH), are not appreciably altered by advancing age.[30,31] However, a delayed natriuretic response after sodium loading and plasma volume expansion and a diminished renal response to ADH secretion have been reported in elderly persons.[31]

PULMONARY SYSTEM

Many of the changes in the pulmonary system that occur with aging are reflected in pulmonary function tests and include changes in thoracic wall expansion and respiratory muscle strength, morphology of alveolar parenchyma, and decreases in arterial oxygen tension (PaO_2)[32] (Table 7-2). These changes occur progressively as age advances and should not alter the elderly person's ability to breathe effort-lessly. However, factors such as repeated exposure to envi-ronmental pollutants, cigarette smoking, and frequent pulmonary infections can accelerate age-related changes, thereby making it difficult to identify the age-associated changes in pulmonary function.

Thoracic Wall and Respiratory Muscles

Upper airway changes include weakening support of upper and lower cartilage, predisposing elderly persons to obstruc-tive changes. Submucosal glands decrease production of mucus, leading to dryness and thickened secretions.[33] With advancing age the chest wall (thoracic skeleton) and verte-brae undergo a small degree of osteoporosis, and at the same time the costal cartilages that connect the rib cage together become calcified and stiff. These changes may produce kyphosis and reduce chest wall compliance, respec-tively.[32,34,35] The functional effect is a decrease in thoracic wall excursion. Other factors, such as an increase in abdomi-nal girth and change in posture, also decrease thoracic excursion. These anatomic changes are reflected by an increase in residual volume and decrease in vital capacity.

The strength of the respiratory muscles (diaphragm, external/internal intercostal muscles) gradually decreases. Respiratory muscle weakness begins as early as age 55 years.[36] During aging, skeletal muscle progressively atro-phies and its energy metabolism decreases, which may par-tially explain the declining strength of the respiratory muscles.[37,38] In addition, an age-associated decrease occurs in the effectiveness of the cough reflex, possibly caused by a decrease in ciliary responsiveness and motion.[39]

Alveolar Parenchyma

With advancing age a diminished recoil (or increased com-pliance) of the lung occurs.[40] The reduced recoil results from the increase in the ratio of elastin to collagen content that occurs with advancing age.[41] Collagen, elastin, and reticulin are the primary connective tissue proteins of the lung tissue.[42,43] They are responsible for the elasticity and performance of the airways of the lung. Whereas total lung collagen remains unaltered, the amount of elastin increases with age in the interlobular septa and pleura and possibly within the bronchi and their vessels. These anatomic changes are reflected by an increase in residual volume and a decrease in forced expiratory volume. With changes in carti-lage the trachea and bronchi become stiffer and less compli-ant.[33] Also, the size of the alveolar ducts increases after age 40 years.[32] The bronchial enlargement displaces inhaled air volume away from the alveoli that line the alveolar ducts (Figure 7-1).

Ventilation and oxygen/carbon dioxide exchange (diffu-sion) depend on numerous factors, including the surface area available for diffusion. A displacement of inhaled air volume away from the alveoli limits the surface area avail-able for gas exchange. This may partly explain the progres-sive and linear decrease in the pulmonary diffusion capacity, which depends on both surface area and capillary blood vol-ume. Capillary blood volume and surface area have been reported to decrease with advancing age.[44]

Pulmonary Gas Exchange

PaO_2 decreases with age, such that the median PaO_2 for healthy persons older than 60 years is 74.3 mm Hg, com-pared with 94 mm Hg for younger adults. In contrast, arterial carbon dioxide tension ($PaCO_2$) does not change with

Table **7-2**	Progressive Changes in Arterial Oxygen Tension (PaO_2) and Carbon Dioxide ($PaCO_2$) Tension (Partial Pressure)	
Age-Group (years)	**PaO_2 (mm Hg)**	**$PaCO_2$ (mm Hg)**
<30	94	39
31-40	87	38
41-50	84	40
51-60	81	39
>60	74	40

Data from Sorbini CA et al: *Respiration* 25:3, 1968.

advancing age (see Table 7-2).[45] Decreased alveolar surface along with a decreased capillary network leads to less gas-exchange ability.[33]

Lung Volumes and Capacities

With advancing age, total lung capacity and tidal volume do not change.[34] Residual volume (RV) increases with age, paralleling the decrease in chest wall compliance and reduced strength of the respiratory muscles. The increase in RV may also add to the diminished strength of the inspiratory muscles by stretching the diaphragm and altering the tension-length relationship.

RENAL SYSTEM

Aging produces changes in renal structure and function, many of which begin at approximately 30 to 40 years of age.[46] One of the prominent changes is a decrease in the number and size of the *nephrons*, which begins in the cortical regions and progresses toward the medullary portions of the kidney. The decrease in the number of nephrons corre-

sponds to a 20% decrease in the weight of the kidney between 40 and 80 years of age. Initially, this loss of nephrons does not appreciably alter renal function because of the large renal reserve; the kidney contains 2 to 3 million nephrons, all of which are not needed to maintain adequate fluid and acid-base homeostasis. Over time, however, the geriatric patient loses this renal reserve as well.[47] Nephron loss is caused by a gradual reduction in blood flow to the glomerular capillary tuft.[48]

Total renal blood flow declines after the fourth decade of life[46] because of hyaline arteriolosclerosis.[48,49] The etiology of this vascular lesion within the glomerular tuft is unknown. By the eighth decade of life, 50% of the glomeruli are lost as a result of this arteriolar hyalinization.[47]

Fluid Filtration

GFR decreases with advancing age.[46,47] In elderly persons the decrease in GFR is most likely caused by the decrease in nephron number as well as decreased renal blood flow.[46]

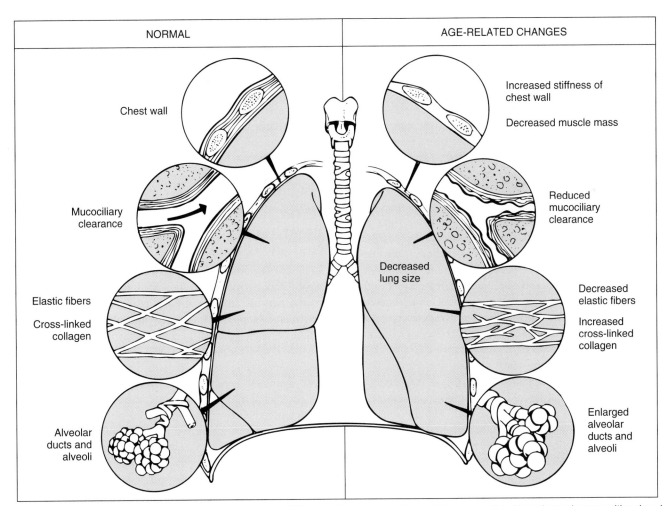

Figure 7-1 Age-related changes in human respiratory system. With advancing age, compliance of the chest wall and lung tissue changes, with reduced clearance of mucus by cilia that line the pulmonary tree and enlargement of alveolar ducts and alveoli.

Even though the remaining nephrons adapt to the loss of nephrons by glomerular hyperfiltration and increased solute load per nephron, the reduced GFR predisposes the elderly patient to adverse drug reactions and drug-induced renal failure. Some drugs are excreted unchanged in the urine, whereas other drugs have active or nephrotoxic metabolites that are excreted in the urine. In addition, the senescent kidney is more susceptible to injury by hypotensive episodes because of the age-related decrease in renal blood flow and reduced pressure gradient across the afferent arteriole.[50]

Age-related changes also occur in tubular function. The age-related changes in tubular function become apparent when extreme changes occur in the body fluid composition or acid-base balance. For example, with systemic acidosis the rate and amount of total acid excretion (bicarbonate, titratable acid, ammonium) are reduced.[46,50] This predisposes the elderly patient to metabolic acidosis, volume depletion, and hyperchloremia. At a normal pH level, however, the kidney of an elderly person can maintain acid-base homeostasis.

The senescent kidney has diminished capability to excrete a free water load, conserve water during periods of dehydration, and conserve sodium during periods of low salt intake.[46] Elderly persons are at high risk for dehydration because of these renal changes, along with decreased overall total body water, decreased concentrating ability, and decreased thirst perception.[51] Age-related changes also occur in extrarenal mechanisms, such as the decreased activity and responsiveness of the senescent kidney to the sympathetic nervous system and renin-angiotensin-aldosterone system, which are important in integrating overall fluid homeostasis and maintaining blood pressure in response to changes in body position.[29]

GASTROINTESTINAL SYSTEM

Age-related gastrointestinal changes occur in the processes of swallowing, motility, and absorption.[52,53] Swallowing may be difficult for the elderly person because of incomplete mastication of food.[53] Deteriorating dentition, diminished lubrication (secondary to salivary dysfunction), and poorly fitting dentures result in insufficient mastication of food within the oral cavity, predisposing the elderly patient to aspiration.[52] In addition, the number and velocity of the peristaltic contractions of the elderly person's esophagus decrease, and the number of nonperistaltic contractions increases.[53]

These changes in esophageal motility are referred to as *presbyesophagus*. These changes may predispose the patient to erosion of the esophageal wall (recurrent esophagitis) because food remains in the esophagus longer. In addition, bed rest and reclining in a supine position for a prolonged period can cause esophageal reflux, which also can lead to esophagitis.

The aging process produces thinning of the smooth muscle within the gastric mucosa.[54] The epithelial layer of the gastric mucosa, which contains the chief and parietal cells, undergoes a modest degree of atrophy, resulting in the hyposecretion of pepsin and acid, respectively.[55]

Mucin secretion from the mucus cells decreases, thereby altering the protective function of the gastric mucosal (bicarbonate) barrier. Because of this, the stomach wall is more susceptible to acid injury, thus increasing the incidence of gastric ulcerations.[56] Aging does not appreciably alter gastric emptying of solid foods. Alterations within the small intestine include a decrease in intestinal weight after age 50 and a flattening and shortening of jejunal villi.[57] Age produces no change in the small intestine's absorption of fats and proteins; however, decreased carbohydrate absorption has been reported.[58,59] There is essentially no change in vitamin or mineral absorption, except for a decrease in calcium absorption from the aged duodenum.[53]

Liver

With advancing age, both hepatocyte number and liver weight decrease.[60] Total liver blood flow decreases by 50% between 25 and 65 years of age.[60-62] The liver has many complex functions, including carbohydrate storage, ketone body formation, reduction/conjugation of adrenal and gonadal steroid hormones, synthesis of plasma proteins, deamination of amino acids, storage of cholesterol, urea formation, and detoxification of toxins and drugs. Despite changes in hepatocyte number and blood flow, however, liver function is not appreciably altered.[62] Several liver function tests, including serum bilirubin, alkaline phosphatase, and aspartate aminotransferase (AST) levels, are not altered with advancing age. However, because of the decrease in total liver blood flow, first-pass clearance of drugs is somewhat reduced. The most important age-related change in liver function is the decrease in the liver's capacity to metabolize drugs.[63,64] Although liver function tests do not reflect this change in metabolism, it is well recognized that drug side effects and toxic effects occur more frequently in older adults than in young adults.[64]

CENTRAL NERVOUS SYSTEM
Cognitive Functioning

Cognitive functioning involves the process of transforming, synthesizing, storing, and retrieving sensory input. Additional components include perception, attention, thinking, memory, and problem solving. For the aging individual, cognition is altered by the speed at which information is processed and retrieved.[65] Performance on timed tests declines slowly after age 20 years. Intelligence remains fairly stable after age 30 until the mid-80s. Although the rate at which complex tasks are completed may be diminished, these age-related changes are not synonymous with cognitive impairment.

Marked deterioration of any component of cognitive functioning is not a normal expectation of the aging process.[66] Cognitive impairment in older adults more often results from acute and chronic etiologies. Acute problems such as infection, electrolyte imbalance, and pharmacologic toxicity are generally reversible once identified. Long-term chronic impairment develops from more organic causations, such as multi-infarct dementia or Alzheimer's disease.[67]

Changes in Structure and Morphology

The brain decreases approximately 20% in size between 25 and 95 years of age (Figure 7-2).[68] The reduced brain weight may be related in part to the overall decrease in the number of neurons that occurs with advancing age. Neurons are lost from the hippocampus, amygdala, and cerebellum and from areas of the brain stem such as the locus ceruleus, dorsal motor nucleus of vagus nerve, and substantia nigra.[65] In contrast, very few neurons disappear with advancing age in areas such as the hypothalamus.[67] In addition, portions of the cerebral cortex atrophy, principally the frontal (superior frontal gyrus) and temporal (superior temporal gyrus) cortical association areas.[68]

The cerebral ventricles enlarge and develop an asymmetric appearance. Cerebrospinal fluid (CSF) also accumulates in the ventricles, although total brain CSF is not increased.[69] Accompanying the loss of neurons are changes in the ultrastructure and intracellular structures of the neuron.[70] Also, neuron shrinkage and degenerative changes in the cell bodies and axons of certain acetylcholine-secreting neurons have been reported. These changes may explain alterations in processing and receiving information.[67]

In the senescent brain, synaptogenesis (synaptic regeneration) still occurs after partial nerve degeneration. After a nerve fiber is damaged, neighboring undamaged neurons often sprout new fibers and form new connections. However, synaptogenesis occurs at a slower rate in the older brain.[70]

Cerebral Metabolism and Blood Flow

Cerebral blood flow decreases with advancing age. This decrease parallels the decrease in brain weight and is most likely caused by the reduction in neuron number and metabolic needs of the cerebral tissue.[71]

IMMUNE SYSTEM

Several changes in immune function render the elderly person more susceptible to infections.[72-77] Infections in the elderly population are associated with higher rates of mortality. Common infections in elderly patients include bacterial pneumonia, urinary tract infection, intra-abdominal

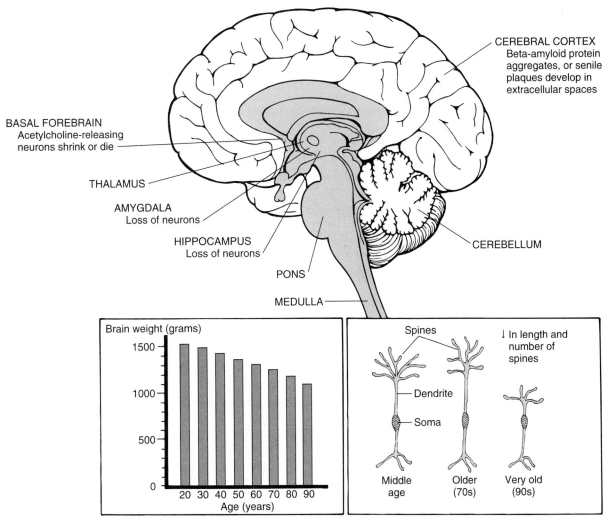

Figure 7-2 Summary of age-related changes in the brain. (From Selkoe DJ: *Sci Am* 267:135, 1992.)

infections, gram-negative bacteremia, and decubitus ulcers.[77] The many reasons for the increased susceptibility include changes in cell-mediated and humoral-mediated immunity, a breakdown in physical barriers (e.g., skin, oral mucosa), and changes in nutrition.

Cell-Mediated and Humoral-Mediated Immunity

Immune system function depends on many cell types with distinct functions. *T cells* are the primary effectors of cell-mediated immunity, whereas bone marrow–derived *B cells* produce antibodies that are the effectors of humoral-mediated immunity.[72,75] With aging, cell-mediated immunity declines. Even though the total number of T cells remains unchanged with advancing age, T cell function decreases.[74,76]

INTEGUMENTARY AND MUSCULOSKELETAL SYSTEMS

The loss of elastic and connective tissue causes the skin to wrinkle; both skin wrinkles and sagging may be found over many areas of the body. Underlying structures, such as the veins and muscles, are more visible because of the transparency of the skin.

Multiple ecchymotic areas may result from decreased protective subcutaneous tissue layers, increased capillary fragility, and flattening of the capillary bed, all of which predispose elderly persons to developing ecchymosis.[78-81] In conjunction with frequent aspirin use, these physiologic factors result in increased bleeding tendencies and the appearance of ecchymotic areas. However, areas of unexplained ecchymosis may also indicate elder abuse.

Changes that occur in the musculoskeletal system are a decrease in lean body mass, compression of the spinal column resulting from the thinning of cartilage between verte-bra, and a decrease in the mobility of skeletal joints.[82] Muscle rigidity increases, especially in the neck, shoulders, hips, and knees,[83] possibly causing changes in range of motion.

Bone demineralization affects both men and women as they age but occurs four times more often in women than men. *Bone demineralization* refers to an increase in osteoblast and osteoclast activity, which decreases calcium absorption into the bone.[82] Osteoporosis produces bones that are more "porous" or fragile. With extensive bone demineralization, an elderly patient may sustain multiple fractures.

CHANGES IN PHARMACOKINETICS AND PHARMACODYNAMICS

There are many age-related changes in drug pharmacokinetics, or how the body absorbs, distributes, metabolizes, and excretes a drug.[65,84] The aging process is associated with changes in gastric acid secretion, which can alter a drug's ionization or solubility and thus its absorption.[64,84]

Drug distribution depends on body composition as well as the drug's physiochemical properties. With advancing age, fat content increases while lean body mass and total body water decrease, which can alter the drug disposition.[84]

Because the senescent liver is less able to metabolize drugs, clearance of some drugs is also affected. For example, clearance of loop diuretics is reduced in elderly patients, which decreases the peak plasma concentration of the diuretic as well as the magnitude of the diuretic response.[84] Other drugs, such as angiotensin II–converting enzyme (ACE) inhibitors, have delayed excretion, increased serum concentration, and more prolonged duration of action because their excretion parallels GFR, which decreases with age[86] (Tables 7-3 and 7-4).[50,85-91]

Table 7-3 Age-Related Changes in Pharmacokinetics

Action	Definition	Changes
Absorption	Receptor-coupled or diffusional uptake of drug into tissue	Decreased absorptive surface area of small intestine Decreased splanchnic blood flow Increased gastric acid pH Decreased gastrointestinal motility
Distribution	Theoretic space (tissue) or body compartment into which free form of drug distributes	Decreased lean body mass and total body water Increased total body fat Decreased serum albumin level Increased α_1-acid glycoprotein
Metabolism	Chemical change in drug that renders it active or inactive	Decreased liver mass Decreased activity of microsomal drug-metabolizing enzyme system Decreased total liver blood flow
Excretion	Removal of drug through an eliminating organ, often the kidney; some drugs are excreted in bile or feces, in saliva, or through the lungs	Decreased renal blood flow and glomerular filtration rate Decreased distal renal tubular secretory function

Data from Gilman AG et al, editors: *Goodman and Gilman's the pharmacological basis of therapeutics*, ed 8, London, 1990, Pergamon; Vestal RE, Cusack BJ: In Schneider EL, Rowe JW, editors: *Handbook of the biology of aging*, San Diego, 1990, Academic Press.

Table 7-4   Pharmacologic Management of Gerontologic Patients

Agent	Actions	Adverse Effects*	Nursing Interventions/Considerations
ANGIOTENSIN-CONVERTING ENZYME (ACE) INHIBITORS			
Captopril	Inhibits conversion of angiotensin I to angiotensin II	Hypotension, especially in patients taking diuretics	Monitor heart rate and blood pressure
Enalapril		Hypokalemia	Monitor serum creatinine level Monitor serum K^+ level Excreted by kidney, so dosage reduced if GFR reduced
DIURETICS			
Bumex	Inhibits Na^+ and Cl^- absorption from proximal tubule and loop of Henle	Hypokalemia	Reduced rate of clearance and magnitude of diuretic response
Lasix		Volume depletion	
CARDIAC GLYCOSIDES			
Digoxin	Inhibits the sarcolemmal Na^+/K^+-ATPase	Digitalis toxicity	Monitor heart rate and serum K^+ and serum digoxin levels
Dopamine	α_1-Adrenergic agonist, dopaminergic agonist	Ectopic beats, hypotension	Verapamil, quinidine, and amiodarone increase digoxin levels
Dobutamine	Sympathomimetic, β_1-adrenergic agonist		
ANTIDYSRHYTHMICS			
Procainamide	Decreases myocardial conduction velocity and excitability and prolongs myocardial refractoriness	Procainamide toxicity	Converted to its active metabolite, NAPA, which may accumulate in liver and cause side effects, even though procainamide plasma level within therapeutic range
Lidocaine	Decreases automaticity (especially in Purkinje fibers) and prolongs conduction and refractoriness	Dizziness, paresthesia, and drowsiness at lower plasma concentrations	Can be administered only parenterally
CALCIUM CHANNEL BLOCKERS			
Verapamil	Blocks entry of Ca^{++} through voltage-dependent Ca^{++} channels and decreases SA automaticity and AV conduction	Constipation May alter liver function	Monitor liver function tests Contraindicated in heart failure, sick sinus syndrome, and first-degree AV block
Nifedipine		Headaches, tachycardia, palpitations, flushing, ankle edema	Produces less of the negative inotropic effect of this drug class compared with verapamil
Diltiazem		Constipation	Monitor liver function tests Contraindicated in heart failure, sick sinus syndrome, and first-degree AV block
NARCOTIC ANALGESICS			
Meperidine	Blocks transmission of pain and inhibits release of substance P; site of action in CNS	Respiratory depression, oversedation Tremors and muscle twitches related to effects of the metabolite normeperidine	Accumulation of normeperidine can produce CNS hyperexcitability
Morphine	Synthetic analgesic; mechanism similar to meperidine	Respiratory depression, oversedation	Small volume of distribution; thus plasma/tissue levels are greater at a specific plasma concentration

Data from Creasy WA et al: *J Clin Pharmacol* 26:264, 1986; Gilman AG et al, editors: *Goodman and Gilman's the pharmacological basis of therapeutics*, London, 1990, Pergamon; Hockings N, Ajayi AA, Reid JL: *Br J Pharmacol* 21:341, 1986; Lynch RA, Horowitz LN: *Geriatrics* 46:41, 1991; Pederson KE: *Acta Med Scand* 697(suppl 1):1, 1985; Vidt GD, Borazanian RA: *Geriatrics* 46:28, 1991; Wall RT: *Clin Geriatr Med* 6:345, 1990; Watters JM, McClaran JC: In Wilmore DW et al, editors: *Care of the surgical patient*, New York, 1990, Scientific American.

Ca^{++}, Intracellular free calcium; K^+, potassium; Na^+, sodium; Cl^-, chloride; *GFR*, glomerular filtration rate; *SA*, sinoatrial; *AV*, atrioventricular; *CNS*, central nervous system; *ATPase*, adenosine triphosphatase; *NAPA*, *N*-acetyl-procainamide.

*Not all side effects are listed for each drug.

Table 7-5 Age-Related Physiologic Changes and Clinical Considerations

Changes/Effects	Clinical Considerations
CARDIOVASCULAR SYSTEM → Inotropic and chronotropic response of myocardium to catecholamine stimulation ↑ Myocardial collagen content ↓ Baroreceptor sensitivity Prolonged rate of relaxation ↓ Compliance of blood vessels	Increase in cardiac output during stress or exercise achieved by increase in diastolic filling (increased dependence on Starling's law of heart) Leads to decrease in compliance of ventricle (higher filling pressures needed to maintain stroke volume) ↑ Tendency for orthostatic hypotension after prolonged bed rest, or if patient taking antihypertensive or has systolic hypertension May predispose elderly patient to hemodynamic derangements in presence of tachydysrhythmias, hypertension, or ischemic heart disease ↑ Peripheral vascular resistance and blood pressure
RESPIRATORY SYSTEM ↓ Strength of respiratory muscles, recoil of lungs, chest wall compliance, and efficiency and number of cilia in airways ↓ Arterial oxygen tension (Pao_2) level	↑Susceptibility to aspiration, atelectasis, and pulmonary infection Patient may require more frequent deep breathing, coughing, and position change ↓ Ventilatory response to hypoxia and hypercapnia ↑ Sensitivity to narcotics
RENAL SYSTEM ↓ Glomerular filtration rate ↓ Ability to concentrate and conserve water ↓ Ability to excrete salt and water loads, as well as urea, ammonia, and drugs ↓ Response to an acid load	Careful observation of patient when administering aminoglycosides, antibiotics, and contrast dyes May predispose patient to development of dehydration and hypernatremia, especially if patient is fluid restricted and insensible losses are high (e.g., during mechanical ventilation or fever) Observe for clinical manifestations of fluid overload and drug reactions After an acid load (i.e., metabolic acidosis), elderly patient may be in state of uncompensated metabolic acidosis for longer period
LIVER ↓ Total liver blood flow	Adverse drug reactions, especially with polypharmacy
GASTROINTESTINAL SYSTEM Diminished ability to swallow Impaired esophageal motility Delayed emptying of liquids ↓ Stool weight and transit time	May predispose elderly patient to aspiration pneumonia Assess for proper fit of dentures and ability to chew Flex head forward 45 degrees Develop awareness for complaints of food or medications "sticking in throat" Assess for complaints of heartburn and epigastric discomfort Avoid prolonged supine position Examine abdomen for distention Investigate complaints of anorexia Obtain thorough bowel history; note routine use of laxatives Increase intake of dietary fiber; assess for fecal incontinence and impaction
NEUROLOGIC SYSTEM ↑ Cranial dead space ↓ Number of neurons/dendrites and length of dendrite spines Delay in rate of synaptogenesis Changes in neurotransmitter turnover	Elderly persons may sustain significant hemorrhage before symptoms are apparent Delayed or impaired processing of sensory and motor information May cause desynchronization of neurotransmission

Modified from Rebenson-Piano M: *Crit Care Q* 12:1, 1989.

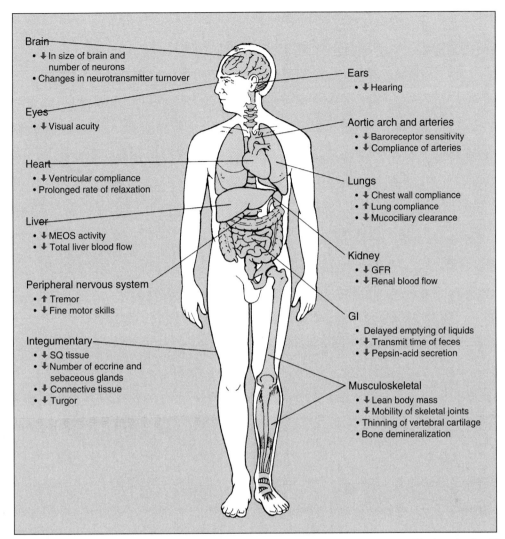

Figure 7-3   Summary of physiologic changes that occur in all systems and that the critical care nurse must consider in caring for elderly patients in the critical care unit. *MEOS*, Microsomal enzyme oxidative system; *GFR*, glomerular filtration rate; *GI*, gastrointestinal; *SQ*, subcutaneous.

Box **7-1**	Effects of Aging on Various Laboratory Values

VALUES THAT DO NOT CHANGE WITH AGE	VALUES THAT CHANGE WITH AGE AND HAVE CLINICAL SIGNIFICANCE
Hemoglobin/hematocrit Platelet count White blood cell count with differential Serum electrolytes Coagulation profile Liver function tests Thyroid function tests ↔ or ↓ Blood urea nitrogen ↔ or ↓ Creatinine	↓ Erythrocyte sedimentation rate ↓ Arterial oxygen tension (partial pressure) ↑ Blood glucose ↓ or ↑ Serum lipid profile ↓ Albumin
VALUES THAT CHANGE WITH AGE BUT HAVE LITTLE CLINICAL SIGNIFICANCE ↓ Calcium ↑ Uric acid	

From Duthie EH, Abbasi AA: *Geriatrics* 46:41, 1991.
↔, No change; ↓, decreased; ↑, increased.

SUMMARY

The elderly patient requires more intense observation and consideration in the critical care unit. The patient's system has become less adaptable to stress and illness, and changes in laboratory values may be clinically significant[92,93] (Box 7-1). The major changes in the various systems require specific clinical considerations (Table 7-5).[94] Many physiologic changes occur with advancing age, and each change may render a particular system less adaptable to stress (Figure 7-3). In addition, a change in one system may affect another system in the presence of disease.

REFERENCES

1. Abrass IB: Biology of aging. In Wilson JD et al: *Harrison's principles of internal medicine*, ed 12, New York, 1991, McGraw-Hill.
2. Weisfeldt ML, Lakatta EG, Gerstenblith G: Aging and the heart. In Braunwald E, editor: *Heart disease*, Philadelphia, 1992, Saunders.
3. Eghbali M et al: Collagen accumulation in heart ventricles as a function of growth and aging, *Cardiovasc Res* 23:723, 1989.
4. Wegelius O, von Knorring J: The hydroxyproline and hexosamine content in human myocardium at different ages, *Acta Med Scand Suppl* 412:233, 1964.
5. Katz AM: Heart failure. In Fozzard HA et al, editors: *The heart and cardiovascular system*, New York, 1991, Raven.
6. Gerstenblith G et al: Echocardiographic assessment of normal adult aging population, *Circulation* 56:273, 1977.
7. Walsh RA: Cardiovascular effects of the aging process, *Am J Med* 82:34, 1987.
8. Opie LH: *The physiology of the heart and metabolism*, New York, 1991, Raven.
9. Lakatta EG et al: Prolonged contraction duration in the aged myocardium, *J Clin Invest* 55:61, 1975.
10. Spurgeon HA, Steinbach MF, Lakatta EG: Prolonged contraction duration in senescent myocardium is prevented by exercise, *Am J Physiol* 244:H513, 1983.
11. Froehlich JP et al: Studies of sarcoplasmic reticulum function and contraction in young and aged rat myocardium, *J Mol Cell Cardiol* 10:427, 1978.
12. Cinelli P et al: Effects of age on mean heart rate variability, *Ageing* 10:146, 1987.
13. Ribera JM et al: Cardiac rate and hyperkinetic rhythm disorders in healthy elderly subjects: evaluation by ambulatory electrocardiographic monitoring, *Gerontology* 35:158, 1989.
14. Lakatta EG: Heart and circulation. In Schneider EL, Rowe JW, editors: *Handbook of the biology of aging*, San Diego, 1990, Academic Press.
15. Bonow RO et al: Effects of aging on asynchronous left ventricular regional function and global ventricular filling in normal human subjects, *J Am Coll Cardiol* 11:50, 1988.
16. Miller TR et al: Left ventricular diastolic filling and its association with age, *Am J Cardiol* 58:531, 1986.
17. Davidson WR, Fee WC: Influence of aging on pulmonary hemodynamics in a population free of coronary artery disease, *Am J Cardiol* 65:1454, 1990.
18. Bachman S, Sparrow D, Smith LK: Effect of aging on the electrocardiogram, *Am J Cardiol* 48:513, 1981.
19. Horwitz LN, Lynch RA: Managing geriatric arrhythmias. I. General considerations, *Geriatrics* 46:31, 1991.
20. Docherty JR: Cardiovascular responses in ageing: a review, *Pharmacol Rev* 42:103, 1990.
21. Smith JJ et al: The effect of age on hemodynamic response to graded postural stress in normal men, *J Gerontol* 42:406, 1987.
22. Dambrink JHA, Wieling W: Circulatory response to postural change in healthy male subjects in relation to age, *Clin Sci* 72:335, 1987.
23. Applegate WB et al: Prevalence of postural hypotension at baseline in the Systolic Hypertension in the Elderly Program (SHEP) cohort, *J Am Geriatr Soc* 39:1057, 1991.
24. Stanley JA: Congestive heart failure in the elderly, *Geriatr Nurs* 20:180, 2000.
25. Bierman EL: Arteriosclerosis and aging. In Finch CE, Schneider EL, editors: *Handbook of the biology of aging*, New York, 1985, Van Nostrand Reinhold.
26. Schoenberger JA: Epidemiology of systolic and diastolic systemic blood pressure elevation in the elderly, *Am J Cardiol* 57:45, 1986.
27. Rowe JW: Clinical consequences of age-related impairments in vascular compliance, *Am J Cardiol* 60:68, 1987.
28. Rose BD: *Clinical physiology of acid-base and electrolyte disorders*, New York, 1989, McGraw-Hill.
29. Hall JE, Coleman TG, Guyton AC: The renin-angiotensin system: normal physiology and changes in older hypertensives, *J Am Geriatr Soc* 37:801, 1989.
30. Crane MG, Harris JJ: Effect of aging on renin activity and aldosterone excretion, *J Lab Clin Med* 87:947, 1976.
31. Sica DA, Harford A: Sodium and water disorders in the elderly. In Zawada ET, Sica DA, editors: *Geriatric nephrology and urology*, Littleton, Mass, 1985, PSG.
32. Webster JR, Kadah H: Unique aspects of respiratory disease in the aged, *Geriatrics* 46:31, 1991.
33. Sheahan SL, Musialowski R: Clinical implications of respiratory system changes in aging, *J Gerontol Nurs* 27(5):26, 2001.
34. Levitzky MG: Effects of aging on the respiratory system, *Physiologist* 27:102, 1984.
35. Mittman C et al: Relationship between chest wall and pulmonary compliance and age, *J Appl Physiol* 20:1211, 1965.
36. Anderson WM, Tockman MS: Aging and the lungs. In Beers MH, Berkow R, editors: *Merck manual of geriatrics*, http://www.merck.com/pubs/mm_geriatrics.
37. Rizzato G, Marazzine L: Thoracoabdominal mechanisms in elderly men, *J Appl Physiol* 28:457, 1970.
38. Gutmann E, Hanzlikova V: Fast and slow motor units in ageing, *Gerontology* 22:280, 1976.
39. Pontoppidan HH, Beecher HK: Progressive loss of protective reflexes in the airway with advance of age, JAMA 1974:229, 1960.
40. Knudson RJ et al: Changes in the normal maximal expiratory flow-volume curve with growth and aging, *Am Rev Respir Dis* 127:725, 1983.
41. Turner JM, Mead J, Wohl ME: Elasticity of human lungs in relation to age, *J Appl Physiol* 25:664, 1968.
42. Pierce JA, Hocott JB: Studies on the collagen and elastin content of the human lung, *J Clin Invest* 39:8, 1960.
43. Pierce JA, Ebert RV: Fibrous network of the lung and its change with age, *Thorax* 20:469, 1965.
44. Semmens M: The pulmonary artery in the normal aged lung, *Br J Dis Chest* 64:65, 1970.
45. Sorbini CA et al: Arterial oxygen tension in relation to age in healthy subjects, *Respiration* 25:3, 1968.
46. Weder AB: The renally compromised older hypertensive: therapeutic considerations, *Geriatrics* 46:36, 1991.
47. Gilbert BR, Vaughan ED: Pathophysiology of the aging kidney, *Clin Geriatr Med* 6:12, 1990.
48. Kasiske BL: Relationship between vascular disease and age-associated changes in the human kidney, *Kidney Int* 31:1153, 1987.
49. Anderson S, Brenner BM: Effects of aging on the renal glomerulus, *Am J Med* 80:435, 1986.

50. Watters JM, McClaran JC: The elderly surgical patient. In Wilmore DW et al, editors: *Care of the surgical patient.* Vol VII. Special problems, New York, 1990, Scientific American.

51. Bennett JA: Dehydration: Hazards and benefits, *Geriatr Nurs* 21:84, 2000.

52. Brandt LJ: Gastrointestinal disorders in the elderly. In Rossman I, editor: *Clinical geriatrics*, ed 3, Philadelphia, 1986, Lippincott.

53. Williams SA, Fogel RP: Common gastrointestinal problems in the elderly, *JAMA* 87:29, 1989.

54. Altman DF: Changes in gastrointestinal, pancreatic, biliary and hepatic function in aging, *Gastroenterol Clin North Am* 19:227, 1990.

55. Thomson AB, Keelan M: The aging gut, *Can J Physiol Pharmacol* 64:30, 1986.

56. Bansal SK et al: Upper gastrointestinal hemorrhage in the elderly: a record of 92 patients in a joint geriatric/surgical unit, *Age Ageing* 16:279, 1987.

57. Schuster MM: Disorders of the aging GI system, *Hosp Pract* 11:95, 1976.

58. Curran J: Overview of geriatric nutrition, *Dysphagia* 5:72, 1990.

59. Ausman LM, Russel RM: Nutrition and aging. In Schneider EL, Rowe JW, editors: *Handbook of the biology of aging*, San Diego, 1990, Academic Press.

60. Sato TG, Miwa T, Tauchi H: Age changes in the human liver of the different races, *Gerontology* 16:368, 1970.

61. Bach B et al: Disposition of antipyrine and phenytoin correlated with age and liver volume in man, *Clin Pharmacokinet* 6:389, 1981.

62. Kampmann JP, Sinding J, Moller-Jorgensen I: Effect of age on liver function, *Geriatrics* 30:91, 1975.

63. Schmucker DL, Wang RK: Age-related changes in liver drug metabolism: structure versus function, *Proc Soc Exp Biol Med* 165:178, 1980.

64. Vestal RE, Cusack BJ: Pharmacology and aging. In Schneider EL, Rowe JW, editors: *Handbook of the biology of aging*, San Diego, 1990, Academic Press.

65. Katzman R: Human nervous system. In Masoro EJ, editor: *Handbook of physiology: aging*, New York, 1995, Oxford University Press.

66. Foreman MD, Grabowski R: Diagnostic dilemma: cognitive impairment in the elderly, *J Gerontol Nurs* 18:5, 1992.

67. Arriagada P et al: Neurofibrillary tangles but not senile plaques parallel duration and severity of Alzheimer's disease, *Neurology* 42:631, 1992.

68. Selkoe DJ: Aging brain, aging mind, *Sci Am* 267:134, 1992.

69. Morris JC, McManus DQ: The neurology of aging: normal versus pathologic change, *Geriatrics* 46:47, 1991.

70. Lytle LD, Altar A: Diet, central nervous system, and aging, *Fed Proc* 38:2017, 1979.

71. Gottstein U, Held K: Effects of aging on cerebral circulation and metabolism in man, *Acta Neurol Scand Suppl* 72:54, 1979.

72. Cotman CW, Kahle JS, Korotzer AR: Maintenance and regulation in brain of neurotransmission, trophic factors and immune responses. In Masoro EJ, editor: *Handbook of physiology: aging*, New York, 1995, Oxford University Press.

73. Hiller JM, Fan L-Q, Simon EJ: Alterations in opioid receptor levels in discrete areas of the neocortex and in the globus pallidus of the aging guinea pig: a quantitative autoradiographic study, *Brain Res* 614:86, 1993.

74. Miller RA: Immune system. In Masoro EJ, editor: *Handbook of physiology: aging*, New York, 1995, Oxford University Press.

75. Terpenning MS, Bradley SF: Why aging leads to increased susceptibility to infection, *Geriatrics* 46:77, 1991.

76. Miller RA: The aging immune system: primer and prospectus, *Science* 273:70, 1996.

77. McClure CL: Common infections in the elderly, *Am Fam Physician* 45:2691, 1992.

78. Jones PL, Millman A: Wound healing and the aged patient, *Nurs Clin North Am* 25:263, 1990.

79. Kelly L, Mobily PR: Iatrogenesis in the elderly, *J Gerontol Nurs* 17(9):24, 1991.

80. Shenefelt PD, Fenske NA: Aging and the skin: recognizing and managing common disorders, *Geriatrics* 45(10):57, 1990.

81. Wenger NK: Cardiovascular disease in the elderly, *Curr Probl Cardiol*, October 1992, p 611.

82. Kalu DN: Bone. In Masoro EJ, editor: *Handbook of physiology: aging*, New York, 1995, Oxford University Press.

83. Exton-Smith AN: Mineral metabolism. In Finch CE, Schneider EL, editors: *Handbook of the biology of aging*, New York, 1985, Van Nostrand Reinhold.

84. Yuen GJ: Altered pharmacokinetics in the elderly, *Clin Geriatr Med* 6:257, 1990.

85. Gilman AG et al, editors: *Goodman and Gilman's the pharmacological basis of therapeutics*, ed 8, London, 1990, Pergamon.

86. Mooradian AD: An update of the clinical pharmacokinetics, therapeutic monitoring techniques and treatment recommendations, *Clin Pharmacokinet* 18:165, 1988.

87. Creasy WA et al: Pharmacokinetics of captopril in elderly healthy male volunteers, *J Clin Pharmacol* 26:264, 1986.

88. Hockings N, Ajayi AA, Reid JL: Age and the pharmacodynamics of angiotensin-converting enzyme inhibitors, enalapril and enalaprilat, *Br J Pharmacol* 21:341, 1986.

89. Pederson KE: Digoxin interactions: the influence of quinidine and verapamil on the pharmacokinetics and receptor binding of digitalis glycosides, *Acta Med Scand* 697(suppl 1):1, 1985.

90. Lynch RA, Horowitz LN: Managing geriatric arrhythmias. II. Drug selection and use, *Geriatrics* 46:41, 1991.

91. Vidt GD, Borazanian RA: Calcium channel blockers in geriatric hypertension, *Geriatrics* 46:28, 1991.

92. Cavalieri TA et al: When outside the room is normal: interpreting lab data in the aged, *Geriatrics* 47(5):66, 1992.

93. Kane RL et al: *Essentials of clinical geriatrics*, ed 3, New York, 1994, McGraw-Hill.

94. Rebenson-Piano M: The physiologic changes that occur with aging, *Crit Care Q* 12:1, 1989.

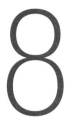

LYNNE JETT

Pain
Management

Objectives

- Explain the physiology of pain.
- Discuss how to perform a pain assessment in the critically ill patient.
- Identify patient and health care professional barriers to a pain assessment.
- Describe pharmacologic and nonpharmacologic interventions for pain management.
- Describe nursing interventions that are essential in the treatment of acute pain.

Pain is defined in a number of ways. Pain is a warning signal from the body that an injury has occurred. Unlike other sensations, pain is the protective signal for a threat to survival.[1] Pain is an unpleasant sensory experience associated with actual and potential tissue damage. Pain is not simply a pure physiologic response to an injury but is associated with an emotional response to the sensation.[2] Pain is an extremely complex set of responses to a physical stimulus. The definition with the most clinical significance is that pain is whatever the person experiencing it says it is, and that pain occurs when that person says it does.[3,4] Pain is a common thread that binds critical care patients together. Whether the pain is from an elective procedure or trauma, its presence is ubiquitous.[5] Studies examining the ability of the critically ill surgical patient to sleep identified pain and the inability "to get comfortable" as the most frequently cited barriers to sleep.[6]

With the frequency of the diagnosis of pain and the professional responsibility to manage pain, the critical care nurse must understand the mechanisms, assessment technique, and appropriate therapeutic measures to manage the pain state. Unfortunately, studies of pain management reflect that critical care patients are often undermedicated. On average the nurse administers only 30% to 36% of the maximum opioid dose ordered.[7] Critically ill patients reported that the second most common memory of their illness was that of a painful, uncomfortable experience.[8] A multisite study revealed that critical care patients, although reporting satisfaction with pain management, also reported moderate to severe pain.[9]

PHYSIOLOGY OF PAIN

Peripheral Nervous System

The peripheral nervous system (PNS) contains a multitude of free nerve endings. The sensation of pain requires the activation of some nerve endings. Similar free nerve endings are responsible for the transmission of touch, pressure, and warmth. The specialized nerve endings responsible for pain, the *nociceptors*, do not adapt to repeated painful stimuli because the role of pain in the body is protective. On the contrary, repeated stimulation heightens their sensitivity. The supersensitive state lowers the threshold for stimulation and increases the response to stimulation.[2,3] This phenomenon, known as *hyperalgesia*, is responsible for the hypersensitive state of many critically ill patients. In this hypersensitive state the slightest painful stimulus is interpreted as very painful.[10] Nociceptors are present in numerous organs but primarily in the skin, joints, muscle, fascia, viscera, and arterial wall smooth muscle. These nerve endings are activated by thermal, mechanical, and chemical stimuli.[11]

Two types of afferent nerve fibers transmit painful stimuli from the site of injury through distinct neural pathways (Table 8-1). The *Aδ fiber* conducts the rapid acute pain sensation described as prickling, sharp, and fast (Figure 8-1). The Aδ fiber is activated by mechanical and thermal stimuli. The second type of nociceptor, the polymodal *C fiber*, is implicated in the transmission of pain described as dull, diffuse, prolonged, and delayed. These fibers are activated by chemicals and released when cell damage occurs.[1-3,11] These chemical transmitters are responsible for irritating the nerve endings and for activating the PNS to transmit other neurotransmitters that are active in the inhibition of pain transmission. These mediators are released when there is tissue damage of any type. Depending on which of the mediators is active, associated reactions (e.g., vasoconstriction, vasodilation, altered capillary permeability) occur at the site of injury.[11]

Both the Aδ fibers and the C fibers have roots in the dorsal horn of the spinal column. These fibers are the afferent arm of the ascending spinal pathways of pain. In the dorsal horn at the laminae, the nociceptor neurons release *substance P*, which has as excitatory effect on the spinal cord and enhances the transmission of pain.[12] This is the point of integration of the peripheral and central nervous systems for the transmission of the pain impulse.

Central Nervous System

The central nervous system (CNS) has two components used in the pain response: the ascending, or conducting, pathways and the descending, or modulating, pathways.

Table **8-1**   Nerve Fibers for Pain Transmission

Nerve Fiber (Description)	General Location	Type of Pain Transmitted	Patient Descriptors	Rate of Transmission
Aδ fibers (thinly myelinated)	Skin, cutaneous tissue	Mechanical or thermal stimulus; easily localized	Sharp, pricking, electric, acute	Rapid, within 0.1 second; velocity 6-30 meters per second (m/sec)
C fibers (primitive, unmyelinated)	Subcutaneous tissue, fascia, tendons, joints, ligaments, muscles	Mechanical, chemical, or thermal stimulus; difficult to localize	Throbbing, aching, burning, gnawing, chronic	Slow, 1+ second, increases slowly; velocity 0.5-2.0 m/sec

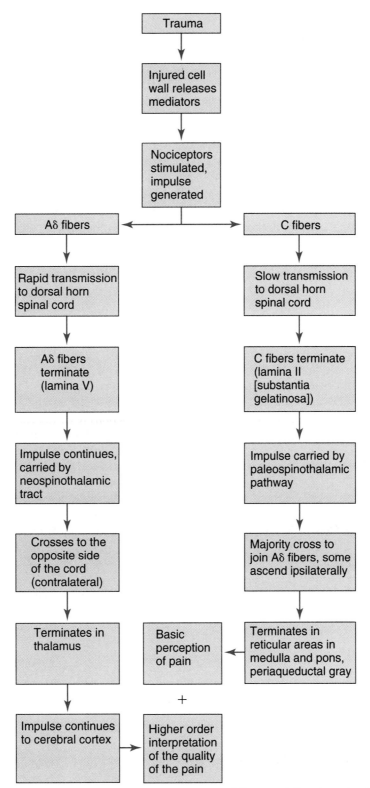

Figure 8-1 Dual pathways of pain transmission using Aδ fibers and C fibers for nociception.

Ascending Pain Pathways

The ascending tracts synapse with primary Aδ and C afferent nerve fibers that terminate in the spinal cord. The sensations are transmitted via the *spinothalamic* tract. Two other tracts are responsible for the transmission of nociceptor messages. The *spinoreticular* tract transmits to the brain stem reticular formation and terminates in the thalamus. The third nociceptor tract, the *spinomesencephalic* tract, terminates in the midbrain reticular formation and the midbrain periaqueductal gray. This area of the brain is also responsible for strong inhibitory responses to the pain transmission. Nociception continues to the somatosensory cortex of the brain. Cortical interpretation of the stimulus is necessary to finalize the perception of the pain— discretely locating it, identifying its intensity, and interpreting its meaning— and to add the emotional component. This cortical process underlies the individual patient's unique perception of the pain.[11]

Descending Pain Pathways

The other CNS component of pain is the descending analgesia system. This *endogenous pain modulation system* is responsible for the body's attempt to manage the pain intrinsically.[11] The system consists of a series of neurons in the brain and spinal cord that synapse with the ascending neurons (Figure 8-2). In the brain the cortex and hypothalamus activate the periaqueductal gray, which influences fibers in the dorsal horns to release neurotransmitters that inhibit the action of the neurons that transmit pain impulses.[11]

The neurotransmitters that inhibit or modulate the transmission of pain are produced in the body at sites along the neural synapses. The sites are located in both the brain and the descending pathways. These neurotransmitters are the endogenous opioid peptides known as *endogenous opioids* and are similar to morphine.[13]

On release, the endogenous opioids bind to the nerve receptor sites located throughout the ascending pain transmission system and significantly modify the transmission of pain. The binding sites, or receptors, are generally classified as the mu (μ) effect, kappa (κ) effect, and delta (δ) effect. Each receptor type acts differently when stimulated.[11] A knowledge of the individual responses contributes to the interpretation of physiologic findings in the assessment of pain and pain management responses; some of the effects are quantifiable (Table 8-2). Different levels of these pain-modifying endorphins in individuals are responsible for the difference in response to the same painful stimulus among individuals.

β-Endorphin, the most morphine-like endorphin, is located primarily in the hypothalamus and the midbrain. β-Endorphin is released during acupuncture and transcutaneous stimulation[2] and in response to stress, fear, restraint, hypertension, and hypoglycemia. Endorphin release is well documented during labor and delivery and exercise.[12] Endorphin release during stress accounts for a person's ability to perform normally or supranormally with an apparent unawareness of pain after an injury. This response is referred to as *stress analgesia*.

The *enkephalins* are located primarily in the limbic system and the hypothalamus, as well as periaqueductal gray. The endings of many of the nerves in these areas secrete enkephalins. In an associated response, fibers originating in the same area but with their endings in the dorsal horn secrete serotonin. The serotonin in turn acts on yet another set of neurons to incite the release of additional enkephalins. The enkephalins block the presynaptic transmission of both Aδ and C fibers.[12] This inhibition can last from minutes to hours, providing analgesia for that period.

The *dynorphins* are found in minute quantities in the nervous system, primarily in the periaqueductal gray and the spinal cord. Dynorphins are extremely powerful opiates, with as much as 200 times the pain-killing effect of morphine.[12]

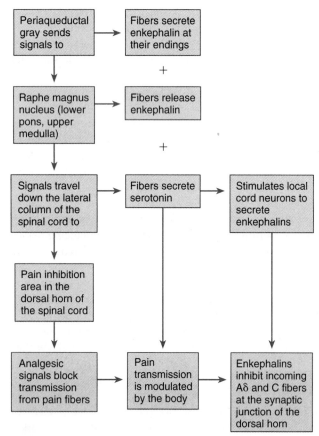

Figure 8-2 The human body's endogenous pain modification, or analgesia, system.

Table **8-2**	Opiate Receptor Classification and Actions	
Affected Area	**μ Effect**	**δ Effect**
Pupils	Miosis	Mydriasis
Respiratory system	Stimulates, then depresses	Stimulates
Heart	Bradycardia	Tachycardia
Temperature	Hypothermia	—
Gastrointestinal	Constipation	Nausea

Modified from Williams J: In Cardona D et al, editors: *Trauma nursing: from resuscitation through rehabilitation*, ed 2, Philadelphia, 1994, Saunders.

A second, less-discussed inhibitory pathway contributes to pain modification. This pathway, the *monoamine system*, is a nonopioid form of endogenous analgesia. The primary neurotransmitters involved in this system are serotonin and norepinephrine. Serotonin is a major pain-inhibiting factor from the medulla to the spinal cord descending pathway.[2,11,12] At the dorsal horn, serotonin is responsible for the release of enkephalins. Norepinephrine's role in pain modulation is in its attachment to α_2-adrenergic receptors and the resulting inhibition of nociception.[2]

TYPES OF ACUTE PAIN

Although all pain uses primarily the same nociception, pain experts describe pain in a number of different groupings. Occasionally the types of pain are grouped by differentiating the *location* of the fibers that are sensitized. The fibers are grouped as cutaneous, somatic, visceral, and deafferentation.

Cutaneous Pain

Cutaneous or *superficial* pain, sometimes grouped with somatic pain, begins with injury at the skin (e.g., incision, needle insertion). This tissue trauma activates the nociceptors on the skin. The mediators histamine, bradykinin, potassium, and hydrogen ion are released into the extracellular fluid around the wound. The cell wall injury causes the release of serotonin from platelets, prostaglandins, and substance P. All the active mediators will sensitize and activate the cutaneous fibers to transmit the noxious stimuli to the CNS.[1-3] The cutaneous Aδ fibers are now sensitive to noxious stimuli that would not ordinarily be interpreted as painful, such as touch, pressure, or stretch. Normally the patient can discretely locate this type of pain.[11]

Somatic Pain

Somatic pain originates in the subcutaneous tissue, joints, tendons, muscles, and fascia.[3] It is also associated with muscle ischemia and spasm.[2] Bradykinin and histamine release are associated with somatic pain, and C fibers are responsible for its transmission. Somatic pain is difficult for the patient to locate and can be dull, aching, or diffuse.[1,2,13] In addition, deep somatic pain is associated with an autonomic nervous system (ANS) response that may cause nausea, vomiting, and cold clammy skin.

Visceral Pain

In general the viscera have only sensory receptors for pain. The unique characteristic of visceral pain is that highly localized stimulation of pain receptors in the viscera can cause minimal discomfort. However, diffuse stimulation of multiple receptors can cause extreme pain.[3,9] Visceral pain results from compression, distention, or stretching of the viscera in the thoracic or abdominal cavity. The pain of myocardial ischemia or infarction is considered visceral. Visceral pain is described as pressure, deep, and squeezing. It

is sometimes difficult to localize and is associated with referred pain. The visceral pain fibers are unique in that they travel to the spinal cord with the fibers of the sympathetic nervous system (SNS). This may account for the intense SNS response often seen with visceral pain.[2,3]

Deafferentation Pain

Deafferentation pain is considered *neuropathic* pain rather than nociceptive pain and is seen most often in cancer patients. The mechanism of deafferentation pain is an injury to a CNS or PNS component from the disease or its treatment. The injury usually results from tumor invasion and thermal damage or chemical injuries from radiation.[1] Deafferentation is also considered the type of pain stemming from chronic pain syndromes, in which case the origin of the pain may be peripheral or central. Neuralgia and phantom pain are peripheral deafferentation pains in which thalamic lesions related to cerebrovascular accidents cause central deafferentation pain.[14]

PAIN ASSESSMENT

Adequate assessment of pain in the critically ill patient is made more difficult by the complexity of the critical care experience. Altered communication may be a complicating factor, for example, or the patient may be unconscious and unable to communicate pain. Pain assessment in the critically ill population has three major components: assessment technique, patient barriers to assessment, and nurse/physician barriers to complete or accurate assessment. The complexity of assessment requires the use of multiple strategies by critical care practitioners.

Multidimensional Assessment

Because it is a multidimensional phenomenon, pain requires a multidimensional assessment. Complete assessment involves the collection of subjective and objective data about the patient's physiologic, cognitive, and emotional responses to the pain.[10] Because of the life/death immediacy of most actions in the critical care environment, assessment is typically one dimensional.[15] The critical care environment includes the complex task of balancing hemodynamic considerations with the management of the patient's pain state.[16]

The evaluation of pain includes type, location, intensity, aggravating factors, and alleviating factors. The most important consideration in assessment is that pain is an entirely subjective experience. Pain is whatever the patient says it is and however the patient describes it.[3] In the assessment of pain type, the verbal patient can give descriptive terms.[17] The patient may describe the pain as dull, aching, or sharp and stabbing. This provides the nurse with data regarding the type of pain the patient is experiencing (e.g., visceral or cutaneous).

The differentiation between types of pain may contribute to the determination of cause and management. A patient who has had defibrillation and cardiopulmonary resuscitation (CPR) after a heart attack may complain of chest pain that is prickling or stinging. This information would lead the nurse to investigate for cutaneous injuries, such as defibrillation burns. The same patient may describe a dull, aching pain with radiation that might lead the nurse to consider a visceral anginal pain from myocardial ischemia. A verbal description of pain also provides a baseline description, allowing the critical care nurse to monitor changes in the type of pain, which could indicate a change in the underlying pathology.

Pain Assessment Tools

Intensity or severity of pain is a measurement that has undergone much recent investigation. The consistent use of a visual tool aids both the patient and the practitioner in correctly identifying the intensity of the patient's pain.[3,8,18,19] Multiple visual analog scales are available, as well as numeric pain intensity scales frequently used in the critical care environment (Figure 8-3).[20] Many critical care units have identified a specific tool to be used. The use of a single tool provides consistency of assessment and documentation. The employment of a pain grading scale is also useful in the critical care environment.[15] Asking the patient to grade the pain on a scale of 1 to 10 is a consistent method and aids the nurse in objectifying the subjective nature of the patient's pain. The pain grading scale is also useful in establishing a baseline for comparison of future episodes of pain. A unique part of the assessment of pain is the need to have the patient identify exactly what amount or level of pain allows functionality and is *acceptable* to the patient.[20] This level of acceptable pain is the target for subsequent pain management techniques.[3,18]

Pain Location

The next area of evaluation is the location of the patient's pain. Location is normally easy for the patient to identify, although visceral pain is more difficult for the patient to localize.[3,17] If patients have difficulty naming the location, they should be asked to point to the location on their body or on a simple anatomic drawing. This technique is also helpful in identifying multiple sites of pain.[16]

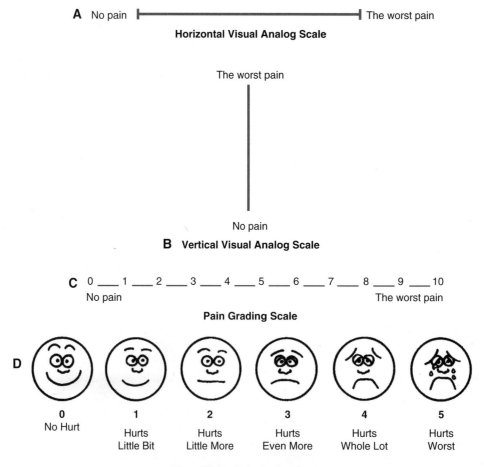

Figure 8-3 Visual analog scales. **A,** Horizontal visual analog scale. **B,** Vertical visual analog scale. **C,** Pain grading scale. **D,** Wong-Baker FACES Pain Rating Scale. (**D** from Wong DL: *Whaley & Wong's essentials of pediatric nursing,* ed 5, St Louis, 1997, Mosby.)

Asking the patient to identify factors that moderate pain is an important evaluation component for the critical care nurse. Position or movement as a component of pain may contribute significantly to the final evaluation of the pain occurrence, as with deep breathing intensifying chest pain because of pericarditis. Factors that reduce the pain or discomfort are also important findings. The moderation of pain continues after the patient leaves the critical care environment. A knowledge of any alleviation activities contributes to the patient's plan of care throughout the continuum of care.

The subjective data of intensity, type, location, and moderating factors form a single component of pain assessment. The critical care nurse also completes a physiologic assessment on any patient who reports pain. Lack of a physiologic response to pain does not mean that the patient is reporting pain that does not exist.[3,8,13,16] A number of factors may explain the lack of a physiologic response. Many therapies employed in the critical care area are designed to block the SNS response to stress, also successfully blocking the SNS response to pain. If there is a response to pain, the nurse assesses for (1) tachycardia, (2) hypertension, (3) tachypnea, (4) increased muscle tone in the area of pain, (5) sweating, (6) pallor, and (7) hypervigilance. Any of the body's responses to SNS stimulation might be expected. Complicating this finding in the critical care patient is the possibility of the original illness or injury as the cause of the sympathetic response.[2,8]

Some critical care patients respond to pain or painful stimuli by simply withdrawing from the painful stimuli. These patients are able to perceive the pain, but the higher somatosensory cortical contribution of interpretation of the pain is absent. Other patients do not respond to painful stimuli. These patients may lack integrity in the nociceptive system and may be unable to perceive the pain. These phenomena are usually associated with brain or spinal cord pathology that interrupts the system.

Behavioral Assessment

Certain behaviors may be manifested in the patient with pain. It is important to remember that not all patients have an observable behavioral response. Diligent observation of the patient experiencing pain may uncover behavioral cues (Table 8-3). Behaviors may indicate pain or an attempt to control pain with types of distraction.[13,15,16]

Patient Barriers
Communication

The most obvious patient barrier to the assessment of pain in the critical care population is an alteration in the ability to communicate. The intubated patient is unable to verbalize a description of the pain. If able to communicate in any manner, the patient may report the pain in that form. If able to write a description, the patient may describe the pain in writing. The nurse relies most on nonverbal clues or behav-

Table 8-3	Behaviors Associated with Pain
Type	**Examples**
Expression	Grimacing, frowning, eyes squeezed closed, withdrawn expression, staring, crying, teeth clenched, wrinkled brow
Noises	Groaning, moaning, sighing, sobbing, grunting
Speech	Cursing, shouting, praying, calling for help, chanting
Body movements	Rocking, thrashing, tossing/turning
Behaviors	Guarding, protective posturing, massaging or applying pressure, reading, watching TV, wandering

Modified from Salerno E, Willens J: *Pain management handbook*, St Louis, 1996, Mosby.

iors to assess for pain and its intensity in the nonverbal patient. Eye movement or leg movement up and down may indicate pain in the intubated patient.

The nurse cannot rely on predictable pain behaviors only and therefore must address other sources of assessment. The patient's family can contribute significantly in the assessment of behavioral clues to pain. The family is familiar with the patient's normal responses to pain and can assist the nurse in identifying such clues.[21] If no observable evidence supports a diagnosis of pain, the practitioner must use the concept that if the trauma, disease, injury, or procedure is a painful one for most patients, it is painful for this patient.[3]

Altered Level of Consciousness

The presence of delirium, dementia, or altered mentation related to psychoactive therapies or disease states presents a unique pain assessment barrier. It has been erroneously thought that the confused patient would be unable to perceive pain. Research now supports that the patient with altered cognitive abilities is able to report pain accurately when questioned or on occurrence of the painful event. However, this population has limited pain recall and limited ability to integrate the pain experience over time.[6] The critical care nurse needs to assess for pain frequently in cognitively impaired patients and not anticipate that these patients will initiate a pain discussion. If the patient is unable to use a numeric rating scale, the nurse should consider using a "faces" scale (see Figure 8-3).

The patient in a coma presents a dilemma for the critical care nurse. Because pain relies on cortical response to provide recognition, one theory states that the patient without higher cortical functioning has no perception of pain.[1,22] Conversely, the inability to interpret the nociceptive transmission does not negate the transmission. The critical care nurse can initiate a discussion with other health care team members to formulate a plan of care for the coma patient's comfort.

Cultural Influences

Another barrier to accurate pain assessment is the cultural influences on pain and pain reporting.[10,19,23,24] The cultural influences may be compounded by the patient who speaks a different language than the health team. The first consideration in assessing a patient from a different cultural group is to avoid the assumption that the patient will have a specific response to pain or exhibit a particular behavior because of culture. Patients are uniquely individual in their response to pain, and the practitioner might unjustly assign or expect behaviors that a patient will not exhibit.

A second consideration that is often overlooked is the role of pain in the patient's life. The nurse must communicate with the patient or family to ascertain this role. Some cultures believe that "God's test" or "punishment" takes the form of pain. Persons of such cultures would not necessarily believe that the pain should be relieved. Other cultures perceive pain as being associated with an imbalance in life (e.g., in hot/cold). Persons of these cultures believe they need to manipulate the environment to restore balance to accomplish pain control.[24]

The complexities and intricacies of cultural beliefs require much greater discussion. Many critical care units have established references or resources for dealing with cultural diversity in the critically ill patient. It is important for the nurse to support, whenever possible, the special beliefs and needs of the patient and family to provide the most therapeutic environment for healing.

Knowledge Deficit

A relatively overlooked patient barrier to accurate pain assessment is the public knowledge deficit regarding pain and pain management. Many patients and families are concerned about the risk of addiction to pain medication. Some fear that addiction will occur if the patient is medicated frequently or with sufficient amounts of opiates necessary to relieve the pain. Programs (e.g., "Just Say No to Drugs" campaign) that increase the public's concern regarding drugs compound this belief. The concern is powerful enough for some that they will deny or deliberately underreport the frequency or intensity of pain. Another inaccurate belief is the expectation that unrelieved pain is part of a critical illness or procedure.[25] Many patients have no memory of an explanation of their pain management plan.[19] As part of the patient plan for pain management, the critical care nurse must teach both the family and the patient the importance of pain control and the use of opioids in treating the critically ill patient.[26]

Health Professional Barriers

The health professional's beliefs and attitudes about pain and pain management are often a barrier to accurate and adequate assessment of pain that can lead to poor management practices.[3,7,8,13] The study of pain assessment and management is lacking in most schools of nursing as well as in nursing textbooks.[8,16,25] Multiple studies have documented nurses' misconceptions or lack of knowledge regarding addiction, physiologic dependence, drug tolerance, and respiratory depression.[3] The most problematic misconception on the part of nurses is the belief that the patient must have a physiologic and behavioral response to pain that matches the nurse's notion of what a patient in pain "looks like" (e.g., patient must have marked change in vital signs and be moaning, writhing, and crying to be "truly" in pain). This hampers appropriate management of the patient's pain. The critical care nurse must remember that pain is *what the patient states it is* and that no additional finding is necessary to treat the patient's pain.[3] When a patient is denied pain management based on the misconception that there is a certain behavior that always accompanies pain, an ethical conflict arises.[25,27,28]

Nursing concerns with addiction can contribute to misinterpretation of signs during the pain assessment process. Addiction rates for patients in acute pain who receive opioid analgesics are less than 1%.[3] Some false beliefs about addiction result from lack of knowledge about the terms addiction and tolerance. *Addiction* is defined as as "a pattern of compulsive drug use that is characterized by an incessant longing for a drug and the need to use the drug for effects other than pain control."[18] *Tolerance* is defined as a decreasing duration of opioid action.[3] Physical dependence and tolerance to opioids may develop if the drugs are given over a long period. If this is an anticipated problem, withdrawal may be avoided by simply weaning the patient from the opioid slowly to allow the brain to reestablish neurochemical balance in the absence of the opioid.[2] Tolerance to an opioid is a rare phenomenon in the critical care patient.

Health care professionals are also concerned that aggressive management of pain with opiates will cause critical respiratory depression.[3,18,29] Opioids can cause respiratory depression, but this rarely occurs in critically ill patients. As with addiction, the incidence is less than 1%. Respiratory depression from the administration of opioids, although a concern, can be managed with diligent assessment practices.

PAIN MANAGEMENT

The management of pain in the critically ill patient is as multidimensional as the assessment and is a multidisciplinary task (Box 8-1). The control of pain can be pharmacologic, nonpharmacologic, or a combination of the two therapies. The most common course for pain control in critical care is through the pharmacologic domain.

Pharmacologic Management

The pharmacologic management of pain takes a variety of forms in the critical care unit. Pharmacologic agents for pain are divided into the following four categories according to action:

- Opioid agonists: morphine, hydromorphone, fentanyl, meperidine

Box 8-1 COLLABORATIVE Management

1. Assess the patient's pain.
   - Location
   - Description
   - Intensity
   - Duration
   - Alleviating and aggravating factors
   - Associative factors
2. Select appropriate drugs based on efficacy in pain relief.
3. Recognize drug side effects.
4. Initiate nonpharmacologic techniques to manage pain.
   - Heat or cold
   - Positioning or external support
   - Massage
   - Guided imagery
   - Relaxation
5. Monitor patient to evaluate effectiveness of pain interventions.

- Partial agonists and agonist-antagonists: buprenorphine, pentazocine
- Nonopioids: acetaminophen, nonsteroidal antiinflammatory drugs (NSAIDs)
- Adjuvants: anticonvulsants, antidepressants

The way the pain is approached and managed involves progressive or combination therapy with the available agents and depends on the type of pain and the patient's response to therapy (Table 8-4).[18,30-35]

Delivery Methods

The most common route for drug administration is the intravenous (IV) route through continuous infusion, bolus administration, or patient-controlled analgesia (PCA). The traditional choice has been IV bolus administration. The benefits of this method are the rapid onset of action and the ease of titration. The major disadvantage is the rise and fall of the serum level of the opioid, leading to periods of pain control with periods of breakthrough pain.[36]

Continuous infusion of the opioids via infusion pump provides constant blood levels of the ordered opioid, promoting a consistent level of comfort. Continuous infusion is particularly helpful during sleep because the patient awakens with an adequate level of pain relief.[37] It is important that the patient be given the loading dose that relieves the pain and raises the circulating dose of the drug. After the basal rate is established, the patient maintains a steady state of pain control, unless there is additional pain from a procedure, an activity, or a change in the patient's condition. Orders for additional boluses of opioid need to be available.

Patient-Controlled Analgesia. PCA is a method of delivery via infusion pump that allows the patient to self-administer small doses of analgesics. PCA allows the patient to control the level of pain and sedation and to avoid the peaks and valleys of intermittent dosing by the health care professional. The patient can self-administer a bolus of medication the moment the pain begins, thus acting preemptively.[38]

Although a variety of routes can be used, PCA is traditionally administered intravenously. Certain patients are not candidates for PCA. Alterations in the level of consciousness or mentation preclude an understanding of how to use the equipment. Elderly patients and those with renal or hepatic insufficiency may require careful screening for PCA.[38]

Allowing the patient to self-administer opioid doses does not diminish the role of the critical care nurse in pain management. The nurse advises for necessary changes to the prescription and continues to monitor the effects of the medication and doses. The patient is closely monitored during the first 2 hours of therapy and after every change in the prescription. If the patient's pain does not respond within the first 2 hours of therapy, a total reassessment of the pain state is essential. The nurse monitors the number of boluses the patient delivers. If the patient is administering boluses more often than the prescription, the dose may be insufficient to maintain pain control. Naloxone must be readily available to reverse adverse opiate respiratory effects. Ideally, the patient undergoing an elective procedure requiring opioid analgesia postoperatively is instructed in the use of PCA during preoperative teaching. This allows the patient to become comfortable with the concept of self-medication before use.[38]

Intraspinal Pain Control. Intraspinal anesthesia uses the concept that the spinal cord is the primary link in nociceptive transmission. The goal is to mimic the body's endogenous opioid pain modification system by interfering with the transmission of pain by providing an opiate receptor–binding agent directly into the spinal cord. The benefits of the intraspinal route include good-to-excellent pain control with typically lower doses of opioids, increased patient mobility, minimal sedation, and, typically, increased patient satisfaction.[36] Also, little change occurs in the paient's hemodynamic status. Intraspinal anesthesia is particularly appropriate for pain in the thorax, upper abdomen, and lower extremities.

The two intraspinal routes are intrathecal and epidural.[39] Regardless of the route, the effects of the opioid agonist used will be the same, so assessment parameters are similar to those used for other routes.

Intrathecal analgesia. Intrathecal (subarachnoid) opioids are placed directly into the cerebrospinal fluid (CSF) and attach to spinal cord receptor sites. Opioids introduced at this site act quickly at the dorsal horn. The dural sheath is punctured, eliminating any barrier for pathogens between the environment and the CSF. This creates the risk for serious infections. The intrathecal route is usually reserved for intraoperative use. Single-bolus dosing provides short-term relief for pain that is short lived; the pain of labor and delivery, for example, is well managed using this regimen. Side

Table 8-4	Pharmacologic Management of Pain		
Drug	**Dosage**	**Action**	**Special Considerations**
Amitriptyline (Elavil)	PO 10 mg/day	Blocks reuptake of serotonin	Can be sedating
Bupivacaine (Marcaine)	Epidural 1-5 mg/hr	Local hydrophilic anesthetic; blocks C and Aδ fiber transmission	May be given alone or with an opioid; monitor carefully for hypotension and respiratory depression
Butorphanol (Stadol)	IM or slow IV infusion 1-2 mg q 3-4hr	Agonist-antagonist	Psychometric effects, anxiety, hallucinations, nightmares
Capsaicin	Topical 3 or 4 times/day	Causes release and depletion of substance P	Effective for peripheral neuropathies and neuralgias
Codeine	PO 15-30 mg q 4hr	Weak μ agonist	Effective for minor pain; constipating
Diazepam (Valium)	IV 2-5 mg PO 2.5-10 mg	Adjuvant agent for pain; antilytic	Must not be given directly with an opioid, which can increase side effects; sedation
Fentanyl	IV 0.1 mg Epidural 25-250 mcg or 10-25 mcg/hr	Moderate-dose analgesia High-dose anesthesia opioid agonist	80 times as potent as morphine Transdermal onset 72 hours
Hydromorphone (Dilaudid)	PO 2 mg q 4hr IM 1.5 mg	μ Agonist	Shorter duration of action than morphine
Ibuprofen (Advil, Motrin)	PO 200-600 mg q 6hr	NSAID	Gastrointestinal disturbances; prolonged bleeding time
Ketorolac (Toradol)	IM 15-30 mg qid	Parenteral NSAID; prevents production of prostaglandins	Platelet aggregation interrupted; inhibits maintenance of gastric mucosa
Meperidine (Demerol)	IM 75-150 mg q 4hr	μ Agonist	Short half-life; extremely neurotoxic; limited use advised
Methadone (Dolophine)	PO 20 mg q 4hr IV 5-10 mg	μ Agonist	PO route highly efficient; accumulates with multiple dosing, causing serious sedation (2-5 days)
Oxycodone (Percocet, with acetaminophen; Percodan, with aspirin)	PO 2 tabs (10 mg total) q 4hr	Moderately strong μ agonist	Blocks both peripheral and central pathways
Pentazocine (Talwin)	PO 50-100 mg q 3-4hr SQ/IM 30-60 mg q 3-4hr IV 30 mg	Mixed agonist-antagonist, blocks μ and activates κ receptors; considered weak	Has ceiling effect; increases cardiac workload
Propoxyphene (Darvocet-N)	PO 1 or 2 tabs q 4hr	Weak μ agonist	Central nervous system toxic metabolite; for minor pain or short-term use
Morphine	IV 2-15 mg/hr bolus IV infusion 1-10 mg/hr IM 5-15 mg q 3-4hr SQ 5-15 mg q 3-4hr Epidural bolus 1-5 mg/hr, infusion 0.5-2.0 mg/hr PO 8-20 mg q 4hr	Analgesia, antianxiety, opioid agonist	Respiratory depression, hypotension, nausea, vomiting, sedation, pruritus; titrate to effect

PO, Oral; *IM,* intramuscular; *IV,* intravenous; *SQ,* subcutaneous; *q 3-4hr,* every 3 to 4 hours; *qid,* four times a day; *NSAID,* nonsteroidal antiinflammatory drug.

effects of intrathecal pain control include postdural puncture headache and infection.[39]

Epidural analgesia. Epidural analgesia is often used in the critical care unit after major abdominal surgery, nephrectomy, thoracotomy, and major orthopedic procedures.[39,40] Conditions that preclude the use of epidural pain control include systemic infection, anticoagulation, and increased intracranial pressure. Epidural delivery of opiates provides longer-lasting pain relief with less dosing of opiates. When delivered into the epidural space, 5 mg of morphine may be effective for 6 to 24 hours, versus 3 to 4 hours when delivered intravenously.

Opioids infused in the epidural space are more unpredictable than those administered intrathecally. The epidural space is filled with fatty tissue and is external to the dura mater. The fatty tissue interferes with uptake, and the dura acts as a barrier to diffusion, making diffusion rate difficult to predict. The rapidity of drug diffusion is determined by the type of drug used. *Hydrophilic* drugs (e.g., morphine) are water soluble and penetrate the dura slowly, giving these agents a longer onset and duration of action. *Lipophilic* drugs (e.g., fentanyl) are lipid soluble; these agents penetrate the dura rapidly and therefore have a rapid onset of action and a shorter duration of action.[40] The dura itself acts as a physical barrier and delays diffusion; compared with the intrathecal route, this allows more drug to be absorbed in the systemic circulation, requiring greater doses for pain relief.[39] Epidural drugs may be delivered by bolus or continuously infused.

Epidural analgesia is increasingly used in the critical care environment and requires careful monitoring. The nurse must assess the patient for respiratory depression using the unit protocol. This phenomenon may occur early in the therapy or as late as 24 hours after initiation. The epidural catheter also puts the patient at risk for infection. The efficiency of epidural pain control and the increased mobility of the patient does not diminish the nurse's responsibility to monitor and evaluate the outcomes of the pain management protocol in use.

Equianalgesia

At some point in the patient's recovery, strong opioids are replaced by more moderate agents. In doing any conversion, the goal is to provide equal analgesic effects with the new agents, referred to as *equianalgesia*. The critical care nurse is the practitioner most likely to convert the patient from parenteral to oral medication in preparation for a change in the level of care or for discharge. Studies have identified that nurses lack knowledge regarding equal doses between IV and oral administration. A common misconception is that when a patient is able to take oral medication, the pain is less severe. The change to oral medications does not indicate a need for less medication. The nurse needs to practice equianalgesia when converting the patient. Because of the variety of agents and routes, professional pain organizations have developed equianalgesia charts for use by the health care professional.[18] All critical care units need to have a chart posted for easy referral (Table 8-5).

Nonpharmacologic Methods

Numerous methods of pain management other than drugs appear in the critical care literature.[41] In most cases these therapies augment and enhance the pharmacologic management of the patient's pain. Stimulating other nonpain sensory fibers present in the periphery modifies pain transmission. These fibers are stimulated by *thermal changes* (e.g., application of heat/cold), simple *massage*, and *transcutaneous electrical nerve stimulation* (TENS). Massage, a mainstay in the nursing management of the patient in pain, is appropriate for most critically ill patients.

The use of TENS has contraindications in the critical care unit. Because the patient controls the device, mentation must be intact. TENS is also contraindicated in patients with pacemakers and automatic implantable defibrillators because these devices may recognize and erroneously interpret the TENS electrical signal. TENS therapy is efficient, patient-controlled pain management for orthopedic, obstetric, and some postoperative pain states.

Using the cortical interpretation of pain as the foundation, interventions known to reduce the patient's pain report include cognitive techniques such as patient teaching, relaxation, distraction, guided imagery, music therapy, and hypnosis.[3,41]

Relaxation is a well-documented method for reducing the distress associated with pain. Although not a substitute for pharmacology, relaxation is an excellent adjunct to control pain. Relaxation decreases oxygen consumption and muscle tone and can decrease heart rate and blood pressure. Relaxation gives the patient a sense of control over the pain and reduces muscle tension and anxiety. For patients not interested in relaxation therapy, *deep-breathing exercises* may be helpful and frequently lead to relaxation.[3]

Guided imagery uses the imagination to provide control over pain and can be used to distract or relax. Guiding a patient to a place that is pain-free and relaxing requires a considerable time commitment by the nurse. Although this may be difficult in the critical care environment, guiding patients to a place in their imagination that is free from pain can be done rapidly and may be very beneficial.[41]

Music therapy is often used for relaxation. Music that is pleasing to the patient may have extremely soothing effects.[42] Ideally the music should be supplied by a small set of lightweight headphones. This method also serves to minimize the distracting and anxiety-producing noises of a critical care unit.[43] It is important to educate the patient and family regarding the role of music in relaxation and pain control and to provide music of the patient's choice.

The patient and family may provide information about other sources of distraction for the patient. Determining the distraction therapies typically used by the patient may suggest an approach that might work during the illness. Some persons are distracted by television, whereas TV is a source of increased anxiety for others. The critical care nurse should not assume that the patient does or does not want to watch TV until the nurse determines whether TV will be beneficial or harmful to the patient.

The key to success with any of these therapies is to understand their mechanism of action so that the therapy matches the needs of the patient. All the previously mentioned interventions require the patient's cooperation, and the patient must have some degree of commitment to the treatment. When handled efficiently, nonpharmacologic tools can assist in pain management.

An increasing number of therapies are appearing in the critical care research. It is important for the practitioner to be aware of the current literature to provide the most effective and current interventions to manage the patient's pain. The current health care environment mandates that

Table 8-5

Equianalgesic Chart: Approximate Equivalent Doses of Opioids for Moderate to Severe Pain

Analgesic	Parenteral Route (IM, SC, IV)[1,2]	Oral (PO) Route[1]	Comments
MU OPIOID AGONISTS			
Morphine	10 mg	30 mg	Standard for comparison. Multiple routes of administration; available in IR and CR formulations. Active metabolite M6G can accumulate with repeated dosing in renal failure.
Codeine	130 mg	200 mg	IM route has unpredictable absorption and high side-effect profile. PO route used for mild to moderate pain. Usually combined with a nonopioid (e.g., Tylenol #3).
Fentanyl	100 mcg/hr parenterally and transdermally ≅ 4 mg/hr morphine parenterally; 1 mcg/hr transdermally ≅ 2 mg/24 hr morphine PO	Not recommended	Short half-life, but at steady state, slow elimination from tissues can lead to prolonged half-life (up to 12 hours). Start opioid-naive patients on no more than 25 mcg/hr transdermally. Transdermal fentanyl is not recommended for acute pain management. Available by oral transmucosal route.
		—	
Hydromorphone (Dilaudid)	1.5 mg	7.5 mg	Useful alternative to morphine. No evidence that metabolites are clinically relevant; shorter duration than morphine. Available in high-potency parenteral formulation (10 mg/ml) useful for SC infusion; 3 mg rectal ≅ 650 mg aspirin PO. With repeated dosing (e.g., PCA), it is more likely that 2-3 mg parenteral hydromorphone = 10 mg parenteral morphine.
Levorphanol (Levo-Dromoran)	2 mg	4 mg	Longer acting than morphine when given repeatedly. Long half-life can lead to accumulation within 2-3 days of repeated dosing.
Meperidine	75 mg	300 mg	No longer preferred as a first-line opioid for management of acute or chronic pain because of potential toxicity from accumulation of metabolite, normeperidine. Normeperidine has half-life of 15-20 hours and is not reversed by naloxone. Not recommended by continuous IV infusion or in elderly patients or those with impaired renal function.
		Not recommended	
Methadone (Dolophine)	10 mg	20 mg	Longer acting than morphine when given repeatedly. Long half-life can lead to delayed toxicity from accumulation in 3-5 days. Start PO dosing on as-needed (prn) schedule; in opioid-tolerant patients converted to methadone, start with 10%-25% of equianalgesic dose.
Oxycodone	—	20 mg	Used for moderate pain when combined with a nonopioid (e.g., Percocet, Tylox). Available as single entity in IR and CR formulations (e.g., OxyContin); can be used similar to PO morphine for severe pain.
Oxymorphone (Numorphan)	1 mg	10 mg rectal	Used for moderate to severe pain. No PO formulation.

[1]Duration of analgesia is dose dependent; the higher the dose, usually the longer the duration.
[2]Intravenous (IV) boluses may be used to produce analgesia that lasts approximately as long as intramuscular (IM) or subcutaneous (SC) doses. Of all routes of administration, however, IV produces highest peak concentration of drug, and peak concentration is associated with highest level of toxicity, e.g., sedation. To decrease peak effect and lower level of toxicity, IV boluses may be administered more slowly, e.g., 10 mg of morphine over 15 minutes, or smaller doses may be administered more often, e.g., 5 mg of morphine every 1 to 1½ hours.
≅, Approximately equal to; *IR,* immediate-release; *CR,* controlled-release; *M6G,* morphine-6-glucuronide; *PCA,* patient-controlled analgesia.

Approximate Equivalent Doses of Opioids for Moderate to Severe Pain

Analgesic	Parenteral Route (IM, SC, IV)[1,2]	Oral (PO) Route[1]	Comments
AGONIST-ANTAGONIST OPIOIDS*			
Buprenorphine (Buprenex)	0.4 mg	—	Not readily reversed by naloxone.
Butorphanol (Stadol)	2 mg	—	Not recommended for laboring patients.
Dezocine (Dalgan)	10 mg	—	Available in nasal spray.
Nalbuphine (Nubain)	10 mg	—	
Pentazocine (Talwin)	60 mg	180 mg	

*Not recommended for severe, escalating pain. If used in combination with mu agonists, may reverse analgesia and precipitate withdrawal in opioid-dependent patients. For more complete information and additional references, see Pasero C, Portenoy RK, McCaffery M: Opioid analgesics. In McCaffery M, Pasero C: *Pain: clinical manual*, St Louis, 1999, Mosby, p 241.
American Pain Society: *Principles of analgesic use in the treatment of acute and cancer pain*, ed 3, Glenview, Ill, 1992, The Society.
Lawlor P et al: Dose ratio between morphine and hydromorphone in patients with cancer pain: a retrospective study, *Pain* 72(1/2):79, 1997.
Manfredi PL et al: Intravenous methadone for cancer pain unrelieved by morphine and hydromorphone: clinical observations, *Pain* 70:99, 1997.
Portenoy RK: Opioid analgesics. In Portenoy RK, Kanner RM, editors: *Pain management: theory and practice*, Philadelphia, 1996, Davis, p 249.

Approximate Equivalent Doses of PO Nonopioids and Opioids for Mild to Moderate Pain

Analgesic	Oral (PO) Dose
NONOPIOIDS	
Acetaminophen	650 mg
Aspirin (ASA)	650 mg
OPIOIDS[†]	
Codeine	32-60 mg
Hydrocodone[‡]	5 mg
Meperidine (Demerol)	50 mg
Oxycodone[§]	3-5 mg
Propoxyphene (Darvon)	65-100 mg

[†]Often combined with acetaminophen; avoid exceeding maximum total daily dose of acetaminophen (4000 mg/day).
[‡]Combined with acetaminophen, e.g., Vicodin, Lortab.
[§]Combined with acetaminophen, e.g., Percocet, Tylox. Also available alone as CR OxyContin and IR formulations.

A GUIDE TO USING EQUIANALGESIC CHARTS

- *Equianalgesic* means approximately the same pain relief.
- The equianalgesic chart is a guideline. Doses and intervals between doses are titrated according to individual's response.
- The equianalgesic chart is helpful when switching from one drug to another, or switching from one route of administration to another.
- Dosages in the equianalgesic chart for moderate to severe pain are not necessarily starting doses. The doses suggest a ratio for comparing the analgesia of one drug to another.
- For elderly patients, initially reduce the recommended adult opioid dose for moderate to severe pain by 25% to 50%.
- The longer the patient has been receiving opioids, the more conservative the starting doses of a **new** opioid.

For more complete information and additional references, see McCaffery M, Pasero C, Portenoy RK: Nonopioids: acetaminophen and nonsteroidal anti-inflammatory drugs. In McCaffery M, Pasero C: *Pain: clinical manual*, St Louis, 1999, Mosby, p 133.
American Pain Society: *Principles of analgesic use in the treatment of acute pain and cancer pain*, ed 3, Glenview, Ill, 1992, The Society.
Kaiko R et al: Analgesic efficacy of controlled-release (CR) oxycodone and CR morphine, *Clin Pharmacol Ther* 59:130, 1996.
From McCaffery M, Pasero C: *Pain: clinical manual*, St Louis, 1999, Mosby.

patients experience positive outcomes as rapidly as possible. Because pain is a major barrier to early mobility and rapid return to a preillness state, pain management is of paramount importance to the critical care nurse. The critically ill patient is the most difficult patient to assess and manage, and the critical care nurse must develop the skill and intervention techniques necessary to manage the most difficult of the pain states. **As patient advocate, the nurse assumes the responsibility for establishing pain control as a priority for the health care team.**[44]

REFERENCES

1. Caillet R: *Pain: mechanisms and management*, Philadelphia, 1993, Davis.
2. Puntillo K: Physiology of pain and its consequences in critically ill patients. In Puntillo K, editor: *Pain in the critically ill: assessment and management*, Gaithersburg, Md, 1991, Aspen.
3. McCaffery M, Pasero C: *Pain: clinical manual for nursing practice*, ed 2, St Louis, 1999, Mosby.
4. Wallace KG: The pathophysiology of pain, *Crit Care Nurs Q* 15(2):1, 1992.
5. Carson MM, Barton DM, Morrison CG: Managing pain during mediastinal chest tube removal, *Heart Lung* 23:500, 1994.
6. Simpson T, Lee E, Cameron C: Patients' perceptions of environmental factors that disturb sleep after cardiac surgery, *Am J Crit Care* 5:173, 1996.
7. Sun X, Weissman C: The use of analgesics and sedatives in the critically ill patient: physicians, order versus medication administered, *Heart Lung* 23:169, 1994.
8. Alpen M, Titler M: Pain management in the critically ill: what do we know and how can we improve? *AACN Clin Issues Crit Care Nurs* 5:159, 1994.
9. Carroll K et al: Pain assessment and management in the critically ill postoperative and trauma patient, *Am J Crit Care* 8:20, 1999.
10. Jurf J, Nirschl A: Acute postoperative pain review and update, *Crit Care Nurs Q* 16:8, 1993.
11. Edwards AD: Physiology of pain. In St Marie B, editor: *Core curriculum for pain management nursing*, Philadelphia, 2002, Saunders.
12. Guyton AC, Hall JE: *Textbook of medical physiology*, ed 10, Philadelphia, 2000, Saunders.
13. Willens J: Introduction to pain management. In Salerno E, Willens J, editors: *Pain management handbook: an interdisciplinary approach*, St Louis, 1996, Mosby.
14. Maxam-Moore V, Wilkie D, Woods S: Analgesics for cardiac surgery patients in critical care: describing current practice, *Am J Crit Care* 3:31, 1994.
15. McGuire D: Comprehensive and multidimensional assessment and measurement of pain, *J Pain Symptom Manage* 7:312, 1992.
16. Voight L, Paice J, Pouilot J: Standardized pain flowsheet: impact on patient reported experiences after cardiovascular surgery, *Am J Crit Care* 4:308, 1995.
17. St Marie B: Assessment. In St Marie B, editor: *Core curriculum for pain management nursing*, Philadelphia, 2002, Saunders.
18. Jacox A et al: *Acute pain management: operative or medical procedures and trauma*. Clinical practice guidelines, Pub No 92-0032, Rockville, Md, 1992, Agency for Health Care Policy and Research, US Department of Health and Human Services.
19. Villaire M: Pain: assessment, treatment and the coming thunder, *Crit Care Nurse* 12:159, 1995 (interview with Kathleen Puntillo).
20. Stranik-Hutt J: Pain management in the critically ill, *Crit Care Nurse* 18:85, 1998.
21. Kwekkebom KL: Assessment of pain in the critically ill, *Crit Care Nurs Clin North Am* 13:181, 2001.
22. Halloran T, Pohlman A: Managing sedation in the critically ill patient, *Crit Care Nurse* 5(4 suppl):1, 1995.
23. Bozeman M: Cultural aspects of pain management. In Salerno E, Willens J, editors: *Pain management handbook: an interdisciplinary approach*, St Louis, 1996, Mosby.
24. Lasch KE: Culture, pain and culturally sensitive pain care, *Pain Manage Nurse* 1(3):S16, 2000.
25. Ulmer J: Identifying and preventing pain mismanagement. In Salerno E, Willens J, editors: *Pain management handbook: an interdisciplinary approach*, St Louis, 1996, Mosby.
26. Standard D et al: Clinical judgment and management of postoperative pain in the critical care patient, *Am J Crit Care* 5:433, 1996.
27. Faucett J: Care of the critically ill patient. In Puntillo K, editor: *Pain in the critically ill: assessment and management*, Gaithersburg, Md, 1991, Aspen.
28. Puntillo K et al: Relationship between behavioral and physiologic indicators of pain, critical care patients self-report, and opioid administration, *Crit Care Nurse* 25:1159, 1997.
29. Watt-Watson J: Misbeliefs about pain. In Watt-Watson J, Donovan M, editors: *Pain management: nursing perspective*, St Louis, 1992, Mosby.
30. Salerno E: Pharmacologic approaches to pain. In Salerno E, Willens J, editors: *Pain management handbook: an interdisciplinary approach*, St Louis, 1996, Mosby.
31. Paice J: Pharmacologic management. In Watt-Watson J, Donovan M, editors: *Pain management: nursing perspective*, St Louis, 1992, Mosby.
32. American Society of Hospital Pharmacists: *American Hospital Formulary Service drug information '02*, Bethesda, Md, 2002, The Society/Service.
33. Mather I, Denson D: Pharmacokinetics of systemic opioids for the management of pain. In Sinatra R et al, editors: *Acute pain*, St Louis, 1992, Mosby.
34. Wild L: Intravenous methods of analgesia for pain in the critically ill. In Puntillo K, editor: *Pain in the critically ill: assessment and management*, Gaithersburg, Md, 1991, Aspen.
35. Glen VL, St Marie B: Overview of pharmacology. In St Marie B, editor: *Core curriculum for pain management nursing*, Philadelphia, 2002, Saunders.
36. McKenry L, Salerno E, editors: *Mosby's pharmacology in nursing*, ed 21, St Louis, 2003, Mosby.
37. Collins P, Spunt A, Huml M: Symptom management. In Salerno E, Willens J, editors: *Pain management handbook: an interdisciplinary approach*, St Louis, 1996, Mosby.
38. Etches RC: Patient-controlled analgesia, *Surg Clin North Am* 72:297, 1999.
39. Dyble K: Epidural and intrathecal methods of analgesia in the critically ill. In Puntillo K, editor: *Pain in the critically ill: assessment and management*, Gaithersburg, Md, 1991, Aspen.
40. Puntillo K: Dimensions of procedural pain and its analgesic management in critically ill surgical patients, *Am J Crit Care* 3:116, 1994.
41. Gujol M: A survey of pain assessment and management practices among critical care nurses, *Am J Crit Care* 3:123, 1994.
42. Courts N: Nonpharmacologic approaches to pain. In Salerno E, Willens J, editors: *Pain management handbook: an interdisciplinary approach*, St Louis, 1996, Mosby.
43. Edgar L, Smith-Hanrahan C: Nonpharmacologic pain management. In Watt-Watson J, Donovan M, editors: *Pain management: nursing perspective*, St Louis, 1992, Mosby.
44. Meehan D et al: Analgesic administration, pain intensity, and patient satisfaction in cardiac surgical patients, *Am J Crit Care* 4:435, 1995.

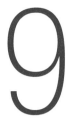

Sedation Assessment and Management

Objectives

- Explain the differences among light, moderate, and deep levels of sedation.
- Describe the role of standardized assessment tools to determine sedation requirements.
- Compare and contrast pharmacologic and nonpharmacologic interventions used to provide sedation.
- Discuss medical and nursing interventions essential for management of the patient receiving sedation therapy.

evolve Be sure to check out the free exercises on-line at *http://evolve.elsevier.com/Urden/priorities/*

PATIENT AGITATION AND NEED FOR SEDATION/ANALGESIA

One of the challenges facing clinicians is how to provide a therapeutic environment for patients in the alarm-filled, emergency-focused critical care unit. Rest and relaxation can be difficult to find. Up to 74% of critical care patients demonstrate some degree of agitation during their critical care hospitalization.[1] Many report upsetting dreams, hallucinations, nightmares, and flashbacks once they are recovered. The many causes of this agitation include painful procedures, invasive tubes, sleep deprivation, fear, anxiety, and the stress associated with critical illness. Some patients experience a "posttraumatic stress disorder" syndrome after prolonged hospitalization.[1]

The goal of recent clinical practice guidelines is to increase the awareness of these issues within the medical and nursing community.[2] When the sedation assessment, as with the pain assessment, is recognized as a *fifth vital sign*, nurses may be able to decrease the incidence of agitation and delirium in critically ill patients.[1]

The need for analgesics and sedatives to maintain patient safety and comfort is important, but it is increasingly recognized that excessive sedation can prolong the duration of mechanical ventilation, create physical and psychologic dependence, and increase the length of the hospital stay.[2] The goal is to find a balance between providing compassionate patient care and avoiding oversedation.

ASSESSING LEVEL OF SEDATION
Sedation Scales

The use of scoring systems to assess and record levels of sedation and agitation are now strongly recommended.[2] Three frequently used scales are the Ramsey Scale, Riker Sedation-Agitation Scale (SAS), and Motor Activity Assessment Scale (MAAS) (Table 9-1). Frequent assessment of the patient's motor activity and sedation level is helpful to titrate continuous infusions of sedatives such as propofol or lorazepam. Collaboratively, the critical care team must decide which level of sedation is most appropriate for an individual patient.[2,3]

Sedative levels are standardized by using "light," "moderate," and "deep" to describe the level of sedation (Box 9-1).[2,3] *Light sedation*, or "minimal" sedation, is used when the goal of sedative therapy is to relieve anxiety and ensure patient comfort while allowing the patient to remain responsive to the environment. A recent research survey of critical care nurses found most believe that treating patient's anxiety is both beneficial and important.[4] *Moderate sedation*, also called "conscious" or "procedural" sedation, is used in conjunction with analgesia to ensure patient comfort during a painful or invasive procedure (e.g., bronchoscopy). *Deep sedation* is used when the patient must be unresponsive so that care may be delivered safely. For example, in the diagnosis of acute respiratory distress syndrome (ARDS) deep sedation and analgesia may be required to achieve ventilator synchrony.[2] By contrast, when a patient is weaning from the ventilator, only light sedation may be necessary. During ventilator-weaning trials, it is more reasonable to limit sedation so that the patient is comfortable and arousable to voice while avoiding the twin perils of agitation and oversedation.

The first step in assessing the agitated patient is to rule out any sensations of pain.[2] Clinical assessment is more challenging when the patient is obtunded or has an artificial airway in place. If the patient can communicate, the 1 to 10 verbal pain scale is very useful. If the patient is intubated and cannot vocalize, assessing pain becomes considerably more complex. Once medication for pain has been provided, the next step is to determine the minimum level of sedation required. If deep or moderate sedation is being applied, it is essential that all individuals are qualified and have appropriate credentials to manage these medications and any potential patient complications that arise.[2,3]

Continuous Nervous System Monitoring

One of the challenges with deep sedation is recognizing whether a patient is effectively sedated and pain-free. Two clinicians evaluating the same patient may not agree about whether the level of applied sedation and analgesia is appropriate; one may describe the patient as "oversedated," and the other may describe the patient as "inadequately sedated."[5] Clinical parameters such as heart rate and blood pressure are not always reliable because these can be changed by other conditions.

In an attempt to clarify clinical assessment of depth of consciousness, some hospitals use continuous monitoring of the electroencephalogram (EEG) for sedated mechanically ventilated patients.[5] Two monitoring systems are currently approved by the United States Food and Drug Administration (FDA). The first system to be used in critical care units was the bispectral index (BIS).[5] The BIS system uses sensor electrodes on a single band placed on the patient's forehead. The BIS analyzes the patient's EEG signals to detect the effect of sedatives and anesthetics on the brain. The other continuous monitoring system is the Physiometrix PSA 4000, which also continuously monitors the EEG via an electrode array placed on the forehead. These technologies have been successfully used in the operating room when the patient is under general anesthesia. Both systems calculate a number from 0 to 99-100. A value greater than 95 indicates wakefulness, and a value less than 50-60 indicates the patient is unconscious or deeply sedated with a low probability of mental recall of events.[2,5] Both systems incorporate an electromyelogram (EMG) sensor to filter out erroneous muscle movement that may distort the numeric sedation value.

Continuous nervous system monitoring via EEG definitely has a role for the most critically ill patients who are deeply sedated, receiving opiate analgesia, and are pharmacologically paralyzed, although research outside the operating room is limited at this time.[5] Research is non-existent on

Table 9-1   Sedation Scales

Score	Description	Definition
RIKER SEDATION-AGITATION SCALE (SAS)		
7	Dangerous agitation	Pulls at endotracheal tube (ETT), tries to remove catheters, climbs over bedrail, strikes at staff, thrashes side-to-side
6	Very agitated	Does not calm despite frequent verbal reminding of limits, requires physical restraints, bites ETT
5	Agitated	Anxious or mildly agitated, attempts to sit up, calms down to verbal instructions
4	Calm and cooperative	Calm, awakens easily, follows commands
3	Sedated	Difficult to arouse, awakens to verbal stimuli or gentle shaking but drifts off again, follows simple commands
2	Very sedated	Arouses to physical stimuli, but does not communicate or follow commands, may move spontaneously
1	Unarousable	Minimal or no response to noxious stimuli, does not communicate or follow commands
MOTOR ACTIVITY ASSESSMENT SCALE (MAAS)		
6	Dangerously agitated	No external stimulus required to elicit movement; is uncooperative, pulls at tubes/catheters, thrashes side-to-side, strikes at staff, tries to climb out of bed, does not calm down when asked
5	Agitated	No external stimulus required to elicit movement; attempts to sit up or move limbs out of bed, does not consistently follow commands (e.g., will lie down when asked, but soon reverts back to attempts)
4	Restless and cooperative	No external stimulus required to elicit movement; picks at sheets/tubes or uncovers self, follows commands
3	Calm and cooperative	No external stimulus required to elicit movement; adjusts sheets/clothes purposefully, follows commands
2	Responsive to touch or name	Opens eyes, raises eyebrows, or turns head toward stimulus; or moves limbs when touched or when name loudly spoken
1	Responsive only to noxious stimulus	Opens eyes, raises eyebrows, or turns head toward stimulus; or moves limbs with noxious stimulus
0	Unresponsive	Does not move with noxious stimulus*
RAMSEY SCALE		
1	Awake	Anxious and agitated or restless, or both
2		Cooperative, oriented, and tranquil
3		Responds only to commands
4	Asleep	Brisk response to light glabellar tap or loud auditory stimulus
5		Sluggish response to light glabellar tap or loud auditory stimulus
6		No response to light glabellar tap or loud auditory stiumulus

Modified from Jacobi J et al: *Crit Care Med* 30(1):119-141, 2002.

*Noxious stimulus indicates suctioning or 5 seconds of vigorous orbital, sternal, or nailbed pressure.

Box **9-1** Levels of Sedation

LIGHT SEDATION (MINIMAL SEDATION, ANXIOLYSIS)

Drug-induced state during which patients respond normally to verbal commands. Although cognitive function and coordination may be impaired, ventilatory and cardiovascular functions are unaffected.

MODERATE SEDATION WITH ANALGESIA (CONSCIOUS SEDATION)

Drug-induced depression of consciousness during which patients respond purposefully to verbal commands, either alone or accompanied by light tactile stimulation. No interventions are required to maintain a patent airway, and spontaneous ventilation is adequate. Cardiovascular function is usually maintained.

DEEP SEDATION AND ANALGESIA

Drug-induced depression of consciousness during which patients cannot be easily aroused but respond purposefully

after repeated or painful stimulation. The ability to maintain ventilatory function independently is impaired. Patients require assistance in maintaining a patent airway, and spontaneous ventilation may be inadequate. Cardiovascular function is usually maintained.

GENERAL ANESTHESIA

Drug-induced loss of consciousness during which patients are not arousable, even by painful stimulation. The ability to maintain ventilatory function independently is impaired, and assistance to maintain a patent airway is required. Positive-pressure ventilation may be required because of depressed spontaneous ventilation or drug-induced depression of neuromuscular function. Cardiovascular function may be impaired.

Data from Joint Commission on Accreditation of Healthcare Organizations: *Comprehensive accreditation manual for hospitals,* Oakbrook Terrace, Ill, 2000, The Commission; and Jacobi J et al: *Crit Care Med* 30(1):119-141, 2002.

the role of continuous EEG monitoring for the moderately or lightly sedated patient but this may change as continuous EEG monitoring becomes more widely used in the critical care setting.

It is recommended that all critically ill, intubated, mechanically ventilated patients have a stated goal for analgesia and sedation (Figure 9-1).[2] Once the sedation goal is articulated and documented, the ongoing use of a validated assessment scale is recommended to facilitate consistency between the various health care practitioners (see Table 9-1).

COMPLICATIONS OF SEDATION

Oversedation is recognized as a state of unintended patient unresponsiveness in which the patient resides in a state of suspended animation that resembles general anesthesia.[6] Prolonged deep sedation is associated with significant complications of immobility, including pressure ulcers, thromboemboli, gastric ileus, nosocomial pneumonia, and delayed weaning from mechanical ventilation.

Too little sedation is equally hazardous. Most nurses have experienced the challenge of caring for a patient who unexpectedly removes the endotracheal or nasogastric tube. Unplanned extubation in restless, anxious, agitated patients occurs in 8% to 10% of intubated patients after an average of 3.5 days in the critical care unit. Six percent of self-extubations cause significant complications, including aspiration, dysrhythmias, bronchospasm, and bradycardia.[6]

SELECTING MEDICATIONS FOR SEDATION

Several categories of sedatives are commercially available. None of these medications has any analgesic properties. Therefore, if the patient is experiencing pain, analgesia must be administered in addition to any sedative agents. Sedative

agents include the benzodiazepines, anesthetic agents such as propofol, and the central α agonists (Table 9-2).[2]

Benzodiazepines

Benzodiazepines are sedative-hypnotics with powerful amnesic properties that inhibit reception of new sensory information.[2,6] Benzodiazepines do not have analgesic properties. The most frequently used critical care benzodiazepines are *diazepam* (Valium), *midazolam* (Versed), and *lorazepam* (Ativan). Midazolam is recommended for control of acute short-term agitation because of an intravenous (IV) onset of action of under 3 minutes.[2,6] However, when midazolam is administered for longer than 24 hours as a continuous infusion, the sedative effect is prolonged by active metabolites.[2]

When long-term sedation is required, converting to a continuous infusion of lorazepam is recommended (see Figure 9-1). One advantage of lorazepam for long-term sedation is that it does not have active metabolites that contribute to the overall sedative effect. Lorazepam has a slow onset, which makes it unsuitable for the treatment of acute agitation, but it is also very potent.

The major clinical side effects associated with the benzodiazepines are dose-related respiratory depression and hypotension.[6] If needed, *flumazenil* (Romazicon) is the antidote used to reverse benzodiazepine overdose in symptomatic patients.[6] Flumazenil should be avoided in patients with benzodiazepine dependence because rapid withdrawal can induce seizures.[6]

Anesthetic Agents

Propofol (Diprivan) is an IV general anesthetic agent.[2,7] At high doses, propofol is used with other agents to produce a

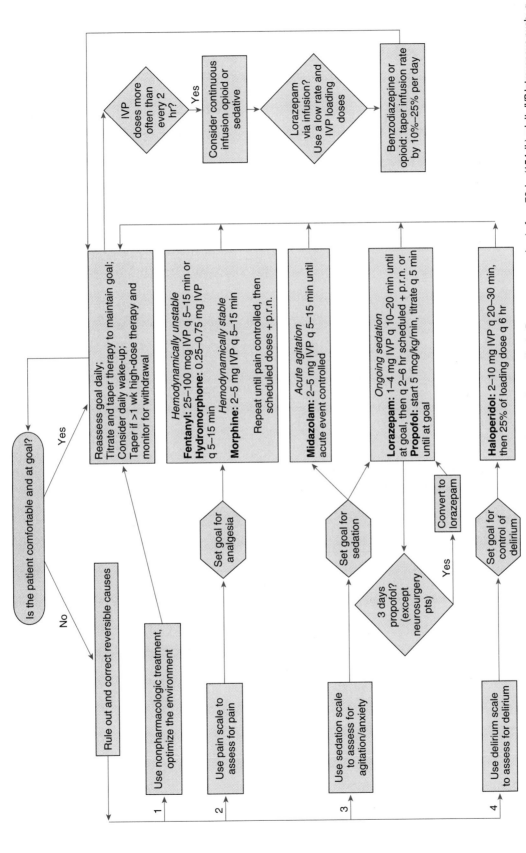

Figure 9-1   General guidelines for sedation and analgesia management of mechanically ventilated critical care patients. Doses are approximate for a 70-kg (154-lb) adult. *IVP,* Intravenous push; *q,* every; *prn,* as needed; *mg,* milligrams; *mcg,* micrograms; *min,* minute; *hr,* hour. (From Jacobi J et al: *Crit Care Med* 30(1):119-141, 2002.)

Table **9-2** Pharmacology of Select Sedatives

Agent	Onset after IV Dose	Half-life of Parent Compound	Metabolic Pathway	Active Metabolite	Unique Adverse Effects	Intermittent IV Dose*	Infusion Dose Range (Usual)
Diazepam	2-5 min	20-120 hr	Desmethylation Hydroxylation	Yes (prolonged sedation)	Phlebitis	0.03-0.1 mg/kg every 0.5-6 hr	
Lorazepam	5-20 min	8-15 hr	Glucuronidation	None	Solvent-related acidosis/renal failure at high doses	0.02-0.06 mg/kg every 2-6 hr	0.01-0.1 mg/kg/hr
Midazolam	2-5 min	3-11 hr	Oxidation	Yes (prolonged sedation, especially with renal failure)		0.02-0.08 mg/kg every 0.5-2 hr	0.04-0.2 mg/kg/hr
Propofol	1-2 min	26-32 hr	Oxidation	None	Elevated triglycerides, pain on injection		5-80 mcg/kg/min
Haloperidol†	3-20 min	18-54 hr	Oxidation	Yes (EPS)	QT-interval prolongation	0.03-0.15 mg/kg every 0.5-6 hr	0.04-0.15 mg/kg/hr

Modified from Jacobi J et al: *Crit Care Med* 30(1):119-141, 2002.
*More frequent doses may be needed for management of acute agitation in mechanically ventilated patients.
†Used in management of delirium. Sedation is an unintended side effect.
IV, Intravenous; *min*, minute; *hr*, hour; *EPS*, extrapyramidal symptoms; *mg*, milligrams; *mcg*, micrograms; *kg*, kilogram.

state of general anesthesia in the operating room. In the critical care unit, propofol is prescribed to induce a state of deep sedation. The advantage of propofol is its very short half-life. It is especially suitable for management of the agitated neurologic patient with brain injury. Propofol slows cerebral metabolism and decreases elevated intracranial pressure.

With short-term administration the drug infusion can be turned off, and the patient can be fully alert within 30 minutes. If propofol is infused for several days, the wake-up time is prolonged, although propofol does not have active metabolites.[7] Propofol is not a reliable amnesic, and patients sedated with only propofol can have vivid recollections of their experiences. It is therefore important to add a narcotic such as *fentanyl* to ensure adequate amnesia.[7]

Significant disadvantages of propofol are mainly related to the high lipid content. It comes packaged in a glass container and has the appearance of milk. Propofol is emulsified in a soybean intralipid emulsion that delivers 1.1 kilocalories per milliliter (kcal/ml) as fat. These calories must be taken into account when assessing nutritional intake. Propofol can elevate serum triglyceride levels and has been associated with pancreatitis. The lipid emulsion can also act as a medium for bacterial growth, although a preservative is added to reduce this complication.[2] Administration requires a dedicated IV line, and all IV solution and tubing must be changed every 12 hours.[7] Propofol shares with other sedatives the propensity for hypotension when delivered rapidly. Propofol is prescribed only for intubated patients.

Central α Agonists

Two central α-adrenergic agonists are available for sedation: clonidine: (often prescribed as a Catapres patch) and dexmedetomidine (Precedex as a continuous infusion). *Clonidine* is prescribed for patients experiencing withdrawal syndromes. *Dexmedetomidine* is a newer α-2 agonist recently approved for use as a short-term sedative (<24 hours) for the mechanically ventilated patient. It is prescribed in some hospitals to wean patients from short-term ventilation after cardiac surgery. At this time there is not enough information to determine whether dexmedetomidine will have a wider role in long-term sedation therapy.[2]

The choice of sedative is very patient and situation specific. If the need is for *short-term* sedation (<24 hours) the most frequently used sedatives are midazolam and propofol.[2,6,7] Both these drugs may be combined with a short-acting opioid analgesic (e.g., fentanyl). If the need is for *intermediate-term* sedation (1 to 3 days), the most frequently prescribed drugs again are propofol and midazolam, plus an opiate. If the need is for *long-term* sedation, the recommended agent is lorazepam.[2]

MANAGING DRUG DEPENDENCE AND WITHDRAWAL

The question of which drugs to use for prolonged sedation is complex. Long-term patients are frequently mechanically ventilated and often seriously ill for weeks or months. To tolerate the ventilator and other procedures, patients must receive sedation and analgesia. When it is time to decrease the sedation, many patients become physically and psychologically dependent, and as the drug dosage is reduced, they become highly agitated.

Physical symptoms of agitation can include increased heart rate, blood pressure, and respiratory rate. Other notable symptoms include lack of self-awareness, unawareness of surroundings, very-short-term memory for information, irritability, anxiety, confusion, delirium, and even seizures.[2] The patient may pull at the tubes, attempt to climb out of bed, and represent a danger to themselves, the nurse, and family visitors. The temptation to resedate is powerful because it is painful to watch a patient experience the stages of withdrawal. During this period the patient does not sleep well, even when sedation provides the appearance of sleep.

One innovative strategy to avoid pitfalls of sedative dependence and withdrawal is a planned "daily drug holiday." This means that all sedative and analgesic agents are turned off once a day.[7] The patient is carefully monitored, and when consciousness and awareness are attained, an assessment of level of consciousness and neurologic function is performed. Reportedly, when regular "daily wake-up periods" and drug infusions are scheduled, patients experience less agitation and a shortened stay on the ventilator. When using protocols that incorporate daily interruption of sedative infusions, it is imperative that accurate assessment be performed and documented during the wake-up period.[8] Also, if the patient becomes agitated, it is essential that a protocol exists that permits the nurse to restart the sedatives, plus opiates if applicable.

One protocol scheduled the daily interruption of sedatives in the morning and, after a full assessment, recommended restarting the sedative and opiate infusions at 50% of the previous morning dose and adjusting upward until the patient was comfortable. Initially it was believed that patients would be highly agitated during each interruption. However, because the patients had less sedative and opiate medication accumulated, they were less restless in the wake-up period.[8]

An important nursing responsibility is to prevent the patient from coming to harm during drug withdrawal (Table 9-3). Some movement in bed is expected, but extreme restlessness increases myocardial oxygen consumption and work of breathing and activates the sympathetic nervous system. If the patient is seriously agitated, it is vital to consult with the physician and pharmacist to establish an effective treatment plan that will allow weaning from these agents without harm. The approach to avoidance of drug dependence and withdrawal symptoms is not yet fully delineated but clearly requires a multidisciplinary effort with ongoing evaluation using an established assessment scale (see Table 9-1).

Table **9-3** Signs and Symptoms of Sedative/Analgesic Drug Withdrawal*

System	Opiate Withdrawal	Benzodiazepine Withdrawal†
Neurologic	Delirium, tremors, seizures	Agitation, anxiety, delirium, tremors, myoclonus, headache, seizures, fatigue, paresthesias, sleep disturbances
Hemodynamic	Tachycardia, hypertension (SNS stimulation)	Tachycardia, hypertension (SNS stimulation)
Sensory	Dilation of pupils, teary eyes, irritability, increased sensitivity to pain, sweating, yawning	Increased sensitivity to light/sound, sweating
Musculoskeletal	Cramps, muscle aches	Muscle cramps
Gastrointestinal	Vomiting, diarrhea	Nausea, diarrhea
Respiratory	Tachypnea	Tachypnea

*Data on propofol is limited, but withdrawal symptoms after prolonged use similar to those of the benzodiazepines.[2]
†Not all symptoms are seen in all patients.[2,9]
SNS, Sympathetic nervous system.

ASSESSING FOR DELIRIUM

Delirium is described as a reversible global impairment of cognitive processes, usually of sudden onset, coupled with disorientation, impaired short-term memory, altered sensory perceptions (hallucinations), abnormal thought processes, and inappropriate behavior.[9] Delirium is probably more prevalent than generally recognized and is difficult to diagnose in the critically ill patient. The incidence ranges from 30% to 70% in medical-surgical critical care patients[2] (Box 9-2).[9]

It is challenging to recognize when a patient has moved from being simply restless, or mildly confused but easily oriented, to a state of delirium. The delirious patient is not always agitated. In fact, it is more difficult to detect delirium when the patient is apparently calm.[2,9] The major categories to assess include (1) acute onset of mental status changes or fluctuating course, (2) inattention, (3) disorganized thinking, and (4) altered level of consciousness, which can include any level of consciousness other than "alert" (vigilant, lethargic, stupor, coma). Routine assessment for the presence of delirium is recommended in critical care patients. Specific scoring scales are available to assess for delirium, and an experienced psychiatric consultant can be helpful.

SELECTING MEDICATIONS FOR MANAGING DELIRIUM

Unfortunately, the medications typically prescribed for sedation and analgesia may exacerbate the symptoms of delirium. Sedatives make delirious patients confused, less responsive, and more obtunded.[9] This situation can also lead to a paradoxical increase in agitation. The neuroleptic drug *haloperidol* (Haldol) is frequently prescribed. This antipsychotic agent stabilizes cerebral function by blocking dopamine-mediated neurotransmission at the cerebral synapses and in the basal ganglia. Delirium is reduced, but the patient tends to have a flat affect, diminished interest in surroundings, and with higher doses becomes sedated.

Box **9-2** Causes of Delirium in Critically Ill Patients

METABOLIC
Acid-base disturbance
Electrolyte imbalance
Hypoglycemia

INTRACRANIAL
Epidural/subdural hematoma
Intracranial hemorrhage
Meningitis
Encephalitis
Cerebral abscess
Tumor

ENDOCRINE
Hyperthyroidism/hypothyroidism
Addison's disease
Hyperparathyroidism
Cushing's syndrome

ORGAN FAILURE
Liver encephalopathy
Uremic encephalopathy
Septic shock

RESPIRATORY
Hypoxemia
Hypercarbia

DRUG RELATED
Alcohol withdrawal
Drug induced
Heavy metal poisoning

Data from Szokol JW, Vender JS: *Crit Care Clin* 17(4):821–842, 2001.

Electrocardiographic (ECG) monitoring is recommended because neuroleptic agents produce dose-dependent QT-interval prolongation, with an increased incidence of ventricular dysrhythmias.[6]

PREVENTING AGITATION AND DELIRIUM

Agitation and delirium are common in critically ill patients.[2,9] Causes are multifactorial, but *sleep deprivation* is experienced by almost all these patients. Even when patients are apparently "sleeping," if the sleep is induced by sedatives, analgesics, neuromuscular blockade, or neuroleptics, it is unlikely that this represents true rapid eye movement (REM) sleep. Similar to pain assessment, self-report of sleep deprivation is considered the most accurate measure.

The *nonpharmacologic* strategies used to prevent agitation and delirium are similar to those used to control pain. These methods include back massage, music therapy, noise reduction in the environment, decreasing lights at night to promote sleep, clustering nursing care to provide some uninterrupted rest periods, and speaking in a calm, quiet, and gentle voice.[2,3,5-8]

CONCLUSION: COLLABORATIVE MANAGEMENT

The goal of making the critical care unit a therapeutic healing environment is shared by patients, families, and health care practitioners alike.[1] Critical care nurses remain challenged by limitations in the medications and monitoring tools currently available.[10] Sedatives for short-term use are fairly well delineated, but no ideal agent is available for long-term sedation. New clinical practice guidelines have resulted in a renewed emphasis on finding appropriate levels of sedation, both to provide comfort and to avoid oversedation.[2]

The role of the critical care nurse is pivotal to act as a patient advocate so that all aspects of patient comfort are considered the "fifth vital sign." Collaborative management of anxiety, agitation, and sedation is a responsibility shared by all members of the health care team (Box 9-3). Recognition of the problem is the first step toward a solution to establish a more effective standard of patient care in sedation/analgesia management.

Box 9-3 COLLABORATIVE Management

Sedation/Analgesia for Critical Care Patients
- Assess patient and determine if sedation and analgesia are required.
- Use sedation scale and analgesia scale to document goal and purpose of therapy.
- Communicate sedation and analgesia goals to all caregivers.
- Consider "daily wake-up" period from sedative agents once patient is stable.
- Provide nonpharmacologic interventions to increase patient comfort (bath, change of position, massage, calm voice, music, calm environment, calm visits from significant people in patient's life).
- When weaning from sedative/opiate agents, monitor for signs and symptoms of withdrawal.
- Educate patient's family about the plan of care and the role of sedative/analgesic agents.

REFERENCES

1. Fraser GL, Riker RR: Monitoring sedation, agitation, analgesia, and delirium in critically ill adult patients, *Crit Care Clin* 17(4):967-987, 2002.
2. Jacobi J et al: Clinical practice guidelines for the sustained use of sedatives and analgesics in the critically ill adult, *Crit Care Med* 30(1):119-141, 2002.
3. Joint Commission on Accreditation of Healthcare Organizations: Standards and intents for sedation and analgesia care in the revisions to anesthesia care standards. In *Comprehensive accreditation manual for hospitals*, Oakbrook Terrace, Ill, 2000, The Commission.
4. Frazier SK et al: Critical care nurses' beliefs about reported management of anxiety, *Am J Crit Care* 12(1):19-27, 2003.
5. McGaffigan P: Advancing sedation assessment to promote patient comfort, *Crit Care Nurs* 22(1 suppl):29-36, 2002.
6. Young CC, Prielipp RC: Benzodiazepines in the intensive care unit, *Crit Care Clin* 17(4):843-862, 2001.
7. Angelini G, Ketzler JT, Coursin DB: Use of propofol and other nonbenzodiazepine sedatives in the intensive care unit, *Crit Care Clin* 17(4):863-880, 2001.
8. Kress JP, Pohlman AS, O'Connor MF, Hall JB: Daily interruption of sedative infusions in critically ill patients undergoing mechanical ventilation, *N Engl J Med* 342(20):1471-1477, 2000.
9. Szokol JW, Vender JS: Anxiety, delirium, and pain in the intensive care unit, *Crit Care Clin* 17(4):821-842, 2001.
10. Arbour R, Continuous nervous system monitoring, EEG, the bispectral index, and neuromuscular transmission, *AACN Clinical Issues* 14(2); 185-207, 2003.

UNIT THREE

CARDIOVASCULAR ALTERATIONS

MARY E. LOUGH

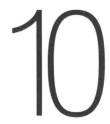

Cardiovascular Assessment and Diagnostic Procedures

Objectives

- Identify the components of a cardiovascular history.
- Describe inspection, palpation, percussion, and auscultation of the patient with cardiovascular dysfunction.
- Discuss the clinical significance of selected laboratory tests used in the assessment of cardiovascular disorders.
- Describe key diagnostic procedures used in assessment of the patient with cardiovascular dysfunction.
- Discuss the nursing management of a patient undergoing a cardiovascular diagnostic procedure.
- Illustrate the proper placement of the electrodes for accurate bedside electrocardiographic (ECG) monitoring.
- Outline the steps in analyzing an ECG rhythm strip.
- Explain the ECG findings and nursing actions for significant atrial, ventricular, and junctional dysrhythmias.
- Describe the use of arterial, central venous, and pulmonary artery catheters for bedside monitoring.

evolve Be sure to check out the free exercises on-line at *http://evolve.elsevier.com/Urden/priorities/*

Physical assessment of the cardiovascular patient is a skill that must not be lost amidst the technology of the critical care setting. Data collected from a thorough, thoughtful history and examination contribute to both the nursing and the medical decisions for therapeutic interventions.

HISTORY

The patient history is important for providing data that contribute to the cardiovascular diagnosis and treatment plan. For a patient in acute distress, the history is curtailed to just a few questions about the patient's chief complaint, precipitating events, and current medications. For a patient without obvious distress, the history focuses on the following four areas:

1. Review of the patient's present illness
2. Overview of the patient's general cardiovascular status, including previous cardiac diagnostic studies, interventional procedures, cardiac surgeries, and current medications (cardiac, noncardiac, herbal)[1]
3. Examination of the patient's general health status, including family history of coronary artery disease (CAD), hypertension, diabetes, and cerebrovascular accident (CVA, stroke)
4. Survey of the patient's lifestyle, including risk factors for CAD

One of the unique challenges in cardiovascular assessment is identifying when "chest pain" is of cardiac origin and when it is not.[2] The following safety information should always be considered:

- If there is any evidence of CAD or risk of heart disease, assume that the chest pain is caused by myocardial ischemia until proven otherwise.[3,4]
- There may be little correlation between the severity of chest discomfort and the gravity of its cause. This is a result of the subjective nature of pain and the unique presentation of ischemic disease in women, elderly patients, and individuals with diabetes.[5,6]
- There is poor correlation between the location of chest discomfort and its source because of *referred pain*. For example, patients with esophageal spasm and gastroesophageal reflux disease (GERD) also present with visceral substernal chest pain that radiates to the left arm and jaw. GERD is also relieved with nitroglycerin. The only differentiating characteristic between angina and esophageal spasm is the longer duration of esophageal pain.[7-9]

Other common symptoms that may signal cardiac dysfunction are dyspnea, palpitations, cough, fatigue, edema, leg pain, nocturia, syncope, and cyanosis.

PHYSICAL EXAMINATION

A comprehensive physical assessment is fundamental to achievement of an accurate diagnosis. The nurse who has developed the skills of inspection, palpation, and auscultation will be confident when assessing patients with cardiovascular disease.

Inspection

The priorities for inspection of the patient with cardiovascular dysfunction are (1) assessing the patient's general appearance, (2) evaluating jugular veins, (3) observing the apical impulse, and (4) examining the extremities.

Assessing General Appearance

The weight in proportion to the height is assessed to determine whether the patient is obese or cachectic. The face is observed for the color of the skin (cyanotic, pale, or jaundiced) and for apprehensive or painful expressions. Body posture can indicate the amount of effort it takes to breathe. For example, sitting upright to breathe may be necessary for the patient with acute heart failure, and leaning forward may be the least painful position for the patient with pericarditis. The patient is also observed for diaphoresis, confusion, or lethargy, each of which could indicate hypotension or low cardiac output (CO).

The skin, lips, tongue, and mucous membranes are inspected for pallor or cyanosis. *Central cyanosis* is a bluish discoloration of the tongue and sublingual area. Multiracial studies indicate that the tongue is the most sensitive site for observation of central cyanosis, which must be recognized and treated as a medical emergency. Pulse oximetry, arterial blood gas analysis, and treatment with 100% oxygen must be instituted immediately.[3]

Evaluating Jugular Veins

The jugular veins of the neck are inspected for a noninvasive estimate of intravascular volume and pressure. The external jugular veins are observed for jugular vein distention (Figure 10-1 and Box 10-1). *Jugular venous distention* occurs when central venous pressure is elevated, which occurs with fluid volume overload and right ventricular dysfunction.[10] The right internal jugular vein can be used for measurement of central venous pressure in centimeters of water (cm H_2O) (Figure 10-2 and Box 10-2).

Observing Apical Impulse

The anterior thorax is inspected for the *apical impulse*, sometimes referred to as the *point of maximal impulse* (PMI). The apical impulse occurs as the left ventricle contracts during systole and rotates forward, causing the left ventricular apex of the heart to hit the chest wall. The apical impulse is a quick, localized, outward movement normally located just lateral to the left midclavicular line at the fifth intercostal space in the adult patient (Figure 10-3). The apical impulse is the only normal pulsation visualized on the chest wall. In the patient without cardiac disease, PMI may not be noticeable.

Examining Extremities

The last area of inspection focuses on the extremities. The nailbeds are inspected for signs of discoloration or peripheral cyanosis. *Peripheral cyanosis* indicates reduction of peripheral blood flow as a result of vascular disease or decreased

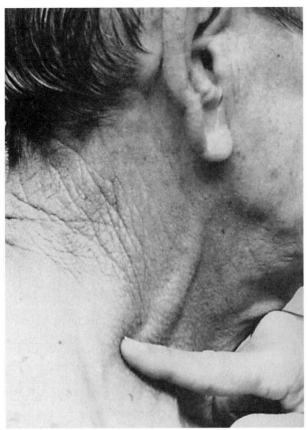

Figure 10-1   Assessment of jugular vein distention (JVD). Applying light finger pressure over sternocleidomastoid muscle, parallel to clavicle, helps identify external jugular vein by occluding flow and distending it. Release finger pressure, and observe for true distention. In the patient without heart failure, when the patient's trunk is elevated 30 degrees or more, JVD should not be present.

CO. The arms and legs are assessed for signs of vascular disease (Table 10-1).

Palpation

The priorities for palpation of the patient with cardiovascular dysfunction are (1) assessing arterial pulses, (2) evaluating capillary refill, (3) estimating edema, (4) observing for signs of deep vein thrombosis, and (5) evaluating thoracic and abdominal pulsations.

Assessing Arterial Pulses

Seven major arterial pulses are palpated. The examination incorporates bilateral assessment of the carotid, brachial, radial, ulnar, popliteal, dorsalis pedis, and posterior tibial arteries. The pulses are palpated separately and compared bilaterally to check for consistency. Pulse volume is graded on a scale of 0 to 3+ (Box 10-3). A diminished or absent pulse may indicate low CO or the presence of arterial stenosis or occlusion proximal to the site of the examination. An abnormally strong or bounding pulse suggests the presence of an aneurysm or an occlusion distal to the examination site. If a distal pulse cannot be palpated using light finger pressure, a Doppler ultrasound stethoscope is often helpful (Box 10-4). It is important to mark the location of the audible signal with an indelible ink marker pen for future evaluation of pulse quality.

Evaluating Capillary Refill

Capillary refill assessment is a maneuver using the nailbeds to evaluate both arterial circulation to the extremity and overall perfusion. The nailbed is compressed to produce blanching, and the release of the pressure should result in a return of blood flow and baseline nail color in less than 3 seconds. The severity of arterial insufficiency is directly proportional to the amount of time necessary to reestablish flow and color.

Estimating Edema

Edema is fluid accumulated in the extravascular spaces of the body. The dependent tissues within the legs and sacrum are particularly susceptible. Note whether the edema is dependent, unilateral or bilateral, pitting or nonpitting. The amount of edema is quantified by measuring the circumference of the limb or by pressing the skin of the feet, ankles, and shins against the underlying bone. Edema is a symptom associated with several diseases and further diagnostic evaluation is required to determine the cause. Although no universal scale for pitting edema exists, typical scales use a 0 to 4+ system (Table 10-2).

Box **10-1**   Procedure for Assessing Jugular Vein Distention (JVD)

1. Patient reclines at a 30- to 45-degree angle.
2. Examiner stands on patient's right side and turns patient's head slightly toward the left.
3. If jugular vein is not visible, light finger pressure is applied across sternocleidomastoid muscle just above and parallel to clavicle. This pressure will fill external jugular vein by obstructing flow (see Figure 10-1).
4. Once location of vein has been identified, pressure is released and presence of JVD assessed.

5. Because inhalation decreases venous pressure, JVD should be assessed at end-exhalation.
6. Any fullness in the vein extending more than 3 cm above sternal angle is evidence of increased venous pressure. Generally the higher the sitting angle of the patient when JVD is visualized, the higher the central venous pressure.
7. *Documentation*: JVD is reported by including angle of the head of the bed at the time JVD was evaluated (e.g., "presence of JVD with head of bed elevated to 45 degrees").

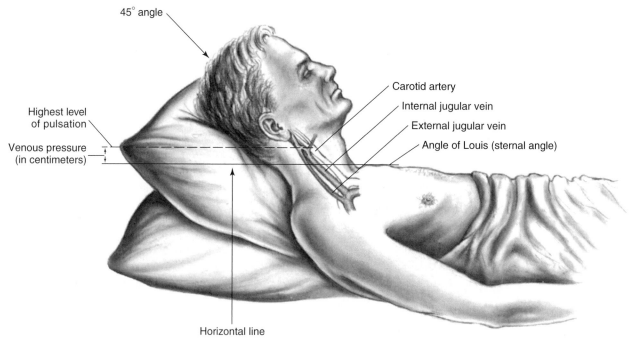

45° angle

Carotid artery

Internal jugular vein

External jugular vein

Angle of Louis (sternal angle)

Highest level
of pulsation

Venous pressure
(in centimeters)

Horizontal line

Figure 10-2 Position of internal and external jugular veins. Pulsation in internal jugular vein can be used to estimate central venous pressure. (Modified from Thompson JM et al: *Mosby's clinical nursing,* ed 5, St Louis, 2002, Mosby.)

Box **10-2**	**Procedure for Assessing Central Venous Pressure (CVP)**

1. Patient reclines in bed. Highest point of pulsation in the internal jugular vein is observed during exhalation.
2. Vertical distance between this pulsation (at top of fluid level) and the sternal angle is estimated or measured in centimeters (cm).
3. This number is then added to 5 cm for an estimation of CVP. The 5 cm is the approximate distance of sternal angle above level of right atrium (see Figure 10-2).
4. *Documentation*: Degree of elevation of patient is included in report (e.g., "CVP estimated at 13 cm, using internal jugular vein pulsation, with head of bed elevated 45 degrees").

Observing for Signs of Deep Vein Thrombosis

Deep vein thrombosis (DVT) predisposes patients with many different diagnoses to pulmonary emboli. Although fewer than 23% to 50% of patients with DVT have signs or symptoms, almost 50% of all patients with documented DVT were found to have pulmonary embolism, underscoring the importance of DVT detection. Symptoms that may indicate DVT include intermittent or constant pain, tenderness, and a tight or heavy sensation, as well as temperature changes in the affected extremity and a low-grade fever. The most common physical finding is the development of edema in only one extremity. Testing for *Homans sign* is a traditional although unreliable tool. Almost 80% of patients with DVT exhibit a negative Homans sign. Patients considered at risk for DVT include those with a history of DVT (30% will experience a recurrence), those hospitalized with heart disease, and individuals older than 40 years of age who have had major surgery or myocardial infarction (MI).[11-16]

Evaluating Thoracic and Abdominal Pulsations

The chest wall is palpated for the apical impulse. The entire precordium is then assessed for additional pulsations, vibrations, heaves, or thrills (see Figure 10-3). The abdomen is palpated for pulsations of the femoral arteries and the descending aortic artery. The femoral arteries are palpated by pressing deeply into the groin beneath the inguinal ligament, approximately midway between the anterior superior iliac spine and the symphysis pubis on both right and left sides. The aortic pulsation is normally located in the epigastric area and can be felt as a forward movement by using firm fingertip pressure above the umbilicus. If prominent or diffuse, the pulsation may indicate an abdominal aneurysm.

Auscultation

The priorities for auscultation of the patient with cardiovascular dysfunction are (1) measuring blood pressure, (2) detecting bruits, (3) assessing normal heart sounds, and (4) identifying abnormal heart sounds, murmurs, and pericardial friction rubs.

Measuring Blood Pressure

Blood pressure is measured in both arms to rule out aortic or subclavian stenosis. Normally the blood pressure between

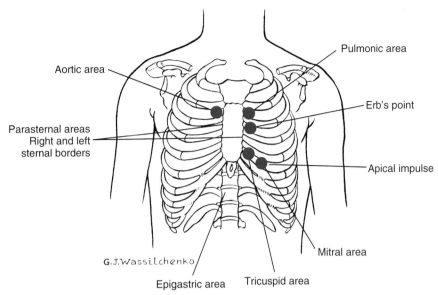

Figure 10-3   Thoracic palpation and auscultation points.

Table **10-1**	Inspection and Palpation of Extremities: Arterial Disease versus Venous Disease	
Characteristic	**Arterial Disease**	**Venous Disease**
Hair loss	Present (minimal leg hair)	Absent (normal leg hair)
Skin texture	Thin, shiny, dry	Flaking, stasis, dermatitis, mottled
Ulceration	Located at pressure points; painful, pale, dry with little drainage; well demarcated with eschar or dried; surrounded by fibrous tissue; scant, pale granulation tissue	Usually at the ankle; painless, pink, moist with large amount of drainage; irregular, dry, scaly; surrounded by dermatitis; healthy granulation tissue
Skin color	Elevational pallor, dependent rubor	Brawny, brown, cyanotic when dependent
Nails	Thick, brittle	Normal
Varicose veins	Absent	Present
Temperature	Cool	Warm
Capillary refill	>3 seconds	<3 seconds
Edema	None or mild, usually unilateral	Usually present foot to calf, unilateral or bilateral
Pulses	Weak or absent (0 to 1+)	Normal, strong, symmetric

Modified from Krenzer ME: *AACN Clin Issues* 6:631, 1995.

both arms varies only 5 to 10 millimeters of mercury (mm Hg). A difference of 20 mm Hg or more suggests arterial obstruction on the side with the lower pressure.[17,18] Asymmetry is documented so that all subsequent measurements are made on the arm with the higher pressure. Evaluation of orthostatic blood pressure changes may also be necessary (Box 10-5).

Box **10-3**	Pulse Palpation Scale
0	Not palpable
1+	Faintly palpable (weak and thready)
2+	Palpable (normal pulse)
3+	Bounding (hyperdynamic pulse)

Detecting Bruits

The carotid and femoral arteries are auscultated for bruits. A *bruit* is a high-pitched "sh-sh" extracardiac vascular sound that vacillates in volume with systole and diastole. An abnormal bruit is produced as blood flows through a partially occluded vessel. The auscultation of a bruit can expedite the diagnosis of suspected arterial obstruction in combination with inspection and palpation of the lower extremities.

Assessing Normal Heart Sounds

Auscultation of the heart is the most challenging part of the cardiac physical examination and, in an era of increasing technologic demands, is daunting to new clinicians.[19] Normal heart sounds are referred to as the *first heart sound*

| Box **10-4** | Use of Doppler Ultrasound Stethoscope |

1. Liberally apply ultrasound gel to the pulse point.
2. Insert tip of probe into gel at a 45- to 60-degree angle to blood vessel, applying light pressure.
3. Ultrasound waves do not pass through air, so use adequate gel to exclude air.
4. Water-soluble lubricating gel can be substituted, but never use ECG electrode gel because it will damage the probe.
5. Activate the stethoscope by turning it on or pressing the activation button.
   Doppler ultrasonography, a velocity detector, detects the shift in ultrasound frequency that results when the transmitted

beam is reflected off moving particles within blood vessels. It can detect arterial signals in a vessel with a pressure as low as 20 mm Hg. Signals are generated by both arteries and veins, each with distinct characteristic patterns. Normal peripheral arteries have a biphasic or triphasic pulsatile sound. With a partially obstructed sound, one or more components are lost, but the sound remains pulsatile. A *normal* venous signal is a low-frequency sound resembling a windstorm that varies with respiration. Venous signals can be absent during Valsalva maneuver. A *positive* Doppler signal indicates presence of blood flow but not adequacy of perfusion.

From Krenzer ME: AACN Clin Issues Crit Care Nurs 6:631, 1995.

| Table **10-2** | Pitting Edema Scale |

		Indentation Depth		
	Edema	Inches	Metric	Time to Baseline
0	None	—	—	—
1+	Trace	0 to ¼	<6.5 mm	Rapid
2+	Mild	¼ to ½	6.5-12.5 mm	10-15 seconds
3+	Moderate	½ to 1	12.5 mm-2.5 cm	1-2 minutes
4+	Severe	>1	>2.5 cm	2-5 minutes

(S_1) and the *second heart sound* (S_2). S_1 is the sound associated with mitral and tricuspid valve closure and is heard most clearly in the mitral and tricuspid areas. S_2 (aortic and pulmonic closure) can be heard best at the second intercostal space to the right and left of the sternum (see Figure 10-3). Both sounds are high pitched and heard best with the diaphragm of the stethoscope. Each sound is loudest in an auscultation area located "downstream" from the actual valvular component of the sound.

Identifying Abnormal Heart Sounds, Murmurs, and Pericardial Rubs

The abnormal heart sounds are labeled as the *third heart sound* (S_3) and *fourth heart sound* (S_4) and are referred to as *gallops* when auscultated during a tachycardia.[20] These low-pitched sounds occur during diastole and are best heard with the bell of stethoscope positioned lightly over the apical impulse. The presence of S_3 may be normal in children and young adults because of rapid filling of the ventricle in a young, healthy heart. However, an S_3 in the presence of cardiac symptoms is an indication of increased end-systolic volume suggestive of heart failure with fluid overload.[21,22] Auscultation of an S_4 also leads the examiner to suspect heart failure and decreased ventricular compliance.

Heart valve murmurs are prolonged extra sounds that occur during systole or diastole. The sounds are vibrations caused by turbulent blood flow through cardiac chambers or valves. Murmurs are characterized by their timing (systolic/diastolic), location and radiation, quality (blowing, grating, harsh), pitch (high or low), and intensity, with

| Box **10-5** | Measurement of Postural (Orthostatic) Vital Signs |

GUIDELINES
1. Record blood pressure (BP) and heart rate (HR) in each position.
2. Do not remove cuff between measurements.
3. Record all associated signs and symptoms.
4. Clearly document patient position.

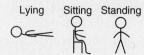

Lying   Sitting   Standing

TECHNIQUE
1. Keep patient as flat as possible for 10 minutes before initial assessment.
2. Obtain supine BP and HR measurements.
3. Patient sitting with legs hanging: measure immediately and after 2 minutes.

4. Patient standing: measure immediately and after 2 minutes.
   • If BP and HR stable but orthostasis suspected, BP and HR can be repeated every 2 minutes.
   • Note that this is rarely practical for the critically ill patient.

RESULTS
Normal Changes
• HR increases by 5 to 20 beats/min (transiently).
• Systolic BP drops 10 mm Hg.
• Diastolic BP drops 5 mm Hg.

Positive Orthostatasis
• Drop in systolic BP >20 mm Hg.
• Drop in diastolic BP >10 mm Hg within 3 minutes.

loudness graded on a scale of I to VI (Box 10-6). When auscultating murmurs, the examiner visualizes the cardiac anatomy, specifically the location of the heart valves and the direction of sound transmission with valve closure and specific murmur in mind. Generally the systolic valvular murmurs radiate downstream from the valve that is narrowed (stenotic), and the diastolic valvular murmurs (indicating a backflow of blood through an incompetent valve) are auscultated best directly over the area of the valve[23-25] (Table 10-3).

Box 10-6 Grading of Cardiac Murmurs

I/VI	Very faint; may be heard only in a quiet environment
II/VI	Quiet, but clearly audible
III/VI	Moderately loud
IV/VI	Loud; may be associated with a palpable thrill
V/VI	Very loud; thrill easily palpable
VI/VI	Very loud; may be heard with stethoscope off the chest. Thrill palpable and visible

Table 10-3 Characteristics of Heart Murmurs

Defect	Timing in Cardiac Cycle	Pitch, Intensity, Quality	Location, Radiation
SYSTOLIC MURMURS			
Mitral regurgitation	S_1 — S_2	High / Harsh / Blowing	Mitral area / May radiate to axilla
Tricuspid regurgitation	S_1 — S_2	High / Often faint, but varies / Blowing	Tricuspid RLSB, apex, LLSB, epigastric areas / Little radiation
Ventricular septal defect	S_1 — S_2	High / Loud / Blowing	Left sternal border
Aortic stenosis	S_1 — S_2	Chhhh hh / Medium / Rough, harsh	Aortic area to suprasternal notch, right side of neck, apex
Pulmonary stenosis	S_1 — S_2	Low to medium / Loud / Harsh, grinding	Pulmonic area / No radiation
DIASTOLIC MURMURS			
Mitral stenosis	S_2 — Atrial kick — S_1	Low / Quiet to loud with thrill / Rough rumble	Mitral area / Usually no radiation
Tricuspid stenosis	S_2 — Atrial kick — S_1	Medium / Quiet; louder with inspiration / Rumble	Tricuspid area or epigastrium / Little radiation
Aortic regurgitation	S_2 — S_1	High / Faint to medium / Blowing	Aortic area to LLSB and aorta / Erb's point
Pulmonic regurgitation	S_2 — S_1	Medium / Faint / Blowing	Pulmonic area / No radiation

RLSB, Right lower sternal border; *LLSB*, left lower sternal border.

A *pericardial friction rub* is a sound that can occur within 2 to 7 days of an MI. A rub occurs in about 5% of patients who receive thrombolytic agents or other interventional procedures for acute MI.[26] The friction rub results from pericardial inflammation (*pericarditis*). Classically, a pericardial friction rub is a grating or scratching sound that is both systolic and diastolic, corresponding with cardiac motion within the pericardial sac. It is often associated with chest pain, which can be aggravated by deep inspiration, coughing, swallowing, and changing position. It is important to differentiate pericarditis from acute myocardial ischemia, and the detection of the pericardial friction rub through auscultation can assist in this differentiation, leading to effective diagnosis and treatment.[26]

LABORATORY ASSESSMENT

The priorities for laboratory assessment for the patient with cardiovascular dysfunction focus on (1) **interpreting serum electrolytes and safely replacing electrolyte deficiencies,** (2) **monitoring cardiac enzyme levels,** (3) **trending hematologic studies,** (4) **assessing coagulation values,** and (5) **evaluating the serum lipid profile.**

Interpreting Serum Electrolytes
Potassium
During depolarization and repolarization of nerve and muscle fibers, potassium and sodium exchange occurs intracellularly and extracellularly. The potassium gradient across the cell membrane determines conduction velocity and helps confine pacing activity to the sinus node. Excess or deficiency of potassium can alter myocardial muscle function. Normal serum potassium levels are 3.5 to 5.5 milliequivalents per liter (mEq/L).

Hyperkalemia. Hyperkalemia is an elevated serum potassium level of greater than 5.5 mEq/L. Hyperkalemia can be caused by a variety of conditions, including excess potassium administration, extensive skeletal muscle destruction (rhabdomyolysis), potassium-sparing diuretics, and renal failure.[27-31] Hyperkalemia elicits significant changes in the electrocardiogram (ECG) as the serum level rises above 5.5 mEq/L. Peaked T waves are usually, although not uniquely, associated with early hyperkalemia and are followed by a widening of the QRS complex and prolongation of the P wave and PR interval (Figure 10-4, A). With untreated severe hyperkalemia, either ventricular fibrillation or cardiac standstill will result. This life-threatening condition can be acutely managed with an intravenous (IV) insulin/glucose infusion that drives the potassium inside the cell and temporarily out of the serum. Potassium is permanently removed from the serum by diuretics, cation-exchange resin products (e.g., Kayexalate) for the gastrointestinal (GI) tract, and hemodialysis.

Hypokalemia. Hypokalemia is a low serum potassium level of less than 3.5 mEq/L. Hypokalemia is typically caused by GI losses, diuretic therapy with insufficient replacement,

or chronic steroid therapy. Hypokalemia is also reflected by changes on the ECG (Figure 10-4, B). The earliest ECG change is often premature ventricular contractions (PVCs), which can deteriorate into ventricular tachycardia/fibrillation (VT/VF) without appropriate potassium replacement.[32,33] Severe hypokalemia produces a prominent U wave (a positive deflection following the T wave on the ECG). The U wave is not totally unique to hypokalemia, but its presence is a signal for the clinician to check the serum potassium level. If concomitant hypomagnesemia exists, successful replenishment of potassium deficit cannot be accomplished until the hypomagnesemia is reversed.

Calcium
Calcium is an important mediator of many cardiovascular functions because of its effect on vascular tone, myocardial contractility, and cardiac excitability. The most common blood test for calcium levels is total serum calcium; normal range is 8.5 to 10.5 milligrams per deciliter (mg/dl). The biologically active portion of the total calcium is called the *ionized* calcium. Ionized calcium is primarily responsible for the pathophysiologic effects of hypercalcemia and hypocalcemia. The normal serum concentration of ionized calcium is maintained within very narrow limits (4 to 5 mg/dl).

Hypercalcemia. Hypercalcemia is an increase of ionized calcium (greater than 4.8 mg/dl) or an increase of total serum calcium (greater than 10.5 mg/dl). Serum calcium levels are increased by bone tumors, some endocrine disorders, hypomagnesemia, and excessive intake of vitamin D.[34] This condition has the cardiovascular effect of strengthening contractility and shortening ventricular repolarization. The ECG demonstrates the shortened repolarization with a shortened QT interval. Rhythm disturbances may include bradycardia; first-, second-, and third-degree heart block; and bundle branch block. Hypercalcemia can potentiate the effects of digitalis, precipitate digitalis toxicity, and cause hypertension.[35,36]

Hypocalcemia. Hypocalcemia is defined as an ionized calcium level less than 4.0 mg/dl or a total serum calcium level less than 8.5 mg/dl, with a normal albumin level and normal serum pH. Hypocalcemia is common in critically ill and postsurgical patients because of fluid shifts, blood transfusions (the citrate used as an anticoagulant in bank blood binds to the calcium), and magnesium depletion. The cardiovascular effects of hypocalcemia include decreased myocardial contractility, reduced cardiac output, decreased cardiac responsiveness to digitalis, and hypotension. Hypocalcemia lengthens the ST segment and QT interval on the ECG. Rhythm disturbances are variable, ranging from bradycardia to VT and asystole. When the ionized calcium is less than 3.2 mg/dl, the ECG typically demonstrates a prolonged QT interval. An ionized calcium level this low is considered a medical emergency and requires immediate reversal with an IV infusion of calcium.[37]

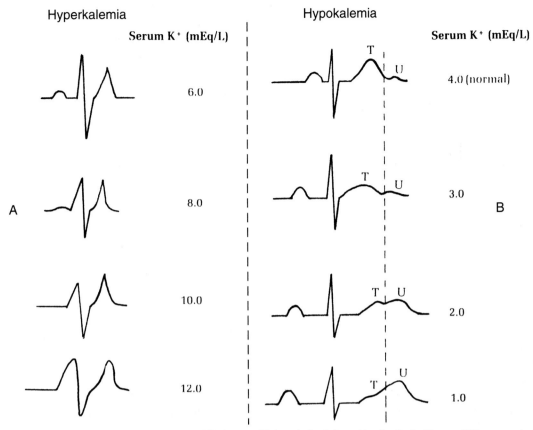

Figure 10-4   **A,** Hyperkalemia. Earliest electrocardiogram (ECG) change with hyperkalemia is peaking (tenting) of T wave. With progressive increases in serum potassium level, QRS complexes widen, P waves disappear, and finally, ventricular fibrillation occurs. **B,** Hypokalemia. Variable ECG patterns may be seen, ranging from slight T-wave flattening to appearance of U waves, sometimes with ST-segment depressions or T-wave inversions.

Magnesium

Magnesium is essential for many enzyme, protein, lipid, and carbohydrate functions in the body and is critical for the production and use of energy. In the bloodstream, magnesium is found predominantly within the cells, although an adequate serum level (extracellular) is essential to normal cardiac and skeletal muscle function. Serum magnesium can be reported either in mEq/L or mg/dl depending on the laboratory running the analysis. The normal serum range is 1.8 to 2.4 mg/dl (1.5 to 2.0 mEq/L) and varies slightly depending on the methods and reference values used by each laboratory.

Hypermagnesemia. The incidence of hypermagnesemia is rare compared with hypomagnesemia. Hypermagnesemia is most often seen with renal insufficiency or iatrogenic overtreatment.[38]

Hypomagnesemia. Hypomagnesemia is low serum magnesium concentration of less than 1.8 mg/dl (or less than 1.5 mEq/L). It is often associated with other electrolyte imbalances, most notably potassium, sodium, calcium, and phosphorus. Hypomagnesemia can be caused by insufficient intake in the diet or in total parenteral nutrition (TPN), chronic alcohol abuse, diuresis, diarrhea, or rapid adminis-

tration of citrated blood products, which causes the citrate to bind to the magnesium (citrate chelation).[39-41]

Both hypokalemia and hypocalcemia are likely to be unresponsive to replacement therapy until the hypomagnesemia is corrected.[33] Cardiac changes with hypomagnesemia include hypertension and vasospasm, including coronary artery spasm. Several studies have linked magnesium depletion to sudden cardiac death, increased incidence of acute MI, and ventricular dysrhythmias.[42] Dysrhythmias associated with hypomagnesemia may not respond to usual antidysrhythmic drugs but often respond well to magnesium infusions. IV magnesium sulfate is the treatment of choice for torsades de pointes.[41,43] It is advised to evaluate renal function when administering magnesium to avoid precipitating hypermagnesium states.[38]

Safely Replacing Electrolyte Deficiencies

Recognizing electrolyte deficiencies and safely replacing the depletion is an important critical care nursing responsibility. Unfortunately, several patients have died as a result of rapid administration of concentrated electrolyte solutions. As a result, several health care organizations have recommended that concentrated potassium solutions not be stored directly on nursing units but rather come prediluted from the pharmacy (Box 10-7).

Monitoring Cardiac Enzymes

Cardiac enzymes are proteins that are released from irreversibly damaged myocardial tissue cells. Enzymes can be divided into *cardiac-specific* enzymes that are present only in cardiac muscle and *nonspecific* enzymes present in many muscles of the body. The enzymes that are routinely measured include the cardiac-specific enzymes troponin I (TnI), troponin T (TnT), and *creatine kinase–myocardial band* (CK-MB) as well as the nonspecific muscle enzymes *myoglobin* and *creatine kinase* (CK)[44,45] (Table 10-4).

---

patient safety Box **10-7**

Goals for Medication Administration

1. **Improve the accuracy of patient identification.**
   - Use at least two patient identifiers (not patient's room number) whenever taking blood samples or administering medications or blood products. Examples include: patient name, date of birth, and hospital record number.
2. **Improve the effectiveness of communication among caregivers.**
   - Hospitals should have (or implement) a process for taking verbal or telephone orders that requires a verification "read-back" of the complete order by the person receiving the order.

Because thousands of brand name and generic drugs are available, there is always potential for error. Similar drug names, either written or spoken, account for approximately 15% of all medication error reports to the *U.S. Pharmacopeia* (USP) Medication Errors Reporting program.

In March 2001 the USP released "Use Caution, Avoid Confusion," an updated list highlighting hundreds of confusing drug name sets and identifying more than 750 unique drug names that have been reported to the Medication Errors Reporting program. A poster and a laminated, quick-reference card are available for health care professionals free of charge from the USP by contacting USP's Practitioner and Product Experience department at 800-487-7776, or the list may be accessed from USP's website at *www.usp.org/reporting/review/*.

An organizational method to decrease number of medication errors is the use of *computerized physician order entry* (CPOE), as advocated by the Leapfrog group: *www.leapfroggroup.org*.

   - Standardize the abbreviations, acronyms, and symbols used throughout the organization, including a list of abbreviations, acronyms, and symbols not to use.

Examples of problematic abbreviations include "U" for "units" and "μg" for "micrograms." When handwritten, "U" can be mistaken for a zero; in numerous case reports, an insulin dosage in "U" was interpreted as "0." Using the abbreviation "μg" instead of "mcg" for micrograms is also problematic; when handwritten, the symbol "μ" can look like an "m."

Use of "trailing zeros" (e.g., 2.0 vs. 2) and a "leading decimal point without a leading zero" (e.g., .2 instead of 0.2) are also dangerous prescription-writing practices. Misinterpretation of such abbreviations has caused and could lead to 10-fold dosing errors.

Information on similar medication issues is available on the web pages of the Joint Commission for the Accreditation of Healthcare Organizations (JCAHO): *www.JCAHO.org*.

3. **Improve the safety of using high-alert medications.**
   - Remove concentrated electrolytes (including but not limited to potassium chloride, potassium phosphate, and hypertonic sodium chloride) from patient care units.
   - Standardize and limit the number of drug concentrations available in the organization.

In the first 2 years after enacting a "sentinel event" reporting mechanism, the most common category was medication errors, and the most frequently implicated drug was potassium chloride (KCl). JCAHO reviewed 10 incidents of patient death resulting from misadministration of KCl. Eight were the result of direct infusion of concentrated KCl. In six of the eight cases the KCl was mistaken for another medication, primarily due to similarities in packaging and labeling. Most often, KCl was mistaken for sodium chloride, heparin, or furosemide (Lasix).

JCAHO suggests that health care organizations NOT make concentrated KCl available outside the pharmacy unless appropriate, specific safeguards are in place.

4. **Improve the safety of using infusion pumps.**
   - Ensure free-flow protection on all general-use and patient-controlled analgesia (PCA) intravenous (IV) infusion pumps used in the organization.

Infusion pumps that do not provide protection from the free flow of IV fluid or medication into the patient are hazardous. USP reported six cases in which a patient died because an IV pump did not provide protection from free flow of the IV solution. (October 1991 to November 1999: four additional cases resulted in near-death.)

Free flow occurs when IV solution flows freely, under force of gravity, without being controlled by the infusion pump. Free flow typically occurs after the administration set is temporarily removed from the pump to transfer a patient to another area, change a patient's gown, or place a patient on a radiography table. Clinicians can greatly reduce this risk by using administration sets with set-based anti–free-flow mechanisms that prevent gravity free flow by closing off the IV tubing to prohibit flow when the administration set is removed from the pump.

The information in this safety box can be accessed on the web pages of the following three safety organizations: Joint Commission on Accreditation of Healthcare Organizations (*www.JCAHO.org*); U.S. Pharmacopeia (*www.usp.org*); The Leapfrog Group (*www.leapfroggroup.org*).

Table 10-4	Serum Markers after Acute Myocardial Infarction (MI)*		
Marker	**Earliest Increase**	**Peak**	**Return to Normal**
Total CK	3-6 hours	24-36 hours	3 days
CK-MB	4-8 hours	15-24 hours	3-4 days
Myoglobin	2-3 hours	6-9 hours	12 hours
Troponin T	4-6 hours	10-24 hours	10-15 days
Troponin I	4-6 hours	10-24 hours	10-15 days

*Time periods represent average reported values. There is a range of reported values because different studies use different time periods after onset of symptoms, different benchmarks for establishing the diagnosis, and different patient populations.
CK, Creatine kinase.

Serum Creatine Kinase

The traditional "gold standard" for diagnosing MI is the rise and fall of the serum MB fraction of CK. The CK-MB serum levels elevate 4 to 8 hours after MI, peak at 15 to 24 hours, and remain elevated for 2 to 3 days. Serial samples are drawn routinely every 6 to 12 hours, and three samples are usually sufficient to support or rule out the diagnosis of MI.

Troponin

The troponins are a structurally related group of proteins found in both cardiac and skeletal muscle and are termed *cardiac troponin I* (cTnI) and *cardiac troponin T* (cTnT). Because of the specific cardiac nature of TnI and TnT, both are used as markers of acute MI, both in centralized laboratory tests [44-46] and in bedside point-of-care testing.[47,48] Several different methods of laboratory assay are currently in clinical use, which means that "normal" serum levels will vary between different clinical settings, although serum cardiac TnI and TnT levels are very low in the absence of myocardial muscle damage.

Myoglobin

Myoglobin is a nonspecific indicator of myocardial cell damage because it is identical in both cardiac and skeletal muscle. Myoglobin is useful because it is the enzyme that rises earliest in the serum, about 2 hours after myocardial injury. It is never used alone but can be used in conjunction with other, more cardiac-specific enzyme markers.[45]

Trending Hematologic Studies

Hematologic laboratory studies routinely ordered for the management of patients with altered cardiovascular status include red blood cell (RBC), hemoglobin (Hgb), hematocrit (Hct), and white blood cell (WBC) concentrations.

Red Blood Cells

The normal amount of RBCs present varies with age, gender, altitude, and exercise. *Anemia* is a clinical condition in which insufficient RBCs are available to carry oxygen to the tissues. *Polycythemia* occurs when excess RBCs are produced.

Hemoglobin and Hematocrit

Normal Hgb levels are 14 to 18 grams per deciliter (g/dl) in males and 12 to 16 g/dl in females. The Hct is the percentage of RBCs in whole blood: 40% to 54% for men and 38% to 48% for women.

White Blood Cells

Most inflammatory processes (e.g., rheumatic fever, endocarditis, MI) that produce necrotic tissue within the heart muscle increase the WBC count. The normal WBC level for both men and women is 5000 to 10,000 cells/mm^3.

Assessing Blood Coagulation Values

Coagulation studies are ordered to determine effectiveness of blood clotting. Anticoagulants, most notably heparin, warfarin, and platelet inhibitory agents (e.g., GPIIb/IIIa agents, aspirin), are administered to decrease MI extension and to reduce the incidence of reocclusion after successful coronary artery reperfusion, as well as for management of patients with unstable angina and non–ST-segment elevation acute MI.[3,49,50] Patients who have stasis of blood, valvular heart disease, atrial fibrillation, or a history of thrombosis are at risk for developing a thrombus and usually require anticoagulation.[23,51] Coagulation studies are required to guide dosage of antithrombotic drugs (Table 10-5).

Prothrombin Time and International Normalized Ratio

Most coagulation study results are reported as the length of time in seconds it takes for blood to form a clot in the laboratory test tube. The *prothrombin time* (PT) is also reported as an *international normalized ratio* (INR). The INR was developed by the World Health Organization (WHO) in an attempt to standardize PT results among clinical laboratories worldwide. The PT and INR are used to determine therapeutic dosage of warfarin (Coumadin) necessary to achieve anticoagulation.[52,53]

Table 10-5	Adult Coagulation Values	
Test	**Normal Value**	**Therapeutic Value**
PT	11-16 seconds*	1.5-2.5 times normal
INR	<1.0	Chronic atrial fibrillation 2.0-3.0
		Treatment of DVT/PE 2.0-3.0
		Mechanical heart valve(s) 2.5-3.5
aPTT	28-38 seconds	1.5-2.5 times normal
PTT	60-90 seconds	1.5-2.0 times normal
ACT†	70-120 seconds	150-190 seconds
		>300 seconds post-PCI

*May vary by 2 seconds among different laboratories.
†Normal, therapeutic, and postprocedure values may vary with type of anticoagulant used.
PT, Prothrombin time; INR, international normalized ratio; aPTT, activated partial thromboplastin time; PTT, partial thromboplastin time; ACT, activated coagulation time; DVT, deep vein thrombosis; PE, pulmonary embolism.

Partial Thromboplastin Time and Activated Coagulation Time

The *partial thromboplastin time* (PTT) and *activated partial thromboplastin time* (aPTT) are used to measure the effectiveness of heparin administration. An additional test of heparin effect is the *activated coagulation time* (ACT). The ACT can be performed outside the laboratory setting in the cardiac catheterization laboratory, operating room, and specialized critical care units (see Table 10-5).

Evaluating Serum Lipid Profile

Four primary blood lipid levels are important in evaluating an individual's risk of developing CAD or experiencing progressive CAD: total cholesterol, low-density lipoprotein (LDL) cholesterol, triglycerides, and high-density lipoprotein (HDL) cholesterol When LDLs and triglycerides are elevated or HDLs are low, the patient is considered "at risk" for developing or having progressive CAD[49,50,54-56] (Table 10-6).

Total Cholesterol

Cholesterol is a fatlike substance (lipid) present in cell membranes, is a precursor of bile acids and steroid hormones, and is produced by the liver. The cholesterol level in the blood is determined partly by genetics and partly by acquired factors such as diet, calorie balance, and level of physical activity. Cholesterol in excess amounts (greater than 200 mg/dl) in the serum fosters the progression of atherosclerosis.[54-56]

Low-Density Lipoproteins

About 60% to 70% of the total serum cholesterol is transported in the bloodstream complexed as LDL cholesterol. Both the LDL cholesterol and total serum cholesterol levels are directly correlated with risk for CAD, and high levels of each are significant predictors of future MI. LDL cholesterol is the major atherogenic lipoprotein and thus is the primary target for cholesterol-lowering efforts.[54-56]

Table **10-6** Desirable Lipid Levels	
Lipid	**Desirable Level**
Total cholesterol	<200 mg/dl
LDL-C	<130 mg/dl without CAD
	<100 mg/dl with CAD
Triglycerides	<150 mg/dl
HDL-C	>40 mg/dl

Data from Third Report of National Cholesterol Education Program (NCEP) Expert Panel on Detection, Evaluation, and Treatment of High Blood Cholesterol in Adults (Adult Treatment Panel III), *JAMA* 285:2486-2497, 2001.
LDL-C, Low-density lipoprotein cholesterol; *HDL-C,* high-density lipoprotein cholesterol; *CAD,* coronary artery disease.

Very-Low-Density Lipoproteins and Triglycerides

The very-low-density lipoproteins (VLDLs) contain 10% to 15% of the total serum cholesterol along with most of the triglycerides in fasting serum. Elevated triglyceride levels are also often associated with reduced HDL cholesterol levels.[54]

High-Density Lipoproteins

HDL cholesterol particles carry 20% to 30% of the total serum cholesterol. A low HDL cholesterol level (less than 35 mg/dl) is another independent, significant risk factor for coronary artery disease.[49] A high HDL cholesterol level protects against atherosclerotic CAD (see Table 10-6).

DIAGNOSTIC PROCEDURES

An overview of the various diagnostic procedures used to evaluate the patient with cardiovascular dysfunction is provided in Table 10-7.

Nursing Management

The nursing management of a patient undergoing a diagnostic procedure involves a variety of interventions. **Nursing priorities are directed toward (1) preparing the patient psychologically and physically for the procedure, (2) obtaining informed consent, (3) monitoring the patient's physiologic responses, and (4) assessing the patient after the procedure.**

Preparing the patient includes teaching about the procedure, answering questions, and ensuring that the patient is informed about the diagnostic procedure. If the procedure is invasive the medical professional that will perform the procedure must discuss risks, benefits, and potential complications with the patient to ensure that informed consent is obtained. The critical care nurse may assist with transport or positioning of the patient for the procedure. Monitoring the patient's responses during diagnostic procedures includes observing for signs of pain, anxiety, and hemorrhage and monitoring vital signs. Assessing the patient after the procedure includes monitoring for complications and medicating the patient for any postprocedural anxiety, pain, or discomfort. Evidence of bleeding or chest pain should be immediately reported to the physician and emergency measures undertaken to maintain circulation and increase myocardial oxygen supply.

ELECTROCARDIOGRAPHY

The critical care nurse considers many clinical factors when interpreting bedside electrocardiography, which records electrical changes in heart muscle. The electrocardiogram (ECG) does not record the mechanical contraction, which usually immediately follows electrical depolarization.

ECG Leads

All electrocardiographs use a system of one or more leads. The basic lead system consists of three electrodes: positive

Table 10-7   Cardiovascular Diagnostic Procedures

Procedure	Evaluation	Comments
Aortography	Aortic valve insufficiency Aneurysms or dissection of ascending aorta Coarctation of aorta Injuries to aorta and major branches	Contrast medium used: check for allergy to iodine, shellfish, and dye; ensure hydration after procedure. Monitor for clinical indications of anaphylaxis (flushing, urticaria, stridor). Monitor puncture site.
Cardiac biopsy	Effect of cardiotoxic drugs Evidence of cardiac transplant rejection Inflammatory heart disease Tumors Cardiomyopathy	Observe closely for signs of cardiac perforation and cardiac tamponade.
Cardiac catheterization and coronary angiography	Severity of coronary artery stenosis Cardiac muscle function Pressures within heart Cardiac output, ejection fraction Arterial blood gas analysis within chambers Allows angioplasty, atherectomy, intracoronary stents, or lasers to reduce coronary artery obstruction	*Before test,* check for allergy to iodine, shellfish, and dye (contrast medium used). *After test:* Ensure hydration (contrast medium used). Keep affected extremity immobilized in a straight position for 6-12 hours. Monitor arterial puncture point for hemorrhage or hematoma. Monitor neurovascular status of affected limb. Note complaints of back pain and vital sign changes (may indicate retroperitoneal hemorrhage). Inquire about possibility of pregnancy.
Chest radiography	Cardiac size and shape Pulmonary congestion or pleural effusion Thoracic aneurysm or aortic calcification Position of pulmonary artery and cardiac catheter, pacemaker, wires	
Computed tomography (CT)	Left ventricular wall motion Cardiac tumors MI Pericardial effusion Aortic aneurysm/dissection	May be done with or without contrast medium. If contrast medium used, check for allergy to iodine, shellfish, and dye; ensure hydration after procedure.
Digital subtraction angiography	Vascular disease Degree of occlusion	Contrast medium used: check for allergy to iodine, shellfish, and dye; ensure hydration after procedure. Monitor for clinical indications of anaphylaxis (flushing, urticaria, stridor). Monitor puncture site.
Doppler ultrasonography	Vascular disease Degree of occlusion	
Echocardiography • *M mode:* single ultrasound beam • *2D:* planar ultrasound beam; wider view of heart, structures	Chamber size and wall thickness Valve functioning Papillary muscle functioning Prosthetic valve functioning	TEE is better choice if patient is obese or has COPD, chest wall deformity, chest trauma, or thick chest dressings.

Continued

Table **10-7** Cardiovascular Diagnostic Procedures—cont'd

Procedure	Evaluation	Comments
• *Doppler:* flow of blood through heart • *Color flow:* Doppler image superimposed on 2D image • *Stress:* images before, during, and after exercise or pharmacologic stress • *TEE:* transducer placed in esophagus	Ventricular wall motion abnormalities Intracardiac masses Pericardial fluid Intracardiac pressures (Doppler) Ejection fraction, cardiac output (Doppler) Valve gradients (Doppler) Intracardiac shunts (Doppler) Thoracic aneurysm (TEE)	
Electrocardiography (ECG)	Dysrhythmias Conduction defects, including intraventricular blocks Electrolyte imbalance Drug toxicity MI, myocardial ischemia/injury Chamber hypertrophy	List drugs the patient is receiving on ECG request. Be alert to electrical safety hazards.
Electrophysiologic studies (EPS)	Dysrhythmias under controlled circumstances Best therapy for control of dysrhythmia: drug/dosage, pacemaker, catheter ablation	Patient may have near-death experience during EPS; encourage expression of fears, concerns, and anxieties. Monitor puncture site.
Holter monitoring	Suspected dysrhythmias over 24-hour period Pacemaker function Silent ischemia	Instruct patient on importance of keeping diary.
Intravascular ultrasound (IVUS)	Coronary artery size/patency Vessel wall structure Coronary stent position/patency Aorta; aneurysms, aneurysm dissections	As for cardiac catheterization.
Magnetic resonance imaging (MRI)	Three-dimensional view of heart Anatomy/structure of heart and great vessels, including cardiomyopathy, congenital defect, masses, and aneurysms Changes in chemistry of tissues before structural changes occur	Does not involve radiation or dyes. Cannot be used in patients with any implanted metallic device, including pacemakers, defibrillators, metallic heart valves, and intracranial aneurysm clips.
Multiple-gated acquisition (MUGA) scan (radionuclide angiography)	Ventricular size/wall motion Cardiac output, cardiac index, end-systolic volume, end-diastolic volume, ejection fraction Intracardiac shunts	Assure patient that amount of radioactive material is minimal.
Pericardiocentesis and pericardial fluid analysis	Blood, pus, pathogens, malignancy Emergency relief of cardiac tamponade	Observe closely for signs of cardiac tamponade.
Peripheral angiography	Atherosclerotic plaque Occlusion Aneurysm Traumatic injury	*Before test,* check for allergy to iodine, shellfish, and dye (contrast medium used). *After test:* Ensure hydration (contrast medium used).

Procedure	Findings	Nursing Considerations
Phonocardiography	Extra heart sounds and murmurs in relation to cardiac cycle and ECG	
Positron emission tomography (cardiac PET scan)	Severity of coronary artery stenosis Collateral circulation Patency of bypass grafts Size/location of infarcted tissue	Rarely used at present. Assure patient that amount of radioactive material is minimal.
Stress electrocardiography	High-risk patients, patients with known CAD, or postsurgical patients for ischemia with exercise or pharmacologic agents (e.g., adenosine, dipyridamole, dobutamine) Exercise-induced dysrhythmias	≥1 mm of transient ST-segment depression 80 msec after J point suggests CAD. Monitor closely for exercise-induced hypotension and ventricular dysrhythmias.
Technetium-99 pyrophosphate scan	Size and location of acute MI; infarcted areas show increased uptake of radioactivity (hot spots) 1-7 days after MI.	Assure patient that amount of radioactive material is minimal. Peak accuracy at 12-48 hours after initial symptoms.
Thallium stress electrocardiography	Myocardial ischemia during exercise; ischemic areas show decreased uptake of radioactivity (cold spots).	Assure patient that amount of radioactive material is minimal.
Thallium-201 scan	Myocardial ischemia; ischemic areas show decreased uptake of radioactivity (cold spots).	Assure patient that amount of radioactive material is minimal.
Vectorcardiography	Chamber hypertrophy Bundle branch blocks/hemiblocks Myocardial ischemia or infarction	
Venography (ascending contrast phlebography)	Deep leg veins, DVT Competence of deep vein valves Location of suitable vein for arterial bypass graft	Contrast medium used: check for allergy to iodine, shellfish, and dye; ensure hydration after procedure. Monitor for clinical indications of anaphylaxis (flushing, urticaria, stridor). Monitor puncture site.
Ventriculography	Ventricular wall motion/thickness Ventricular aneurysm Mitral valve motion Left ventricular end-diastolic volume, end-systolic volume, stroke volume, ejection fraction Intracardiac shunt	Keep affected extremity immobilized in a straight position for 6-12 hours. Monitor arterial puncture point for hemorrhage or hematoma. Monitor neurovascular status of affected limb. Monitor for indications of systemic emboli. Contrast medium used: check for allergy to iodine, shellfish, and dye; ensure hydration after procedure. Monitor for clinical indications of anaphylaxis (flushing, urticaria, stridor). Monitor puncture site.

From Dennison RD: *Pass CCRN!*, ed 2, St Louis, 2000, Mosby.
MI, Myocardial infarction; *2D*, two dimensional; *TEE*, transesophageal echocardiography; *COPD*, chronic obstructive pulmonary disease; *CAD*, coronary artery disease; *DVT*, deep vein thrombosis.

electrode, negative electrode, and ground electrode. The function of the ground electrode is to prevent the display of background electrical interference on the ECG tracing. Leads do not transmit any electricity to the patient; leads only sense and record electrical impulses. During continuous cardiac monitoring, adhesive pre-gelled electrodes are placed on the patient to obtain the ECG tracing for a visual display of one, two, or more leads simultaneously. Emergency defibrillators use a three-lead system (Figure 10-5, A). Most modern bedside systems use at least five leads (Figure 10-5, B), and some systems use a set of precordial (chest) leads similar to the 12-lead ECG.[57-59]

ECG Analysis

ECG paper records the speed and magnitude of electrical impulses on a grid composed of small and large boxes (Figure 10-6). Every large box has five small boxes in it. At a standard paper speed of 25 millimeters per second (mm/sec), on the horizontal axis one small box (1 mm) is equivalent to 0.04 second, and one large box (5 mm) represents 0.20 second. Distances along the horizontal axis represent *speed* and are stated in seconds rather than in millimeters or number of boxes. The vertical axis represents the magnitude, or *force*, of the electrical signal. The vertical scale is standardized to a specific calibration as well. One small box equals 0.1 mm on the vertical scale. The standard ECG calibration is 1 millivolt (mV) equal to 10 mm (or 10 small boxes) on the vertical ECG scale.[59]

Waveforms

Analysis of waveforms and intervals provides the basis for ECG interpretation (Figure 10-7).

P Wave. The P wave represents *atrial depolarization.* Mechanical contraction follows electrical depolarization.

QRS Complex. The QRS complex represents *ventricular depolarization.* It is referred to as a *complex* because it actually consists of several different waves. The letter *Q* is used to describe an initial negative deflection; in other words, only if the first deflection from the baseline is negative will the wave be labeled a Q wave. The letter *R* applies to any positive deflection. A second positive deflection within the same complex is termed *R prime* (R'). The letter *S* refers to any subsequent negative deflection. Any combination of these deflections can occur and is collectively called the QRS complex (Figure 10-8). The QRS duration is normally less than 0.10 second (2½ small boxes on the horizontal scale).

T Wave. The T wave represents *ventricular repolarization.* The onset of the QRS to approximately the midpoint or peak of the T wave represents an *absolute refractory period*, during which the heart muscle cannot respond to another stimulus regardless of the strength of that stimulus (Figure 10-9). From the midpoint to the end of the T wave, the heart muscle is in the *relative refractory period.* The heart muscle has not yet fully recovered, but it could be depolar-

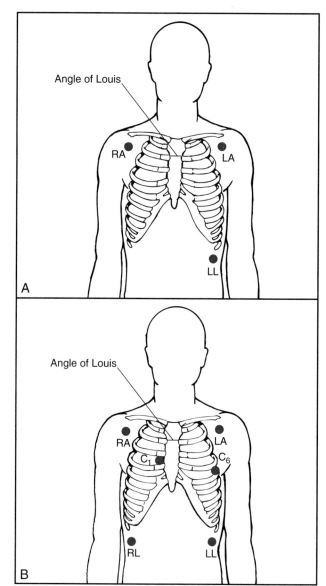

Figure 10-5 A, Three electrodes and lead-wire cables allow monitoring of three ECG limb leads (I, II, and III) and can also be rearranged to monitor MCL$_1$ and MCL$_6$. **B,** Multilead monitoring system. Five electrodes and lead-wire cables allow monitoring of any of six standard limb leads (I, II, III, aV$_R$, aV$_L$, and aV$_F$) and one precordial (chest) lead, V$_1$ or V$_6$. C_1 indicates proper position of chest electrode for monitoring lead V$_1$. C_6 indicates proper position of chest electrode for monitoring V$_6$. Cable attachments are color-coded for quick identification and placement. Accurate electrode placement is essential.

ized again if a sufficiently strong stimulus were received. This can be a particularly dangerous time for ventricular ectopy to occur, especially if any portion of the myocardium is ischemic, because the ischemic muscle takes even longer to repolarize fully. This sets the stage for disorganized, self-perpetuating depolarizations known as *ventricular fibrillation.*

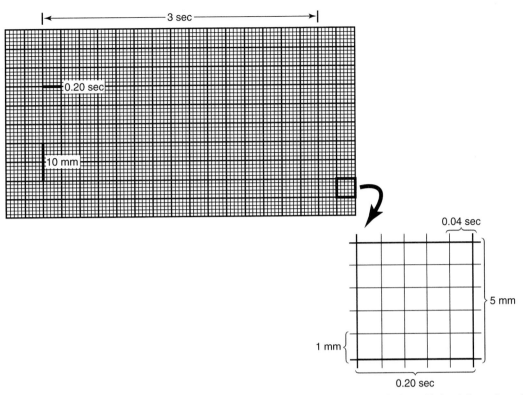

Figure 10-6   ECG graph paper. Horizontal axis represents time, and vertical axis represents magnitude of voltage. Horizontally, each small box is 0.04 second and each large box 0.20 second. Vertically, each large box is 5 mm. Markings are present every 3 seconds at top of paper for ease in calculating heart rate.

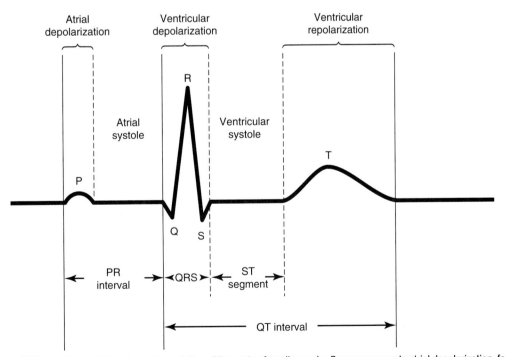

Figure 10-7   Normal ECG waveforms, intervals, and correlation with events of cardiac cycle. *P wave* represents atrial depolarization, followed immediately by atrial systole. *QRS* represents ventricular depolarization, followed immediately by ventricular systole. *T wave* represents ventricular repolarization. *PR interval*, measured from beginning of P wave to beginning of QRS, corresponds to atrial depolarization and impulse delay in atrioventricular (AV) node. *QT interval*, measured from beginning of QRS complex to end of T wave, represents the time from initial depolarization of ventricles to end of ventricular repolarization.

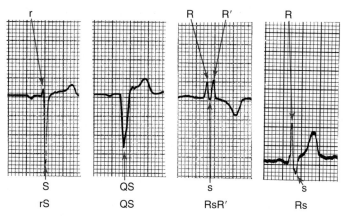

Figure 10-8 Examples of QRS complexes. Small deflections are labeled with lowercase letters, and uppercase letters are used for larger deflections. A second upward deflection is labeled *R′* ("R prime").

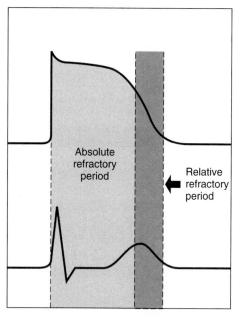

Figure 10-9 Absolute and relative refractory periods correlated with cardiac muscle's action potential and with ECG tracing.

Intervals between Waveforms

The intervals between ECG waveforms are also evaluated (see Figure 10-7).

PR Interval. The PR interval is measured from the beginning of the P wave to the beginning of the QRS complex. Normally, the PR interval is 0.12 to 0.20 second in length and represents the time between sinus node discharge and the beginning of ventricular depolarization. Because most of this period results from delay of the impulse in the atrioventricular (AV) node, the PR interval is an indicator of AV nodal function.

ST Segment. The ST segment is the portion of the wave that extends from the end of the QRS to the beginning of the T wave. Its duration is not measured. Instead, its shape and location are evaluated. The ST segment is normally flat and at the same level as the isoelectric baseline. Any change from baseline is expressed in millimeters and may indicate myocardial ischemia (one small box equals 1 mm on the vertical scale). ST-segment elevation (increase greater than 1 mm) is associated with acute myocardial injury. ST-segment depression (decrease from baseline of more than 1 mm) is associated with myocardial ischemia.[58] The measurement of ST elevation or depression is made using the *J point* in relation to the baseline isoelectric line (Figure 10-10).

QT Interval. The QT interval is measured from the beginning of the QRS complex to the end of the T wave and indicates the total time from the onset of depolarization to the completion of repolarization.[59] The corrected QT (QTc) interval is less than 0.44 second. A prolonged QT interval is significant because it can predispose the patient to the development of polymorphic VT, known also as *torsades de pointes*.[58-60] A long QT interval can occur secondary to electrolyte imbalance and antidysrhythmic drug therapy[43] and also some non-antidysrhythmic medications.[61]

Dysrhythmia Interpretation

In clinical practice the terms "dysrhythmia" and "arrhythmia" often are used interchangeably. Both are correct, and either may be used in practice; this text favors "dysrhythmia." A *dysrhythmia* is any disturbance in the normal cardiac conduction pathway. Dysrhythmias can be detected on a 12-lead ECG but often occur only sporadically. For this reason, patients in a critical care unit are monitored continuously, using a single or multilead system, and rhythm strips are recorded routinely as well as any time the patient's rhythm changes.[59]

Heart Rate Determination

The first element to assess when evaluating a rhythm strip is the ventricular rate. Regardless of the dysrhythmia involved, the ventricular rate holds the key to whether the patient can tolerate the dysrhythmia (i.e., maintain adequate blood pressure, CO, and mentation). If the ventricular

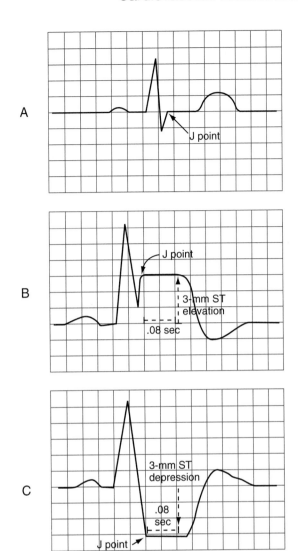

Figure 10-10   A, Normal position of J point. **B**, 3-mm ST elevation. **C**, 3-mm ST depression. ST changes are measured 60 to 80 msec (0.06-0.08 second) after the J point.

Rhythm Determination

The term *rhythm* refers to the regularity with which the P waves or R waves occur. Calipers assist in determining rhythm. One point of the calipers is placed on the beginning of one R wave while the other point is placed on the next R wave. Leaving the calipers "set" at this interval, each succeeding RR interval is checked to ensure it is the same width.

In describing the rhythm, three terms are used. If the rhythm is *regular*, the RR intervals are the same (plus/minus 10%). If the rhythm is *regularly irregular*, the RR intervals are not the same, but some pattern is involved, which could be grouping, rhythmic speeding up and slowing down, or any other consistent pattern. If the rhythm is *irregularly irregular*, the RR intervals are not the same, and no pattern can be found.

P-Wave Evaluation. The P wave is analyzed by determining (1) if it is present or absent and (2) if it is related to the QRS complex. One P wave should be in front of every QRS, and two, three, or four P waves may be in front of every QRS at times. If this pattern is consistent, the P wave and QRS are still related, although not on a 1:1 basis.

PR-Interval Evaluation. The duration of the PR interval, which normally is 0.12 to 0.20 second, is measured first. This is measured from the start of a visible P wave to the beginning of the following QRS. Next, all PR intervals on the strip are verified to ensure they have the same duration as the original interval.

QRS-Complex Evaluation. The entire ECG strip must be evaluated to ascertain that the QRS complexes are consistently the same shape and width. The normal QRS duration is 0.06 to 0.10 second. If more than one QRS shape is on the strip, each QRS must be measured. The QRS is measured from where it leaves the baseline to where it returns to the baseline.

rate is consistently greater than 200 or less than 30 beats/min, emergency measures must be started to correct the rate. A detailed analysis of the underlying rhythm disturbance can proceed later when the immediate crisis is over. The following three methods are used for calculating heart rate (Figure 10-11):

Method 1: Number of RR intervals (in 6 seconds) × 10. ECG paper is usually marked at the top in 3-second increments, making a 6-second interval easy to identify.

Method 2: Number of large boxes between QRS complexes divided into 300.

Method 3: Number of small boxes between QRS complexes divided into 1500.

In the healthy heart, the atrial rate and the ventricular rate are the same. In many dysrhythmias, however, the atrial and ventricular rates are different, and therefore both must be calculated. To find the atrial rate, the PP interval, instead of the RR interval, is used in one of the three methods.

Dysrhythmias

Normal Sinus Rhythm (Figure 10-12)

RATE: 60 to 100 beats/min.   P WAVE: Present, all the same shape, with only one preceding each QRS complex.

RHYTHM: Regular (±10%).   PR INTERVAL: 0.12 to 0.20 second.
   QRS DURATION: 0.06 to 0.10 second.

QRS COMPLEX: Shape and whether deflection is positive or negative vary depending on lead placement. For example, in lead II the normal complex is positive (strip A) and in MCL_1 or V_1 the normal complex is negative (strip B).

ETIOLOGY: Normal conduction.

TREATMENT: None required.

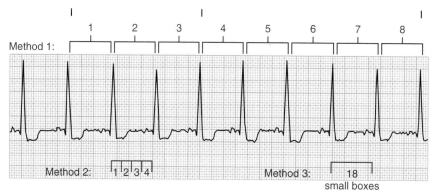

Figure 10-11   Calculation of heart rate if the rhythm is regular. *Method 1*: number of RR intervals in 6 seconds multiplied by 10 (e.g., 8 × 10 = 80/min). *Method 2*: number of large boxes between QRS complexes divided into 300 (e.g., 300 ÷ 4 = 75/min). *Method 3*: number of small boxes between QRS complexes divided into 1500 (e.g., 1500 ÷ 18 = 84/min).

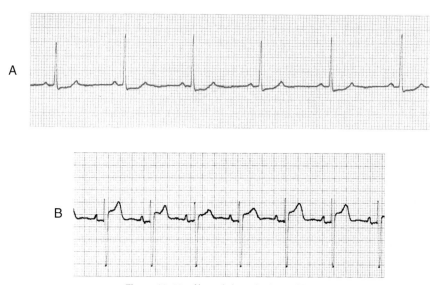

Figure 10-12   Normal sinus rhythm (NSR).

Sinus Bradycardia (Figure 10-13)

RATE: Less than 60 beats/min.

RHYTHM: Regular.

QRS COMPLEX: Same as NSR. Narrow complex QRS.

P WAVE: Present, all the same shape, with only one preceding each QRS complex.

PR INTERVAL: 0.12 to 0.20 second.

QRS DURATION: 0.06 to 0.10 second.

ETIOLOGY: Vagal stimulation, increased intracranial pressure (ICP), or ischemia of sinus node Sinus bradycardia is also normal in well-conditioned, healthy athletes at rest.

TREATMENT: Only treated if accompanied by symptoms of hypoperfusion (e.g., hypotension, dizziness, chest pain, decreased level of consciousness). If patient becomes symptomatic, advanced cardiac life support (ACLS) measures (e.g., atropine, transcutaneous pacing) will be required.

Sinus Tachycardia (Figure 10-14)

RATE: Greater than 100 beats/min. Rates may be as high as 180 in young healthy adults during strenuous exercise. In critically ill patients, a heart rate above 150 beats/min is usually caused by other dysrhythmias.

P WAVE: Present, all the same shape, with only one preceding each QRS complex.

PR INTERVAL: 0.12 to 0.20 second.

QRS DURATION: 0.06 to 0.10 second.

RHYTHM: Regular.

QRS COMPLEX: Same as NSR. Narrow complex QRS.

ETIOLOGY: Pain, fever, hemorrhage, shock, and acute heart failure. Many medications used in the critical care unit cause sinus tachycardia (ST), including aminophylline, dopamine, hydralazine, nitroglycerin, epinephrine, and atropine.

PHYSIOLOGY: Tachycardia is detrimental to patients with ischemic heart disease. The rapid heart rate (HR) shortens

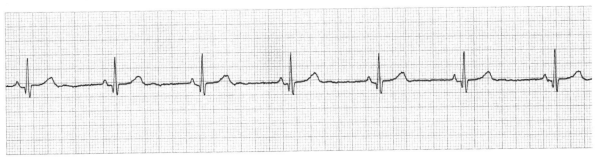

Figure 10-13   Sinus bradycardia (SB).

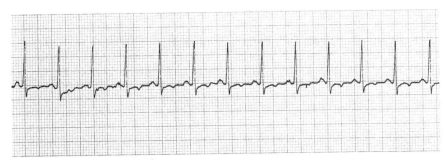

Figure 10-14   Sinus tachycardia (ST).

the time for ventricular filling, decreasing both stroke volume (SV) and cardiac output (CO). This increases myocardial oxygen demand while decreasing oxygen supply because of decreased coronary artery filling time.

TREATMENT: Treatment varies according to the cause. If the cause of ST is evident (fever or pain), the cause should be treated rather than treating the HR directly. If the problem is cardiac related, both calcium channel blockers and β-blockers are widely used to decrease rapid HRs. However, clinical assessment is required before these drugs are administered. CO is determined by HR and SV. If an injured heart can no longer maintain an adequate SV, the body increases HR to maintain CO and supply an adequate blood flow to vital body tissues. If a drug is administered to force the sinus node to slow down and the heart cannot increase SV, sudden severe heart failure can result.

Sinus Dysrhythmia (Figure 10-15)

RATE: 60 to 100 beats/min.

RHYTHM: Irregular, varying with respiratory cycle. Increases with inhalation, and decreases with exhalation.

P WAVE: Present, all the same shape, with only one preceding each QRS complex.

QRS COMPLEX: Same as with NSR. Narrow complex QRS.

PR INTERVAL: 0.12 to 0.20 second.

QRS DURATION: 0.06 to 0.10 second.

ETIOLOGY: Normal variant. Also frequently called *sinus arrhythmia*.

TREATMENT: None required.

Premature Atrial Contraction (Figure 10-16)

RATE: Determined by underlying rhythm, which is usually sinus related.

RHYTHM: Variable. Underlying rhythm may be regular, but premature atrial contractions (PACs) create irregularity.

P WAVE: Present, different shape from other P waves, may be inverted. Early P wave may be buried in preceding T wave.

PR INTERVAL: 0.12 to 0.20 second. PR interval may be different from

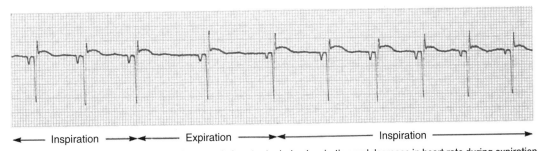

←——— Inspiration ———→←——— Expiration ———→←———— Inspiration ————→

Figure 10-15   Sinus dysrhythmia. Note increase in heart rate during inspiration and decrease in heart rate during expiration.

PR interval of a sinus beat in the same patient.

QRS DURATION: 0.06 to 0.10 second.

QRS COMPLEX: Usually has normal appearance because conduction through AV node and ventricular conduction system is normal (strip A). Exceptions, do occur (strip C).

ETIOLOGY: Can occur normally. Often accentuated by emotional disturbances, caffeine, nicotine, digitalis, mitral valve prolapse, and heart failure.

PHYSIOLOGY: Originates from an ectopic focus in the atria, somewhere other than the sinus node. Ectopic impulse occurs prematurely before normal sinus impulse is due to occur.

- Usually the premature P wave initiates a normal QRS complex (strip A).
- If the beat is so early that AV node remains refractory to stimuli, a pause resulting from a nonconducted PAC is seen (strip B).
- Occasionally the early ectopic P wave can be conducted through AV node, but part of this conduction pathway through ventricles is blocked. This appears as an early, abnormal P wave on ECG, followed by an abnormally wide QRS (strip C). This is termed *aberrant conduction*.

PACs are also known to start and stop reentrant bursts of supraventricular tachycardia.[62]

TREATMENT: None if infrequent. If frequent and patient is symptomatic, treat the cause. For example, reduce stress, eliminate caffeine and nicotine, modify digitalis dosage, and treat symptoms of heart failure.

Paroxysmal Supraventricular Tachycardia (Figure 10-17)

RATE: Atrial rate 150 to 250 beats/min.

RHYTHM: Regular.

P WAVE: Present, may have an abnormal shape. Not all P waves may be conducted to the ventricle.

PR INTERVAL: 0.12 to 0.20 second.

QRS DURATION: 0.06 to 0.10 second.

QRS COMPLEX: Usually narrow and normal in appearance.

ETIOLOGY: Paroxysmal supraventricular tachycardia (PSVT) has causal factors similar to those of PACs, but PSVT has greater clinical significance. PSVT refers to the sudden interruption of sinus rhythm by an atrial ectopic focus that fires repetitively and rapidly and is sustained by a reentry or circular movement. It eventually stops as suddenly as it began. *Paroxysmal* means starting and stopping abruptly.

TREATMENT: Usually responds rapidly to medical treatment. IV *adenosine* (Adenocard) is the drug of choice to slow conduction through the AV node and unmask the ectopic P waves; often PSVT will return to normal sinus rhythm because of a well-timed spontaneous PAC.[62] Other options include vagal maneuvers, calcium channel blockers, digitalis, and cardioversion.

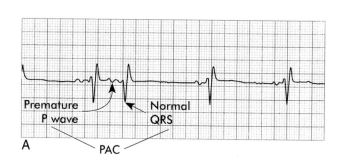

A PAC

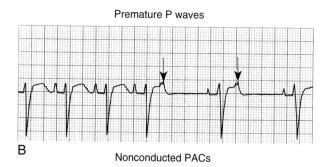

Premature P waves

B Nonconducted PACs

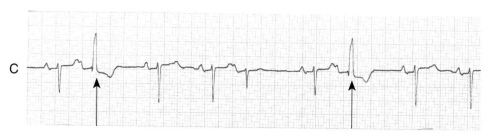

C PAC with aberrant conduction

Figure 10-16 Premature atrial contraction (PAC).

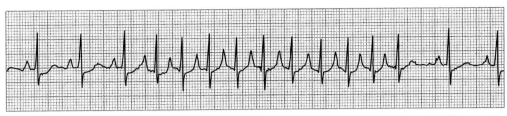

Figure 10-17 Paroxysmal supraventricular tachycardia (PSVT). Note that atrial rate during tachycardia is 158 beats/min. The run starts and stops abruptly.

Atrial Flutter (Figure 10-18)

RATE: Atrial rate 250 to 350 beats/min.

When evaluating rate of atrial flutter, both atrial and ventricular rates must be calculated. The atrial rate is faster.

RHYTHM: Regular flutter waves. Ventricular response (QRS complexes) may be regular or irregular.

P WAVE: Flutter (F) waves.

PR INTERVAL: No longer applies; instead a conduction ratio of P waves to QRS complexes (e.g., 2:1, 3:1, or 4:1) is used. The conduction ratio is clearly visible in strip A. At times, however, F waves are hidden by QRS complex or T wave (strip B).

QRS COMPLEX: Shape is usually narrow and normal.

PHYSIOLOGY: Believed to be caused by a circular reentry pathway through which the wave of depolarization is continually moving. At this rapid rate, individual P waves form the classic sawtooth pattern (strip A).

TREATMENT: May be difficult to identify F waves, especially if the conduction ratio is 2:1.[63] Vagal maneuvers or IV adenosine do not usually terminate atrial flutter but frequently aid in diagnosis. Drugs used to slow conduction through the AV node and protect the ventricles from the rapid atrial rate include ibutilide, calcium channel blockers (verapamil, diltiazem), digoxin, amiodarone, and β-blockers. Pharmacologic conversion using *ibutilide* (Corvert) is effective in approximately 70% of patients; if this does not succeed, electrical cardioversion usually will restore sinus rhythm.[64-67] If the flutter has been present for more than 72 hours, thrombi may be present in the atria, and anticoagulation may be required before either pharmacologic ther-

apy or electrical cardioversion.[51] Permanent, nonpharmacologic termination of atrial flutter can be achieved by *radiofrequency catheter ablation* (RFA), which creates a line of conduction block across the reentry pathway. Most frequent location for RFA is between inferior vena cava and tricuspid annulus.[63]

Atrial Fibrillation (Figure 10-19)

RATE: Atrial rate 350 to 600 fibrillatory waves per minute.

Ventricular rate 60 to 100 (controlled by medication), greater than 100 (uncontrolled by medication).

RHYTHM: Irregularly irregular ventricular rhythm.

P WAVE: Replaced by fibrillating baseline or waves.

PR INTERVAL: Absent. Replaced by fibrillating baseline.

QRS DURATION: 0.06 to 0.10 second.

QRS COMPLEX: Usually normal because pathway through ventricles is unchanged once impulse leaves AV node.

ETIOLOGY: Small sections of atrial muscle are activated individually, resulting in quivering of atrial muscle without effective contraction. The sinoatrial (SA) node is rendered ineffective becoming one of many competing atrial sites.

PHYSIOLOGY: When numerous sites in atria fire spontaneously and rapidly, an organized spread of depolarization can no longer take place, and atrial fibrillation results. AF can be acute or chronic.

TREATMENT: Two approaches: (1) convert atrial fibrillation back to sinus rhythm using electrical cardioversion or chemical cardioversion with pharmacologic agents or (2) allow atrial fibrillation to exist and use pharmacologic

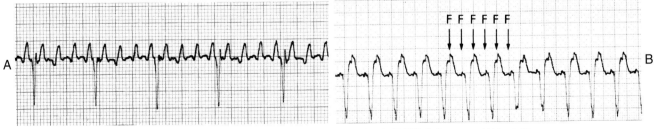

Figure 10-18 Atrial flutter. **A,** With 4:1 conduction through AV node. **B,** With flutter waves hidden in T waves.

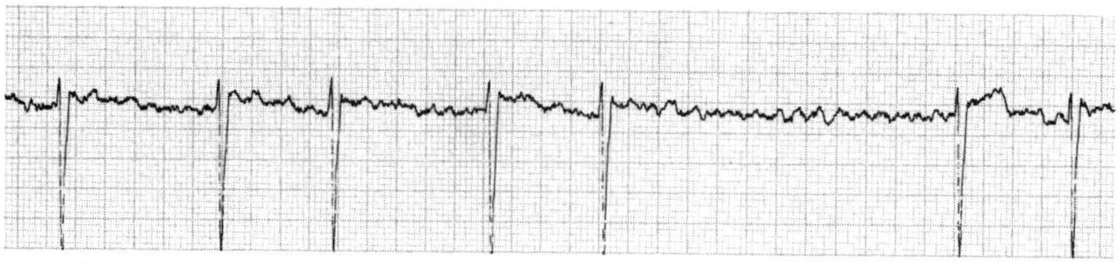

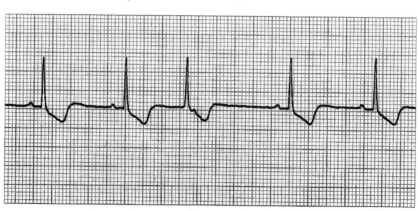

Figure 10-19   Atrial fibrillation (AF). Note irregularly irregular ventricular rhythm.

measures to control ventricular response rate.[68] *Electrical cardioversion* may be successful in converting the rhythm to sinus if attempted within a few days or weeks of the onset of atrial fibrillation. Cardioversion also carries the threat of precipitating emboli. During atrial fibrillation the atria do not contract and blood may pool, promoting thrombus formation (mural thrombi) within atria. If cardioversion is successful and normal sinus rhythm is restored, atria again contract forcibly and, if thrombus formation has occurred, clots may be sent traveling through the pulmonary or systemic circulation. To prevent this, patients in atrial fibrillation for 3 or more days should be anticoagulated for 3 weeks before elective cardioversion.[51] *Transesophageal echocardiography* (TEE) may help in identifying atrial thrombi, although thrombi may be missed or transient. Inability to visualize thrombi on echocardiography does not negate the need for anticoagulation.[51] TEE is sometimes used as a screening tool before elective cardioversion. Amiodarone, calcium channel blockers, β-blockers, and digoxin are the drugs most often used to control the ventricular response rate in atrial fibrillation.[69-71] Other options include a surgical cure known as the "maze procedure," although this option is normally limited to younger patients with well-preserved ventricular function.[72-74] Investigations are also exploring use of "atrial pacemakers" to "convert" the atria to a sinus rhythm.[75-77]

Premature Junctional Contraction
(Figure 10-20)

RATE: Depends on underlying rhythm, usually NSR.

P WAVE: May be entirely absent, may be seen in T wave, or may be inverted

RHYTHM: On ECG, rhythm is regular from sinus node except for early QRS complex (PJC) of normal shape and duration.

with PR interval less than 0.12 second.

PR INTERVAL: Usually absent. Lack of normal PR interval is a defining characteristic of junctional rhythms.

QRS DURATION: 0.06 to 0.10 second.

QRS COMPLEX: Usually narrow and normal.

ETIOLOGY: Premature junctional contraction (PJC) is a single ectopic impulse that originates in AV junctional area.

PHYSIOLOGY: Only certain areas of AV node have the property of automaticity. The entire area around the AV node is collectively called the *junction*; impulses generated there thus are called *junctional*. After arising in junction, ectopic impulse spreads in two directions at once. One wave of depolarization spreads upward into atria, depolarizes atria, and causes a P wave that is usually seen after QRS. At the same time, another wave of depolarization spreads downward into ventricles through normal conduction pathway and results in a normal QRS complex.

TREATMENT: Usually none required. PJCs have virtually the same clinical significance as PACs. If the patient is receiving digoxin, however, digitalis toxicity at least should be suspected. Although digoxin slows conduction through AV node, it also increases automaticity in junction.

Junctional Escape Rhythm (Figure 10-21)

RATE: At times, junction becomes dominant pacemaker of heart.

P WAVE: Same as for PJC.
PR INTERVAL: Usually absent.

Figure 10-20   Premature junctional contraction (PJC).

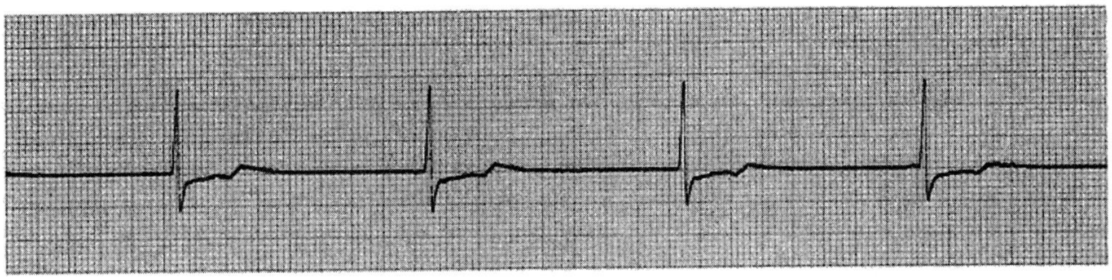

Figure 10-21 Junctional escape rhythm. Ventricular rate is 38 beats/min. P waves are absent, and QRS complex is of normal width.

Intrinsic rate of junction is 40 to 60 beats/min.
QRS DURATION: 0.06 to 0.10 second.

RHYTHM: Regular.

QRS COMPLEX: Usually narrow and normal because impulse originates above ventricles.

ETIOLOGY: Originates in AV junction after failure of sinus node.

PHYSIOLOGY: Under normal conditions, the AV junction never is able to "escape" and depolarize the heart because it is overridden by the faster sinus node. If the sinus node fails, however, the AV node junctional impulses can depolarize and pace the heart. This junctional escape rhythm is a protective mechanism to prevent asystole in the event of sinus node failure.

TREATMENT: Generally a junctional escape rhythm is well tolerated hemodynamically, although efforts should be directed toward restoring sinus rhythm. Sometimes a pacemaker is inserted as a protective measure because of concern that the AV junction may fail completely.

Accelerated Junctional Rhythm (Figure 10-22)

RATE: 60 to 100 beats/min. Junctional tachycardia: greater than 100 beats/min.
P WAVE: Same as for PJC.
PR INTERVAL: Usually absent.
QRS DURATION: 0.06 to 0.10 second.

RHYTHM: Regular.

QRS COMPLEX: Usually narrow and normal.

ETIOLOGY: Rapid AV node junctional rhythms may indicate irritability caused by AV nodal ischemia or digitalis toxicity.

PHYSIOLOGY: Accelerated junctional rhythms are usually well tolerated hemodynamically by patients, because the HR is within normal range. Junctional tachycardia may not be so well tolerated, depending on the patient's hemodynamic tolerance of the rapid rate.

TREATMENT: No treatment if patient has good blood pressure and no unusual symptoms. If this is a recent rhythm change and patient is receiving digoxin, digitalis toxicity should be suspected because digoxin enhances automaticity of AV node.

Premature Ventricular Contraction (Figure 10-23)

RATE: Depends on underlying HR, usually NSR.
P WAVE: Absent or after early QRS complex.
PR INTERVAL: Absent.

RHYTHM: Early QRS complexes interrupt underlying rhythm.
QRS DURATION: Greater than 0.12 second. Prolonged width of QRS is diagnostic for ventricular ectopy.

QRS COMPLEX: Wide, with bizarre shape.

Unifocal premature ventricular contractions (PVCs): All ventricular ectopic beats look the same in a particular lead. Unifocal PVCs probably all result from the same irritable focus (strip A).

Multifocal PVCs: Ventricular ectopic beats have various shapes in the same lead. More serious than unifocal PVCs, multifocal PVCs indicate that a greater area of irritable myocardium is involved. Multifocal PVCs are more likely

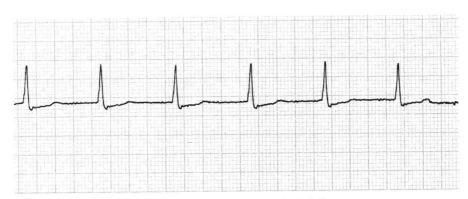

Figure 10-22 Accelerated junctional rhythm.

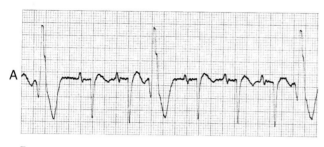

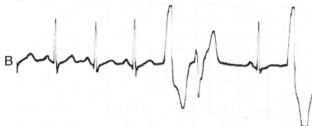

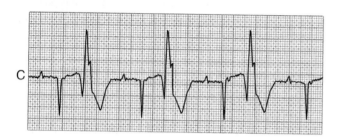

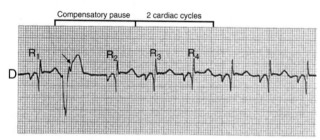

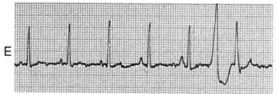

Figure 10-23 Premature ventricular contraction (PVC). **A**, Unifocal PVCs. **B**, Multifocal PVCs. **C**, Ventricular bigimeny. **D**, PVC with full compensatory pause. **E**, Interpolated PVC.

to deteriorate into ventricular tachycardia/fibrillation (strip *B*).

Fusion beats: If a ventricular ectopic impulse and a sinus beat depolarize simultaneously and meet in the middle of a depolarization, a fusion beat results. Fusion beats are narrower than ventricular beats and look like a cross between patient's sinus QRS and ventricular ectopic QRS.

Ventricular bigimeny: PVC follows each normal beat (strip *C*).

Couplet: Two consecutive PVCs.

Triplet: Three consecutive PVCs.

Compensatory pause: The apparently long "pause" following a PVC. However, the time-interval from the last normal QRS preceding the PVC to the QRS following the PVC is equal to two complete cardiac cycles (strip *D*). The compensatory pause allows the sinus node to resume the normal pattern.

Interpolated PVC: PVC falls between two normal QRS complexes without disturbing the rhythm. RR interval between sinus beats remains the same (strip *E*).

R on T: If a PVC occurs on the T wave during the relative refractory period (latter half of T wave) when only part of the muscle is repolarized, individual segments of muscle can depolarize separately from each other, resulting in ventricular fibrillation.

ETIOLOGY: Myocardial ischemia, electrolyte imbalances, hypoxia, acidosis, heart disease (e.g., cardiomyopathy, ventricular aneurysm, previous MI), and prodysrhythmic medications.

PHYSIOLOGY: Ventricular dysrhythmias result from ectopic focus in any portion of ventricular myocardium. Usual conduction pathway through ventricles is not used, and the wave of depolarization spreads from cell to cell.

DOCUMENTATION: Underlying rhythm must always be described first (e.g., sinus bradycardia with frequent unifocal PVCs, atrial fibrillation with occasional multifocal PVCs).

TREATMENT: Not all ventricular ectopy requires treatment. In patients with no significant heart disease, PVCs do not increase the risk for sudden death and are considered benign. If possible, the cause of the PVCs should be treated; for example, PVCs caused by hypokalemia and hypomagnesemia are managed by potassium/magnesium administration. Patients with hypoxia receive oxygen, ventilation if required, and have acidosis corrected.

Idioventricular Rhythm (Figure 10-24)

RATE: 20 to 40 beats/min. Accelerated rhythm: 40 to 100 beats/min.	P WAVE: Present, but not associated with QRS complex.
RHYTHM: Regular.	PR INTERVAL: Absent.
	QRS DURATION: Greater than 0.12 second.

QRS COMPLEX: Wide and bizarre because complexes originate in ventricles.

ETIOLOGY: SA and AV nodes may be damaged by degenerative heart disease or acute MI or depressed by drug toxicity.

PHYSIOLOGY: At times an ectopic focus in the ventricles can become the dominant pacemaker of the heart. If both SA node and AV junction fail, ventricles will depolarize at own intrinsic rate of 20 to 40 times/min (idioventricular rhythm). When a ventricular focus assumes control of heart at a rate greater than 40 beats/min, an accelerated idioventricular rhythm occurs.

TREATMENT: Rather than trying to abolish ventricular beats, aim of treatment is to increase effective HR and reestablish a higher pacing site (e.g., SA node, AV junction). HR may be increased pharmacologically with infusion

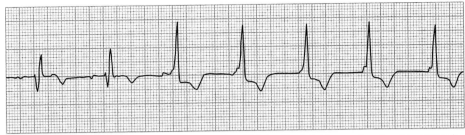

Figure 10-24 Accelerated idioventricular rhythm (AIVR) after third complex. QRS duration is 0.14 second, and ventricular rate is 65 beats/min. , P waves are not synchronied with widened QRS suring AIVR.

of isoproterenol (Isuprel). More often a transvenous temporary pacemaker is inserted and the heart is paced at a faster rate until underlying problems that caused failure of faster pacing sites can be resolved. Drugs such as lidocaine are contraindicated in treatment of idioventricular rhythms because if the ventricular ectopic focus is abolished, patients could become asystolic.

Ventricular Tachycardia (Figure 10-25)

RATE: Greater than 100 beats/min.

RHYTHM: Mostly regular. May have some irregularities.

P WAVE: Not related to QRS. Sinus node usually is unaffected and will continue to depolarize atria on schedule, so P waves may be seen on ECG and even may conduct a normal impulse to ventricles if timing is right.

PR INTERVAL: Absent.

QRS DURATION: Greater than 0.12 second.

QRS COMPLEX: Wide, with bizarre shape compared with sinus QRS (strip A).

Nonsustained ventricular tachycardia (VT): Three or more consecutive PVCs, rate greater than 110 beats/min, lasts less than 30 seconds without hemodynamic collapse, and self-terminates.[78]

Torsades de pointes ("twisting of the points"): Specific form of VT that refers to twisting appearance of VT on ECG (strip B). It may be precipitated by antidysrhythmics that prolong QT interval (e.g., quinidine) and ventricular refractory period.

ETIOLOGY: Same factors that cause PVCs; myocardial ischemia, digitalis toxicity, electrolyte disturbances, adverse side effect of certain antidysrhythmic drugs. Some antidysrhythmics can cause more serious dysrhythmias than those the drugs were intended to treat.

PHYSIOLOGY: VT results from repeating ectopic focus in ventricular myocardium. Usual conduction pathway through ventricles is bypassed, and wave of depolarization spreads from cell to cell.

TREATMENT: Pharmacologic, or electrical cardioversion/defibrillation.

Acute sustained VT: If patient is pulseless, ACLS measures such as immediate defibrillation, epinephrine, and cardiopulmonary resuscitation (CPR) are required. If patient has a pulse but is unstable (e.g., chest pain, shortness of breath,

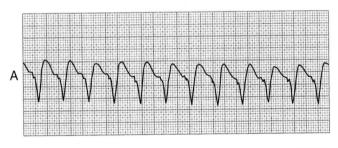

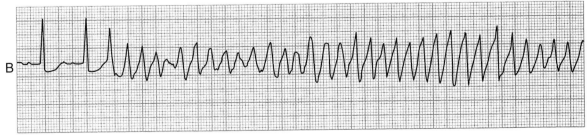

Figure 10-25 **A,** Ventricular tachycardia (VT). **B,** Torsades de pointes.

decreased level of consciousness, hypotensive), ACLS measures such as immediate synchronized cardioversion, amiodarone, and lidocaine are required.[71,79,80] If patient has a pulse and is stable, ACLS measures such as amiodarone, lidocaine, and procainamide are required.[79, 80] If hypoxia, acidosis, electrolyte imbalance, or drug toxicity is the cause, this must also be corrected to prevent recurrence of VT.

Chronic VT: Many patients with underlying heart disease from cardiomyopathy or past MI have frequent PVCs and episodes of VT. Traditionally these patients have been treated aggressively with oral antidysrhythmics. However, the *Cardiac Arrhythmia Suppression Trial* (CAST) indicated that treatment of this ventricular ectopic activity may increase the risk of sudden cardiac death. Another option for treatment of chronic VT is an implantable cardioverter/defibrillator (ICD).[81,82]

Ventricular Fibrillation (Figure 10-26)

RATE: Indeterminable.

RHYTHM: Irregular, wavy baseline without recognizable QRS complexes.

P WAVE: Absent. Cannot be distinguished from fibrillating ventricular baseline.

PR INTERVAL: Absent.

QRS DURATION: Absent. No QRS complexes present.

QRS COMPLEX: Normal QRS is missing. ECG appears as wavy baseline. *Coarse* ventricular fibrillation (VF) is seen on ECG as large, erratic undulations of the baseline, whereas in *fine* VF the ECG baseline exhibits only a mild tremor. In either case, patients have no pulse or blood pressure and are unconscious.

ETIOLOGY: VT is most common precursor of VF. Therefore all the factors that predispose patients to VT apply.

PHYSIOLOGY: VF is a result of electrical impulses from single or multiple ventricular foci that prevent ventricles from contracting. Ventricles merely quiver, with no forward flow of blood.

TREATMENT: Defibrillation is the emergency treatment of choice. Epinephrine may be used to try to change fine VF to coarse VF and facilitate defibrillation attempts. Antidysrhythmics (e.g., IV amiodarone, lidocaine) are also given if initial defibrillation attempts fail. As with any cardiac arrest situation, supportive measures (e.g., CPR, intubation, correction of metabolic abnormalities) are performed concurrently with definitive therapy.[83]

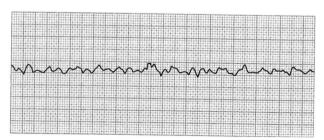

Figure 10-26 Ventricular fibrillation (VF).

First-Degree Atrioventricular Block
(Figure 10-27)

RATE: Depends on underlying rhythm, usually NSR.

RHYTHM: Regular if NSR.

P WAVE: Present, normal shape.

PR INTERVAL: Greater than 0.20 second.

QRS DURATION: 0.06 to 0.10 second.

QRS COMPLEX: Unaffected.

ETIOLOGY: All atrial impulses that should be conducted to ventricles are conducted, but PR interval is prolonged.

TREATMENT: None required. Many older patients have first-degree AV block as a chronic condition associated with aging of AV junction.

Acute myocardial infarction: Patients with acute MI should be monitored for degeneration into more serious forms of AV block.

Drug side effect: If development of first-degree AV block is new and related to recent antidysrhythmic administration, the medication regimen must be evaluated.

Second-Degree Atrioventricular Block Type I
(Figure 10-28)

RATE: Atrial rate depends on underlying sinus rate. Ventricular rate depends on P wave/QRS ratio.

RHYTHM: Regular, irregular pattern. P waves regular. As part of Mobitz I pattern, R-to-R intervals become progressively shorter until sinus P wave is not conducted, resulting in a pause. After the pause, cycle repeats itself.

P WAVE: Normal shape.

PR INTERVALS: Progressively lengthen until a P wave is not conducted to ventricles and therefore is not followed by QRS complex.

QRS DURATION: 0.06 to 0.10 second.

QRS COMPLEX: Conducted complexes are normal.

ETIOLOGY: Anatomic site of block is at level of AV node. If associated with acute inferior wall MI, block is caused by ischemia and is usually transient.

PHYSIOLOGY: AV conduction time lengthens until P wave not conducted to ventricles.

DOCUMENTATION: P wave/QRS complex ratio. For example, if four P waves are conducted to ventricles and

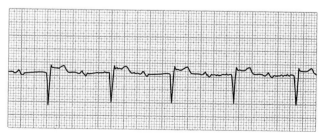

Figure 10-27 First-degree atrioventricular (AV) block. PR interval is prolonged to 0.44 second.

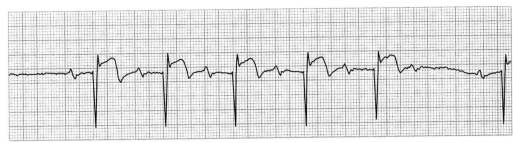

Figure 10-28 Second-degree AV block, type I (Mobitz I or Wenckebach). Note that PR intervals gradually increase from 0.36 to 0.46 second until finally a P wave is not conducted to ventricles.

fifth wave is not, a 5:4 conduction ratio is present (five P waves to four QRS complexes).

TREATMENT: No treatment required if ventricular rate is sufficient to sustain hemodynamic stability. In certain clinical conditions, such as acute MI, possibility of progression to more serious conduction disturbance exists, and patient is closely monitored. If hemodynamic compromise is present or deemed likely, temporary transvenous pacemaker may be inserted.

Second-Degree Atrioventricular Block Type II
(Figure 10-29)

RATE: Atrial rate usually 60 to 100 beats/min. Ventricular rate slower and depends on number of conducted P waves.

RHYTHM: Regular if AV node consistently conducts every second or third P wave. Irregular if P waves conducted inconsistently.

P WAVE: Normal in shape. More P waves than QRS complexes.

PR INTERVAL: 0.12 to 0.20 second. Constant for P waves that conduct to ventricles.

QRS DURATION: 0.06 to 0.10 second. Wider if bundle branch block (BBB) present.

QRS COMPLEX: May be narrow and normal or widened due to coexisting BBB.

ETIOLOGY: Usually indicates block below AV node, either in bundle of His or in both bundle branches. Mobitz II most frequently occurs when one bundle branch is blocked and other is ischemic. Mobitz II is more ominous clinically than Mobitz I block and often progresses to complete AV block.

PHYSIOLOGY: Occurs in presence of long absolute refractory period with virtually no relative refractory period, resulting in an "all or nothing" situation. Sinus P waves may

be conducted. When conduction does occur, all PR intervals are the same.

TREATMENT: Mobitz II can be serious and often precedes complete AV block. Use of temporary transvenous pacemaker is usually necessary, but its insertion can be elective if patient remains hemodynamically stable.

Third-Degree Atrioventricular Block
(Figure 10-30)

RATE: Depends on underlying rhythm.

RHYTHM: Usually regular.

P WAVE: Normal shape.

PR INTERVAL: P waves are not related to QRS complexes, so PR interval varies widely.

QRS DURATION: Greater than 0.10 second.

QRS COMPLEX: If *junctional* focus is pacing heart, complex looks normal but is not related to P waves. If *ventricular* focus is pacing heart, QRS is wide and unrelated to P waves.

ETIOLOGY: Degeneration of AV node caused by underlying heart disease or acute MI. Blockage of AV node is side effect of some antidysrhythmic drugs.

PHYSIOLOGY: In third-degree, or *complete*, AV block, no atrial impulses can conduct through AV node to cause ventricular depolarization. Opportunity for conduction is optimal but does not occur. Ideally a junctional or ventricular focus depolarizes spontaneously at its intrinsic rate of 20 to 60 beats/min, and ventricular contraction continues. If not, asystole occurs, the pulse stops, and death results if intervention is not immediate.

TREATMENT: Almost always requires a pacemaker. If patient hemodynamically unstable, external pacemaker can be used to maintain an adequate ventricular rate until temporary transvenous pacemaker can be inserted.[84,85]

Nursing Management

Nursing priorities for the patient with bedside ECG monitoring focus on (1) positioning electrodes correctly to obtain specific lead views, (2) selecting the optimal monitoring lead based on the patient's clinical status, (3) documenting significant changes in the patient's heart rhythm,

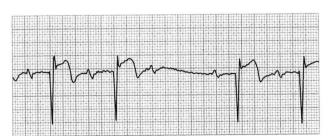

Figure 10-29 Second-degree AV block, type II (Mobitz II). PR intervals of conducted beats remain constant.

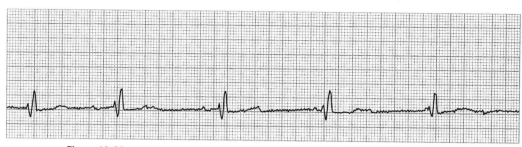

Figure 10-30 Third-degree AV block, with ventricular escape rhythm (QRS >0.10 second).

and (4) **initiating emergency measures to treat dysrhythmias when required.**

BEDSIDE HEMODYNAMIC MONITORING

Intensity levels of hemodynamic monitoring differ depending on the patient's clinical needs. The simplest level includes monitoring heart rhythm, central venous pressure (CVP), and arterial blood pressure, a combination often used after uncomplicated general surgery. If the patient has a low CO after an acute MI, a more intense level of surveillance may be necessary, including use of a thermodilution pulmonary artery catheter, which provides hemodynamic information that includes intracardiac pressures and measurement of CO.

Equipment

A hemodynamic monitoring system has the following four parts (Figure 10-31):

1. Invasive catheter and high-pressure tubing connect the patient to the transducer.
2. Transducer receives the physiologic signal through the catheter and tubing and converts it into electrical energy.
3. Flush system maintains patency of the fluid-filled system and catheter.
4. Bedside monitor contains the amplifier/recorder, which increases the volume of the electrical signal and displays it on an oscilloscope and on a digital scale (mm Hg).

Although many different types of invasive catheters can be inserted to monitor hemodynamic pressures, all are similarly connected. Equipment consists of a bag of 0.9% normal saline solution (some centers use 5% dextrose or lactated Ringer's solution), usually containing 1 unit of heparin (range 0.25 to 2.0 units) per milliliter of solution depending on institutional protocol (some hospitals do not use heparin at all); a pressure infusion cuff inflated to 300 mm Hg; IV tubing; three-way stopcocks; and in-line flow device attached for both continuous fluid infusion and manual flush. The high-pressure tubing connects the invasive catheter to the transducer to prevent *damping* (flattening) of the waveform. The most common transducers are disposable, use a silicon chip, and are extremely accurate.[86,87]

Nursing Management

Nursing priorities for the patient with hemodynamic monitoring focus on (1) accurately calibrating the hemodynamic equipment, (2) recognizing normal values, (3) establishing safe monitor alarm limits, (4) accommodating changes in patient position, and (5) troubleshooting monitoring system problems.

Calibrating Hemodynamic Equipment

To ensure accuracy of hemodynamic pressure readings, two baseline measurements are necessary: calibrating the system to atmospheric pressure ("zeroing" the transducer) and determining the phlebostatic axis for transducer height placement ("leveling" the transducer).[88]

Zeroing the Transducer. To calibrate the equipment to atmospheric pressure, the three-way stopcock nearest the transducer is turned to simultaneously open the transducer to air (atmospheric pressure) and to close it to the patient and the flush system. The monitor is adjusted so that "0" is displayed, which equals atmospheric pressure. Atmospheric pressure is not actually "0" but 760 mm Hg at sea level; using zero to represent current atmospheric pressure provides a convenient baseline for hemodynamic measurement purposes. Some monitors also require calibration of the upper scale limit while the system remains open to air. At the end of the calibration procedure, the stopcock is returned to the closed position, and a closed cap is placed over the open port. At this point the patient's waveform and hemodynamic pressures are displayed. Disposable transducers are now so accurate that once they are calibrated to atmospheric pressure, drift from the zero baseline is minimal. Although in theory this means that repeated calibration is unnecessary, clinical protocols in many units require the nurse to calibrate the transducer at the beginning of each shift for quality control and safety.

Leveling the Transducer. Leveling the transducer is different from zeroing and aligns the disposable transducer with the tip of the invasive catheter. Some critical care units use a carpenter's level for this purpose. The transducer air-reference stopcock is leveled with the phlebostatic axis reference point. The *phlebostatic axis* is a physical reference point on the chest used as a baseline for consistent transducer height placement. To obtain the axis, a theoretic line is drawn from

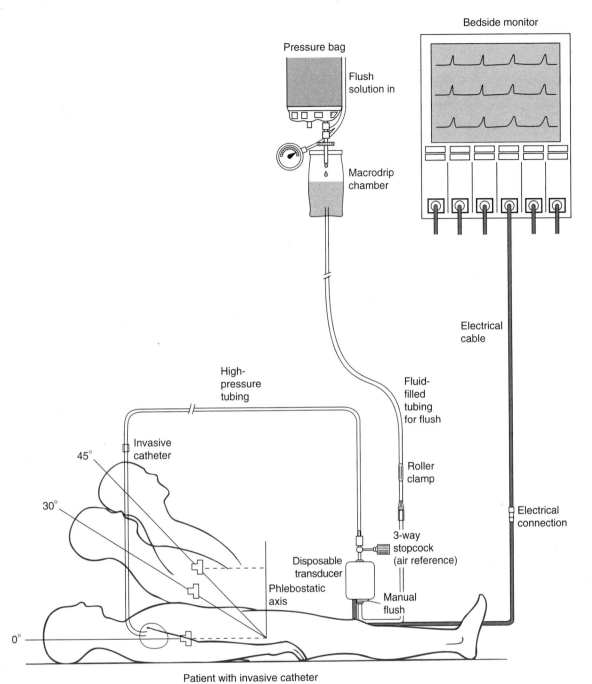

Figure 10-31   Four parts of hemodynamic monitoring system include invasive catheter attached to high-pressure tubing for connection to the transducer; transducer; flush system, including a manual flush; and bedside monitor. 0, 30 and 45 degree head of bed positions demonstrate different positions of the phlebostatic axis for transducer levelling.

the fourth intercostal space, where it joins the sternum, to a midaxillary line on the side of the chest. This point approximates the level of the atria (see Figure 10-31). It is used as the reference mark for both CVP and pulmonary artery catheter transducers. In other words, the level of the transducer "air reference stopcock" approximates the level of the tip of the invasive catheter.

Recognizing Normal Values

Once the system is correctly calibrated, the clinical team uses the known normal values as a reference when evaluating clinical patient outcomes and response to interventions (Table 10-8).

Table **10-8** Hemodynamic Pressures and Calculated Hemodynamic Values

Hemodynamic Pressure	Definition/Explanation	Normal Range*
Mean arterial pressure (MAP)	Average perfusion pressure created by arterial blood pressure during cardiac cycle. Normal cardiac cycle is one-third systole and two-thirds diastole. Three components divided by 3 to obtain average perfusion pressure for entire cardiac cycle.	70-100 mm Hg
Central venous pressure (CVP)	Pressure created by volume in right side of heart. When tricuspid valve open, CVP reflects filling pressures in right ventricle. Clinically, CVP often used as guide to overall fluid balance.	2-5 mm Hg 3-8 cm H_2O
Pulmonary artery pressure (PAP) PA systolic (PAS) PA diastolic (PAD) PA mean (PAM)	Pulsatile pressure in pulmonary artery, measured by indwelling catheter.	PAS 20-30 mm Hg PAD 5-10 mm Hg PAM 10-15 mm Hg
Pulmonary artery occlusion pressure (PAOP) (wedge)	Pressure created by volume in left side of heart. When mitral valve open, PAOP reflects filling pressures in pulmonary vasculature, and pressures in left side of heart are transmitted back to catheter "wedged" into a small pulmonary arteriole.	5-12 mm Hg
Cardiac output (CO)	Amount of blood pumped out by a ventricle. Clinically, CO can be measured using the thermodilution method (liters per minute).	4-6 L/min (at rest)
Cardiac index (CI)	CO divided by body surface area (BSA), tailoring CO to individual body size. BSA conversion chart is necessary to calculate CI, which is considered more accurate than CO because CI is individualized to height and weight (liters per minute per square meter BSA).	2.2-4.0 L/min/m²
Stroke volume (SV)	Amount of blood ejected by ventricle with each heartbeat. Hemodynamic monitoring systems calculate SV by dividing CO (L/min) by heart rate, then multiplying answer by 1000 to change liters to milliliters.	60-130 ml/beat
Stroke volume index (SI)	SV indexed to BSA (milliliters per square meter BSA).	40-50 ml/m²
Systemic vascular resistance (SVR)	Mean pressure difference across systemic vascular bed, divided by blood flow. Clinically, SVR represents resistance (created by systemic arteries, arterioles) against which *left* ventricle must pump to eject its volume. As SVR increases, left ventricular CO falls. Measured in units or dynes/sec/cm⁻⁵. If number of units multiplied by 80, value is converted to dynes/sec/cm⁻⁵	800-1400 dynes/sec/cm⁻⁵ for noncardiac patients; 800-1200 dynes/sec/cm⁻⁵ for patients with cardiovascular disease
Pulmonary vascular resistance (PVR)	Mean pressure difference across pulmonary vascular bed, divided by blood flow. Clinically, PVR represents resistance (created by pulmonary arteries, arterioles) against which *right* ventricle must pump to eject its volume. As PVR increases, right ventricular CO decreases. Measured in units or dynes/sec/cm⁻⁵. PVR is normally one sixth of SVR.	100-250 dynes/sec/cm⁻⁵
Left ventricular stroke work index (LVSWI)	Amount of work the left ventricle performs with *each heartbeat*. Hemodynamic formula represents pressure generated (MAP) multiplied by volume pumped (SV). A conversion factor is used to change ml/mm Hg to *gram-meter* (g-m). Always represented as an indexed volume. LVSWI increases or decreases because of changes in pressure (MAP) or volume pumped (SV).	50-62 g-m/m²
Right ventricular stroke work index (RVSWI)	Amount of work the right ventricle performs with *each heartbeat*. Hemodynamic formula represents pressure generated (PAP mean) multiplied by volume pumped (SV). A conversion factor is used to change mm Hg to g-m. Always represented as an indexed value (BSA chart). RVSWI increases or decreases because of changes in pressure (PAP mean) or volume pumped (SV).	7.9-9.7 g-m/m²

*The formulas for these hemodynamic values are listed in the Appendix.

Establishing Safe Monitor Alarm Limits

All bedside hemodynamic monitoring systems have alarm limits that are preset to ensure patient safety.[94,95] The alarms must be sufficiently distinctive and audible to be heard over the noise of a typical critical care unit. Patient safety guidelines are designed to promote clinical alarm goals (Box 10-8). Some clinical situations create special challenges with respect to alarm safety. Nursing care actions that cause the patient to move in the bed will often trigger the alarms. Temporarily silencing the sound for 1 to 3 minutes while continuing to observe the bedside monitor is appropriate. The real challenge occurs when a patient is restless or fidgeting with IV tubing or electrodes, resulting in the alarms bring constantly triggered because the monitor is unable to evaluate the ECG rhythms and hemodynamic waveforms effectively. It is tempting to "silence" these "nuisance alarms" permanently.[95] The alarms should not be turned off because the patient is left in a vulnerable position if a dysrhythmia or hemodynamic complication arises. Clinical interventions to ameliorate the root cause of the problem (e.g., restlessness) are more appropriate.

Accommodating Changes in Patient Position

Patient position in the hemodynamically monitored patient would not be an issue if critical care patients were always flat in the bed. However, lying flat is not always a comfortable position, especially if the patient is alert or if the head of the bed needs to be elevated to decrease the work of breathing. Nurse researchers have determined that the CVP, pulmonary artery pressure (PAP), and pulmonary artery occlusion pressure (PAOP), also called pulmonary artery wedge pressure (PAWP), can be reliably measured at head-of-bed positions from 0 degrees (flat) to 60 degrees if the patient is lying on his or her back (supine). In general, if the patient is normovolemic and hemodynamically stable, raising the head of the bed does not affect hemodynamic pressure values. The majority of patients do not need the head of the bed to be lowered to "0" to obtain accurate CVP, PAP, or PAOP (wedge) readings.[89,90]

Troubleshooting Monitoring System Problems

Typical problems with hemodynamic bedside monitoring are addressed in Table 10-9.

Intraarterial Blood Pressure Monitoring
Indications

Intraarterial blood pressure monitoring is indicated for any major medical or surgical condition that compromises CO, tissue perfusion, or fluid volume status.[91] The system is designed for continuous measurement of three blood pressure parameters: systole, diastole, and mean arterial blood pressure. In addition, the direct arterial access is helpful in the management of patients with acute respiratory failure who require frequent arterial blood gas measurements.

Catheters

The size of the catheter used is proportionate to the diameter of the cannulated artery. In small arteries (e.g., radial, dorsalis pedis) a 20-gauge, nontapered Teflon catheter is used most often. If the larger femoral or axillary

---

patient safety   Box 10-8

Goals for Clinical Alarm Systems

IMPROVE EFFECTIVENESS OF CLINICAL ALARM SYSTEMS
1. Implement regular preventive maintenance and testing of alarm systems.
2. Ensure that alarms are activated with appropriate settings and are sufficiently audible with respect to distances and competing noise within the unit.

IMPROVE CLINICAL ALARM SAFETY
Alarm Identification
1. Audible and visual indication should be present for any condition that poses a risk to the patient. Indicator should be visible from at least 10 feet (3 meters).
2. Cause of the alarm must be easily identifiable by health care practitioner.
3. Life-threatening conditions should be clearly differentiated from noncritical alarm situations.
4. High-priority alarms should override low-priority alarms.
5. Alarm must be sufficiently loud or distinctive to be heard over environmental noise of a busy critical care unit.

6. It should never be possible to turn the volume control to "off."

Disabling and Silencing
1. Alarm silence must have visual indicator to clearly show it is disabled.
2. Critical alarms should not be permanently overridden (turned "off").
3. New, life-threatening alarm condition should override a silenced alarm.

Power
Battery units should initiate an alarm before a unit stops working effectively.

Alarm Limits
1. Alarm limits can be adjusted to meet clinical needs of patient. The system should default to standard settings between patients.
2. Alarm limits should preferably be displayed on the monitor.

Data from www.JCAHO.org and Health Devices 31:397-412, 2002.

Table **10-9** Nursing Measures to Ensure Patient Safety and to Troubleshoot Problems with Hemodynamic Monitoring Equipment

Problem	Prevention	Rationale	Troubleshooting
Overdamping of waveform	Provide continuous infusion of solution containing heparin through in-line flush device (1 unit of heparin for each milliliter of flush solution).	To ensure that recorded pressures and waveform are accurate because a damped waveform gives inaccurate readings.	Before insertion, completely flush line/catheter. In a line attached to patient, back-flush through system to clear bubbles from tubing/transducer.
Underdamping ("overshoot" or "fling")	Use short lengths of noncompliant tubing. Use "fast-flush square wave" test to demonstrate optimal system damping. Verify arterial waveform accuracy with cuff blood pressure.	If monitoring system is underdamped, both systolic and diastolic values will be overestimated by both waveform and digital values. Falsely high systolic values may lead to clinical decisions based on erroneous data.	Perform "fast-flush square wave" test to verify optimal damping of monitoring system.
Clot formation at end of catheter	Provide continuous infusion of solution containing heparin through in-line flush device (1 unit of heparin for each milliliter of flush solution).	Any foreign object placed in body can cause local activation of patient's coagulation system as a normal defense mechanism. Clots that are formed may be dangerous if they break off and travel to other parts of body.	If clot in catheter is suspected because of a damped waveform or resistance to forward flushing of system, gently aspirate line using small syringe inserted into proximal stopcock. Then flush line again once clot is removed, and inspect waveform, which should return to normal pattern.
Hemorrhage	Use Luer-Lok (screw) connections in line setup. Close and cap stopcocks when not in use. Ensure that catheter is sutured or securely taped in position.	Loose connection or open stopcock creates low-pressure sump effect, causing blood to back into line and into open air. If catheter is accidentally removed, vessel can bleed profusely, especially with arterial line or if patient has abnormal coagulation factors (from heparin in line) or has hypertension.	Once blood leak is recognized, tighten all connections, flush line, and estimate blood loss. If catheter has been inadvertently removed, put pressure on cannulation site. When bleeding has stopped, apply sterile dressing, estimate blood loss, and inform physician. If patient is restless, an armboard may protect lines inserted in arm.
Air emboli	Ensure that all air bubbles are purged from a new line setup before attachment to an indwelling catheter.	Air can be introduced at several times, including when central venous pressure (CVP) tubing comes apart, when new line setup is attached, or when new CVP or pulmonary artery (PA) line is inserted. During insertion of CVP or PA line, patient may be asked to hold breath at specific times to prevent drawing air into chest during inhalation.	Because it is impossible to retrieve air once it has been introduced into bloodstream, prevention is the best cure.

Problem	Prevention	Rationale	Correction/Intervention
	Ensure that drip chamber from bag of flush solution is more than half full before using in-line fast-flush system. Some sources recommend removing all air from bag of flush solution before assembling system.	In-line fast-flush devices are designed to permit clearing of blood from line after withdrawal of blood samples. If chamber of IV tubing is too low or empty, rapid flow of fluid will create turbulence and cause flushing of air bubbles into system and into bloodstream.	If detected, air bubbles must be vented through in-line stopcocks, and drip chamber must be filled. Left atrial pressure (LAP) line setup is the only system that includes an air filter specifically to prevent air emboli.
Normal waveform with *low* digital pressure	Ensure that system is calibrated to atmospheric pressure. Ensure that transducer is placed at level of phlebostatic axis.	To provide a "0" baseline relative to atmospheric pressure. If transducer has been placed *higher* than phlebostatic level, gravity and lack of hydrostatic pressure will produce falsely *low* reading.	Recalibrate equipment if transducer drift has occurred. Reposition transducer at level of phlebostatic axis. Misplacement can occur if patient moves from bed to chair or if bed is placed in a Trendelenburg position.
Normal waveform with *high* digital pressure	Ensure that system is calibrated to atmospheric pressure. Ensure that transducer is placed at level of phlebostatic axis.	To provide a "0" baseline relative to atmospheric pressure. If transducer has been placed *lower* than phlebostatic level, weight of hydrostatic pressure on transducer will produce falsely *high* reading.	Recalibrate the equipment if transducer drift has occurred. Reposition transducer at level of phlebostatic axis. This situation can occur if head of bed was raised and transducer was not repositioned. Some centers require attachment of transducer to patient's chest to avoid this problem.
Loss of waveform	Always have the hemodynamic waveform monitored so that changes or loss can be quickly noted.	Catheter may be kinked, or a stopcock may be turned off.	Check line setup to ensure that all stopcocks are turned in correct position and that tubing is not kinked. At times, catheter migrates against a vessel wall, and having patient change position restores waveform.

arteries are used, a 19- or 20-gauge Teflon catheter is used. Teflon catheters are preferred because of their lower risk of thrombosis.

The catheter insertion is usually percutaneous, although the technique varies with vessel size. Cannulas are most often inserted in the smaller arteries, using a "catheter-over-needle" unit in which the needle is used as a temporary guide for catheter placement. With this method, once the unit has been inserted into the artery, the needle is withdrawn, leaving the supple plastic cannula in place. Insertion of a cannula into a larger artery usually necessitates use of the *Seldinger technique*. This procedure involves (1) entry into the artery using a needle, (2) passage of a supple guidewire through the needle into the artery, (3) removal of the needle, (4) passage of the catheter over the guidewire, and (5) removal of the guidewire, leaving the cannula in the artery

Insertion

Several major peripheral arteries are suitable for receiving a cannula and for long-term hemodynamic monitoring. The most frequently used site is the radial artery. If this artery is not available, the femoral, dorsalis pedis, axillary, or brachial artery may be used.

Allen Test

The major advantage of the *radial artery* is that collateral circulation to the hand is provided by the ulnar artery and the palmar arch in most of the population; thus other avenues of circulation are available if the radial artery becomes blocked after catheter placement. Before radial artery cannulation, collateral circulation must be assessed using flow Doppler imaging or the Allen test.[92] In the Allen test the radial and ulnar arteries are compressed simultaneously. The patient is asked to clench and unclench the hand until it blanches. One of the arteries is then released, and the hand should immediately flush from that side. The same procedure is repeated for the remaining artery.[92]

Nursing Management

Nursing priorities for the patient with intraarterial monitoring focus on (1) assessing arterial perfusion pressures, (2) interpreting the accuracy of the arterial pressure waveform, and (3) troubleshooting monitoring system problems.

Assessing Arterial Perfusion Pressures. Intraarterial blood pressure monitoring is designed for continuous assessment of arterial perfusion to the major organ systems of the body. *Mean arterial pressure* (MAP) is the clinical parameter most often used to assess perfusion because MAP represents perfusion pressure throughout the cardiac cycle. Because one third of the cardiac cycle is spent in systole and two thirds in diastole, the MAP calculation must reflect the greater amount of time spent in diastole.

The formula for calculating MAP is [(Diastole × 2) + Systole] ÷ 3. Thus a blood pressure of 120/60 mm Hg produces a MAP of 80 mm Hg [(120 + 120) ÷ 3].

A MAP greater than 60 mm Hg is the minimum value necessary to perfuse the coronary arteries, brain, and kidneys. A MAP of 70 to 90 mm Hg is ideal for the cardiac patient to decrease left ventricular workload. After carotid endarterectomy or neurologic surgery, a MAP of 90 to 110 mm Hg may be the most appropriate to increase cerebral perfusion pressure. Systolic and diastolic pressures are monitored in conjunction with the MAP as a further guide to the accuracy of perfusion. Should cardiac output decrease, the body compensates by constricting peripheral vessels to maintain the blood pressure. In this situation the MAP may remain constant but the pulse pressure (difference between systolic and diastolic pressures) narrows.

For example, *Mr. A* has BP of 90/70 mm Hg and MAP of 76 mm Hg, and *Mr. B* has BP of 150/40 mm Hg and MAP of 76 mm Hg. Both these patients have a mean perfusion pressure of 76 mm Hg, but clinically they are very different. *Mr. A* is peripherally vasoconstricted, as demonstrated by the narrow pulse pressure. His skin is cool to touch, and he has weak peripheral pulses. *Mr. B* has a wide pulse pressure, warm skin, and normally palpable peripheral pulses. Thus nursing assessment of the patient with an arterial line includes comparison of clinical findings with arterial line readings, including perfusion pressure and MAP.

Interpreting Accuracy of Arterial Pressure Waveform. As the aortic valve opens, blood is ejected from the left ventricle and is recorded as an increase of pressure in the arterial system. The highest point recorded is called *systole*. After peak ejection (systole), the ejection force is decreased and the pressure drops. A notch may be visible on the downstroke of this arterial waveform, representing closure of the aortic valve; this *dicrotic notch* signifies the beginning of diastole. The remainder of the downstroke represents diastolic runoff of blood flow into the peripheral arterial vasculature.[88] The lowest point recorded is termed *diastole*. In a normal arterial pressure tracing, electrical stimulation (QRS) is always first, and the arterial pressure tracing follows the initiating QRS (Figure 10-32).

Troubleshooting Monitoring System Problems. Major complications associated with arterial pressure monitoring are rare.[93] The most life-threatening risk is exsanguination if the Luer-Lok connections are not tight or if an in-line stopcock is inadvertently opened to air. Pressure monitor alarms must always be "on" with alarm limits (high and low) set at a safe, audible warning range for each patient.[94,95] When the arterial monitor displays a low blood pressure digital reading, it is a nursing responsibility to determine whether this is a true patient problem or a problem with the monitoring equipment. A *damped waveform* occurs when communication from the artery to the transducer is interrupted and produces false values on the monitor and oscilloscope. Troubleshooting techniques are used to find the origin of the problem and to remove the cause of damping (see Table 10-9).

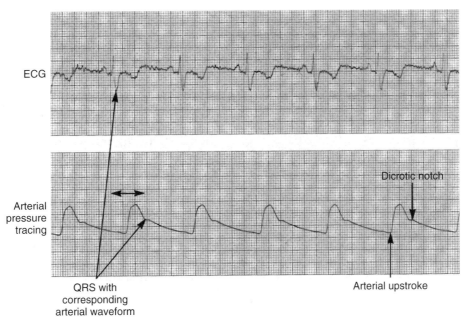

Figure 10-32 Simultaneous ECG and normal arterial pressure tracing.

Central Venous Pressure Monitoring

Indications

CVP monitoring is indicated whenever a patient has significant alteration in fluid volume. The CVP can be used as a guide in fluid volume replacement in hypovolemia and to assess the impact of diuresis after diuretic administration in the case of fluid overload. In addition, when a major IV line is required for volume replacement, a *central venous catheter* (CVC) is a good choice because large volumes of fluid can easily be delivered.

Catheters

CVCs are available as single-, double-, or triple-lumen infusion catheters, depending on the specific needs of the patient. Made of polyvinyl chloride, CVCs are soft and flexible.

Insertion

The large veins of the upper thorax—the subclavian (SC) or internal jugular (IJ) veins—are typically used for percutaneous CVC insertion. Insertion is guided by physical landmarks in the neck and shoulder area or by ultrasound for difficult catheter insertion.[96] During insertion using the SC or IJ veins, the patient may be placed in the Trendelenburg position. Placing the head in a dependent position causes the IJ veins in the neck to become more prominent, facilitating line placement. To minimize the risk of air embolus during the procedure, the patient may be asked to "take a deep breath and hold it" any time the needle or catheter is open to air. The tip of the catheter is designed to remain in the vena cava and should not migrate into the right atrium.

If the IJ or SC veins are not available, the femoral veins can be used for central venous access. The femoral veins are further away from the heart, so for accurate CVP measure-

ments, the tip of the catheter must be advanced into the inferior vena cava close to the right atrium. The femoral site is associated with a higher rate of nosocomial infection.[97] Prevention of intravascular catheter-related infections is a major safety issue in critical care units[98,99] (Box 10-9).

Because many patients are awake and alert when a CVC is inserted, a brief explanation about the procedure will minimize patient anxiety and result in cooperation during the insertion. This cooperation is important because insertion is a sterile procedure and the Trendelenburg position may not be comfortable for many patients. When possible, the ECG should be monitored during CVC insertion because of the associated risk of dysrhythmias.[100] After CVC placement a chest radiograph is obtained to verify placement and the absence of an iatrogenic hemothorax or pneumothorax. Other suitable insertion sites include the antecubital fossae veins.

Nursing Management

Nursing priorities for the patient with CVP monitoring focus on (1) assessing fluid volume status, (2) accommodating changes in patient position, (3) preventing catheter-related complications, and (4) accurately interpreting the CVP waveform and digital pressures.

Assessing Fluid Volume Status. The CVP catheter is used to measure the filling pressures of the right side of the heart. During diastole, when the tricuspid valve is open and blood is flowing from the right atrium to the right ventricle, the CVP accurately reflects fluid volume pressures in the right ventricle. The normal CVP is 2 to 5 mm Hg.

Low Central Venous Pressure. A low CVP often occurs in the hypovolemic patient and suggests that insufficient blood volume is filling the right ventricle to produce an ade-

Box **10-9**

Guidelines for Prevention and Management of Central Venous Catheter (CVC) Infections

1. Use effective handwashing.
2. Educate and train health care providers who insert and maintain CVCs.
3. Use maximal sterile barrier precautions during CVC insertion.
4. Use 2% chlorhexidine preparation for skin antisepsis.
5. Avoid routine replacement of CVCs as a strategy to prevent infection.
6. Insert antiseptic/antibiotic-impregnated short-term CVCs if rate of infection is high despite adherence to other strategies (education/training, maximal sterile barrier precautions, 2% chlorhexidine).
7. Confirm clinical suspicion of infection by taking cultures of blood and catheter samples.
8. Initially treat intravascular catheter infection with IV antimicrobial therapy, considering severity of patient's acute illness, underlying disease, and potential pathogens. Once the catheter-related pathogen is documented, narrow focus of antimicrobial therapy to treat specific organism(s).
9. Remove CVC if infected.

Data from O'Grady NP et al: *Am J Infect Control* 30:476-489, 2002; and Boyce JM, Pittet D: *Am J Infect Control* 30:1-46, 2002.

quate stroke volume. Thus, to maintain normal CO, the heart rate must increase. This increase produces the tachycardia often observed in hypovolemic states. CVP is used in combination with MAP and other clinical parameters to assess hemodynamic stability. In the hypovolemic patient, CVP falls before MAP decreases significantly because peripheral vasoconstriction keeps the MAP normal. Thus the CVP is an excellent early-warning system for the patient who is bleeding, vasodilated, receiving diuretics, or being rewarmed after cardiac surgery.

High Central Venous Pressure. An elevated CVP occurs in cases of fluid overload and heart failure. To circulate the excess blood volume, the heart must greatly increase its contractile force to move the increased volume of blood. This increases the cardiac workload and increases myocardial oxygen consumption. The critical care nurse follows the trend of the CVP measurements to determine subsequent interventions for optimal fluid volume management.

Accommodating Changes in Patient Position. To achieve accurate CVP measurements, the phlebostatic axis is used as a reference point on the body and the transducer zero must be level with this point. If the phlebostatic axis is used and the transducer is correctly aligned, any head-of-bed position of up to 60 degrees may be accurately used for CVP readings for most patients. Elevating the head of the bed is especially helpful for the patient with respiratory or cardiac problems who will not tolerate a flat position.[89]

Preventing Catheter-Related Complications

Air Embolus. The risk of air embolus, although uncommon, is always present for the patient with a central venous line in place. Air can enter during insertion, through a disconnected or broken catheter, or along the path of a removed CVC. This is more likely if the patient is in an upright position, because air can be pulled into the venous system with the increase in negative intrathoracic pressure during spontaneous inhalation. If a large volume of air (20 to 30 ml) is infused rapidly, it may become trapped in the right ventricular outflow tract (RVOT), stopping blood flow from the right side of the heart to the lungs. The patient may experience respiratory distress and cardiovascular collapse. Treatment involves administering 100% oxygen and placing the patient on the left side with the head downward (left lateral Trendelenburg position). This position displaces the air from the RVOT to the apex of the heart, where it can be either reabsorbed or aspirated. Precautions to prevent an air embolism in a CVP line include using only Luer-Lok connections, avoiding long loops of IV tubing, and using screw caps on three-way stopcocks.

Infection. Infection related to the use of CVCs is a major problem. It is estimated that more than 50,000 infections related to catheter use occur annually in the United States, with a 10% to 20% associated mortality. Risk factors include extremes of age, impaired host defense mechanisms, severe illness, malnutrition, and presence of other invasive lines. Generalized manifestations of infection are often present, although inflammation at the catheter site may be absent. To determine whether the catheter is contaminated, after removal the tip is placed in a sterile container and cultured. The CVC is left in place until there is evidence of infection. No decrease in infections was found when catheters were routinely changed to prevent infectious complications, and this practice is no longer recommended.[98] Catheters changed over guidewires usually have a higher rate of infection.

Prevention is the best defense against complications resulting from infections. Because most infections are transmitted through the skin, the physician should use good handwashing,[98] clean the patient's skin with 2% chlorhexidine, use optimal sterile technique during catheter insertion, and maximize barrier precautions[98] (Box 10-9).

Nurses are to follow aseptic procedures during site care and any time they enter the system to withdraw blood, give medications, or change tubing.[98,99] Incidence of infection is higher with use of transparent occlusive dressings that do not allow removal of moisture. Therefore nonocclusive moisture-permeable dressings are recommended. Site dressings with antimicrobial properties are being developed to lower infection rates. New developments in catheter design may also help to reduce CVC infection. Some catheters are now impregnated with an antimicrobial substance or have an attached silver-impregnated cuff to act as a tissue barrier.[98]

Interpreting Central Venous Pressure Waveform. The normal right atrial (CVP) waveform has three positive deflections, called *a*, *c*, and *v* waves, that correspond to specific atrial events in the cardiac cycle (Figure 10-33). The *a wave* reflects atrial contraction and follows the P wave seen on the ECG. The downslope of the *a* wave is called the *x descent* and represents atrial relaxation. The *c wave* reflects the bulging of the closed tricuspid valve into the right atrium during ventricular contraction. The *c* wave is small and not always visible but corresponds to the QRS-T interval on the ECG. The *v wave* represents atrial filling and increased pressure against the closed tricuspid valve in early diastole. The downslope of the *v* wave is named the *y descent* and represents the fall in pressure as the tricuspid valve opens and blood flows from the right atrium to the right ventricle.

Pulmonary Artery Pressure Monitoring

The pulmonary artery (PA) catheter, also known as a "right heart" catheter or *Swan-Ganz catheter*, is the most invasive of the critical care monitoring catheters. Routine use of PA catheters is controversial. Various reports describe a range of clinical outcomes for patients with a PA catheter in place, including a reduction in new-onset organ failure,[101] an increase in morbidity,[102] and no benefit as a guide to clinical interventions compared with less invasive methods.[103] The most important clinical advice is not to insert the PA catheter as a routine measure in every patient, but rather determine whether the individual's clinical condition and management require this level of intense monitoring.[104]

The PA catheter can simultaneously assess several hemodynamic parameters, including PA systolic and diastolic pressures, pulmonary MAP, and PAOP (wedge pressure). The PA catheter also measures CO, which is then be used to calculate other hemodynamic parameters.

Catheters

The traditional PA catheter, invented by Swan and Ganz, has four lumens for measurement of right atrial pressure (RAP or CVP), PA pressures, PAOP (wedge), and CO (Figure 10-34, A). Multifunction catheters have additional lumens that are frequently used to optimize care for critically ill patients. Extra lumens include additional atrial lumens for IV infusion (Figure 10-34, B), a fiberoptic lumen to measure continuous mixed-venous oxygen saturation (SvO_2), plus lumens dedicated to right ventricular volumetric measurement and continuous CO (Figure 10-34, C). Other PA catheters include transvenous pacing electrodes to pace the heart if needed. The PA catheter is 110 cm in length, and the most common size is 7.5 or 8.0 French (Fr). Each of the four lumens exits into the heart at a different point along the catheter length.

Right Atrial Lumen. The proximal lumen is situated in the right atrium and is used for IV infusion, CVP measurement,

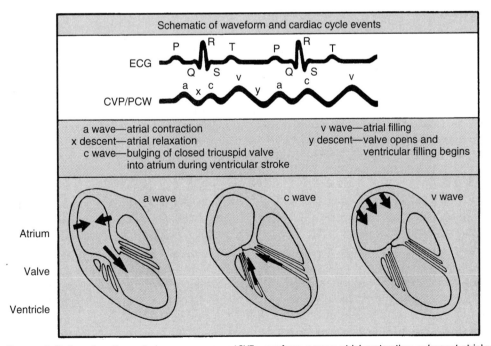

Figure 10-33   Cardiac events that produce the central venous pressure (*CVP*) waveform: *a wave*, atrial contraction; *x descent*, atrial relaxation; *c wave*, bulging of closed tricuspid valve into right atrium during ventricular systole; *v wave*, atrial filling; *y descent*, opening of tricuspid valve and filling of ventricle.

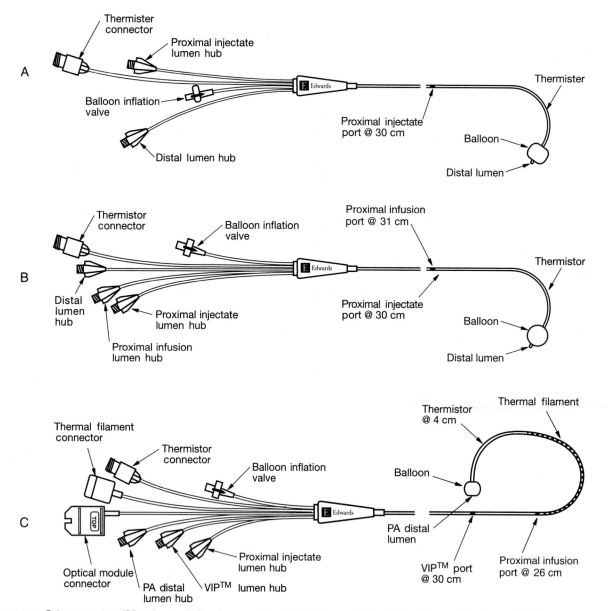

Figure 10-34 Pulmonary artery (*PA*) catheters. **A,** Four-lumen catheter. **B,** Five-lumen catheter that includes additional venous infusion port (*VIP*) into right atrium. **C,** Seven-lumen catheter that includes a VIP port and two additional lumens for continuous cardiac output (CCO) and thermal filament, and continuous mixed-venous oxygen saturation monitoring (optical module connector). An additional option is to combine use of CCO filament and thermistor response time to calculate continuous end-diastolic volume (CEDV) monitoring.(Courtesy Edwards Lifesciences LLC, 2001.)

withdrawal of venous blood samples, and injection of fluid for CO determinations. This port is often described as the *right atrial port* (RAP), also called the *CVP port*.

Pulmonary Artery Lumen. The distal PA lumen is located at the tip of the PA catheter and is situated in the pulmonary artery. It is used to record PA pressures and can be used for withdrawal of blood samples to measure SvO_2.

Balloon Lumen. The third lumen opens into a balloon at the end of the catheter that can be inflated with 0.8 (7.0 Fr) to 1.5 (7.5 Fr) ml of air. The balloon is inflated during catheter insertion once the catheter reaches the right atrium to assist in forward flow of the catheter and to minimize right

ventricular ectopy from the catheter tip. It is also inflated to obtain PAOP measurements when the PA catheter is correctly positioned in the pulmonary artery.

Thermistor Lumen. The fourth lumen is a thermistor used to measure changes in blood temperature. It is located near the catheter tip and is used to measure thermodilution CO. The connector end of the lumen is attached directly to the CO computer.

Insertion

If a PA catheter is to be inserted into a patient who is awake, some brief explanations about the procedure are helpful to ensure that the patient understands what will occur. The initial insertion techniques used for placement of a PA catheter are similar to those described for CVP line insertion.[98] In addition, because the PA catheter is positioned within the heart chambers and pulmonary artery on the right side of the heart, catheter passage is monitored using either fluoroscopy or waveform analysis on the bedside monitor (Figure 10-35).

Before inserting the catheter into the vein, and using sterile technique, the physician tests the balloon for inflation and flushes the catheter with normal saline solution to remove any air. The PA catheter is then attached to the bedside hemodynamic line setup and monitor so that the waveforms can be visualized while the catheter is advanced through the right side of the heart. A larger introducer sheath (8.5 Fr), which has the tip positioned in the vena cava and an additional IV side-port lumen, is often used to cannulate the vein first. This introducer sheath is known by several different names in clinical practice, including *sheath*, *cordis*, *introducer*, or *side port*. This introducer sheath remains in place, and the supple PA catheter is threaded through it into the vena cava and into the right side of the heart.

Nursing Management

Nursing priorities for the patient with PA catheter monitoring focus on (1) accurately interpreting PA catheter waveforms, (2) accommodating changes in patient position, (3) recognizing respiratory variation, (4) preventing catheter-related complications, (5) measuring cardiac output, and (6) evaluating hemodynamic performance.

Interpreting Pulmonary Artery Catheter Waveforms. Each chamber of the heart has a distinctive waveform with recognizable characteristics. It is the responsibility of the critical care nurse to recognize each waveform displayed on the bedside monitor, both when the catheter enters the corresponding chamber during insertion and during routine monitoring.[105,106]

Right Atrial Waveform. As the PA catheter is advanced into the right atrium during insertion, a right atrial waveform must be visible on the monitor, with recognizable *a*, *c*, and *v* waves (see Figure 10-35). The normal mean pressure in the right atrium is 2 to 5 mm Hg. Before passage through the tricuspid valve, the balloon at the tip of the catheter is inflated for two reasons. First, the balloon cushions the pointed tip of the PA catheter so that if the tip comes into contact with the right ventricular wall, it will cause less myocardial irritability and thus fewer ventricular dysrhythmias. Second, inflation of the balloon assists the catheter to float with the flow of blood from the right ventricle into the pulmonary artery. Because of these features and the balloon, PA catheters are described as *flow-directional* catheters.

Right Ventricular Waveform. The right ventricular (RV) waveform is pulsatile, with distinct systolic and diastolic pressures. Normal RV pressures are 20 to 30 mm Hg systolic and 0 to 5 mm Hg diastolic. Even with the balloon inflated, some ventricular ectopy may occur during passage through the right ventricle. All patients with a PA catheter inserted must have simultaneous ECG monitoring, with accessible defibrillator and emergency resuscitation equipment.

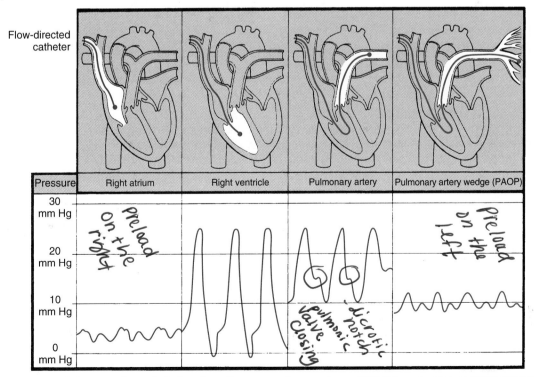

Figure 10-35 Pulmonary artery catheter insertion with corresponding waveforms. *PAOP*, Pulmonary artery occlusion pressure.

Don't Inflate balloon for 710 sec.

Pulmonary Artery Waveform. As the catheter enters the pulmonary artery, the waveform again changes. The diastolic pressure rises. Normal PA pressures range from 20 to 30 mm Hg systolic over 10 mm Hg diastolic. The dicrotic notch, visible on the waveform's downslope, represents closure of the pulmonic valve.

Pulmonary Artery Occlusion Waveform (Wedge). While the balloon remains inflated, the catheter is advanced into the wedge position. This maneuver produces PAOP. The waveform decreases in size and is nonpulsatile, reflecting a normal left atrial tracing with a- and v-wave deflections, described as a *wedge* tracing because the balloon is "wedged" into a small pulmonary vessel. The balloon occludes the pulmonary vessel so that the PA lumen is exposed only to left atrial pressure and is protected from the pulsatile influence of the pulmonary artery. When the balloon is deflated, the catheter should spontaneously float back into the artery. When the balloon is reinflated, the wedge tracing should be visible. The normal PAOP ranges from 5 to 12 mm Hg. The most serious risk associated with repeated balloon inflations is PA rupture.[93]

After insertion, the catheter is sutured to the skin and a chest radiograph is taken to verify placement. If the catheter is advanced too far into the pulmonary bed, the patient is at risk for pulmonary infarction. If insufficiently advanced into the pulmonary artery, the catheter will not be useful for PAOP readings. In many critical care units, however, if the patient's PA diastolic pressure (PADP) and PAOP (wedge) values approximate (within 0 to 3 mm Hg), PADP is used to follow the trend of left ventricular filling pressure (preload). This prevents possible trauma from frequent balloon inflations.[93] When the wedge pressure approximates the PADP, and the wedge is not required for clinical management, the PA catheter may be consciously pulled back into a nonwedging position in the pulmonary artery.

Accommodating Changes in Patient Position. In the supine position, if the transducer is placed at the level of the phlebostatic axis, a head-of-bed position from flat up to 30 degrees is appropriate for most patients. It is important to know that PA and PAOP measurements in the lateral position may be significantly different from those taken when the patient is lying supine.[105] At this point, if there is concern over the validity of pressure readings in a particular patient, it is more reliable to reposition the patient and record the measurements with the patient lying on the back. A stabilization period of only 5 minutes is required before taking pressure readings after a patient changes position.[90,105]

Recognizing Respiratory Variation. All PADP and PAOP tracings are subject to respiratory interference, especially if the patient is on a positive-pressure volume-cycled ventilator.[107] During inhalation the ventilator "pushes up" the PA tracing, which produces an artificially high reading (Figure 10-36, A). During spontaneous respiration, negative intrathoracic pressure "pulls down" the waveform and can produce an erroneously low measurement (Figure 10-36, B). To minimize the impact of respiratory variation, PADP is read at *end-expiration*, the most stable point in the respiratory cycle. If the digital number fluctuates with respiration, a printed readout on paper can be obtained to verify true PADP. In some clinical settings, airway pressure and flow are recorded simultaneously with the PADP/PAOP tracing to identify end-expiration.[105,107]

Positive End-Expiratory Pressure. Some clinical diagnoses, such as acute respiratory distress syndrome (ARDS), require the use of high levels of positive end-expiratory pressure (PEEP) to treat refractory hypoxemia. If a PEEP of greater than 10 cm H_2O is used, PAOP and PA pressures will be artificially elevated. Because of this impact of PEEP, some critical care patients in the past were taken off the ventilator to record PA pressure measurements. This practice has been shown to decrease the patient's oxygenation and may result in persistent hypoxemia. Because patients remain on PEEP for treatment, PEEP is maintained during measurement of PA pressures. In these patients the trend of PA readings is more important than a single measurement.

Preventing Catheter-Related Complications. Potential cardiac complications include ventricular dysrhythmias, endocarditis, valvular damage, cardiac rupture, and cardiac tamponade. Potential pulmonary complications include rupture of a pulmonary artery, PA thrombosis, embolism or hemorrhage, and infarction of a segment of lung.[108,109] The PA tracing is continuously monitored to ensure that the catheter does not migrate forward into a spontaneous wedge or PAOP position. A segment of lung can be infarcted if the wedged catheter occludes an arteriole for a prolonged period. If the catheter is wedged, the critical care nurse can pull it back from the wedge position if the institutional policy allows.[110]

Infection. Infection is always a risk with a PA catheter. The risks are similar to those discussed in the section on CVCs[97,98] (see Box 10-9).

Catheter Removal. PA catheters are routinely removed by the critical care nurse. Removal is not associated with major complications. The most common events are premature ventricular contractions (PVCs) in about 2% of patients as the catheter is pulled through the right ventricle.[111]

Measuring Cardiac Output

Thermodilution Bolus Method. The PA catheter measures CO through the bolus thermodilution method, which can be performed at the bedside and results in CO calculated in liters per minute (L/min). Generally, three CO readings within a 10% mean range are obtained at one time and then averaged to calculate CO.

A known amount (5-ml or 10-ml bolus) of iced or room-temperature normal saline (NS) solution is injected into the proximal lumen of the catheter. The injectate exits into the right atrium and travels with the flow of blood past the thermistor (temperature sensor) located near the distal end of the PA catheter. The injectate can be delivered by hand

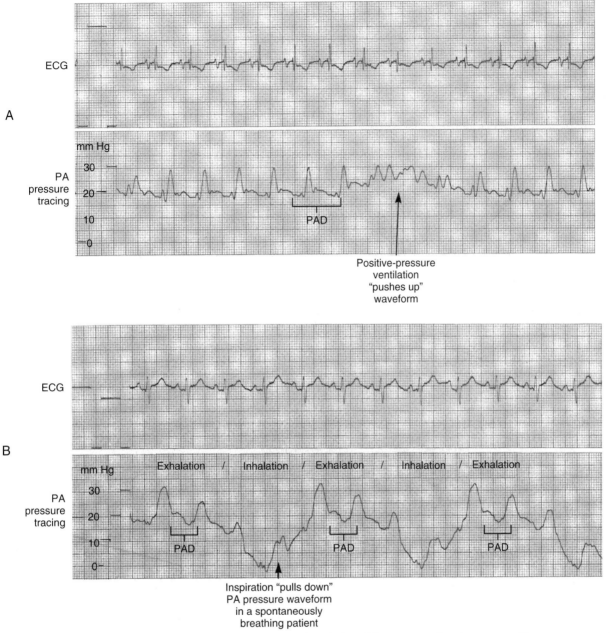

ECG

A

mm Hg

PA
pressure
tracing

30
20
10
0

PAD

Positive-pressure
ventilation
"pushes up"
waveform

ECG

B

mm Hg

PA
pressure
tracing

Exhalation / Inhalation / Exhalation / Inhalation / Exhalation

30
20
10
0

PAD   PAD   PAD

Inspiration "pulls down"
PA pressure waveform
in a spontaneously
breathing patient

Figure 10-36 Pulmonary artery (*PA*) waveforms that demonstrate impact of ventilation of PA pressure readings. For accuracy, PA pressures are read at end-exhalation. **A**, Positive-pressure ventilation. Increase in intrathoracic pressure during inhalation "pushes up" PA pressure waveform, creating a falsely high reading. **B**, Spontaneous breathing. Decrease in intrathoracic pressure during normal inhalation "pulls down" PA waveform, creating a falsely low reading.

injection using individual syringes of NS. More often, how-ever, a closed in-line system attached to a 500-ml bag of NS is used to deliver the individual injections.[112]

The thermodilution CO method uses the *indicator-dilution principle*, in which a known temperature is the indicator. Blood flow can be diagrammatically represented as a CO curve on which temperature is plotted against time (Figure 10-37). Most hemodynamic monitors display this CO curve, which must then be interpreted to determine whether the CO injection is valid. The normal curve has a smooth

upstroke, with a rounded peak and a gradually tapering downslope. A curve with an uneven pattern may indicate faulty injection technique, and the CO measurement is repeated. Patient movement and coughing also alter CO measurement.

If within the normal range, CO is equally accurate whether iced or room-temperature injectate is used. If CO is extremely high or low, however, iced injectate may be more accurate. To ensure accurate readings, the difference between injectate temperature and body temperature must

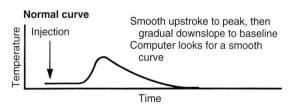

Figure 10-37 Normal cardiac thermodilution bolus output curve.

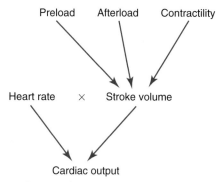

Figure 10-38 Preload, afterload, and contractility all contribute to the heart's stroke volume; stroke volume × heart rate = cardiac output.

be at least 10° C, and the injectate must be delivered within 4 seconds, with minimal handling of the syringe to prevent warming of the solution. This is particularly important if iced injectate is used. With all delivery systems the injectate is delivered at the same point in the respiratory cycle, usually end-exhalation.[113]

Continuous Cardiac Output Measurement. The bolus thermodilution method is reliable but performed intermittently. Continuous CO monitoring using a PA catheter is being used more frequently in clinical practice. One method uses a thermal filament on the PA catheter to emit small energy signals (the indicator) into the bloodstream. These signals are then detected by the thermistor near the tip of the PA catheter, and the equivalent of an indicator curve is created and a CO value calculated from these data.[112,114,115]

Clinical Use of Hemodynamic Information

The function and viability of all body tissues depends on adequate tissue perfusion. The adequacy of the supply is primarily determined by the effectiveness of the pumping action of the heart, adequate hemoglobin, and oxygenation. CO is a measure of the effectiveness of the heart as a pump. CO is the product of heart rate (HR) multiplied by stroke volume (SV). SV is the volume of blood ejected by the heart each beat in milliliters. The normal range for SV is 60 to 130 ml/beat. The clinical factors that contribute to SV are preload, afterload, and contractility (Figure 10-38). All three can be evaluated by using data from the PA catheter to calculate additional hemodynamic parameters. HR is recorded from the bedside ECG.

Preload

Preload is the volume in the ventricles at the end of diastole (filling stage of cardiac cycle when the heart muscle is relaxed). The volume in the ventricle at end-diastole represents the presystolic volume available for ejection for that cardiac cycle. In general, ventricular volume is not measured directly; instead, the pressure created by the volume is measured using either the CVP or PAOP values. When a PA catheter is correctly positioned, there are no valves between the distal tip of the PA catheter and the left atrium (Figure 10-39). When the mitral valve is open (during diastole), the wedged catheter can measure left ventricular end-diastolic pressure. This is the basis for use of the PAOP (wedge) pressure to evaluate left ventricular function.

The preload volume influences myocardial fiber length and stretch, and contributes to the strength of contraction (contractility). The more the muscle fiber is stretched, the more it will shorten in systole and the more force (contractility) will be used. Beyond a certain volume, however, the fibers become overstretched and the force (contractility) is decreased. This concept is often referred to as the *Frank-Starling law of the heart* (Figures 10-40 and 10-41). Causes of *decreased* preload include volume loss (e.g., hemorrhage, third spacing), venous dilation (e.g., hyperthermia, drugs), tachydysrhythmias or atrial fibrillation, increased intrathoracic pressure (e.g., positive-pressure ventilation), and elevated intracardiac pressure (e.g., cardiac tamponade). Causes of *increased* preload include volume overload (e.g., excess IV fluid administration), venous constriction (e.g., hypothermia, drugs), and ventricular failure.

Afterload

Afterload is defined as the pressure the ventricle has to generate (wall tension) to overcome the resistance to ejection created by the arteries and arterioles. It is a calculated measurement derived from information obtained from the PA catheter. As a response to increased afterload, ventricular wall tension rises. After a decrease in afterload, wall tension is lowered. The afterload of the left ventricle is termed *systemic vascular resistance* (SVR), with normal range of 800 to 1200 dynes/sec/cm^{-5}. The afterload of the right side of the heart is called *pulmonary vascular resistance* (PVR), with normal range of 100 to 250 dynes/sec/cm^{-5}. Causes of *decreased* afterload include arterial dilation (e.g., shock, hyperthermia). Causes of *increased* afterload include arterial constriction (e.g., shock, hypothermia, severe hypovolemia).

Pharmacologic manipulation of afterload is often used to improve cardiac performance of critically ill patients. Many drugs are available, with different modes of action. Drugs that vasodilate the arterial system and reduce SVR when given as a continuous infusion include sodium nitroprusside (Nipride) and high-dose nitroglycerin (NTG). Other common vasodilators include IV hydralazine and oral angiotensin-converting enzyme (ACE) inhibitors. If the

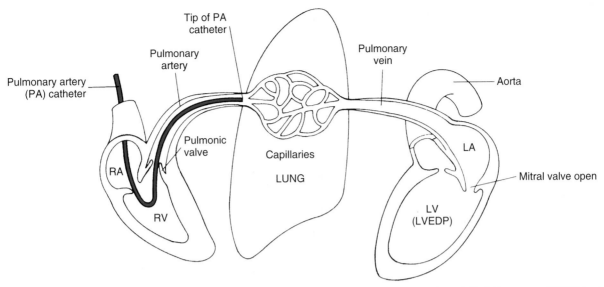

Figure 10-39   Relationship of pulmonary artery occlusion pressure (PAOP, wedge pressure) to left ventricular end-diastolic pressure (*LVEDP*)/preload, illustrating why PAOP accurately reflects LVEDP, or preload, in most clinical situations. During diastole, when mitral valve is open, there are no other valves or other obstructions between catheter tip and left ventricle (*LV*). Thus the pressure exerted by the volume in LV is reflected back through left atrium (*LA*) through pulmonary veins and to pulmonary capillaries. *PA*, Pulmonary artery; *RA*, right atrium; *RV*, right ventricle.

SVR is extremely low (less than 500 dynes/sec/cm^{-5}), medications may be used to "tighten up" the SVR, including high-dose dopamine, epinephrine, and norepinephrine (Levophed) or low-dose vasopressin. In these dose ranges the drugs are known as *vasopressors*. The critical care nurse evaluates the effectiveness of the medication by the increase in SVR into the therapeutic range. Frequent assessment of the peripheral circulation is required with drugs that increase SVR because excessive vasoconstriction can negatively affect tissue perfusion.

Contractility

Contractility, described as the force of myocardial contraction, is related to degree of myocardial fiber stretch (preload) and wall tension (afterload) and influences myocardial oxygen consumption. Increased contractility increases

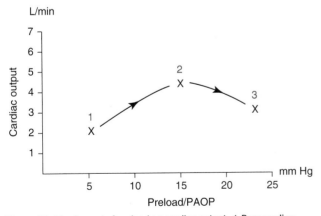

Figure 10-40   Impact of preload on cardiac output. *1*, Poor cardiac output (CO) with low preload as a result of hypovolemia. *2*, Hypovolemia is corrected after administration of 2 L of intravenous (IV) fluid. Preload volume in ventricle is increased, and pulmonary artery occlusion pressure (*PAOP*) has risen. Because of increased fiber stretch secondary to increase in preload, CO has also risen. *3*, After infusion of 2 more liters of IV solution, the myocardial fibers are overdistended, preload (PAOP) has increased, but CO has fallen as volume in left ventricle rises.

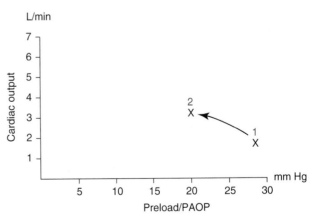

Figure 10-41   Impact of preload and venodilation on cardiac output (CO). *1*, After acute anterior wall myocardial infarction that has created significant LV dysfunction, this patient has LV pump failure with low CO and elevated filling pressures (*PAOP*). One clinical problem faced by this patient is too much preload. *2*, After administration of diuretics to remove volume and nitroglycerin to dilate the venous system, preload is reduced and CO rises.

myocardial workload and thus increases consumption, and vice versa. The contractility of the right side of the heart is measured by the right ventricular stroke work index (RVSWI) and the contractility of the left side of the heart is measured by the left ventricular stroke work index (LVSWI). The normal range for the RVSWI is 7.9 to 9.7 gram-meters (g-m/m^2 and for LVSWI is 50-62 g-m/m^2. Causes of *decreased* contractility include excessive preload or afterload, myocardial damage, drugs that decrease contractility such as β-blockers, and changes in the ionic environment caused by hypoxia, acidosis, or electrolyte imbalances. Increased contractility in the critically ill is mediated by positive inotropic drugs such as dopamine, dobutamine, and epinephrine. Pathologic causes of *increased* contractility include hyperthyroidism and the physiologic response to hypovolemia or fever and inflammation.

CONCLUSION

The range of diagnostic tools available to the bedside critical care nurse will continue to expand. As critical care patient needs become more complex and nursing responsibilities increase, incorporation of sophisticated clinical and technologic diagnostic information into the nursing management plan will become an even more important nursing priority.

REFERENCES

1. Mashour NH, Lin GI, Frishman WH: Herbal medicine for the treatment of cardiovascular disease: clinical considerations, *Arch Intern Med* 158:2225-2234, 1998.
2. Mayou RA, Bass CM, Bryant BM: Management of non-cardiac chest pain: from research to clinical practice, *Heart* 81:387-392, 1999.
3. Ryan TJ et al: 1999 Update: ACC/AHA guidelines for the management of patients with acute myocardial infarction. American College of Cardiology/American Heart Association Task Force on Practice Guidelines, Committee on Management of Acute Myocardial Infarction, *J Am Coll Cardiol* 34:890-911, 1999.
4. Eagle KA et al: ACC/AHA guideline update for perioperative cardiovascular evaluation for noncardiac surgery. American College of Cardiology/American Heart Association Task Force on Practice Guidelines, Committee to Update1996 Guidelines on Perioperative Cardiovascular Evaluation for Noncardiac Surgery, *Circulation* 105:1257-1267, 2002.
5. Milner KA et al: Gender differences in symptom presentation associated with coronary heart disease, *Am J Cardiol* 84:396-399, 1999.
6. Lee WL et al: Impact of diabetes on coronary artery disease in women and men: a meta-analysis of prospective studies, *Diabetes Care* 23:962-968, 2000.
7. Eckardt VF, Stauf B, Bernhard G: Chest pain in achalasia: patient characteristics and clinical course, *Gastroenterology* 116:1300-1304, 1999.
8. Richter JE: Chest pain and gastroesophageal reflux disease, *J Clin Gastroenterol* 30:S39-S41, 2000.
9. Achem SR, DeVault KR: Recent developments in chest pain of undetermined origin, *Curr Gastroenterol Rep* 2:201-209, 2000.
10. Constant J: Using internal jugular pulsations as a manometer for right atrial pressure measurements, *Cardiology* 93:26-30, 2000.
11. Launius BK, Graham D: Understanding and preventing deep vein thrombosis and pulmonary embolism, *AACN Clin Issues Crit Care Nurs* 4:91, 1998.
12. Kelsey LJ, Fry DM, VanderKolk WE: Thrombosis risk in the trauma patient: prevention and treatment, *Hematol Oncol Clin North Am* 14:417-430, 2000.
13. Velmahos GC et al: Prevention of venous thromboembolism after injury: an evidence-based report. Part I. Analysis of risk factors and evaluation of the role of vena caval filters, *J Trauma* 49:132-138, 2000.
14. Velmahos GC et al: Prevention of venous thromboembolism after injury: an evidence-based report. Part II. Analysis of risk factors and evaluation of the role of vena caval filters, *J Trauma* 49:140-144, 2000.
15. Warbel A, Lewicki L, Lupica K: Venous thromboembolism: risk factors in the craniotomy patient population, *J Neurosci Nurs* 31:180-186, 1999.
16. Freedman KB et al: A meta-analysis of thromboembolic prophylaxis following elective total hip arthroplasty, *J Bone Joint Surg* 82A:929-938, 2000.
17. Orme S et al: The normal range for inter-arm differences in blood pressure, *Age Ageing* 28:537-542, 1999.
18. Lloyd-Jones DM et al: Differential impact of systolic and diastolic blood pressure level on JNC-VI staging. Joint National Committee on Prevention, Detection, Evaluation, and Treatment of High Blood Pressure, *Hypertension* 34:381-385, 1999.
19. Woywodt A et al: Cardiopulmonary auscultation: duo for strings—opus 99, *Arch Intern Med* 159:2477-2479, 1999.
20. Lok CE, Morgan CD, Ranganathan N: The accuracy and interobserver agreement in detecting the "gallop sounds" by cardiac auscultation, *Chest* 114:1283-1288, 1998.
21. Tribouilloy CM et al: Pathophysiologic determinants of third heart sounds: a prospective clinical and Doppler echocardiographic study, *Am J Med* 111:96-102, 2001.
22. Drazner MH, Rame JE, Stevenson LW, Dries DL: Prognostic importance of elevated jugular venous pressure and a third heart sound in patients with heart failure, *N Engl J Med* 345:574-581, 2001.
23. Bonow RO et al: ACC/AHA guidelines for the management of patients with valvular heart disease. American College of Cardiology/American Heart Association Task Force on Practice Guidelines, Committee on Management of Patients with Valvular Heart Disease, *J Heart Valve Dis* 6:672-707, 1998.
24. Otto CM: Aortic stenosis—listen to the patient, look at the valve, *N Engl J Med* 343:652-654, 2000.
25. Munt B: Physical examination in valvular aortic stenosis: correlation with stenosis severity and prediction of clinical outcome, *Am Heart J* 137:298-306, 1999.
26. Indik JH, Alpert JS: Post–myocardial infarction pericarditis, *Curr Treat Options Cardiovasc Med* 2:351-356, 2000.
27. Chmielewski CM: Hyperkalemic emergencies: mechanisms, manifestations, and management, *Crit Care Nurs Clin North Am* 10:449-458, 1998.
28. Visweswaran P, Guntupalli J: Rhabdomyolysis, *Crit Care Clin* 15:415-428, 1999.
29. Rush C, Thomas J: A 42-year-old man with rhabdomyolysis from substance abuse and minor trauma, *J Emerg Nurs* 25:7-11, 1999.
30. Pitt B et al: The effect of spironolactone on morbidity and mortality in patients with severe heart failure. Randomized Aldactone Evaluation Study, *N Engl J Med* 341:709-717, 1999.
31. Greenberg A: Diuretic complications, *Am J Med Sci* 319:10-24, 2000.
32. Johnson RG et al: Potassium concentrations and ventricular ectopy: a prospective, observational study in post–cardiac surgery patients, *Crit Care Med* 27:2430-2434, 1999.

33. Rosenberger K: Management of electrolyte abnormalities: hypocalcemia, hypomagnesemia, and hypokalemia, *J Am Acad Nurse Pract* 10:209-217, 1998.
34. Barnett ML: Hypercalcemia, *Semin Oncol Nurs* 15:190-201, 1999.
35. Vella A et al: Digoxin, hypercalcaemia, and cardiac conduction, *Postgrad Med J* 75:554-556, 1999.
36. Ma G, Brady WJ, Pollack M, Chan TC: Electrocardiographic manifestations: digitalis toxicity, *J Emerg Med* 20:145-152, 2001.
37. Koch SM, Warters RD, Mehlhorn U: The simultaneous measurement of ionized and total calcium and ionized and total magnesium in intensive care unit patients, *J Crit Care* 17:203-205, 2002.
38. Schelling JR: Fatal hypermagnesemia, *Clin Nephrol* 53:61-65, 2000.
39. Agus ZS: Hypomagnesemia, *J Am Soc Nephrol* 10:1616-1622, 1999.
40. Innerarity S: Hypomagnesemia in acute and chronic illness, *Crit Care Nurs Q* 23:1-19, 2000.
41. Klevay LM, Milne DB: Low dietary magnesium increases supraventricular ectopy, *Am J Clin Nutr* 75:550-554, 2002.
42. Liao F, Folsom AR, Brancati FL: Is low magnesium concentration a risk factor for coronary heart disease? Atherosclerosis Risk in Communities (ARIC) Study, *Am Heart J* 136:480-490, 1998.
43. Moss AJ: The QT interval and torsade de pointes, *Drug Saf* 21:5-10, 1999.
44. Hillis GS et al: Utility of cardiac troponin I, creatine kinase-MB (mass), myosin light chain 1, and myoglobin in the early in-hospital triage of "high risk" patients with chest pain, *Heart* 82:614-620, 1999.
45. Murphy MJ, Berding CB: Use of measurements of myoglobin and cardiac troponins in the diagnosis of acute myocardial infarction, *Crit Care Nurse* 19:58-66, 1999.
46. Morrow DA et al: Clinical efficacy of three assays for cardiac troponin I for risk stratification in acute coronary syndromes: a Thrombolysis in Myocardial Infarction (TIMI) 11B substudy, *Clin Chem* 46:453-460, 2000.
47. Newman J et al: Prehospital identification of acute coronary ischemia using a troponin T rapid assay, *Prehosp Emerg Care* 3:97-101, 1999.
48. Muller-Bardorff M et al: Quantitative bedside assay for cardiac troponin T: a complementary method to centralized laboratory testing, *Clin Chem* 45:1002-1008, 1999.
49. Braunwald E et al: ACC/AHA 2002 guideline update for the management of patients with unstable angina and non-ST-segment elevation myocardial infarction. American College of Cardiology/American Heart Association Task Force on Practice Guidelines, Committee on Management of Patients with Unstable Angina, *J Am Coll Cardiol* 40:1366-1374, 2002.
50. Scanlon PJ et al: ACC/AHA guidelines for coronary angiography. American College of Cardiology/American Heart Association Task Force on Practice Guidelines, Committee on Coronary Angiography, Society for Cardiac Angiography and Interventions, *J Am Coll Cardiol* 33:1756-1824, 1999.
51. Fuster V et al: ACC/AHA/ESC guidelines for the management of patients with atrial fibrillation. American College of Cardiology/American Heart Association Task Force on Practice Guidelines, European Society of Cardiology Committee for Practice Guidelines and Policy Conferences, Committee to Develop Guidelines for Management of Patients with Atrial Fibrillation, North American Society of Pacing and Electrophysiology, *Circulation* 104:2118-2150, 2001.
52. Galatro KM et al: Bleeding complications and INR control of combined warfarin and low-dose aspirin therapy in patients with unstable angina and non-Q-wave myocardial infarction, *J Thromb Thrombolysis* 5:249-255, 1998.
53. Riley RS, Rowe D, Fisher LM: Clinical utilization of the international normalized ratio (INR), *J Clin Lab Anal* 14:101-114, 2000.
54. Lamendola C: Hypertriglyceridemia and low high-density lipoprotein: risks for coronary artery disease? *J Cardiovasc Nurs* 14:79-90, 2000.
55. Gulanick M, Cofer LA: Coronary risk factors: influences on the lipid profile, *J Cardiovasc Nurs* 14:16-28, 2000.
56. Smith SC Jr et al: AHA/ACC guidelines for preventing heart attack and death in patients with atherosclerotic cardiovascular disease: a statement for healthcare professionals. American Heart Association/American College of Cardiology, *Circulation* 104:1577-1579, 2001.
57. Drew BJ et al: Accuracy of the EASI 12-lead electrocardiogram compared to the standard 12-lead electrocardiogram for diagnosing multiple cardiac abnormalities, *J Electrocardiol* 32:38-47, 1999.
58. Drew BJ, Krucoff MW: Multilead ST-segment monitoring in patients with acute coronary syndromes: a consensus statement for healthcare professionals. ST-Segment Monitoring Practice Guideline International Working Group, *Am J Crit Care* 8:372-386, 1999.
59. Adams-Hamoda MG, Caldwell MA, Stotts NA, Drew BJ: Factors to consider when analyzing 12-lead electrocardiograms for evidence of acute myocardial ischemia, *Am J Crit Care* 12:9-16, 2003.
60. Viskin S: Long QT syndromes and torsade de pointes, *Lancet* 354:1625-1633, 1999.
61. De Ponti F et al: Non-antiarrhythmic drugs prolonging the QT interval: considerable use in seven countries, *Br J Clin Pharmacol* 54:171-177, 2002.
62. Littmann L: The power of PACs, *J Electrocardiol* 33:287-290, 2000.
63. Daoud EG, Morady F: Pathophysiology of atrial flutter, *Annu Rev Med* 49:77-83, 1998.
64. Varriale P, Sedighi A: Acute management of atrial fibrillation and atrial flutter in the critical care unit: should it be ibutilide? *Clin Cardiol* 23:265-268, 2000.
65. Murdock DK et al: Clinical and cost comparison of ibutilide and direct-current cardioversion for atrial fibrillation and flutter, *Am J Cardiol* 85:503-506, 2000.
66. Weiss R et al: Acute changes in spontaneous echo contrast and atrial function after cardioversion of persistent atrial flutter, *Am J Cardiol* 82:1052-1055, 1998.
67. VanderLugt JT et al: Efficacy and safety of ibutilide fumarate for the conversion of atrial arrhythmias after cardiac surgery, *Circulation* 100:369-375, 1999.
68. Wyse DG et al: A comparison of rate control and rhythm control in patients with atrial fibrillation, *N Engl J Med* 347:1825-1833, 2002.
69. Hohnloser SH et al: Pharmacological management of atrial fibrillation: an update, *J Cardiovasc Pharmacol Ther* 5:11-16, 2000.
70. Pinski SL, Helguera ME: Antiarrhythmic drug initiation in patients with atrial fibrillation, *Prog Cardiovasc Dis* 42:75-90, 1999.
71. Roy D et al: Amiodarone to prevent recurrence of atrial fibrillation. Canadian Trial of Atrial Fibrillation, *N Engl J Med* 342:913-920, 2000.
72. Cox JL, Schuessler RB, Boineau JP: The development of the Maze procedure for the treatment of atrial fibrillation, *Semin Thorac Cardiovasc Surg* 12:2-14, 2000.
73. Cox JL, Ad N: New surgical and catheter-based modifications of the Maze procedure, *Semin Thorac Cardiovasc Surg* 12:68-73, 2000.
74. Wood MA et al: Clinical outcomes after ablation and pacing therapy for atrial fibrillation: a meta-analysis, *Circulation* 101:1138-1144, 2000.
75. Gillis AM: Pacing to prevent atrial fibrillation, *Cardiol Clin* 18:25-36, 2000.
76. Swerdlow CD et al: Detection of atrial fibrillation and flutter by a dual-chamber implantable cardioverter-defibrillator. Worldwide Jewel AF Investigators, *Circulation* 101:878-885, 2000.

77. Savelieva I, Camm AJ: Atrial pacing for the prevention and termination of atrial fibrillation, *Am J Geriatr Cardiol* 11:380-398, 2002.
78. Teerlink JR et al: Ambulatory ventricular arrhythmias in patients with heart failure do not specifically predict an increased risk of sudden death. Prospective Randomized Milrinone Survival Evaluation (PROMISE), *Circulation* 101:40-46, 2000.
79. Naccarelli GV et al: Amiodarone: what have we learned from clinical trials? *Clin Cardiol* 23:73-82, 2000.
80. Kudenchuk PJ et al: Amiodarone for resuscitation after out-of-hospital cardiac arrest due to ventricular fibrillation, *N Engl J Med* 341:871-878, 1999.
81. Buxton AE et al: A randomized study of the prevention of sudden death in patients with coronary artery disease. Multicenter Unsustained Tachycardia Trial, *N Engl J Med* 341:1882-1890, 1999.
82. Doe J: Causes of death in the Antiarrhythmics versus Implantable Defibrillators (AVID) Trial, *J Am Coll Cardiol* 34:1552-1559, 1999.
83. Hazinski F, Cummins R: *Handbook of emergency cardiovascular care for healthcare providers,* 2002, American Heart Association.
84. Boyle J, Rost MK: Present status of cardiac pacing: a nursing perspective, *Crit Care Nurs Q* 23:1-19, 2000.
85. Gregoratos G et al: ACC/AHA/NASPE 2002 guideline update for implantation of cardiac pacemakers and antiarrhythmia devices. American College of Cardiology/American Heart Association Task Force on Practice Guidelines, ACC/AHA/NASPE Committee to Update 1998 Pacemaker Guidelines, *Circulation* 106:2145-2161, 2002.
86. Chang MC: Monitoring the critically ill patient, *New Horiz* 7:35-45, 1999.
87. McLane C, Morris L, Holm K: A comparison of intravascular pressure monitoring system contamination and patient bacteremia with use of 48- and 72-hour system change intervals, *Heart Lung* 27:200-208, 1998.
88. Imperial-Perez F, McRae M: Arterial pressure monitoring, *Crit Care Nurse* 19:105-107, 1999.
89. Aitken LM: Reliability of measurements of pulmonary artery pressure obtained with patients in the 60 degrees lateral position, *Am J Crit Care* 9:43-51, 2000.
90. Bridges MEJ et al: Effect of the 30° lateral recumbent position on pulmonary artery wedge pressures in critically ill adult cardiac surgery patients, *Am J Crit Care* 9:262-275, 2000.
91. Petersen D: Managing hypotension after cardiac surgery: an algorithm for treatment, *Crit Care Nurs* 20:36-49, 2000.
92. Cable DG, Mullany CJ, Schaff HV: The Allen test, *Ann Thorac Surg* 67:876-877, 1999.
93. Bowdle TA: Complications of invasive monitoring, *Anesthesiol Clin North America* 20(3):571-588, 2002.
94. Solsona JF et al: Are auditory warnings in the intensive care unit properly adjusted? *J Adv Nurs* 35:402-406, 2001.
95. Critical alarms and patient safety, *Health Devices* 31:395-417, 2002.
96. Keenan SP: Use of ultrasound to place central lines, *J Crit Care* 17:126-37, 2002.
97. Goetz AM et al: Risk of infection due to central venous catheters: effect of site of placement and catheter type, *Infect Control Hosp Epidemiol* 19:842-845, 1998.
98. O'Grady NP et al: Guidelines for the prevention of intravascular catheter-related infections, *Am J Infect Control* 30:476-489, 2002.
99. Boyce JM, Pittet D: Guideline for hand hygiene in health-care settings. Healthcare Infection Control Practices Advisory Committee, HICPAC/SHEA/APIC/IDSA Hand Hygiene Task Force, *Am J Infect Control* 30:1-46, 2002.
100. Matsumoto CG, Drew BJ, Ide B: Why should nurses closely monitor the ECG during insertion or exchange of a central venous catheter? *Prog Cardiovasc Nurs* 15:29, 2000.
101. Ivanov R, Allen J, Calvin JE: The incidence of major morbidity in critically ill patients managed with pulmonary artery catheters: a meta-analysis, *Crit Care Med* 28:615-619, 2000.
102. Connors AF et al: The effectiveness of right heart catheterization in the initial care of critically ill patients. SUPPORT Investigators, *JAMA* 276:889-897, 1996.
103. Sandham JD et al: A randomized, controlled trial of the use of pulmonary artery catheters in high-risk surgical patients, *N Engl J Med* 348:5-14, 2003.
104. Jacka MJ et al: The appropriateness of the pulmonary artery catheter in cardiovascular surgery, *Can J Anaesth* 49:276-282, 2002.
105. Keckeisen M: Monitoring pulmonary artery pressure, *Crit Care Nurs* 19:88-91, 1999.
106. Aitken LM: Expert critical care nurses' use of pulmonary artery pressure monitoring, *Intensive Crit Care Nurs* 16: 209-220, 2000.
107. Tyberg JV et al: Effects of positive intrathoracic pressure on pulmonary and systemic hemodynamics, *J Respir Physiol* 119:171-179, 2000.
108. Stancofski ED, Sardi A, Conaway GL: Successful outcome in Swan-Ganz catheter-induced rupture of pulmonary artery, *Am Surg* 64:1062-1065, 1998.
109. Hofbauer R et al: Thrombus formation on the balloon of heparin-bonded pulmonary artery catheters: an ultrastructural scanning electron microscope study, *Crit Care Med* 28:727-735, 2000.
110. Antle DE: Ensuring competency in nurse repositioning of the pulmonary artery catheter, *Dimens Crit Care Nurs* 19:44-51, 2000.
111. Baldwin IC, Heland M: Incidence of cardiac dysrhythmias in patients during pulmonary artery catheter removal after cardiac surgery, *Heart Lung* 29:155-160, 2000.
112. Gawlinski A: Measuring cardiac output: intermittent bolus thermodilution method, *Crit Care Nurs* 20:118-124, 2000.
113. Groeneveld AB et al: Effect of the mechanical ventilatory cycle on thermodilution right ventricular volumes and cardiac output, *J Appl Physiol* 89:89-96, 2000.
114. Mihm FG et al: A multicenter evaluation of a new continuous cardiac output pulmonary artery catheter system, *Crit Care Med* 26:1346-1350, 1998.
115. Albert NM, Spear BT, Hammel J: Agreement and clinical utility of two techniques for measuring cardiac output in patients with low cardiac output, *Am J Crit Care* 8:464-474, 1999.

MARY E. LOUGH

11

Cardiovascular
Disorders

Objectives

- Describe the etiology and pathophysiology of selected cardiovascular disorders.
- Identify the clinical manifestations of selected cardiovascular disorders.
- Explain the treatment of selected cardiovascular disorders.
- Discuss the nursing priorities for managing a patient with selected cardiovascular disorders.

evolve Be sure to check out the free exercises on-line at *http://evolve.elsevier.com/Urden/priorities/*

Cardiovascular disease remains the leading cause of mortality in the United States, with 2.4 million deaths from cardiovascular causes each year. It is the leading cause of death in both women and men.[1] An understanding of the pathology of cardiovascular disease processes, clinical assessment, and current clinical management allows the critical care nurse to anticipate and plan interventions. This chapter focuses on cardiac disorders often seen in the critical care environment.

CORONARY ARTERY DISEASE

Coronary artery disease (CAD) is a progressive disease that results in coronary artery narrowing or complete occlusion. *Atherosclerosis* is the most prevalent cause of coronary artery narrowing. Atherosclerotic fatty streaks can appear within the aorta during childhood, but symptoms occur only when 75% of a vessel lumen is occluded, usually by late middle age. Research and epidemiologic data collected during the past 50 years have demonstrated an association between nonmodifiable and modifiable risk factors and development of CAD[1] (Box 11-1).

Risk Factors
Age, Gender, and Race

The severe effects of CAD occur as a person ages. In general, CAD symptoms are seen in middle and old age.[1,2] Traditionally, CAD has been regarded as a male disease, but it is increasingly obvious that in modern society it affects both genders equally.[3-7] Nonwhite populations of both genders have higher CAD mortality rates than do white populations.[8-11]

Family History

A positive family history is one in which a close blood relative had a myocardial infarction or stroke before age 60 years. This family history suggests a genetic predisposition to CAD.[1]

Hyperlipidemia

Hyperlipidemia is a leading factor responsible for severe atherosclerosis and the development of CAD. Determining total serum cholesterol and triglyceride levels represents a helpful start in the evaluation process.[12] *Total cholesterol* is subdivided into high-density lipoprotein (HDL), low-density lipoprotein (LDL), and very-low-density lipoprotein (VLDL). *Triglycerides*, an additional and separate CAD risk factor, are serum lipids carried by VLDL cholesterol in the bloodstream.[13] Treatment of hyperlipidemia has advanced beyond the concept of lowering total cholesterol to treatment of specific lipoprotein abnormalities. The current target level for total cholesterol is less than 200 milligrams per deciliter (mg/dl). Specific serum lipids have their own target levels: LDL cholesterol below 100 mg/dl (if patient has CAD) or below 130 mg/dl (if no CAD history) and HDL cholesterol greater than 40 mg/dl. The triglyceride target level is less than 150 mg/dl.[12-15]

High-Fat Diet

A diet rich in saturated fats will lead to elevated cholesterol levels in the blood. The first line of treatment to lower elevated cholesterol is a low-fat high-fiber diet and an increase in physical exercise.[13] If these measures do not lower the total cholesterol and LDL cholesterol levels sufficiently, lipid-lowering drugs are used.[15,16]

Physical Inactivity and Obesity

Obesity is often associated with a sedentary lifestyle. It also increases susceptibility to the development of other risk factors, such as hypertension, decreased insulin sensitivity, and hyperlipidemia, with increased LDL and low HDL cholesterol.[1,17-19] The distribution pattern of fat on the body is a CAD risk factor. The more weight carried in the abdominal area, producing a large waist, the greater is the risk of CAD.[20] Excess abdominal adiposity ("apple" body shape) indicates additional fat around the abdominal organs as compared with individuals who have a smaller waist and larger hips ("pear" shape).[20] Exercise has been shown to lower risk of CAD and to decrease the risk of developing type 2 diabetes.[21,22]

Hypertension

Hypertension is the elevation of either systolic or diastolic blood pressure (BP) above 140/90 millimeters of mercury (mm Hg).[23] Hypertension is a cardiac risk factor because the high intravascular pressure damages blood vessel endothelium and causes pathologic left ventricular hypertrophy. The risk of developing either CAD or heart failure is reduced when BP is less than 140/90 mm Hg.[23] For patients older than 50 years of age, systolic BP above 140 mm Hg is a greater cardiac risk factor than diastolic BP, and beginning

Box **11-1** Coronary Artery Disease Risk Factors
NONMODIFIABLE Age Gender Family history Race **MODIFIABLE** Elevated serum lipids Hypertension Cigarette smoking Impaired glucose tolerance or diabetes mellitus Diet high in saturated fat, cholesterol, and calories Elevated homocystine level Metabolic syndrome Obesity Physical inactivity Postmenopause (*modification is controversial*)

at 115/75 mm Hg, the risk of developing cardiovascular disease doubles with each incremental increase of 20/10 mm Hg. [23] Most patients with hypertension will need two or more oral antihypertensive medications to lower their BP below 140/90 mm Hg. If patients have diabetes or chronic kidney disease the BP goal is lower (130/80 mm Hg), recognizing their greater risk of end-organ damage due to these pre-existing conditions.[23]

Cigarette Smoking

The greater the number of cigarettes smoked per day, the greater is the CAD risk. Cigarette smoking unfavorably alters serum lipid levels, decreasing HDL cholesterol levels and increasing LDL and triglyceride levels. Secondhand smoke exposure also increases CAD risk.[24]

Diabetes Mellitus

Individuals with diabetes mellitus (types 1 and 2) have a higher incidence of CAD than the general population; type 2 (non–insulin-dependent) diabetes is the more common. The recently redefined criteria for diagnosing diabetes may allow more patients to control this important risk factor at an earlier stage. A normal fasting blood glucose level falls between 70 and 110 mg/dl. A fasting blood sugar between 110 and 125 mg/dl represents impaired glucose function and is a risk factor for future development of diabetes.[25,26] A fasting plasma glucose 126 mg/dl suggests a diagnosis of diabetes (see Chapters 23 and 24).

Metabolic Syndrome

An estimated 47 million U.S. residents (23.7%) have *metabolic syndrome*.[1,14] Metabolic syndrome results from the following risk factors, which combine to dramatically increase CAD risk:

1. Waist circumference greater than 40 inches in men and 35 inches in women
2. Serum triglyceride level greater than 150 mg/dl[14]
3. HDL less than 40 mg/dl in men and 50 mg/dl in women[14]
4. BP higher than 130/85 mm Hg[23]
5. Fasting glucose level of 110 mg/dl or higher[25]

Postmenopausal Status

Serious CAD symptoms occur approximately 5 years later in women than men.[6,7] The average age for the first acute myocardial infarction is 65.8 years in men and 70.4 years in women.[1] The incidence of CAD in is two to three times higher in postmenopausal women than premenopausal women.[1] Thus, in the past, it seemed logical to prescribe hormone replacement therapy (HRT) to treat the symptoms of menopause. HRT is no longer recommended for CAD prevention. Recent research trials discovered an increase in cardiovascular events in the first year of HRT (estrogen plus progestin), although cardiac events declined after the first year, as confirmed in subsequent studies.[6,7]

Hyperhomocystinemia

Hyperhomocystinemia, an inborn error of metabolism, is a concern because individuals with high levels of plasma homocystine have a high incidence of atherosclerotic CAD and vascular disease. The risks from elevated homocystine are reduced in women and men who regularly take multivitamin supplements containing folate and vitamin B_6.[27]

Multifactorial Risk

At present, researchers are uncertain why a particular risk factor in one individual may result in serious consequences but may not cause problems for another individual. Studies show that CAD is a multifactorial disease, and as the number of known risk factors increases, the risk of developing the disease increases in an *exponential*, rather than additive, manner.[1,3,4,12]

Pathophysiology

CAD is a progressive atherosclerotic disorder of the coronary arteries that results in narrowing or complete occlusion. Atherosclerosis affects the medium-size arteries that perfuse the heart and other major organs. Normal arterial walls are composed of three layers, the intima, media, and adventitia. Low level vessel inflammation is believed to cause chronic endothelial dysfunction.[28] High sensitivity C-reactive protein (hs-CRP) and other inflammatory markers can be measured using specialized laboratory tests of blood serum to estimate the probability of future acute coronary events.[28-30] Chronic inflammation allows lipoproteins to enter the vessel wall, creating fatty streaks.[30] Over time a connective tissue fibrous cap is laid over a liquid lipid center.[28-30] The abrupt rupture of this cap allows procoagulant lipids to initiate a coronary thrombosis or a heart attack as the clot blocks flow through the coronary artery (Figure 11-1).

Atherosclerotic Plaque Rupture

Deep fissures in the fibrous cap expose procoagulant factors within the plaque core to the blood plasma. When platelets in the bloodstream are exposed to collagen, necrotic debris, von Willebrand factor, and thromboxane, a clot is formed that can occlude the coronary artery. Highly fibrotic plaques do not rupture. The type of atherosclerotic plaque that is prone to rupture has a weak fibrous cap and a large amount of liquid cholesterol within the core.[30]

Plaque Regression

Reduction of blood cholesterol decreases atherosclerotic plaque size by decreasing the amount of cholesterol in the serum and within the plaque core.[14] It will not change the dimensions of the fibrous or calcified portions of the plaque. If diet is not effective in lowering blood cholesterol, lipid-lowering drugs are prescribed to lower the LDL level below 100 mg/dl, to lower triglycerides to less than 150 mg/dl, and to raise HDL-cholesterol above 40 mg/dl.[12-16]

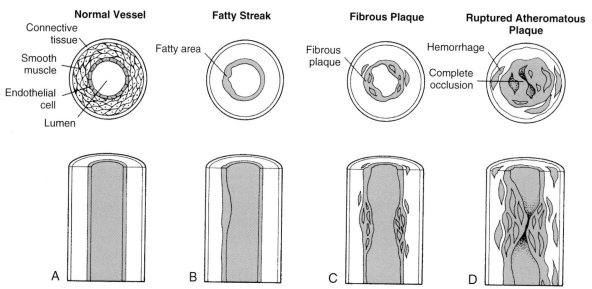

Figure 11-1 Progression of atherosclerosis, longitudinal and cross-sectional views. **A**, Normal vessel. **B**, Fatty streaks. **C**, Fibrous plaque develops. **D**, Advanced (complicated) lesions. Plaque has ruptured and occluded vessel lumen.

Acute Coronary Syndromes

The term *acute coronary syndrome* is used to describe the range of clinical presentations of CAD, from unstable angina to acute myocardial infarction (MI). When an individual comes to the emergency department (ED) complaining of chest pain (angina), clinical interventions are targeted toward the specific acute coronary syndrome manifestation.

Angina

Angina pectoris, or chest pain, caused by myocardial ischemia is not a separate disease but rather a symptom of CAD. It is caused by a blockage or spasm of a coronary artery, leading to diminished myocardial blood supply. The lack of oxygen causes myocardial ischemia, which is felt as chest pain. Angina may occur anywhere in the chest, neck, arms, or back, but the most common location is pain or pressure behind the sternum (Box 11-2). The pain often radiates to the left arm but can also radiate to the arms, back, shoulder, jaw, and neck (Figure 11-2). Angina is classified as stable, unstable, and variant and each type has identifiable characteristics (Box 11-3).

Box **11-2** Characteristics of Angina Pectoris

LOCATION

Beneath sternum, radiating to neck and jaw
Upper chest
Beneath sternum, radiating down left arm
Epigastric
Epigastric, radiating to neck, jaw, and arms
Neck and jaw
Left shoulder, inner aspect of both arms
Intrascapular

DURATION

0.5 to 15 minutes (stable)
Duration longer than 15 minutes without relief from rest or medication indicates unstable angina or preinfarction symptoms.

QUALITY

Sensation of pressure or heavy weight on chest
Feeling of tightness, "like a vise"
Visceral quality (deep, heavy, squeezing, aching)
Burning sensation

Shortness of breath, with feeling of suffocation
Most severe pain ever experienced

RADIATION

Medial aspect of left arm
Jaw
Left shoulder
Right arm

PRECIPITATING FACTORS

Exertion/exercise
Cold weather
Exercising after a large, heavy meal
Walking against the wind
Emotional upset
Fright, anger
Coitus

MEDICATION-INDUCED PAIN RELIEF

Usually within 45 seconds to 5 minutes of sublingual nitroglycerin administration

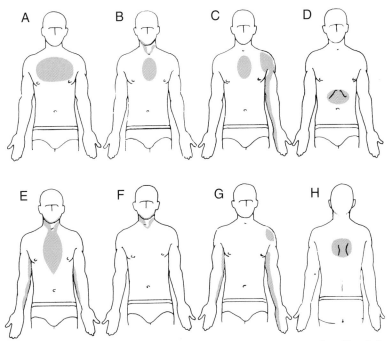

Figure 11-2   Common sites for anginal pain. **A**, Upper part of chest. **B**, Beneath sternum, radiating to neck and jaw. **C**, Beneath sternum, radiating down left arm. **D**, Epigastric. **E**, Epigastric, radiating to neck, jaw, and arms. **F**, Neck and jaw. **G**, Left shoulder. **H**, Intrascapular.

| Box **11-3** | **Factors in Assessment of Chest Pain (Angina Pectoris)** |

Onset (Was pain sudden or gradual?)
Precipitating factors (Did visitors come or leave? Was patient up and moving around?)
Location (Was pain substernal? Was pain located in same area as previous pain?)
Radiation (Did pain radiate to jaw, neck, arm, or shoulder?)
Quality (Was pain similar to previous anginal pain? Less painful or more painful?)
Intensity (On scale of 1 to 10, where would patient rate the pain?)
Duration (Did pain last seconds or minutes? How soon after onset did patient call for help?)
Relieving factors (What made the pain better: changing position, nitroglycerin, oxygen, presence of nurse?)
Aggravating factors (Did factors such as the environment, telephone calls, or waiting for help worsen the pain?)
Associated symptoms (Was pain accompanied by nausea, vomiting, diaphoresis, or dyspnea?)
Emotional response (Did an emotional response intensify the pain: anxiety, fear, anger?)

Stable Angina

Stable angina is predictable and caused by similar precipitating factors each time, such as exercise, emotional upset, and tachycardia. Patients become used to the pattern of this type of angina and may describe it as "my usual chest pain." Pain control is achieved by rest and by sublingual nitroglycerin. Stable angina is the result of fixed lesions (blockages) of more than 75% of the lumen. Ischemia and "chest pain" occur when myocardial demand from exertion exceeds the fixed blood oxygen supply.[31]

Unstable Angina

Unstable angina is defined as a change in a previously established stable pattern of angina. It usually is more intense than stable angina, may awaken the person from sleep, and may necessitate more than nitrates for pain relief. A change in the level or frequency of symptoms requires immediate medical evaluation. Severe angina that persists for more than 15 minutes and is not relieved by three nitroglycerin tablets is called *preinfarction*, or *crescendo*, *angina*. This is a medical emergency, and the person must call emergency medical services (911) immediately.[12] Patients with acute MI who use 911 and are transported to the hospital by ambulance receive initial reperfusion therapies much more quickly than those who self-transport.[32]

Unstable angina indicates atheroslcerotic plaque instability and may indicate plaque rupture, which can precipitate MI. The patient who comes to the ED with recent onset of unstable angina but nonspecific ST-segment changes on the 12-lead electrocardiogram (ECG) may be admitted to the critical care unit to rule out MI. If the symptoms are typical of MI, it is important to treat the patient according to the current guidelines, because not all patients who experience an MI have ST elevation on the 12-lead ECG.[33,34]

Variant Angina

Variant angina, or *Prinzmetal angina*, is caused by spasm of a coronary artery. Spasm can occur with or without atherosclerotic lesions. Variant angina often occurs when the individual is at rest and is often cyclic, occurring at the same time every day. It usually is associated with ST-segment elevation and occasionally with transient abnormal Q waves. Smoking, alcohol, and cocaine use may precipitate spasm. Variant angina is treated with nitroglycerin or calcium channel blockers to vasodilate the coronary arteries.

Medical Management

The change from stable to unstable angina represents a serious problem. If the ST segments are elevated or the 12-lead ECG shows left bundle branch block, the patient is treated for acute MI.[12] If these classic ECG signs are missing, however, and the patient still has significant chest pain, the current pharmacologic treatments of choice are vasodilation by nitroglycerin, intravenous (IV) antiplatelet agents such as the glycoprotein (GP) IIb/IIIa inhibitors, aspirin, and IV heparin.[33] Another option is to take the patient directly to the cardiac catheterization laboratory for direct visualization of the coronary arteries by the cardiologist. Recanalization of the coronary arteries is endorsed provided the institution performs more than 200 procedures annually or the physician performs more than 75 interventional procedures annually.[12,33,34]

Nursing Management

Nursing management of the patient with CAD and angina incorporates a variety of nursing diagnoses (Box 11-4). **Nursing priorities focus on (1) identifying myocardial ischemia, (2) relieving chest pain, (3) assessing for complications, (4) maintaining a calm environment, and (5) providing patient education.**

Identifying Myocardial Ischemia

Complaints of chest discomfort must be evaluated quickly because angina indicates myocardial ischemia (see Box 11-3).

---

nursing diagnosis priorities   Box **11-4**

Coronary Artery Disease and Angina
- Acute Pain related to transmission and perception of cutaneous, visceral, muscular, or ischemic impulses
- Ineffective Cardiopulmonary Tissue Perfusion related to decreased myocardial oxygen supply and/or increased myocardial oxygen demand
- Activity Intolerance related to cardiopulmonary dysfunction
- Powerlessness related to lack of control over current situation
- Anxiety related to threat to biologic, psychologic, and/or social integrity
- Deficient Knowledge: Discharge Regimen related to lack of previous exposure to information

---

The patient is asked to rate the intensity of the chest discomfort on a scale of 1 to 10. The words "chest pain" are not to be used exclusively because some patients describe their angina as "pressure" or "heaviness." It is important to document the characteristics of the pain and the patient's heart rate, rhythm, BP, respirations, temperature, skin color, peripheral pulses, urine output, mentation, and overall tissue perfusion. A 12-lead ECG is used to identify the area of ischemic myocardium. The major concern is that the chest pain may represent preinfarction angina, and early identification is essential so that the patient can be treated immediately, which may include transfer to the cardiac catheterization laboratory for coronary arteriography and opening of a blocked artery using specialized interventional cardiac catheters. If this option is not available, GP-IIb/IIIa receptor blockers may be prescribed to prevent the evolution of the acute MI before transfer[12,34,35] (see Chapter 12).

Relieving Chest Pain

In the critical care unit relief of angina (chest pain) is achieved by a combination of supplemental oxygen, nitrates, analgesia, and surveillance of the effects of pharmacologic therapy on both angina and blood pressure.

Oxygen. All patients with acute ischemic pain are administered supplemental oxygen to increase myocardial oxygenation. Those patients who develop symptoms of acute heart failure may require emergency intubation and mechanical ventilation to correct significant hypoxemia.[12,33]

Nitrates. A combination of IV and sublingual nitroglycerin is used to vasodilate the coronary arteries and decrease chest pain. After nitrate administration the critical care nurse closely observes the patient for relief of angina, return of ST segment to baseline, and development of side effects (e.g., hypotension, headache).[12,33]

Analgesia. Morphine, the analgesic of choice for preinfarction angina, both relieves chest pain and decreases fear and anxiety. After administration the critical care nurse assesses the patient for pain relief and development of side effects (e.g., hypotension, respiratory depression).[12,33]

Maintaining a Calm Environment

Patients admitted to a critical care unit with unstable angina experience extreme anxiety and fear of death. The critical care nurse is faced with the challenge of ensuring that the elements of a calm environment that will alleviate the patient's fear and anxiety are maintained, while being ready at all times to respond to an acute emergency (e.g., cardiac arrest) or to assist with emergency intubation or insertion of hemodynamic monitoring catheters.

Providing Patient Education

In the critical care unit the patient's ability to retain educational information is severely affected by stress and pain.

However, it is essential to teach avoidance of the *Valsalva maneuver*, defined as forced expiration against a closed glottis. This can be explained to the patient as "bearing down" when going to the bathroom or breath holding when repositioning in bed. The Valsalva maneuver causes an increase in intrathoracic pressure, which decreases venous return to the right side of the heart, and is associated with low BP and symptomatic bradycardia.

Once the anginal pain is controlled, longer-term patient and family education can begin. Points to cover include risk factor modification, signs and symptoms of angina, when to call the physician, medications, and dealing with emotions and stress. However, because the acute hospital length of stay for uncomplicated angina is usually less than 3 days, referral to a cardiac rehabilitation program for a controlled exercise program and risk factor modification after discharge may be the most helpful teaching intervention that a critical care nurse can provide (Box 11-5).

MYOCARDIAL INFARCTION

Myocardial infarction (MI) is the irreversible myocardial necrosis (cell death) that results from an abrupt decrease or total cessation of coronary blood flow to a specific area of the myocardium. The three mechanisms primarily responsible for the acute reduction in oxygen delivery to the myocardium are (1) plaque rupture, (2) new coronary artery thrombosis, and (3) coronary artery spasm. Myocardial tissue can be salvaged for up to 12 hours after the onset of anginal symptoms.[12] The earlier the myocardium is revascularized, the better the survival.[35] Unfortunately, many persons do not seek treatment until this phase has passed.[36]

Pathophysiology
Zones (Figure 11-3)
The outer region of the infarcted myocardial area is named the *zone of ischemia*, which is composed of viable cells. Priority interventions target this viable muscle to normalize and save these cells. Repolarization in this zone is temporarily impaired but with adequate perfusion, eventually will be restored to normal. Repolarization of these ischemic cells manifests as T-wave inversion (Figure 11-4, *B*).

The infarcted zone is surrounded by injured but still potentially viable tissue named the *zone of injury*. Cells in this area do not fully repolarize because of deficient blood supply. This is recorded on the ECG as elevation of the ST segment (Figure 11-4, *C*).

The area of necrotic muscle in the myocardium is the *zone of infarction*. These cells are dead and cannot be recovered. On the ECG, evidence of this zone is seen by new pathologic Q waves, which reflect a lack of depolarization from the cardiac surface involved in the MI (Figure 11-4, *D*). As healing takes place, the cells in this area are replaced by scar tissue.

Classification
MIs are classified according to their location on the myocardial surface and the muscle layers affected. A *transmural* (full-thickness) MI, also described as a *Q wave* MI, involves all three layers: endocardium, myocardium, and epicardium. A transmural MI provokes significant ECG changes (see Figures 11-3 and 11-4).

Nontransmural MIs damage part of the wall but do not infarct the full thickness. Because some of the muscle in the

---

Box 11-5 COLLABORATIVE Management

Coronary Artery Disease (CAD) and Angina

1. **Provide comprehensive education.**
   - Emphasis on CAD prevention
   - Risk factor modification
   - Risk of progression to acute coronary syndrome
   - Risk of stroke or peripheral vascular disease
   - Risk of progression to heart failure after acute myocardial infarction
   - Explanation of diagnostic tests
2. **Suggest nonpharmacologic interventions.**
   Diet
   - Low salt, high fiber, fat <30% total calories
   - Multivitamin with B vitamins if homocystine level elevated
   - Decrease in sugary foods to limit calories if overweight
   Exercise
   - Start by walking more and increase from there
   - Refer to cardiac rehabilitation program
   Obesity: Achieve ideal body weight
   Addiction
   - Stop cigarette smoking
   - Limit alcohol intake

Chest pain
- Signs and symptoms of "heart attack"
- When to call 911
3. **Prescribe pharmacologic treatment.**
   Pharmacologic intervention for known risk factors; education on purpose of each medication
   - *Hypertension*: Antihypertensive drugs
   - *Hyperlipidemia*: "Statins" and other drugs
   - *Diabetes mellitus*: Oral hypoglycemic drugs for type 2 diabetes; insulin if indicated
   - *Angina*: Sublingual nitroglycerin
4. **Perform diagnostic tests.**
   - 12-lead electrocardiogram (ECG)
   - Stress echocardiogram or treadmill test
   - Cardiac catheterization and coronary arteriography
5. **Schedule cardiac interventions.**
   - *Percutaneous coronary intervention*: Angioplasty, atherectomy, stenting
   - *Cardiac surgery*: Coronary artery bypass grafting

Data from Smith SC Jr et al: *J Am Coll Cardiol* 38:1581-1583, 2001; and Gibbons RJ et al: *Circulation* 107:149-158, 2003.

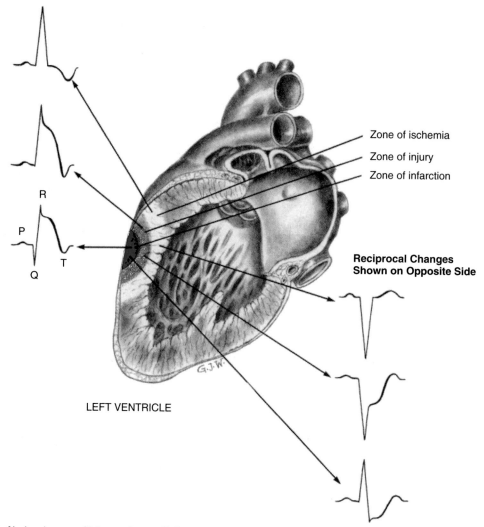

Zone of ischemia
Zone of injury
Zone of infarction

**Reciprocal Changes
Shown on Opposite Side**

LEFT VENTRICLE

Figure 11-3 Zone of ischemia, zone of injury, and zone of infarction, shown through ECG waveforms and reciprocal waveforms corresponding to each zone.

area can still be depolarized, Q waves do not appear. Therefore a nontransmural MI is called a *non–ST-segment elevation myocardial infarction* (NSTEMI),[33] also previously known as a *non–Q-wave* or *subendocardial* MI.

Electrocardiographic Changes

The ECG changes produced by a transmural infarction demonstrate alteration in both myocardial depolarization (QRS complex) and repolarization (ST segment). The changes in repolarization are recognized by the presence of new Q waves. These new pathologic Q waves are deeper and wider than tiny q waves found on the normal 12-lead ECG[12] (Figure 11-4).

Location

The location of an acute MI is determined by correlating the 12-lead ECG leads with new Q waves and acute ST-segment T-wave abnormalities (Table 11-1). Infarction most often occurs in the left ventricle and the interventricular septum;

however, almost 25% of patients who sustain an inferior MI have some right ventricular damage. The ECG manifestations that are used to diagnose an MI and pinpoint the area of damaged ventricle include inverted T waves, ST-segment elevation, and pathologic Q waves.

Anterior Wall Infarction. Anterior wall MI results from occlusion of the proximal left anterior descending (LAD) artery and may involve the left main coronary artery. ST-segment elevation and pathologic Q waves are expected in leads V_1 through V_4 (Figure 11-5). A large anterior wall MI may be associated with left ventricular pump failure, cardiogenic shock, or death.[37] Twelve-lead ECG signs of infarction limited to leads V_1 and V_2 suggest a smaller area of infarction that involves the same coronary arteries but is limited to the interventricular septum (anteroseptal infarction).

Left Lateral Wall Infarction. Left lateral wall infarction occurs as a result of occlusion of the circumflex coronary artery. On a 12-lead ECG, pathologic Q waves and ST-

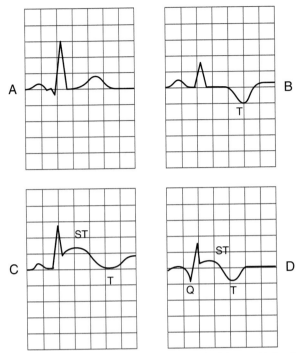

Figure 11-4 ECG changes indicative of ischemia, injury, and infarction (necrosis) of myocardium. **A,** Normal ECG. **B,** Ischemia indicated by inversion of T wave. **C,** Ischemia and injury indicated by T-wave inversion and ST-segment elevation. **D,** Ischemia, injury, and myocardial necrosis. Q wave indicates necrosis of myocardium.

segment T-wave changes are expected in leads I, aV_L, V_5, and V_6.

Inferior Wall Infarction. Inferior wall infarction occurs with occlusion of the right coronary artery (RCA). This infarction is manifested by 12-lead ECG changes in leads II, III, and aV_F. Because the RCA perfuses the sinoatrial node in more than half the population and also perfuses the proximal bundle of His and atrioventricular node in more than 90%, conduction disturbances are expected with an inferior wall MI (Figure 11-6).

Right Ventricular Infarction. Infarction of the right ventricle occurs when there is a blockage in a proximal section of the RCA. This places all of the right ventricle and the inferior wall at risk. Specific ECG leads are placed over the right precordium (chest) to record evidence of right ventricular infarction.

Posterior Wall Infarction. Infarction in the posterior wall can result from blockage in the RCA or circumflex artery because both arteries supply this section of the heart. Posterior wall MI is difficult to detect but may be identified by either specific leads placed in the left scapular area or by very tall R waves in leads V_1 and V_2.

Cardiac Enzymes

Specific cardiac enzymes and isoenzymes are released in the presence of damaged or infarcted myocardial muscle cells. To confirm the diagnosis of acute MI, serum creatine kinase (CK) MB isoenzymes and troponin I or troponin T are measured. With a large anterior MI, the CK-MB level can rise to more than 150 U/L, with a total CK level of more than 1000 U/L.[38]

Complications with Acute MI

Many patients experience complications occurring either early or late in the postinfarction course (Box 11-6). These complications may result from electrical dysfunction or from a pump problem. Electrical dysfunction includes bradycardia, bundle branch blocks, and varying degrees of heart block. Pumping complications cause heart failure, pulmonary edema, and cardiogenic shock.[12]

Sinus Bradycardia/Tachycardia

Sinus bradycardia (heart rate less than 60 beats/min) occurs in approximately 40% of patients who sustain an acute MI and is more prevalent with an inferior wall infarction in the immediate postinfarction period. Symptomatic bradycardia with hypotension and low cardiac output (CO) is treated with atropine 0.5 mg IV push, repeated every 5 minutes to a maximum dose of 2 mg.

Sinus tachycardia (heart rate more than 100 beats/min) most often occurs with anterior wall MIs. Anterior infarctions impair left ventricular pumping ability, thereby reducing the ejection fraction and stroke volume. In an attempt to maintain CO, the heart rate increases. Sinus tachycardia must be corrected because it greatly increases myocardial oxygen consumption, leading to further ischemia.

Table **11-1** Correlations among Ventricular Surfaces, Electrocardiographic Leads, and Coronary Arteries		
Surface of Left Ventricle	**ECG Leads**	**Coronary Artery Usually Involved**
Inferior	II, III, aV_F	Right coronary artery
Lateral	V_5–V_6, I, aV_L	Left circumflex
Anterior	V_2–V_4	Left anterior descending
		Left main coronary artery
Septal	V_1–V_2	Left anterior descending
Posterior	V_1–V_2	Left circumflex or right coronary artery (reciprocal changes)
	V_7–V_9 (direct)	

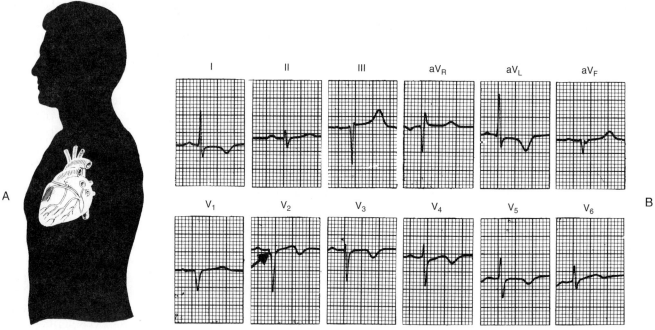

Figure 11-5 **A,** Position of anterior wall infarction. **B,** Anterior wall infarction. Note QS complexes in leads V_1 and V_2, indicating anteroseptal infarction. Characteristic notching (*arrow, V_2*) of QS complex, often seen in infarctions, is present. In addition, note diffuse ischemic T-wave inversions in leads I, aV_L, and V_2 through V_5, indicating generalized anterior wall ischemia. (From Goldberger AL, Goldberger E: *Clinical electrocardiography: a simplified approach*, ed 6, St Louis, 1999, Mosby.)

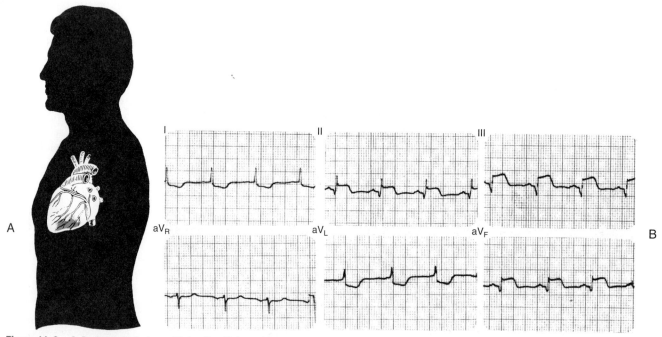

Figure 11-6 **A,** Position of inferior wall infarction. **B,** Acute inferior wall infarction. Note ST elevations in leads II, III, and aV_F, with reciprocal ST depressions in leads I and aV_L. Abnormal Q waves also are seen in leads II, III, and aV_F. Changes are not seen in leads V_4 to V_6, so these leads are not shown. (From Goldberger AL, Goldberger E: *Clinical electrocardiography: a simplified approach*, ed 6, St Louis, 1999, Mosby.)

Box **11-6**   Complications of Myocardial Infarction

Dysrhythmias
Ventricular aneurysm
Ventricular septal defect
Papillary muscle rupture
Pericarditis
Cardiac rupture
Sudden death
Heart failure
Pulmonary edema
Cardiogenic shock

Atrial/Ventricular Dysrhythmias

Premature atrial contractions (PACs) occur frequently in patients who sustain acute MI. *Atrial fibrillation* is also common and may occur spontaneously or be preceded by PACs. With onset of atrial fibrillation the loss of organized atrial contraction decreases CO by up to 25%.

Premature ventricular contractions (PVCs) are seen in almost all patients within the first few hours after MI. They are initially controlled by administering oxygen to reduce myocardial hypoxia and by correcting acid-base or electrolyte imbalances. In the patient with acute MI, PVCs are pharmacologically treated if they are frequent (more than six per minute), closely coupled (R-on-T phenomenon), multiform in shape, and occur in bursts of three or more increasing the risk of sustained ventricular tachycardia. *Ventricular*

fibrillation is a life-threatening dysrhythmia associated with high mortality in patients with acute MI. Increasingly, β-blockers are prescribed after acute MI to decrease mortality from ventricular dysrhythmias.

Atrioventricular Block

Atrioventricular (AV) heart block during MI most often occurs after an inferior wall infarction. Because the RCA supplies the AV node in 90% of the population, RCA occlusion leads to ischemia and infarction of the AV node cells. Symptomatic AV block with hemodynamic compromise is treated by insertion of a transvenous temporary pacemaker.

Ventricular Aneurysm

A ventricular aneurysm is a noncontractile, thinned left ventricular wall that results from acute transmural MI (Figure 11-7). The most common complications of a ventricular aneurysm are acute heart failure, systemic emboli, and ventricular tachycardia. Treatment is directed toward management of these complications and surgical repair by left ventricular aneurysmectomy. Prognosis depends on size of the aneurysm, overall left ventricular function, and severity of coexisting CAD.

Ventricular Septal Defect

Postinfarction rupture of the ventricular septal wall is a rare but potentially lethal complication of an acute anterior wall MI (Figure 11-8). A ventricular septal defect (VSD) is an abnormal communication between the right and left

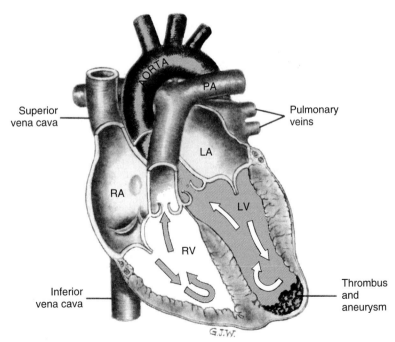

Figure 11-7   Ventricular aneurysm after acute myocardial infarction (MI). *PA*, Pulmonary artery; *LA*, left atrium; *RA*, right atrium; *LV*, left ventricle; *RV*, right ventricle.

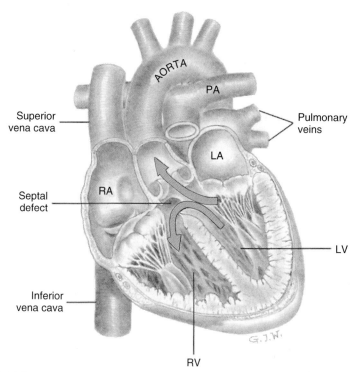

Figure 11-8 Ventricular septal defect after acute MI. *PA*, Pulmonary artery; *LA*, left atrium; *RA*, right atrium; *LV*, left ventricle; *RV*, right ventricle.

ventricles. VSD occurs is less than 5% of acute MI patients (most with symptoms of cardiogenic shock) but carries an extremely high mortality of 87% in the small group affected.[37] VSD manifests as severe chest pain, syncope, hypotension, and sudden hemodynamic deterioration caused by shunting of blood from the high-pressure left ventricle into the low-pressure right ventricle through the new septal opening. A holosystolic murmur can be auscultated and is best heard along the left sternal border. If the murmur is loud it is usually accompanied by a thrill palpable at the left sternal border. Postinfarction VSD can be diagnosed at the bedside using a right heart pulmonary artery catheter or by transesophageal echocardiography. Rupture of the septum is a medical and surgical emergency. The patient's condition is stabilized with vasodilators and an intraaortic balloon pump (IABP) to decrease afterload.[37] The goal of afterload reduction in this patient population is to decrease the amount of blood being shunted to the right side of the heart and thus increase blood flow to the systemic circulation.

Papillary Muscle Rupture

Papillary muscle rupture can occur when the infarct involves the area around one of the papillary muscles that support the mitral valve (Figure 11-9). It is rare but accounts for 1% to 5% of acute MI–related deaths. Infarction of the papillary muscles results in ineffective mitral valve closure, and blood is forced back into the low-pressure left atrium during ventricular systole. The rupture may be partial or complete. Complete rupture is catastrophic and precipitates

severe acute mitral regurgitation, cardiogenic shock, and death. Partial rupture also results in mitral regurgitation, but usually the condition can be stabilized with aggressive medical management using an IABP and vasodilators. Urgent surgical intervention is required to replace the mitral valve.

Cardiac Wall Rupture

From 3% to 4% of deaths after MI can be attributed to cardiac rupture. Rupture typically occurs about the fifth postinfarction day, when leukocyte scavenger cells are removing necrotic debris, thinning the myocardial wall. Onset is sudden and usually catastrophic. Bleeding into the pericardial sac results in cardiac tamponade, cardiogenic shock, pulseless electrical activity (PEA), and death. Survival is rare. If rupture occurs in the hospital, emergency pericardiocentesis is required to relieve the tamponade until surgical repair can be attempted.

Pericarditis

Pericarditis (inflammation of pericardial sac) can occur during an acute transmural MI when the inflammatory damage extends into the epicardial surface of the heart. The damaged epicardium then becomes rough and irritates and inflames the adjacent pericardium, precipitating pericarditis. Pain is the most common symptom of pericarditis, and a pericardial friction rub is the most common initial sign. The friction rub is best heard at the sternal border and is described as a grating, scraping, or leathery scratching. Pericarditis may result in a pericardial effusion. Once the

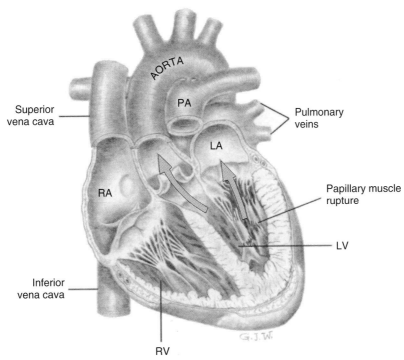

Figure 11-9   Papillary muscle rupture after acute MI. *PA*, Pulmonary artery; *LA*, left atrium; *RA*, right atrium; *LV*, left ventricle; *RV*, right ventricle.

effusion (fluid) occurs, the friction rub may disappear. The patient with pericarditis is treated with nonsteroidal antiinflammatory drugs (NSAIDs).

Nursing Management

Nursing management of the patient with an acute MI incorporates a variety of nursing diagnoses (Box 11-7). Nursing priorities focus on (1) **balancing myocardial oxygen supply and demand**, (2) **preventing complications**, and (3) **providing patient education**.

Balancing Myocardial Oxygen Supply and Demand

In the acute period, if severe myocardial damage has occurred, myocardial oxygen supply is pharmacologically increased by using positive inotropic drugs such as dobutamine, dopamine or milrinone, administering vasodilators such as nitroglycerin, and initially avoiding negative inotropic agents such as β-blockers. Supplemental oxygen is administered to prevent tissue hypoxia. To decrease cardiac work and myocardial oxygen consumption, bed rest with bedside commode privileges are usually prescribed during the first 24 to 48 hours.

Preventing Complications

Assessing for signs of continued ischemic pain is important because angina is a warning sign of myocardium at risk. In response to angina, a 12-lead ECG is taken to determine any extension of the infarct, nitroglycerin is administered, and

nursing diagnosis
priorities   Box **11-7**

Acute Coronary Syndrome and Acute Myocardial Infarction

- Acute Pain related to transmission and perception of cutaneous, visceral, muscular, or ischemic impulses
- Decreased Cardiac Output related to alterations in preload
- Decreased Cardiac Output related to alterations in afterload
- Decreased Cardiac Output related to alterations in contractility
- Decreased Cardiac Output related to alterations in heart rate or rhythm
- Activity Intolerance related to cardiopulmonary dysfunction
- Ineffective Cardiopulmonary Tissue Perfusion related to decreased myocardial oxygen supply and/or increased myocardial oxygen demand
- Disturbed Sleep Pattern related to fragmented sleep
- Anxiety related to threat to biologic, psychologic, and/or social integrity
- Ineffective Coping related to situational crisis and personal vulnerability
- Powerlessness related to lack of control over current situation or disease progression
- Deficient Knowledge: Discharge Regimen related to lack of previous exposure to information

the physician is notified immediately so that interventions may be initiated to limit the size of the MI.

Heart failure is a serious complication after acute MI. If the patient's BP is stable, preferably within 72 hours of the infarct, the vasodilating class of drugs called *angiotensin-converting enzyme* (ACE) *inhibitors* is initiated. These vasodilators are used to prevent the left ventricular remodeling and dilation that occurs in many patients after acute MI.[39] Hypotension is a potential complication of ACE inhibitors, especially with the first dose. It is an important nursing responsibility to monitor blood pressure (BP) and patient symptoms after ACE administration. Surveillance to detect both obvious and subtle signs of bleeding is also a priority because many acute MI patients also receive antiplatelet, anticoagulant, and fibrinolytic medications.[40-45]

In the first 24 hours the stable patient with acute MI may be given only a light diet because appetite is often poor. It is no longer considered necessary to restrict iced fluids or caffeine. While the patient is in bed, an upright position is preferred to foster better lung expansion. Deep breathing decreases the risk of atelectasis. An upright position also decreases venous return, lowers preload, and decreases cardiac work. The patient is taught to avoid increasing intraabdominal pressure (Valsalva maneuver). Stool softeners are given to lessen the risk of constipation from analgesics and bed rest and to decrease the risk of straining. The nurse controls the patient care environment by decreasing noise, diminishing sensory overload, and allowing adequate rest periods.

Providing Patient Education

The person who comes to the emergency department within 12 hours of onset of chest pain immediately receives education about possible therapies to salvage the threatened myocardium. These include fibrinolytic therapy, emergency percutaneous transluminal coronary angioplasty (PTCA) or coronary artery stenting.[40-44] Unfortunately, many people with chest pain delay their arrival at the hospital beyond this period.[32,36] If the person arrives at the hospital after the time window has passed when the myocardium can be saved, the patient is educated to clarify the reasons for critical care unit admission and the importance of avoiding straining when coughing, moving, or using the commode or bathroom.

Once the acute phase has passed, education for the patient and family is focused on risk factor reduction, manifestations of angina, when to call a physician or emergency services, medications, and resumption of physical and sexual activity. If possible, a referral is made to a cardiac rehabilitation program so that this education can be reinforced outside the acute care hospital environment[46] (Box 11-8).

HEART FAILURE

The number of patients with heart failure (HF) is increasing in the United States. Currently, more than 2 million Americans have a diagnosis of HF, and about 500,000 new cases are diagnosed each year. Patients with HF spend more than 6.5 million days in the hospital annually, and 300,000

patients die each year. HF is primarily a disease of elderly persons. Approximately 6% to 10% of people over 65 years of age have HF, and of patients hospitalized, 80% are over 80 years old. About $500 million is spent annually on drugs for HF.[47]

Pathophysiology

HF is a response to cardiac dysfunction, a condition in which the heart cannot pump blood at a volume required to meet the body's needs. Any condition that impairs the ability of the ventricles to fill or eject blood can cause HF. CAD with resultant damage to the left ventricle is the underlying cause of HF in two thirds of all patients.[47] Other precipitating causes of heart failure are listed in Box 11-9.

Assessment and Diagnosis

HF is often classified using the New York Heart Association (NYHA) criteria, which assign patients into groups I through IV depending on the degree of symptoms and the amount of patient effort required to elicit symptoms (Table 11-2). Recent clinical guidelines suggest adding a second level of classification that emphasizes the progressive nature of HF through stages A to D, with increasing symptom distress and intensified clinical interventions (Table 11-3).[47] HF can present in many different ways depending on the degree of ventricular remodeling and dysfunction. HF may be discovered secondary to a known clinical syndrome (e.g., CAD) or because of decreased exercise tolerance, fluid retention, or hospital admission for an unrelated condition.

The first step in diagnosis is to determine the underlying structural abnormality creating the ventricular dysfunction and symptoms. Various imaging tests are available to visualize cardiac anatomy, and laboratory tests can evaluate impact of hormonal or electrolyte imbalances. This permits the cardiologist to design a treatment plan to control symptoms and possibly correct the underlying cause.

Left Ventricular Failure

Failure of the left ventricle is defined as a disturbance of the contractile function of the left ventricle, resulting in a low cardiac output (CO) state that leads to vasoconstriction of the arterial bed (high afterload), and congestion and edema in the pulmonary vascular circulation and alveoli. Clinical manifestations include decreased peripheral perfusion with weak or diminished pulses, cool pale extremities, and peripheral cyanosis (Table 11-4). Over time, with progression of the disease state, the fluid accumulation behind the dysfunctional left ventricle elevates pulmonary vascular pressures and produces dysfunction of the right ventricle, resulting in failure of the right side of the heart.

Right Ventricular Failure

Failure of the right side of the heart is defined as ineffective right ventricular contractile function. Pure failure of the right ventricle may result from an acute condition such as a

Box 11-8 COLLABORATIVE Management

Acute Coronary Syndrome and Acute Myocardial Infarction

1. **Focus on clinical assessment**.
   Chest pain assessment: See Figure 11-2 and Boxes 11-2 and 11-3.
   Vital signs
   - Heart rate, blood pressure, respiratory rate, temperature.
   - Oxygen saturation.
   - Presence of dysrhythmias.
   Clinical findings
   - Assess for warm or cool skin, color, capillary refill, and peripheral pulses.
   - Auscultate heart for cardiac murmur or new S_3 or S_4.
   - Auscultate lungs for air entry as well as crackles and wheezes.
   - Observe for breathlessness and frothy pink sputum (pulmonary edema).
   - Ask patient, family, and significant others for relevant history.
2. **Ensure patient comfort**.
   - Oxygenate myocardium.
     - Oxygen via nasal cannula to maintain oxygen saturation >92%.
     - Sublingual nitroglycerin to vasodilate coronary arteries.
   - Position with head of bed elevated.
   - Obtain intravenous (IV) access and insert two large-bore IV lines.
     - Normal saline to keep vein open.
     - Morphine sulfate for pain.
3. **Perform emergency diagnostic tests**.
   - *12-lead ECG*: Assess for ischemia, injury, and infarction with ST-segment elevation or Q waves (see Figures 11-3, 11-4, 11-5, and 11-6 and Table 11-1).
   - *Laboratory studies*: Hemogram, cardiac enzymes, metabolic panel (electrolytes, glucose, renal and liver function), coagulation panel (if fibrinolytics to be given).
   - *Cardiac catheterization*: Identify blocked coronary artery and wall motion abnormalities.

4. **Select emergency interventions**.
   - *Fibrinolytic drugs*: "Lytic" drugs to "dissolve" clot in coronary artery.
   - *Antiplatelet drugs*: Glycoprotein IIb/IIIa inhibitors, aspirin, other oral agents.
   - *Vasodilator drugs*: Sublingual and IV nitroglycerin (note response).
   - *Pacemaker*: Trancutaneous/transvenous pacemaker available if AV block present.
   - *Percutaneous coronary intervention*: Angioplasty to open occluded vessel; stent to maintain patency of previously occluded vessel.
   - *Cardiac surgery*: For emergency interventions such as papillary muscle rupture, acute ventricular septal defect, and left main coronary artery occlusion; coronary artery bypass grafting alone is uncommon.
   - *Advanced cardiac life support*: ACLS procedures in case of cardiac arrest.
5. **Focus on secondary prevention: administer medications**.
   - ACE inhibitors to prevent ventricular remodeling.
   - β-Blockers to prevent ventricular dysrhythmias.
   - Diuretics if heart failure has developed.
   - Antihyperlipidemics if total cholesterol, LDL cholesterol, or triglycerides elevated.
6. **Provide relevant education**.
   - *Medications*: Written and verbal instructions on dosages, administration, and side effects; provide emergency telephone number for questions.
   - *Risk factor modification*: See Box 11-5.
   - *Referral*: Cardiac rehabilitation sessions will continue process of education and risk factor modification outside acute care environment.

Data from Ryan TJ et al: *Circulation* 100:1016-1030, 1999.
AV, Atrioventricular; *ACE*, Angiotensin-converting enzyme; *LDL*, low-density lipoprotein.

pulmonary embolus or a right ventricular infarction, but it is most commonly caused by failure of the left side of the heart. The common manifestations of right ventricular failure are jugular venous distention, elevated central venous pressure, weakness, peripheral or sacral edema, hepatomegaly, jaundice, and liver tenderness. The patient's appetite is poor, and gastrointestinal symptoms include anorexia, nausea, and a feeling of fullness (see Table 11-4).

Box 11-9 Precipitating Causes of Heart Failure

Reduction or cessation of medication
Dysrhythmias
Systemic infection
Pulmonary embolism
Physical, environmental, and emotional stress
Pericarditis, myocarditis, endocarditis
High–ventricular output states
Development of serious systemic illness
Administration of cardiac depressant or salt-retaining drug
Development of a second form of heart disease

Table 11-2 New York Heart Association Functional Classification of Heart Failure

Class	Definition
I	Normal daily activity does not initiate symptoms.
II	Normal daily activities initiate onset of symptoms, but symptoms subside with rest.
III	Minimal activity initiates symptoms; patients are usually symptom-free at rest.
IV	Any type of activity initiates symptoms, and symptoms are present at rest.

Table **11-3** Progression of Heart Failure

Stage	Structural Heart Disorder	Symptoms	Management	NYHA Class
A	No, but at risk because of: Hypertension CAD Diabetes mellitus	None	Preventive treatment of known risk factors: Hypertension Lipid disorders Cigarette smoking Diabetes mellitus Discourage alcohol and illicit drug use.	I
B	Yes, but without symptoms: Previous MI Family history of CM Asymptomatic valvular disease/CM	None	Treat all risk factors. When indicated, use: ACE inhibitors β-Blockers	II
C	Yes, with prior or current symptoms	Shortness of breath Fatigue Reduced exercise tolerance	Treat all risk factors, plus HF symptoms: Diuretics ACE inhibitors β-Blockers Digitalis Dietary salt restriction	III
D	Yes, with refractory HF symptoms despite maximal specialized interventions (pharmacologic, medical, nursing) Recurrently hospitalized for HF symptoms	Marked symptoms at rest despite maximal medical therapy	Refractory HF requires interventions from previous stages (A-C), plus: Continuous intravenous inotropic support Mechanical assist devices Heart transplantation Hospice care	IV

Data adapted from Hunt SA et al: *Circulation* 104:2996-3007, 2001.
HF, Heart failure; *CAD,* Coronary artery disease; *MI,* myocardial infarction; *CM,* cardiomyopathy; *ACE,* angiotensin-converting enzyme.

Table **11-4** Clinical Manifestations of Right-Sided and Left-Sided Heart Failure

Signs	Symptoms
LEFT VENTRICULAR FAILURE	
Tachypnea	Fatigue
Tachycardia	Dyspnea
Cough	Orthopnea
Bibasilar crackles	Paroxysmal nocturnal dyspnea
Gallop rhythms (S_3 and S_4)	Nocturia
Increased pulmonary artery pressures	
Hemoptysis	
Cyanosis	
Pulmonary edema	
RIGHT VENTRICULAR FAILURE	
Peripheral edema	Weakness
Hepatomegaly	Anorexia
Splenomegaly	Indigestion
Hepatojugular reflux	Weight gain
Ascites	Mental changes
Jugular venous distention	
Increased central venous pressure	
Pulmonary hypertension	

Acute versus Chronic Failure

Acute versus chronic HF refers to the rapidity with which the syndrome develops, the presence and activation of compensatory mechanisms, and the presence or absence of fluid accumulation in the interstitial space (see Table 11-3). Acute HF has a sudden onset, with no compensatory mechanisms. The patient may experience acute pulmonary edema, low CO, or even cardiogenic shock. Patients with chronic HF are hypervolemic, have sodium and water retention, and have structural heart chamber changes such as dilation or hypertrophy.[47] The heart failure is ongoing, with symptoms that may be made tolerable by medication, diet, and a low activity level. Chronic HF is not curable. The deterioration into acute HF can be precipitated by the onset of dysrhythmias, acute ischemia, sudden illness, or cessation of medications. This may necessitate admission to an acute care hospital.

Compensatory Mechanisms

When the heart begins to fail and CO is no longer sufficient to meet the metabolic needs of the tissues, the body activates three major compensatory mechanisms: the sympathetic nervous system (SNS) and the renin-angiotensin-aldosterone system (RAS) that promote development of ventricular hypertrophy (see Table 11-3).

Sympathetic Nervous System. The SNS compensates for low CO by increasing heart rate (HR) and BP. As a result, levels of circulating catecholamines are increased, resulting in peripheral vasoconstriction. In addition to raising BP and HR, catecholamines cause shunting of blood from nonvital organs (e.g., skin) to vital organs (e.g., heart, brain). Although initially helpful, this mechanism may become a negative factor because the elevation of HR increases myocardial oxygen demand while shortening the amount of time for diastolic filling and coronary artery perfusion.

Renin-Angiotensin-Aldosterone System. Activation of the renin-angiotensin system (RAS) promotes vasoconstriction and fluid retention.[48,49] This results in constriction of the renal arterioles, decreased glomerular filtration, and increased reabsorption of sodium from the proximal and distal renal tubules. In addition, diminished hepatic metabolism of aldosterone increases antidiuretic hormone (ADH) level and enhances water retention.[50,51]

Ventricular Hypertrophy. Ventricular hypertrophy is strongly associated with preexisting hypertension. Because myocardial hypertrophy increases the force of contraction, hypertrophy initially helps the ventricle overcome the increase in afterload (vasoconstriction) caused by increased levels of SNS-mediated circulating catecholamines and by activation of the RAS system.

Pulmonary Complications

The clinical manifestations of acute HF result from tissue hypoperfusion and organ congestion. The severity of clinical manifestations progresses as HF worsens.[47]

Shortness of Breath

The patient initially experiences shortness of breath only with exertion, but as HF worsens, symptoms are present at rest as well. Recently a diagnostic blood test has become available to assist clinicians in differentiating whether a patient's shortness of breath is caused by cardiac failure or by pulmonary complications. B-type natriuretic peptide (BNP) is released from the cardiac ventricles in response to increased wall tension. HF increases left ventricular wall tension because of the excess preload in the ventricles. When the BNP blood level is greater than 100 picograms per milliliter (pg/ml), the dyspnea is probably related to cardiac rather than pulmonary failure.[52,53] Breathlessness in HF is described by the following terms:

- *Dyspnea* is the patient's sensation of shortness of breath and results from pulmonary vascular congestion and decreased lung compliance.
- *Orthopnea* describes difficulty in breathing when lying flat because of an increase in venous return that occurs in the supine position.
- *Paroxysmal nocturnal dyspnea* is a severe form of orthopnea in which the patient awakens from sleep gasping for air.
- *Cardiac asthma* is dyspnea with wheezing, a nonproductive cough, and pulmonary crackles that progress to the gurgling sounds of pulmonary edema.

Pulmonary Edema

Pulmonary edema, or fluid in the alveoli, inhibits gas exchange by impairing the diffusion pathway between the alveolus and the capillary (Figure 11-10). Pulmonary edema is a symptom of heart failure and is caused by increased left atrial and ventricular pressures that result in excessive accumulation of serous or serosanguineous fluid in the interstitial spaces and alveoli of the lungs. Pulmonary edema develops in two stages. The first stage is not as severe and is characterized by interstitial edema, engorgement of the perivascular and peribronchial spaces, and increased lymphatic flow. The second stage is characterized by alveolar edema resulting from fluid moving into the alveoli from the interstitium. Eventually, blood plasma moves into the alveoli faster than the lymphatic system can clear it, thereby interfering with diffusion of oxygen, depressing the arterial partial pressure of oxygen (PaO_2), and leading to tissue hypoxia.

HF patients with pulmonary edema are extremely breathless, are anxious, and have a sensation of suffocation. They expectorate pink, frothy liquid and feel as if they are drowning. They may sit rigidly upright, gasp for breath, or thrash about. The respiratory rate is elevated, and accessory muscles of ventilation are used, with nasal flaring and bulging neck muscles. Respirations are characterized by loud inspiratory and expiratory gurgling sounds. Diaphoresis is profuse, and the skin is cold, ashen, and cyanotic, reflecting low CO, increased sympathetic stimulation, peripheral vasoconstriction, and desaturation of arterial blood.

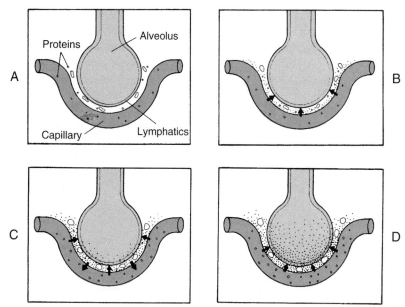

Figure 11-10 As it progresses, pulmonary edema inhibits oxygen and carbon dioxide exchange at the alveolocapillary interface. **A,** Normal relationship. **B,** Increased pulmonary capillary hydrostatic pressure causes fluid to move from vascular space into pulmonary interstitial space. **C,** Lymphatic flow increases in an attempt to pull fluid back into vascular or lymphatic space. **D,** Failure of lymphatic flow and worsening of left-sided heart failure results in further movement of fluid into interstitial space and alveoli.

Arterial blood gas values are variable. In the early stage of pulmonary edema, respiratory alkalosis may be present because of hyperventilation, which eliminates carbon dioxide. As pulmonary edema progresses and gas exchange becomes impaired, acidosis (pH less than 7.35) and hypoxemia ensue. A chest radiograph usually confirms an enlarged cardiac silhouette, pulmonary venous congestion, and interstitial edema.

Medical Management

The goals of medical management of heart failure are to relieve heart failure symptoms, enhance cardiac performance, and identify and correct the precipitating causes of acute heart failure.

Relief of Symptoms and Enhancement of Cardiac Performance

In the acute phase of advanced HF the patient may have a pulmonary artery catheter in place so that left ventricular function can be followed closely. Control of symptoms involves managing fluid overload, improving CO by decreasing systemic vascular resistance, and increasing contractility.

Diuretics are administered to decrease preload and to eliminate excess fluid from the body.[50,51] If pulmonary edema develops, additional diuretics are used. Morphine is given to facilitate peripheral dilation and decrease anxiety. Afterload is decreased by vasodilators (e.g., sodium nitroprusside, nitroglycerin). Nitrates are used to decrease preload and vasodilate the coronary arteries if CAD is an underlying cause of the acute HF. For some patients an IABP is also required.[37]

Contractility is initially increased by continuous infusion of positive inotropic drugs such as dopamine or by combination *inodilators* such as dobutamine or milrinone. Digitalis may be substituted later, especially if atrial fibrillation is present. ACE inhibitors are used to delay or inhibit left ventricular chamber remodeling and slow ventricular dilation and the decline in contractility.[48,49] Low-dosage β-blockers (e.g., carvedilol) may also be prescribed, although strict surveillance is required to anticipate and avoid untoward negative inotropic effects.[54,55] Nesiritide (BNP, Natrecor) is a newer IV drug indicated for the relief of patients with acutely decompensated HF who have dyspnea at rest. Nesiritide lowers pulmonary artery occlusion ("wedge") pressures, resulting in improvement in patient's symptoms of dyspnea.[56]

Nonpharmacologic modalities under investigation include biventricular pacing (right and left ventricles simultaneously) to synchronize the ventricles and improve HF symptoms for patients with a preexisting AV delay.[57,58]

Correction of Precipitating Causes

Once symptoms of HF are controlled, diagnostic studies such as cardiac catheterization, echocardiography, and thallium scanning are undertaken to uncover the cause of HF and thus tailor long-term management. Some structural problems, such as valvular disease, may be amenable to surgical correction.

Nursing Management

Nursing management of the patient with HF incorporates a variety of nursing diagnoses (Box 11-10). **Nursing priorities** focus on (1) **optimizing cardiopulmonary function**, (2) **promoting comfort and emotional support**, (3) **monitoring the effectiveness of pharmacologic therapy**, (4) **providing adequate nutrition**, and (5) **providing patient education**.

Optimizing Cardiopulmonary Function

The patient's ECG is evaluated for any dysrhythmias that may be present or may develop as a result of drug toxicity or electrolyte imbalance. Patients experiencing HF are prone to digoxin toxicity secondary to decreased renal perfusion, as well as to electrolyte imbalances. Breath sounds are auscultated frequently to determine adequacy of respiratory effort and to assess for onset or worsening of pulmonary congestion.[52] Oxygen through a nasal cannula is administered to relieve dyspnea. Diuretics or vasodilators are used to decrease excessive preload and afterload.[50,51,56] If the patient is not hypotensive, morphine may be administered to decrease hyperventilation and anxiety. If the patient's ventilatory status worsens, the nurse must be prepared for endotracheal intubation and mechanical ventilation. Obtaining daily weights is important until the weight stabilizes at a "dry" weight. Generally, the daily weight is used in fluid management and a weekly weight is used for tracking body weight (muscle, fat).

Promoting Comfort and Emotional Support

During periods of breathlessness, activity must be restricted; bed rest usually is prescribed, with the head of the bed elevated to allow for maximal lung expansion. The arms can be supported on pillows so that no undue stress is placed on the shoulder muscles. The legs may be placed in a dependent position to encourage venous pooling, thereby decreasing venous return. Rest periods must be carefully planned

and adhered to, while fostering independence within the patient's activity prescription. Vital signs are recorded before an activity is begun and after it is completed. Signs of activity intolerance, such as dyspnea, fatigue, sustained increase in pulse, and onset of dysrhythmias, are documented and reported to the physician. Activity is gradually increased according to patient tolerance. Skin breakdown is a risk because of the combination of bed rest, inadequate nutrition, edema, and decreased perfusion to the skin and subcutaneous tissue; frequent position changes and mobilization are helpful.

Monitoring Effects of Pharmacologic Therapy

Patients experiencing acute HF require aggressive pharmacologic therapy.[48-56] The nurse must know the action, side effects, therapeutic levels, and toxic effects of the diuretics and venodilators used to decrease preload, the positive inotropic agents used to increase ventricular contractility, the vasodilators used to decrease afterload, and any antidysrhythmics used to control HR and prevent dysrhythmias. The patient's hemodynamic response to these agents is closely monitored. Fluid intake and output balances are tabulated daily or even hourly in the critical care unit.

Providing Nutrition

Because patients with HF often experience decreased appetite and nausea, small frequent meals may be more appropriate than the standard three large meals. Food must be as tasty as possible; favorite foods as well as food from home may be incorporated into the diet as long as the foods are compatible with nutritional restrictions.

Providing Patient Education

The nurse assesses the patient's understanding of conservation of energy in planning activities and collaborates with the patient in organizing the day's schedule. Other topics to cover include the importance of a low-salt diet, daily weight, fluid restrictions, and written information about the multiple medications used to control HF symptoms.[59,60] Achieving the optimal outcomes for HF patients requires contributions from a team of educated health care clinicians[60] (Box 11-11).

CARDIOMYOPATHY

Cardiomyopathy is a disease of the heart muscle: *cardio* (heart), *myo* (muscle), and *pathy* (pathology). Cardiomyopathies are described as primary or secondary. *Primary*, or idiopathic, *cardiomyopathy* is defined as a heart muscle disease of unknown cause, although both viral infections and autoimmune familial disorders have been implicated. *Secondary cardiomyopathy* is defined as severe heart muscle disease resulting from some other systemic cause, such as CAD, valvular heart disease, severe hypertension, alcohol abuse, or known autoimmune disease.

Box **11-11 COLLABORATIVE** Management

Heart Failure

A collaborative heart failure management team provides an integrated approach to care to achieve clinical stability for the patient.

1. **Ensure systematic assessment and management**.
   - To achieve an absence of "congestion" and to stabilize patient's condition at the best "stage" possible when in hospital (see Tables 11-2 and 11-3).
   - To maintain same stability once discharged home and to avoid hospital readmission.
2. **Counsel and educate patient/family after discharge from hospital**. Patients and families should understand the following:
   - Heart failure disease process.
   - Heart failure medications, dosages, medication schedule, drug side effects.
   - Fluid balance related to salt restriction (2-g sodium diet), daily weight, diuretic regimen.
   - When to call health care provider.
   - Risk of additional complications: sudden cardiac death, progressive heart failure, need for other cardiac procedures (pacemaker, ICD, PCI) or cardiac surgery (bypass graft, valve replacement). Some interventions may require a mechanical assist device or heart transplantation (see Chapter 12).
   - Purpose of "advance directive" for health care decisions.
3. **Promote patient compliance with treatment regimen**.
   - Patients need support from concerned companions and health care professionals.
   - Patient should remain physically active and involved with life.
4. **Facilitate hospital discharge; implement outpatient models of health care delivery**.
   - Close communication between inpatient and outpatient health care providers is essential.

Data from Grady KL et al: *Circulation* 102:2443-2456, 2000.
ICD, Implantable cardioverter-defibrillator; *PCI*, percutaneous coronary intervention.

Classification

Cardiomyopathies are further classified on the basis of associated structural abnormalities and, if known, genotype. Cardiomyopathic categories include hypertrophic, restrictive, and dilated (Figure 11-11).

Hypertrophic Obstructive Cardiomyopathy

Hypertrophic cardiomyopathy (HCM) is a genetic disease of the myocardial sarcomere[61] characterized by stiff noncompliant myocardial muscle, with left ventricular hypertrophy and bizarre cellular hypertrophy of the upper ventricular septum.

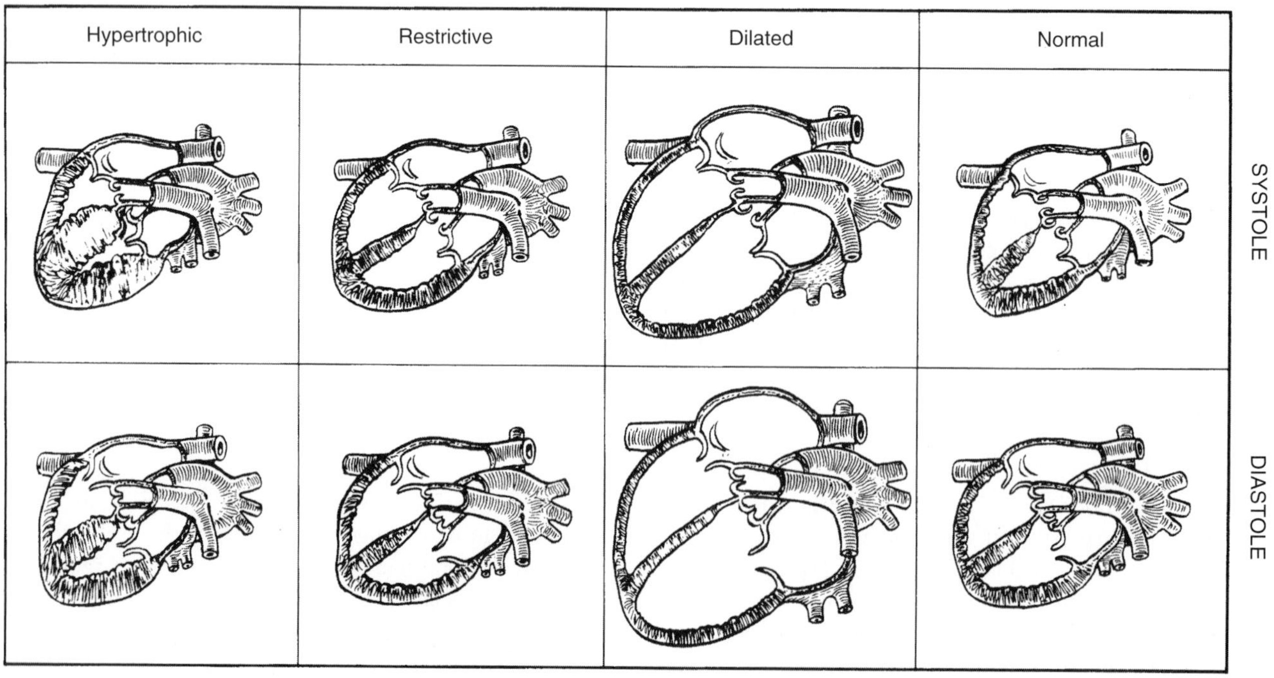

Figure 11-11 Types of cardiomyopathies and differences in ventricular diameter during systole and diastole, compared with normal heart.

This septal hypertrophy results in obstruction of the aortic valve outflow tract (Figure 11-11, A) and pulls the papillary muscle out of alignment, causing mitral regurgitation. This disorder formerly was known as *idiopathic hypertrophic subaortic stenosis* (IHSS); however, because IHSS described only 25% of affected patients, the more general HCM is now used. Symptoms are similar to those seen with HF plus the symptoms of myocardial ischemia, ventricular tachycardia (VT), supraventricular tachycardia (SVT), and syncope. Sudden cardiac death occurs in 2% to 3% of adults with HCM per year. Medical management includes limitation of physical activity, β-blockers, calcium channel blockers, antidysrhythmic therapy, HF treatment, and for some patients an implantable cardioverter defibrillator (ICD), surgical myectomy of the septum, mitral valve replacement, and most recently, percutaneous alcohol ablation of the interventricular septum.

Dilated Cardiomyopathy

Dilated cardiomyopathy is characterized by grossly dilated ventricles without muscle hypertrophy (Fig. 11-11, C). The myocardial muscle fibers contract poorly, resulting in global left ventricular dysfunction, low CO, atrial and ventricular dysrhythmias, blood pooling that leads to ventricular thrombi and embolic episodes, and finally, refractory HF and premature death.[47] The goals of medical management of dilated cardiomyopathy are improvement of pump function, removal of excess fluid, control of HF symptoms, and prevention of sudden cardiac death and other complications.[62]

Restrictive Cardiomyopathy

Restrictive cardiomyopathy, the least common form, results in ventricular wall rigidity as a consequence of myocardial fibrosis (Figure 11-11, B). The overall effect is the obstruction of ventricular filling. Diastolic HF, low CO, dyspnea, orthopnea, and liver engorgement are the most common clinical manifestations of restrictive cardiomyopathy. Medical management is directed toward improvement of pump function, removal of excess fluid, and low-sodium diet.

Nursing Management

Nursing management of the patient with cardiomyopathy incorporates a variety of nursing diagnoses related to the symptoms of HF (see Box 11-10). **Nursing priorities are individualized according to the type of cardiomyopathy and focus on** (1) **maintaining fluid balance**, (2) **monitoring effects of pharmacologic therapy**, (3) **increasing mobility**, (4) **and providing patient education**.

As with HF, a collaborative team of compassionate, knowledgeable professionals is required to provide effective care and education for these challenging patients[59,60] (see Box 11-11).

ENDOCARDITIS

Infective endocarditis (IE) is an infection on the endothelial surface of the heart, specifically thrombotic fibrin vegetations on the cardiac valves. The incidence of IE is rising, with 5000 to 20,000 new cases diagnosed per year. IE is the fourth most common cause of life-threatening infectious syndromes, after urosepsis, pneumonia, and intraabdominal sepsis. The risk of acquiring IE is higher in patients with congenital heart disease, valvular heart disease, or prosthetic heart valves and in intravenous drug abusers. Development of IE depends on two factors: (1) a susceptible lesion in the vascular endothelium and (2) an organism to establish the infection. The source of the organism may be unknown, or it may be traced to an invasive procedure, such as a biopsy, urogenital procedure, or dental work.[63]

Pathophysiology

IE is caused by a bacterial or fungal organism in the bloodstream that successfully colonizes the cardiac endothelium. Bacterial infection is most common. The thrombotic vegetations are colonized by bacteria and encased in a fibrin shell, which protects them from destruction by phagocytic neutrophils. This extensive protective mechanism is why antibiotic therapy must be so intensive and prolonged.[64]

Assessment and Diagnosis

The initial assessment for IE involves an echocardiogram of the heart valves to identify vegetations. Valvular regurgitation is often also evident. Transthoracic echocardiography (TTE) may be performed initially, but transesophageal echocardiography (TEE) is recommended because of the clarity of the heart valve images.[63] Temperature elevation above 38° C is typical, and a positive blood culture identifying the infecting organism is obtained in more than 95% of patients[63] (Box 11-12). Septic emboli may be visible on the fingers and toes. Systemic embolization occurs in 22% to 50% of patients with IE.[63] The risk of death increases with the development of emboli and decreased arterial perfusion to vital organs.

Medical Management

Treatment of IE requires prolonged IV therapy with adequate doses of bactericidal antibiotics. An increasing number of patients are being discharged home earlier and are

---

Box 11-12 Clinical Manifestations of Endocarditis

Fever
Splenomegaly
Hematuria
Petechiae
Cardiac murmurs
Easy fatigability
Osler nodes (small, raised, tender areas most often found in pads of fingers/toes)
Splinter hemorrhages in nailbeds
Roth spots (round or oval spots consisting of coagulated fibrin; seen in retina and lead to hemorrhage)

continuing parenteral therapy through a surgically implanted, long-term central venous catheter.[64]

Nursing Management

Nursing management of the patient with IE incorporates a variety of nursing diagnoses (Box 11-13). **Nursing priorities focus on** (1) **resolving the infection**, (2) **preventing complications**, (3) and **providing patient education**.

Resolving the Infection

IE requires a long course of IV antibiotics, usually 6 weeks, beginning in the hospital and continuing at home with an indwelling central catheter.[64] Nursing assessment includes monitoring for signs of worsening infection, such as persistent temperature elevation, malaise, weakness, easy fatigability, and night sweats.

Preventing Complications

A patient with IE is at risk for embolic events to the brain, lungs, and abdominal organs. Because 20% to 40% of patients with IE develop neurologic complications, the patient's level of consciousness, visual changes, and complaints of headache are frequently assessed. As valvular dysfunction accelerates, acute HF develops. Cardiac assessment includes auscultation of heart sounds to detect the presence of or change in a cardiac murmur. Shortness of breath or chest pain with hemoptysis could be caused by worsening HF or pulmonary emboli and must be reported.[63]

Providing Patient Education

The patient with IE needs to know the manifestations of infection, how to take an oral temperature, and what medical procedures increase risk of an IE recurrence. It is essential that the nurse reinforce the necessity of the patient providing other health care professionals, such as the dentist or podiatrist, with the patient's endocarditis history.[65] Many clinicians collaborate to provide care for the patient with IE (Box 11-14).

VALVULAR HEART DISEASE

Valvular heart disease describes structural and functional abnormalities of a single valve or multiple cardiac valves, which results in alteration in blood flow across the valve(s). The two types of valvular lesions are stenotic and regurgitant.

Usually, the patient admitted to the critical care unit with valve disease is experiencing either acute HF or is being admitted for cardiac surgical valvular replacement. In the past in the United States, most valvular lesions were rheumatic in origin; that is, damage was a direct result of group A β-hemolytic streptococcal pharyngitis. At present, as a result of aggressive antibiotic treatment of "strep-throat," this is rarely a problem.[65] Elderly persons are now more likely to present with symptoms of HF and "degenerative" valve changes.

Pathophysiology
Mitral Valve Stenosis

Mitral stenosis (MS) describes a progressive narrowing of the mitral valve orifice.[65] Symptoms occur when the normal valve size is reduced to less than 2.5 cm^2. Symptoms occur at rest when the valve area is reduced below 1.5 cm^2. Narrowing is caused by aging valve tissue or acute rheumatic valvulitis (Table 11-5, A). The diffuse valve leaflets fibrose and fuse, reducing mobility and thickening the chordae tendineae. As a result, the mitral valve can no longer open or close passively in response to left atrial and ventricular pressure changes. Thus blood flow across the valve is impeded. Atrial fibrillation develops in 30% to 40% of patients who have symptomatic MS. This significantly increases symptoms and may increase the need for surgical replacement of the valve.

Mitral Valve Regurgitation

Mitral regurgitation (MR) may occur secondary to rheumatic disease or aging of the valve or may be caused by endocarditis or papillary muscle dysfunction (Table 11-5, B). In MR the valve annulus, leaflets, chordae tendineae, and papillary muscles may all be dysfunctional, or the dysfunction may be isolated to only one component of the valve. MR results in retrograde flow of blood into the left atrium with each ventricular contraction. MR is always described as either chronic or acute because of the very different impact on the left-sided chambers. With *chronic* MR the left atrium will have *dilated* to accommodate the additional regurgitant volume, whereas the left ventricle will have *hypertrophied* (increased muscle) to maintain an adequate stroke volume and cardiac output. By contrast, *acute* MR is precipitated by papillary muscle rupture secondary to an acute MI; this is a medical emergency. The left atrium cannot accommodate

nursing diagnosis
priorities   Box **11-13**

Endocarditis

- Decreased Cardiac Output related to alterations in preload
- Decreased Cardiac Output related to alterations in afterload
- Decreased Cardiac Output related to alterations in contractility
- Decreased Cardiac Output related to alterations in heart rate or rhythm
- Activity Intolerance related to cardiopulmonary dysfunction
- Acute Pain related to transmission and perception of cutaneous, visceral, muscular, or ischemic impulses
- Risk for Infection risk factor: invasive procedures
- Anxiety related to threat to biologic, psychologic, and/or social integrity
- Deficient Knowledge: Discharge Regimen related to lack of previous exposure to information

Box 11-14 COLLABORATIVE Management

Endocarditis

1. **Detect and treat infecting organism.**
   Blood tests
   - Blood cultures for culture and sensitivity.
     — To determine the infecting organism.
     — To identify the antimicrobial drugs to which organism is sensitive.
   - White blood cell (WBC) count, erythrocyte sedimentation rate (ESR).
   Antimicrobials
   - Administer antimicrobial drugs to combat infection.
   - Choice of antibiotic or antifungal depends on the organism.
   Echocardiogram
   - TEE or TTE to detect intracardiac valvular vegetations or abscesses.
   - Evaluate for valvular regurgitation or stenosis.
2. **Achieve hemodynamic stability.**
   - Follow vital signs closely (blood pressure, heart/respiratory rate, oxygen saturation).
   - Provide continuous intravenous (IV) inotropic support if indicated.
   - Control fever elevation.
   - Treat symptoms of heart failure if present.
   - Manage other embolic complications that may occur.
3. **Consider valve replacement.**
   - If patient has recurrent embolic events from valve vegetations, surgical valvular replacement may be performed.
4. **Continue treatment at home.**
   - Continue IV antimicrobial infusions at home for at least 6 weeks.
   - Treat any concurrent symptoms of heart failure or emboli.
5. **Provide patient/family education.**
   - Rationale and schedule for continued antimicrobial therapy.
   - Information about endocarditis prophylaxis for future reference.

Data from Bayer AS et al: *Circulation* 98:2936-2948, 1998.
TEE, Transesophageal echocardiogram; *TTE,* transthoracic echocardiogram.

the sudden increase in volume and pressure, and use of an IABP and inotropic drug support are often required. Once the patient's condition has stabilized, the incompetent valve is surgically replaced or repaired.

Aortic Valve Stenosis

Aortic stenosis describes a narrowing of the aortic valve area. It can result from aging, calcification of a congenital bicuspid valve, or rheumatic valvulitis (Table 11-5, C). The valve opening must be reduced to a quarter of the normal size before significant changes in the circulation occur.[65] The impedance of left ventricular (LV) ejection into the aorta results in increased LV systolic pressure, LV hypertrophy, and eventually LV dilation. When symptoms such as angina, dyspnea, syncope, and other indicators of HF develop, it is critical to intervene to prevent further damage to the left ventricle. Aortic valve replacement is usually indicated.

Aortic Valve Regurgitation

Aortic regurgitation, also known as *aortic insufficiency,* may result from rheumatic fever, systemic hypertension, Marfan syndrome, syphilis, rheumatoid arthritis, aging valve tissue, or discrete subaortic stenosis (Table 11-5, D). Aortic valve incompetence results in a reflux of blood back into the left ventricle during ventricular diastole. To accommodate this extra volume, the left ventricle initially dilates and then hypertrophies in an attempt to empty more completely and to meet the needs of the peripheral circulation. Aortic valve replacement is recommended for symptomatic patients with well-preserved or moderate LV dysfunction.[66]

Tricuspid Valve Stenosis

Tricuspid stenosis is rarely an isolated lesion (Table 11-5, E). It often occurs in conjunction with mitral or aortic disease. Its origin most often is rheumatic fever or a complication of IV drug abuse and resultant endocarditis.[67] Tricuspid stenosis increases the pressure work of the usually low-pressure right atrium, resulting in right atrial hypertrophy. In addition, the right atrium dilates in an attempt to accommodate the residual right atrial volume and the incoming venous return. As a result, systemic venous congestion occurs, leading to jugular venous congestion, liver failure, hepatomegaly, ascites, and peripheral edema.

Tricuspid Valve Regurgitation

Tricuspid regurgitation usually results from advanced failure of the left side of the heart that eventually affects the right side of the heart; develops secondary to severe pulmonary hypertension; occurs with a right ventricular MI, or develops as a complication of endocarditis[67] (Table 11-5, F).

Pulmonic Valve Disease

Pulmonic valve disease is uncommon in adults. It is most often related to congenital anomalies and produces failure of the right side of the heart.

Mixed Valvular Lesions

Many persons have mixed lesions, with an element of both stenosis and regurgitation. Mixed lesions can accentuate the severity of a condition. For example, combined aortic stenosis and aortic regurgitation increase left ventricular (LV) volume and pressure and multiply the degree of LV work.

Table **11-5** Valvular Dysfunction: Mitral, Atrial, and Tricuspid Stenosis/Regurgitation

	Pathophysiology	Clinical Manifestations	Physical Signs*
A Mitral valve stenosis	**MITRAL VALVE STENOSIS** LA must generate more pressure to propel blood beyond lesion Rise in LA pressure/volume reflected retrograde into pulmonary vessels RV hypertrophy RV failure	Dyspnea on exertion Fatigue, weakness Pronounced respiratory symptoms (orthopnea, paroxysmal nocturnal dyspnea) Mild hemoptysis with bronchial capillary rupture Susceptibility to pulmonary infections	CXR: pulmonary congestion, redistribution of blood flow to upper lobes ECG: atrial fibrillation, other atrial dysrhythmias Aus: diastolic murmur, accentuated S_1, opening snap Cath: elevated pressure gradient across valve; increased LA pressure, PAOP, and PA pressure; low CO
---▶ **indicates stenosis**			
B Mitral valve regurgitation	**MITRAL VALVE REGURGITATION** LV dilation and hypertrophy LA dilation and hypertrophy	Weakness, fatigue Exertional dyspnea Palpitations Severe symptoms precipitated by LV failure, with low CO and pulmonary congestion	CXR: LA/LV enlargement, variable pulmonary congestion ECG: P mitrale, LV hypertrophy, atrial fibrillation Aus: murmur throughout systole Cath: LA opacification during LV injection, V waves, increased LA/LV pressures Variable elevations of PA pressures
indicates backward flow from a valve that is leaking or regurgitant			
C Aortic valve stenosis	**AORTIC VALVE STENOSIS** LV hypertrophy Progressive failure of ventricular emptying Pulmonary congestion Failure of right side of heart, with systemic venous congestion Sudden cardiac death	Exertional dyspnea Exercise intolerance Syncope Angina Heart failure (LV failure)	CXR: poststenotic aortic dilation, calcification ECG: LV hypertrophy Aus: systolic ejection murmur Cath: significant pressure gradient, increased LV end-diastolic pressure
◀--- **indicates stenosis**			

D

AORTIC VALVE REGURGITATION

Aortic valve regurgitation

Increased volume load imposed on left ventricle

LV dilation and hypertrophy

➡ indicates backward flow from a valve that is leaking or regurgitant

Fatigue
Dyspnea on exertion
Palpitations

CXR: boot-shaped elongation of cardiac apex
ECG: LV hypertrophy
Aus: diastolic murmur
Cath: LV opacification during aortic injection
Peripheral signs: hyperdynamic myocardial action, low peripheral resistance

E

TRICUSPID VALVE STENOSIS

Tricuspid valve stenosis

- - -> indicates stenosis

Right atrium must generate higher pressure to eject blood beyond lesion
RA dilation
Systemic venous engorgement
Increased venous pressures

Venous distention
Peripheral edema
Ascites
Hepatic engorgement
Anorexia

CXR: RA enlargement
ECG: RA enlargement (P pulmonale)
Aus: diastolic murmur
Cath: elevated RA pressure with large *a* waves; pressure gradient across tricuspid valve

F

TRICUSPID VALVE REGURGITATION

Tricuspid valve regurgitation

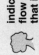 indicates backward flow from a valve that is leaking or regurgitant

RV hypertrophy and dilation

Decreased CO
Neck vein distention
Hepatic engorgement
Ascites
Edema
Pleural effusions

CXR: RA/RV enlargement
ECG: RV hypertrophy, RA enlargement, atrial fibrillation
Aus: murmur throughout systole
Cath: elevated RA pressure and V waves

*CXR, Chest radiograph; ECG, electrocardiogram; Aus, auscultation; Cath, cardiac catheterization. RA, Right atrium/right atrial; LA, left atrium/left atrial; LV, left ventricle/left ventricular; RV, right ventricle/right ventricular; CO, cardiac output; PAOP, pulmonary artery occlusion pressure ("wedge" pressure); PA, pulmonary artery.

This increased workload promotes ventricular hypertrophy that will lead eventually to LV dilation with symptoms of heart failure.

Medical Management

Management of valvular disorders includes pharmacologic therapy to control symptoms of HF and then surgical repair or replacement of the affected valve.[63,68] When surgery is not feasible, balloon dilation is sometimes performed for patients too ill to undergo a major cardiac procedure (see Chapter 12).

Nursing Management

Nursing management of the patient with valvular disease incorporates a variety of nursing diagnoses (Box 11-15). Nursing priorities are focused on (1) **maintaining adequate cardiac output**, (2) **optimizing fluid balance**, and (3) **providing patient education**.

Maintaining Adequate Cardiac Output

Low CO is a common finding in patients with valvular heart disease. It results from decreased forward flow through a stenotic valve, or because of bidirectional flow across an incompetent (regurgitant) valve. Vital signs and the effect of positive inotropic and afterload-reducing agents are assessed and documented. If the patient has hemodynamic catheters inserted, CO and hemodynamic parameters are measured and evaluated. Patient care activities are carefully planned to provide adequate rest periods to prevent fatigue.

Optimizing Fluid Balance

Fluid status is evaluated by auscultation of breath sounds for crackles, heart sounds for presence of an S_3, daily weight to trend a "sudden weight gain," and presence of peripheral edema. The appearance of pulmonary crackles or an S_3 sound confirm volume overload secondary to HF. The jugular vein is assessed for signs of increased distention. Diuretics and vasodilators are administered to counteract excess fluid retention. The patient is weighed daily, and fluid intake/output is monitored and recorded.

Providing Patient Education

Education for the patient with acute or chronic HF secondary to valvular dysfunction includes (1) information related to diet, (2) fluid restrictions, (3) actions and side effects of medications, (4) need for prophylactic antibiotics before undergoing invasive procedures such as dental work, and (5) when to call the health care provider to report a negative change in cardiac symptoms. Many patients also require information about valvular heart surgery.[63] Achieving the optimal outcomes for the patient with valve disease requires contributions from a team of educated health care clinicians (Box 11-16).

CONCLUSION

The number of patients with cardiovascular disease continues to increase.[1] Fortunately, considerable research is being undertaken and clinical progress is being made in the diagnosis and management of cardiac conditions. To be able to participate fully in the collaborative management of

nursing diagnosis priorities   Box 11-15

Valvular Heart Disease

- Decreased Cardiac Output related to alterations in preload
- Decreased Cardiac Output related to alterations in afterload
- Decreased Cardiac Output related to alterations in contractility
- Decreased Cardiac Output related to alterations in heart rate and rhythm
- Activity Intolerance related to cardiopulmonary dysfunction
- Deficient Knowledge: Discharge Regimen related to lack of previous exposure to information

Box 11-16 COLLABORATIVE Management

Valvular Heart Disease

1. **Assess valvular dysfunction.**
   - *Clinical assessment*
     - Auscultation for heart murmurs.
     - Signs/symptoms of heart failure; dyspnea usually the earliest symptom (see Table 11-3).
   - *Echocardiogram*: Valve motion, ventricular wall motion.
   - *Cardiac catheterization*: Valve/ventricular wall motion, ejection fraction.
2. **Consider valve surgery.**
   - If heart failure symptoms appear, surgery is indicated.
   - Valve replacement (see Chapter 12).
3. **Provide patient/family education.**
   - Anticoagulation (if mechanical valve or atrial fibrillation present).
   - Heart failure medications (if present).
   - *Infection prevention*: Endocarditis prophylaxis.
   - *Postoperative*: Specialized education related to sternal incision.

Data from Bonow RO et al: *J Heart Valve Dis* 7:672-707, 1998.

patients with cardiovascular disorders, it is essential that the critical care nurse understand the spectrum of therapy, from basic nursing care procedures to the most recent therapeutic advances.

REFERENCES

1. American Heart Association: *Heart disease and stroke statistics: 2003 update*, Dallas, 2002, American Heart Association, 2002.
2. Aronow WS: The older man's heart and heart disease, *Med Clin North Am* 83:1291-1303, 1999.
3. Mosca L et al: AHA/ACC scientific statement: consensus panel statement. In American Heart Association/American College of Cardiology: Guide to preventive cardiology for women, *J Am Coll Cardiol* 33:1751-1755, 1999.
4. Smith SC Jr et al: AHA/ACC guidelines for preventing heart attack and death in patients with atherosclerotic cardiovascular disease: 2001 update. American Heart Association/American College of Cardiology, *J Am Coll Cardiol* 38:1581-1583, 2001.
5. Hochman JS et al: Sex, clinical presentation, and outcome in patients with acute coronary syndromes. Global Use of Strategies to Open Occluded Coronary Arteries in Acute Coronary Syndromes IIb, *N Engl J Med* 341:226-232, 1999.
6. Hulley S et al: Randomized trial of estrogen plus progestin for secondary prevention of coronary heart disease in postmenopausal women. Heart and Estrogen/Progestin Replacement Study (HERS), *JAMA* 280:605-613, 1998.
7. Grady D et al: Cardiovascular disease outcomes during 6.8 years of hormone therapy. Heart and Estrogen/Progestin Replacement Study follow-up (HERS II), *JAMA* 288:49-57, 2002.
8. Williams JE et al: Racial disparities in CHD mortality from 1968-1992 in the state economic areas surrounding the ARIC study communities. Atherosclerosis Risk in Communities, *Ann Epidemiol* 9:472-480, 1999.
9. Howard BV et al: Rising tide of cardiovascular disease in American Indians: the Strong Heart Study, *Circulation* 99:2389-2395, 1999.
10. Schulman KA et al: The effect of race and sex on physicians' recommendations for cardiac catheterization, *N Engl J Med* 340:618-626, 1999.
11. Rosenberg L et al: Risk factors for coronary heart disease in African-American women, *Am J Epidemiol* 150:904-909, 1999.
12. Ryan TJ et al: ACC/AHA guidelines for the management of patients with acute myocardial infarction: 1999 update. American College of Cardiology/American Heart Association Task Force on Practice Guidelines, Committee on Management of Acute Myocardial Infarction, *Circulation* 100:1016-1030, 1999.
13. Krauss RM et al: AHA dietary guidelines: revision 2000. American Heart Association Nutrition Committee. *Circulation* 102: 2284-2299, 2000.
14. Third Report of National Cholesterol Education Program (NCEP) Expert Panel on Detection, Evaluation, and Treatment of High Blood Cholesterol in Adults (Adult Treatment Panel III), *JAMA* 285:2486-2497, 2001.
15. Rosenson RS, Brown AS: Statin use in acute coronary syndromes: cellular mechanisms and clinical evidence, *Curr Opin Lipidol* 13:625-630, 2002.
16. LaRosa JC, He J, Vupputuri S: Effect of statins on risk of coronary disease: a meta-analysis of randomized controlled trials, *JAMA* 282:2340-2346, 1999.
17. Wilson PW et al: Clustering of metabolic factors and coronary heart disease, *Arch Intern Med* 159:1104-1109, 1999.
18. Mokdad AH et al: Prevalence of obesity, diabetes, and obesity-related health risk factors, 2001, *JAMA* 289:76-79, 2003.
19. Thompson D et al: Lifetime health and economic consequences of obesity, *Arch Intern Med* 159:2177-2183, 1999.
20. Rexrode KM et al: Abdominal adiposity and coronary heart disease in women, *JAMA* 280:1843-1848, 1998.
21. Franklin BA, Swain DP, Shephard RJ: New insights in the prescription of exercise for coronary patients, *J Cardiovasc Nurs*, 18(2):116-123, 2003.
22. Hu FB et al: Walking compared with vigorous physical activity and risk of type 2 diabetes in women: a prospective study, *JAMA* 282:1433-1439, 1999.
23. Chobanian AV, et al: The Seventh Report of the Joint National Committee on Prevention, Detection, Evaluation, and Treatment of High Blood Pressure: The JNC 7 Report, *JAMA* 289(19):2560-2571, 2003.
24. Houterman S, Verschuren WM, Kromhout D: Smoking, blood pressure and serum cholesterol: effects on 20-year mortality, *Epidemiology* 14(1):24-29, 2003.
25. Report of the Expert Committee on the Diagnosis and Classification of Diabetes Mellitus, *Diabetes Care* 26:Suppl 1:S5-S20, 2003.
26. Grundy SM et al: Diabetes and cardiovascular disease: a statement for healthcare professionals from the American Heart Association, *Circulation* 100:1134-1146, 1999.
27. Booth GL, Wang EE: Preventive health care, 2000 update: screening and management of hyperhomocysteinemia for the prevention of coronary artery disease events. Canadian Task Force on Preventive Health Care, *CMAJ* 163:21-29, 2000.
28. Pearson TA et al: Markers of inflammation and cardiovascular disease: application to clinical and public health practice: A statement for healthcare professionals from the Centers for Disease Control and Prevention and the American Heart Association, *Circulation* 107(3):499-511, 2003.
29. Speidl WS et al: High-sensitivity C-reactive protein in the prediction of coronary events in patients with premature coronary artery disease, *Am Heart J* 144:449-455, 2002.
30. Buffon A et al: Widespread coronary inflammation in unstable angina, *N Engl J Med* 347:5-12, 2002.
31. Gibbons RJ et al: ACC/AHA guidelines for the management of patients with chronic stable angina: 2002 update. American College of Cardiology/American Heart Association Task Force on Practice Guidelines, Committee on Management of Patients with Chronic Stable Angina, *Circulation* 107:149-158, 2003.
32. Canto JG et al: Use of emergency medical services in acute myocardial infarction and subsequent quality of care: observations from the National Registry of Myocardial Infarction 2, *Circulation* 106:3018-3023, 2002.
33. Braunwald E et al: ACC/AHA guidelines for the management of patients with unstable angina and non-ST-segment elevation myocardial infarction: 2002 update. American College of Cardiology/American Heart Association Task Force on Practice Guidelines, Committee on Management of Patients with Unstable Angina, *J Am Coll Cardiol* 40:1366-1374, 2002.
34. Boersma E et al: Platelet glycoprotein IIb/IIIa receptor inhibition in non-ST-elevation acute coronary syndromes: early benefit during medical treatment only, with additional protection during percutaneous coronary intervention, *Circulation* 100:2045-2048, 1999.
35. Keeley EC, Boura JA, Grines CL: Primary angioplasty versus intravenous thrombolytic therapy for acute myocardial infarction: a quantitative review of 23 randomised trials, *Lancet* 361(9351):13-20, 2003.
36. Zerwic JJ: Patient delay in seeking treatment for acute myocardial infarction symptoms, *J Cardiovasc Nurs* 13:21-32, 1999.
37. Hochman JS et al: Cardiogenic shock complicating acute myocardial infarction: etiologies, management and outcome. Report from the SHOCK Trial Registry: SHould we emergently revascularize Occluded Coronaries for cardiogenic shocK? *J Am Coll Cardiol* 36(suppl A):1063-1070, 2000

38. Hillis GS: Utility of cardiac troponin I, creatine kinase-MB (mass), myosin light chain 1, and myoglobin in the early in-hospital triage of "high-risk" patients with chest pain, *Heart* 82:614-620, 1999.

39. Moser DK et al: The role of the critical care nurse in preventing heart failure after acute myocardial infarction, *Crit Care Nurse* (suppl):11-15, 1999.

40. Van de Werf F: Incidence and predictors of bleeding events after fibrinolytic therapy with fibrin-specific agents: a comparison of TNK-tPA and rt-PA, *Eur Heart J* 22:2253-2261, 2001.

41. Mehta RH et al: Patient outcomes after fibrinolytic therapy for acute myocardial infarction at hospitals with and without coronary revascularization capability, *J Am Coll Cardiol* 40:1034-1040, 2002.

42. Dracup KA, Cannon CP: Combination treatment strategies for management of acute myocardial infarction, *Crit Care Nurse* (suppl):3-17, April 1999.

43. Keeley EC, Cigarroa JE: Facilitated primary percutaneous transluminal coronary angioplasty for acute ST segment elevation myocardial infarction: rationale for reuniting pharmacologic and mechanical revascularization strategies, *Cardiol Rev* 11:13-20, 2003.

44. Tan WA, Moliterno DJ: Aspirin, ticlopidine, and clopidogrel in acute coronary syndromes: underused treatments could save thousands of lives, *Cleve Clin J Med* 66:615, 1999.

45. Wong GC, Giugliano RP, Antman EM: Use of low-molecular-weight heparins in the management of acute coronary artery syndromes and percutaneous coronary intervention, *JAMA* 289:331-342, 2003.

46. Balady GJ et al: Core components of cardiac rehabilitation/secondary prevention programs: a statement for healthcare professionals from the American Heart Association and the American Association of Cardiovascular and Pulmonary Rehabilitation Writing Group, *Circulation* 102:1069-1073, 2000.

47. Hunt SA et al: ACC/AHA guidelines for the evaluation and management of chronic heart failure in the adult. American College of Cardiology/American Heart Association Task Force on Practice Guidelines, Committee to Revise 1995 Guidelines for Evaluation and Management of Heart Failure, *Circulation* 104:2996-3007, 2001.

48. Michaels AD et al: Early use of ACE inhibitors in the treatment of acute myocardial infarction in the United States: experience from the National Registry of Myocardial Infarction 2, *Am J Cardiol* 84:1176-1181, 1999.

49. Yusuf S et al: Effects of an angiotensin-converting-enzyme inhibitor, ramipril, on cardiovascular events in high-risk patients. Heart Outcomes Prevention Evaluation Study, *N Engl J Med* 342:145-153, 2000.

50. Pitt B et al: The effect of spironolactone on morbidity and mortality in patients with severe heart failure. Randomized Aldactone Evaluation Study, *N Engl J Med* 341:709-717, 1999.

51. Paul S: Balancing diuretic therapy in heart failure: loop diuretics, thiazides, and aldosterone antagonists, *Congest Heart Fail* 8:307-312, 2002.

52. McCullough PA et al: B-type natriuretic peptide and clinical judgment in emergency diagnosis of heart failure: analysis from Breathing Not Properly (BNP) Multinational Study, *Circulation* 106:416-422, 2002.

53. Maisel AS et al: Rapid measurement of B-type natriuretic peptide in the emergency diagnosis of heart failure, *N Engl J Med* 347:161-167, 2002.

54. Meghani SH, Becker D: Beta-blockers: a new therapy in congestive heart failure, *Am J Crit Care* 10:417-429, 2001.

55. Pamboukian SV et al: Carvedilol improves functional class in patients with severe left ventricular dysfunction referred for heart transplantation, *Clin Transplant* 13:426-431, 1999.

56. Burger AJ et al: Effect of nesiritide (B-type natriuretic peptide) and dobutamine on ventricular arrhythmias in the treatment of patients with acutely decompensated congestive heart failure: the PRECEDENT study, *Am Heart J* 144:1102-1108, 2002.

57. Abraham WT et al: Cardiac resynchronization in chronic heart failure, *N Engl J Med* 346:1845-1853, 2002.

58. Abraham WT: Cardiac resynchronization therapy for heart failure: biventricular pacing and beyond, *Curr Opin Cardiol* 17:346-352, 2002.

59. Knox D, Mischke L: Implementing a congestive heart failure disease management program to decrease length of stay and cost, *J Cardiovasc Nurs.* 14:55-74, 1999.

60. Grady KL et al: Team management of patients with heart failure: a statement for healthcare professionals from the Cardiovascular Nursing Council of the American Heart Association, *Circulation* 102:2443-2456, 2000.

61. Barkman A, McCay J: Cardiogenic shock in a patient with hypertrophic obstructive cardiomyopathy after insertion of a pacemaker, *Am J Crit Care* 11:537-542, 2002.

62. Felker GM et al: The spectrum of dilated cardiomyopathy: the Johns Hopkins experience with 1278 patients, *Medicine (Baltimore)* 78:270-283, 1999.

63. Bayer AS et al: Diagnosis and management of infective endocarditis and its complications: American Hospital Association scientific statement, *Circulation* 98:2936-2948, 1998.

64. Andrews MM, von Reyn CF: Patient selection criteria and management guidelines for outpatient parenteral antibiotic therapy for native valve infective endocarditis, *Clin Infect Dis* 33:203-209, 2001.

65. Dajani A et al: Treatment of acute streptococcal pharyngitis and prevention of rheumatic fever: a statement for health professionals. Committee on Rheumatic Fever, Endocarditis, and Kawasaki Disease, Council on Cardiovascular Disease in the Young, American Heart Association, *Pediatrics* 96:758-764, 1995.

66. Hicks GL Jr, Massey HT: Update on indications for surgery in aortic insufficiency, *Curr Opin Cardiol* 17:172-178, 2002.

67. Bonow RO et al: ACC/AHA guidelines for the management of patients with valvular heart disease. American College of Cardiology/American Heart Association Task Force on Practice Guidelines, Committee on Management of Patients with Valvular Heart Disease, *J Heart Valve Dis* 7:672-707, 1998.

68. Frontera JA, Gradon JD: Right-side endocarditis in injection drug users: review of proposed mechanisms of pathogenesis, *Clin Infect Dis* 30:374-379, 2000.

12

Cardiovascular Therapeutic Management

Objectives

- Describe the functions of a temporary pacemaker and an implantable cardioverter-defibrillator.
- Outline the medical and nursing management of a patient undergoing cardiac surgery and cardiac interventional procedures.
- Identify the signs of reperfusion in a patient undergoing thrombolytic therapy.
- List the most important categories of cardiovascular drugs, their intended actions, and major significance.

evolve Be sure to check out the free exercises on-line at *http://evolve.elsevier.com/Urden/priorities/*

A wide variety of therapeutic interventions are employed in the management of the patient with cardiovascular dysfunction. This chapter focuses on the priority interventions used to manage acute cardiovascular disorders in the critical care setting.

TEMPORARY PACEMAKERS

Pacemakers are electronic devices that can be used to initiate the heartbeat when the heart's intrinsic electrical system cannot effectively generate a rate adequate to support cardiac output (CO). Pacemakers can be used temporarily, either supportively or prophylactically, until the condition responsible for the rate or conduction disturbance resolves. Pacemakers also can be used on a permanent basis if the patient's condition persists despite adequate therapy.

Indications

Dysrhythmias that are unresponsive to drug therapy and that compromise hemodynamic status are the primary indication for pacemaker therapy. Temporary pacing is most frequently used to manage symptomatic bradycardia or progressive heart block that develops secondary to myocardial ischemia or drug toxicity. After cardiac surgery, temporary pacing is often used to overcome conduction disturbances and improve CO.[1,2]

Pacemaker System

A pacemaker system is a simple electrical circuit consisting of two main components: a pulse generator and pacing leads (Figure 12-1).

Pulse Generator

The pulse generator is designed to generate an electrical current that travels through the pacing lead and exits through an electrode (exposed portion of the wire) that is in direct contact with the heart. This electrical current initiates a myocardial depolarization. The current then seeks to return to the pulse generator to complete the circuit. The return route will vary according to the specific pacing leads that are used. The power source for a temporary external pulse generator is a standard 9-volt alkaline battery.

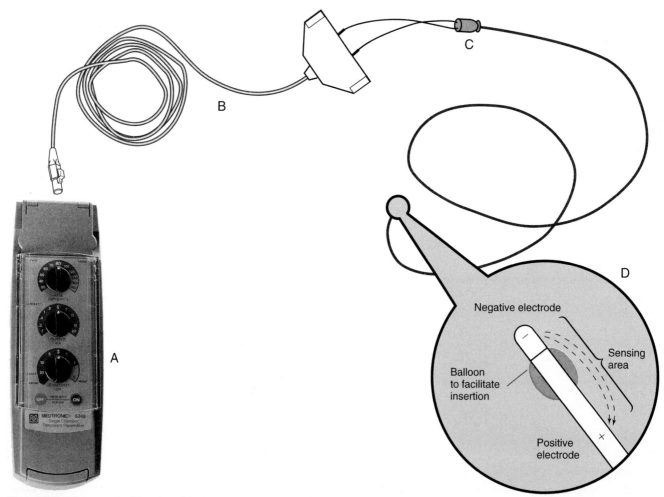

Figure 12-1 Components of temporary bipolar transvenous catheter. **A,** Single-chamber temporary (external) pulse generator. **B,** Bridging cable. **C,** Pacing lead. **D,** Enlarged view of pacing lead tip.

Pacing Leads

Temporary pacing leads have one or more electrodes at the tip. The electrodes are described as either *bipolar* or *unipolar*. In both systems the current flows from the negative terminal of the pulse generator, down the pacing lead to the negative electrode, and into the heart. The current is then picked up by the positive electrode (ground) and flows back up the lead to the positive terminal of the pulse generator.

Bipolar Electrodes. In a bipolar pacing system, two electrodes (positive and negative) are located within the heart. The bipolar lead used in transvenous pacing has two electrodes on one catheter (Figure 12-1, *D*). The distal, or negative, electrode is at the tip of the pacing lead and maintains close or direct contact with the heart, usually inside the right atrium or ventricle. Approximately 1 centimeter (cm) from the negative electrode is a positive electrode. The negative electrode is attached to the negative terminal, and the positive electrode is attached to the positive terminal of the pulse generator, either directly or through a bridging cable. The bipolar system is typically used in temporary pacing systems.

Unipolar Electrode. A unipolar pacing system (epicardial or transvenous) has only one electrode, the negative electrode, making contact with the heart muscle. The positive electrode, also known as "the ground," is not in contact with the heart. This system is infrequently used with temporary pacing.

Pacing Routes
Transcutaneous Pacing

Transcutaneous cardiac pacing involves the use of two large skin electrodes placed on the thorax. One is applied on the front of the chest over the heart or sternum and the other on the back either between the scapula or over the left scapular region. Both electrodes are connected to an external pulse generator and are usually marked "anterior" and "posterior" by the manufacturer to facilitate accurate placement during an emergency. Transcutaneous pacing is a rapid, noninvasive procedure that nurses can perform in an emergency situation. It is recommended as a primary intervention in the advanced cardiac life support (ACLS) algorithm for management of symptomatic bradycardia.[3] Useful as an emergency short-term therapy, transcutaneous pacing is employed until the bradycardia resolves or another route of pacing is established.

Epicardial Pacing

The insertion of temporary epicardial pacing wires is routine during many cardiac surgeries. Ventricular and in many cases atrial pacing wires are loosely sewn to the epicardium. The terminal pins of these wires are pulled through the skin before the chest is closed. Both epicardial leads are in contact with the myocardial tissue, so either wire may be used as the negative, or pacing, electrode. The remaining wire is then used as the positive, or ground, electrode. If both chambers have pacing wires attached, the atrial wires exit subcostally to the right of the sternum, and the ventricular wires exit in the same region but to the left of the sternum. These wires can be removed several days after surgery by gentle traction at the skin surface, with minimal risk of bleeding.[4]

Transvenous Pacing

A transvenous pacing catheter is used for emergency pacing support. This is a specialized catheter with a pacing electrode at the tip. The pacing catheter is inserted into the subclavian, internal jugular, or femoral vein and advanced into the right ventricle. Insertion can be facilitated through direct visualization with fluoroscopy or by the standard electrocardiogram (ECG). In some cases the pacing wire is inserted through a special pulmonary artery catheter through a port that exits in the right ventricle.

Codes and Modes
Three-Letter Pacemaker Code

In 1974 the Inter-Society Commission for Heart Disease (ICHD) adopted a code for describing the various pacing modes. A three-letter code is used to describe temporary pacing modes. The first letter refers to the cardiac chamber that is paced. The second letter designates which chamber is sensed, and the third letter indicates the pacemaker's response to the sensed event.[5]

Five-Letter Pacemaker Code

The five-letter pacemaker code contains the three-letter code categories plus two sections that list additional programming functions (Table 12-1).[5]

Synchronous Pacing Modes

Synchrony implies that the pacemaker only delivers a stimulus when the heart's intrinsic pacemaker fails to function at a predetermined rate. The most physiologic of the synchronous modes are those in which the normal sequential relationship between atrial and ventricular depolarization and contraction is maintained. *Atrioventricular* (AV) *synchrony* increases the volume in the ventricle before contraction and thus improves CO. When atrial-to-ventricular conduction is impaired, as during heart block, AV synchrony can be maintained through dual-chamber (both atrial and ventricular) pacing modes.

DDD Pacing. The most physiologic of the AV pacing modes is the DDD mode.[5] In DDD pacing, atrial and ventricular leads are used for both pacing and sensing. In response to sensed activity, the pacemaker inhibits the pacing stimulus. Therefore a sensed P wave in the atrium will inhibit the atrial pacing stimulus, whereas a sensed R wave in the ventricle will inhibit the ventricular pacing stimulus. DDD pacing is described as "universal pacing" or "true physiologic pacing" (Table 12-2).

| Table **12-1** | NASPE/BPEG Generic (NBG) Pacemaker Code |

Position I* Chamber(s) Paced	II Chamber(s) Sensed	III Response to Sensing	IV Programmability	V Antitachydysrhythmia Function(s)
0 = None A = Atrium	0 = None A = Atrium	0 = None T = Triggered	0 = None P = Simple programmability (rate, output, sensitivity)	0 = None P = Pacing (antitachydysrhythmia)
V = Ventricle D = Dual (A + V) S† = Single (A or V)	V = Ventricle D = Dual (A + V) S = Single (A or V)	I = Inhibited D = Dual (T + I)	M = Multi-programmability C = Communicating R = Rate modulation (rate responsive)	S = Shock D = Dual

Modified from Bernstein AD et al: *Pacing Clin Electrophysiol* 10:794, 1987.
*Positions I through III are used exclusively for antibradydysrhythmia function.
†Used by manufacturer only.
NASPE, North American Society of Pacing and Electrophysiology; *BPEG*, British Pacing and Electrophysiology Group; *NBG*, North American British Generic.

| Table **12-2** | Temporary Pacing Modes |

Mode	Description
FIXED RATE	
AOO	Atrial pacing, no sensing
VOO	Ventricular pacing, no sensing
DOO	Atrial and ventricular pacing, no sensing
DEMAND	
AAI	Atrial pacing, atrial sensing, inhibited response to sensed P waves
VVI	Ventricular pacing, ventricular sensing, inhibited response to sensed QRS complexes
DVI	Atrial and ventricular pacing, ventricular sensing; both atrial and ventricular pacing are inhibited if a spontaneous ventricular depolarization is sensed
UNIVERSAL	
DDD	Both chambers are paced and sensed; inhibited response of pacing stimuli to sensed events in respective chambers; triggered response to sensed atrial activity to allow rate-responsive ventricular pacing

VVI Pacing. The VVI mode is designed to pace the ventricle when the pacemaker does not sense an intrinsic (patient) ventricular depolarization. Other names that are popularly used for this mode include "backup pacing" or "demand pacing" (Table 12-2). VVI pacing is necessary in specific circumstances; the classic example is symptomatic bradycardia with atrial fibrillation (AF). Because AF makes it impossible to pace the atria, one effective intervention is to use VVI pacing to maintain ventricular function.

Asynchronous Pacing Modes

Fixed-rate or asynchronous pacing modes ignore the patient's intrinsic heartbeat. These modes are uncommon with the exception of two situations. Emergency DOO or VOO pacing may be used in asystole as a lifesaving measure. These modes are sometimes used in the operating room, where electromagnetic interference (EMI) from electrocautery and other electrical equipment can interfere with normal pacemaker function.

Pacemaker Settings

The controls on all external temporary pulse generators are similar, and their function must be thoroughly understood to initiate pacing quickly in an emergency situation. In addition, if unexpected problems occur, troubleshooting can be facilitated quickly and effectively.

Rate Control

The rate control regulates the number of impulses that can be delivered to the heart per minute. The rate setting depends on the physiologic needs of the patient, but in general it is maintained between 60 and 80 beats/min.

Output Dial

The output dial regulates the amount of electrical current, measured in milliamperes (mA), that is delivered to the heart to initiate depolarization. The point at which depolarization occurs is termed the *threshold* and is indicated by a myocardial response to the pacing stimulus (capture). The procedure for testing *pacemaker pacing output threshold* in a temporary pacemaker system is described in Box 12-1.

Sensitivity Control

The sensitivity control regulates the ability of the pacemaker to detect the heart's intrinsic electrical activity. Sensitivity, measured in millivolts (mV), determines the size of the intracardiac signal that the generator will recognize. If the sensitivity is adjusted to its most sensitive setting, 1 mV, the pacemaker can respond even to low-amplitude electrical signals coming from the heart. By contrast, turning the sensitivity to its least sensitive setting, 20 mV or to the area labeled "async," blinds the pacemaker to any intrinsic electrical activity and produces pacing at a preset fixed rate. A sense indicator (often a light) on the pulse generator signals each time intrinsic cardiac electrical activity is sensed. The sensing ability of the pacemaker can be quickly evaluated by observing for a change in pacing rhythm in response to spontaneous depolarizations (P wave or QRS complex). A specific procedure for testing *pacing sensitivity thresholds* when a patient is connected to a temporary pacing system is described in Box 12-2.

Atrioventricular Interval Control

The AV interval control (available only on dual-chamber generators) regulates the interval between the atrial and ventricular pacing stimuli. This interval is analogous to the PR interval in the intrinsic ECG. Proper adjustment of this interval to between 150 and 250 milliseconds preserves AV synchrony, permits maximal ventricular stroke volume, and improves CO.

Box **12-1** **Temporary Pacemaker Testing for Pacing Thresholds**

1. Adjust pacemaker rate setting so that patient is 100% paced. It may be necessary to increase the pacing rate to achieve this setting.
2. Gradually decrease output (milliampere, mA) setting until 1:1 capture is lost. Pacing threshold is located where capture is lost.
3. Slowly increase output setting until 1:1 capture is reestablished. With a properly positioned pacing electrode, the pacing threshold should be less than 1.0 mA.
4. Set output (mA) setting two to three times higher than measured threshold because thresholds tend to fluctuate over time.
5. Evaluate pacing thresholds for both atrial and ventricular leads separately if patient is connected to a dual-chamber pulse generator.

Box **12-2** **Temporary Pacemaker Sensitivity Thresholds**

1. Set sensitivity control to its most sensitive setting.
2. Adjust pulse generator rate to 10 beats/min less than patient's intrinsic rate (flash indicator should flash regularly).
3. Reduce generator output to minimal value to prevent risk of competing with intrinsic rhythm.
4. Gradually increase sensitivity value until sense indicator stops flashing and pace indicator starts flashing.
5. Decrease sensitivity until sense indicator begins to flash again; this is the *sensitivity threshold*.
6. Adjust sensitivity setting on generator to half the threshold value; restore generator output and rate to original values.

DDD Controls

Temporary DDD pacemakers have several other digital controls that are unique to this mode. The *lower rate,* or *base rate,* is the rate at which the generator will pace when intrinsic activity falls below the preset pacemaker rate. The *upper rate* determines the fastest ventricular rate the pacemaker will deliver in response to sensed atrial activity. This setting is needed to protect the patient's heart from being paced in response to rapid atrial dysrhythmias. The *pulse width,* which can be adjusted from 0.05 to 2.0 milliseconds, controls the length of time that the pacing stimulus is delivered to the heart. The *atrial refractory period,* programmable from 150 to 500 milliseconds, regulates the length of time after either a sensed or paced ventricular event, during which the pacemaker cannot respond to another atrial stimulus. An *emergency button* is also available on some models to allow for rapid initiation of asynchronous (DOO) pacing during an emergency. Finally, on all temporary pacemakers, an *on/off switch* is provided with a safety feature that prevents the accidental termination of pacing.

Pacing Artifacts

All patients with temporary pacemakers require continuous ECG monitoring. The pacing artifact is the spike that is visible on the ECG tracing as the pacing stimulus is delivered to the heart. A *P wave* is seen following the pacing artifact if the atrium is being paced (Figure 12-2, *A*). Similarly, a *QRS complex* follows a ventricular pacing artifact (Figure 12-2, *B*). With dual-chamber pacing, a pacing artifact precedes both the P wave and the QRS complex (Figure 12-2, *C*).

Pacemaker Malfunctions

Most pacemaker malfunctions can be categorized as abnormalities of either pacing or sensing.

Pacing Malfunctions

Problems with pacing can involve the failure of the pacemaker to deliver the pacing stimulus, a pacing stimulus that

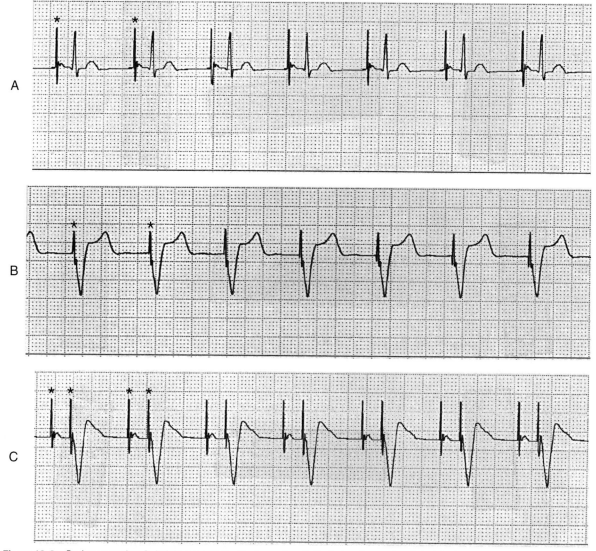

Figure 12-2 Pacing examples. **A**, Atrial pacing. **B**, Ventricular pacing. **C**, Dual-chamber pacing. Asterisks (∗) represent pacemaker impulse.

fails to depolarize the heart, or the incorrect number of pacing stimuli per minute.

Failure to Pace. Failure of the pacemaker to deliver the pacing stimulus results in the disappearance of the pacing artifact, even though the patient's intrinsic rate is less than the set rate on the pacemaker generator (Figure 12-3). This may also be called "failure to fire". It can occur either intermittently or continuously and can be attributed to failure of the pulse generator or its battery or a loose connection between the generator and the pacing leads. Tightening connections, replacing batteries, or replacing the pulse generator itself may restore pacemaker function.

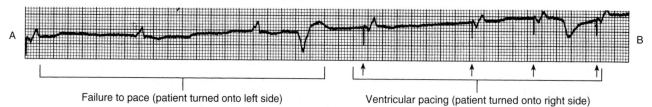

Failure to pace (patient turned onto left side)   Ventricular pacing (patient turned onto right side)

Figure 12-3 Pacemaker malfunction: failure to pace. **A**, Patient with transvenous pacemaker is turned onto left side. Immediately there is a failure to pace (loss of pacer artifacts on ECG). Patient's heart rate is extremely low without pacemaker support. **B**, Nurse turns patient onto right side, the transvenous electrode floats into contact with right ventricular wall, and pacing is resumed. (From Kesten KS, Norton CK: *Pacemakers: patient care, troubleshooting, rhythm analysis*, Baltimore, 1985, Resource Applications.)

Failure to Capture. If the pacing stimulus fires but fails to initiate a myocardial depolarization, a pacing artifact will be present but will not be followed by the expected P wave or QRS complex, depending on the chamber being paced (Figure 12-4). This "loss of capture" most often can be attributed either to displacement of the pacing electrode or to an increase in threshold (electrical stimulus necessary to elicit a myocardial depolarization) as a result of drugs, metabolic disorders, electrolyte imbalance, fibrosis, or myocardial ischemia at the site of electrode placement. In many cases, increasing the output (mA) will elicit capture. For transvenous leads, repositioning the patient to the left side may improve lead contact and restore capture.

Sensing Malfunctions

Undersensing. Undersensing is the inability of the pacemaker to sense spontaneous myocardial depolarizations. This results in competition between paced complexes and the heart's intrinsic rhythm. This malfunction is noted on the ECG as pacing artifacts unrelated to spontaneous complexes (Figure 12-5). Undersensing can be dangerous because it can result in delivery of pacing stimuli into the relative refractory period of the cardiac depolarization cycle. Ventricular pacing stimuli delivered into the downslope of the T wave (R-on-T phenomenon) may precipitate a lethal dysrhythmia. The nurse must act promptly to increase the sensitivity (move the sensitivity dial toward a lower setting). Other possible causes of undersensing include inappropriate asynchronous mode selection, lead displacement or fracture, loose cable connections, and pulse generator failure.

Oversensing. Oversensing is the inappropriate sensing of electrical signals, leading to unnecessary inhibiting of stimulus output. The source of these electrical signals can range from the presence of tall peaked T waves to EMI from equipment in the critical care environment. Oversensing results in unexplained pauses on the ECG tracing as the extraneous signals are sensed and inhibit pacing. Often, simply moving the sensitivity setting slightly toward 20 mV (less sensitive) will stop the pauses.

Medical Management

The physician determines the pacing route based on the patient's clinical situation. Generally, transcutaneous pacing is used in emergent situations until a transvenous lead

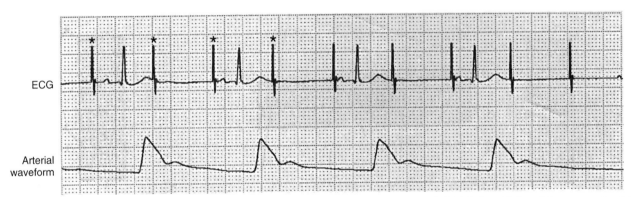

Figure 12-4 Pacemaker malfunction: failure to capture. Atrial pacing and capture occur after pacer spike(s) 1, 3, 5, and 7. Remaining pacer spikes fail to capture the tissue, resulting in loss of the P wave, no conduction to ventricles, and no arterial waveform. Asterisks (∗) represent pacemaker impulse.

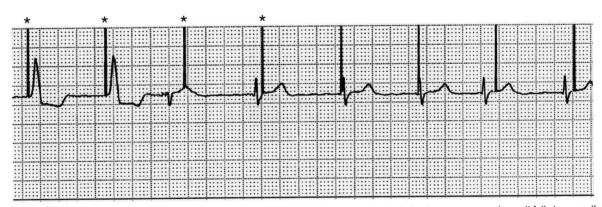

Figure 12-5 Pacemaker malfunction: undersensing. After first two paced beats, a series of intrinsic beats occur; pacemaker unit fails to sense these intrinsic QRS complexes. These spikes do not capture the ventricle because they occur during the refractory period of cardiac cycle. Asterisks (∗) represent pacemaker impulse.

can be secured. If the patient is undergoing heart surgery, epicardial leads may have been electively placed at the end of surgery. Decisions regarding lead placement may limit the pacing modes available to the clinician. For example, to perform dual-chamber pacing, both atrial and ventricular leads must be placed. In an emergency situation, interventions are focused on establishing ventricular pacing, and atrial lead placement may not be feasible. After lead placement the initial settings for output and sensitivity are programmed, the pacing rate and mode are selected, and the patient's response to pacing is evaluated.

Nursing Management

Nursing priorities for the patient connected to a temporary pacemaker focus on (1) preventing pacemaker malfunction, (2) protecting against microshock, (3) monitoring for complications, and (4) providing patient education.

Preventing Pacemaker Malfunction

Continuous ECG monitoring is essential to facilitate prompt recognition of pacemaker malfunction and to initiate appropriate interventions. In addition, proper care of the pacing system will do much to prevent pacing abnormalities.

The temporary pacing lead and bridging cable must be properly secured to the body with tape to prevent the accidental displacement of the pacing electrode, which can result in failure to pace or sense. The external pulse generator can be secured to the patient's waist with a strap or placed in a telemetry bag for the mobile patient. For the patient on a regimen of bed rest, the pulse generator can be suspended with a secure cord from an intravenous (IV) pole mounted overhead on the ceiling.

The nurse inspects for loose connections between the lead(s) and pulse generator on a regular basis. In addition, replacement batteries and pulse generators must always be available on the unit. Although the battery has an anticipated life of 1 month, it probably is sound practice to change the battery if the pacemaker has been operating continually for several days. Newer generators provide a low-battery signal 24 hours before complete loss of battery function to prevent inadvertent interruptions in pacing. The pulse generator must always be labeled with the date that the battery was replaced.

Protecting Patient against Microshock

It is important to be aware of all sources of EMI within the critical care environment that could interfere with the pacemaker's function. Sources of EMI include electrocautery, defibrillation current, radiation therapy, magnetic resonance imaging (MRI) devices, and transcutaneous electrical nerve stimulation (TENS) units. Finding and removing the cause of the EMI always has a high priority to ensure patient safety and accurate pacemaker function in the critical care setting.

Because the pacing electrode provides a direct, low-resistance path to the heart, the nurse takes special care while handling the external components of the pacing system to avoid conducting stray electrical current from other equipment. Even a small amount of stray current transmitted through the pacing lead could precipitate a lethal dysrhythmia. The possibility of "microshock" can be minimized by wearing rubber gloves when handling any exposed sections (terminal pins) of the pacing wires and by proper insulation of terminal pins when not in use. The latter can be accomplished using caps provided by the manufacturer or improvising with a needle cover or section of disposable rubber glove. The wires are to be taped securely to the patient's chest to prevent accidental electrode displacement. Additional safety measures include use of properly grounded electrical equipment that has been verified for safety by the hospital's clinical engineering specialists and permitting the use of only rechargeable or battery operated electrical devices brought in form home.

Monitoring for Complications

Infection at the lead insertion site is a rare but serious complication associated with temporary pacemakers. The insertion site(s) is carefully inspected for purulent drainage, erythema, and edema, and the patient is observed for signs of systemic infection. Site care is performed according to the institution's policy and procedure. Although most infections remain localized, endocarditis can develop if the pacing leads become contaminated. A less common complication associated with transvenous pacing is myocardial perforation, which can result in cardiac tamponade.

Providing Patient Education

Patient teaching for the person with a temporary pacemaker emphasizes prevention of complications. The patient is instructed not to handle any exposed portion of the lead wire and to notify the nurse if the dressing over the insertion site becomes soiled, wet, or dislodged. The patient is advised not to use any electrical devices brought to the hospital from home that might interfere with pacemaker functioning.

IMPLANTABLE CARDIOVERTER-DEFIBRILLATOR

An implantable cardioverter-defibrillator (ICD) is an electronic device used in the treatment of life-threatening tachydysrhythmias. The ICD is capable of identifying and terminating lethal ventricular dysrhythmias. ICD implantation is recommended after cardiac arrest caused by ventricular fibrillation (VF) or ventricular tachycardia (VT), spontaneous sustained VT not responsive to drug therapy, or syncope with hemodynamically compromising VT or VF induced during an electrophysiologic (EP) study.[6] Results from recent clinical trials that compared ICD therapy with class III antidysrhythmic therapy demonstrated improved survival in patients with the ICD.[1] As a result, ICDs are now also indicated for primary prevention of sudden cardiac death in patients with coronary artery disease (CAD), previous myocardial infarction (MI), or left ventricular dysfunction when VT or VF is inducible during an EP study.[7]

ICD System

The ICD system is complex and includes sensing electrodes to recognize lethal dysrhythmias, pacing leads for pace termination, and defibrillation electrodes that can deliver a "shock." Modern defibrillators also are equipped with DDD and VVI backup pacing capabilities. All these electrodes are connected to a generator that is surgically placed in the subcutaneous tissue, usually in the pectoral region (Figure 12-6, A). ICDs combat ventricular dysrythmias with multi-tiered therapy that delivers programmable antitachycardia pacing, low-energy cardioversion, and high-energy defibrillation options (Figure 12-6, D).

Antitachycardia pacing is used as the first line of treatment in most patients with VT. If programmed bursts of pacing do not terminate the VT, the ICD will deliver low-energy synchronous cardioversion to convert the rhythm. If the VT deteriorates into VF, the ICD is programmed to defibrillate at a higher energy level. If the dysrhythmia terminates spontaneously, the device will not discharge. Occasionally the electrical rhythm may deteriorate into asystole or a slow idioventricular rhythm. In such cases a bradycardia backup pacing function (VVI) is activated. Newer ICD generators also contain a dual-chamber pacemaker system, which can provide DDD pacing when required.[8]

Other developments in ICD technology include improved diagnostic and telemetry functions, such as the ability to provide real-time electrograms obtained directly from the ICD electrodes. A new frontier is the development of implantable defibrillators connected to right atrial and coronary sinus defibrillation leads to deliver low-energy shocks to patients in atrial fibrillation to restore sinus rhythm.[9]

ICD Insertion

Transvenous electrode leads are inserted into the subclavian vein and advanced into the right side of the heart, where contact with the endocardium is achieved. The endocardial leads are used for sensing, pacing, and cardioversion-defibrillation. They are connected to the generator by tunneling through the subcutaneous tissue.[10] The ICD generator is connected to the leads and implanted in the pectoral position using a small incision[7] (Figure 12-6, B).

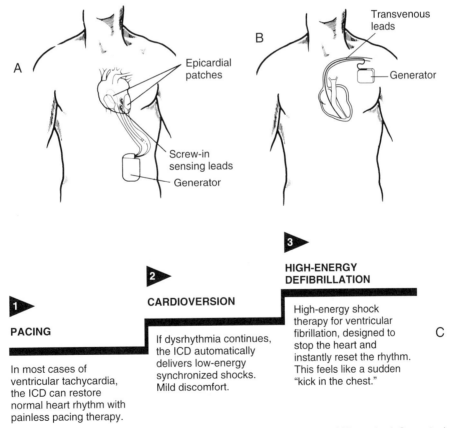

Figure 12-6 **A,** Placement of implantable cardioverter-defibrillator (ICD) and epicardial lead system (older system). Generator is placed in a subcutaneous "pocket" in left upper abdominal quadrant. Epicardial screw-in sensing leads monitor heart rhythm and connect to generator. With this system, leads/patches must be placed during open chest (sternal or thoracotomy) surgery. **B,** In transvenous lead system, open chest surgery is not required. Pacing-cardioversion-defibrillation functions are all contained in a lead (or leads) inserted into right atrium and ventricle. New generators are small enough to place in pectoral region. **C,** Tiered therapy is designed to use increasing levels of intensity to terminate ventricular dysrhythmias. (Courtesy Medtronic Inc, Minneapolis, Minn.)

Medical Management

Medical management of the ICD patient begins before implantation, with a thorough evaluation of the patient's dysrhythmia and underlying cardiac function. Patients identified at risk for sudden cardiac death undergo an EP study to identify the origin of the dysrhythmia and to determine the effect of pharmacologic agents in suppressing or altering the rate of the dysrhythmia. Further assessment of cardiac status is made to determine whether additional interventions (angioplasty/stent, cardiac surgery) are indicated to improve cardiac function and decrease or eliminate ventricular dysrhythmias.

ICD Programming

An electrophysiologist generally performs initial programming of the device at implantation, when defibrillation threshold measurements are obtained. This involves inducing the ventricular dysrhythmia and then evaluating the device's ability to terminate the VT/VF. Once it is determined that the ICD functions adequately, further follow-up is conducted on an outpatient basis to monitor the number of discharges and the battery life of the device.

Nursing Management

Nursing priorities for managing the patient with an ICD focus on (1) maintaining surveillance for complications and (2) providing patient education.

Maintaining Surveillance for Complications

The ICD is not a "cure" for the underlying heart disease. Most patients have a diagnosis of dilated or ischemic cardiomyopathy with consequent heart failure. This leaves them at risk for further episodes of VT or VF. As a result, they require antidysrhythmic medications to decrease the number of "shocks" and to slow the rate of any VT.[11] It is important for the nurse to know why the ICD was implanted, how the device functions, and whether it is activated ("on"). These patients are at high risk for many complications associated with heart failure.

Complications specifically associated with the ICD include infection from the implanted system, broken leads, and the sensing of supraventricular tachydysrhythmias resulting in unneeded discharges.

Providing Patient Education

To facilitate a positive psychologic adjustment to the ICD, education of the patient and family about the device is vital. Preoperative teaching for the ICD patient includes information about how the device works and what to expect during the implantation procedure. After implantation, education is focused on aspects of living with an ICD. Patients need information pertaining to scheduled device follow-up and instructions about what to do if they experience a "shock." Many institutions also successfully use family support groups for this patient population.

THROMBOLYTIC THERAPY

Thrombolytic therapy is an important clinical intervention for the patient experiencing acute MI. This medication allows timely reperfusion of jeopardized myocardium by restoring blood flow to an artery blocked by a new thrombus (clot). The thrombus occurs because of the inflammatory rupture of an atherosclerotic plaque that liberates procoagulant substances into a coronary artery, initiating clot formation. This thrombus is composed of aggregated platelets bound together with fibrin strands. As it occludes the coronary vessel, the thrombus deprives the myocardium of oxygen previously supplied by that artery. The administration of a fibrinolytic agent results in the lysis of the acute thrombus by dissolving the fibrin bonds within the clot, opening the obstructed coronary artery, and restoring blood flow to the affected tissue. Once perfusion is restored, adjunctive measures are taken to prevent further clot formation and reocclusion. Thrombolytic therapy is the general term for this category of drugs, although the more specific term *fibrinolytic therapy* is also used.

Eligibility Criteria
Inclusion Criteria

Certain criteria have been developed, based on research findings, to determine the patient population that would most likely benefit from the administration of thrombolytic (fibrinolytic) therapy. Any patient with recent onset of chest pain (less than 12 hours' duration) and persistent ST elevation (greater than 0.1 mV in two or more contiguous leads) is a candidate for thrombolytic therapy.[11] The patient with a history suggestive of an acute MI who has a bundle branch block that may obscure ST-segment elevation is also a candidate. The earlier the treatment is instituted, the more myocardium can be reperfused. Most clinical protocols strive for administration of thrombolytics within a 6-hour window from the onset of symptoms, although when the fibrinolytics are administered earlier more myocardium is preserved. Time to administrtion is linked to both reducing delays within the emergency department and educating the public about the need to activate the emergency medical services (EMS) earlier by calling 911.[12] Previously, thrombolytic drugs were not administered to patients over age 75 years, but current research has shown that elderly patients can also benefit from fibrinolytic therapy.[13]

Exclusion Criteria

Exclusion criteria are based on the increased risk of bleeding incurred by the use of thrombolytics. Patients who by history are likely to have stable clots are not candidates. A stable clot may exist because of recent surgery, trauma, gastrointestinal bleeding, recent cerebrovascular accident, neoplasm, or known blood dyscrasia.

Thrombolytic Agents

Thrombolytics, more accurately described as *fibrinolytics*, dissolve the fibrin bonds within a clot by converting inactive plasminogen to plasmin, an enzyme responsible for degradation of fibrin (Figure 12-7). The intravenous (IV) or intracoronary (IC) routes can be used for fibrinolytic administration during cardiac catheterization. Many factors influence the choice of IV versus IC administration, including whether the hospital has a cardiac catheterization laboratory and if a cardiologist is available with experience in administering fibrinolytic agents.[14-16]

Intravenous Thrombolytics

Tenecteplase (TNKase) is a genetically engineered fibrinolytic agent that requires only a single bolus injection over 5 seconds to dissolve a clot. It is the agent of choice in the emergency department because of the ease of IV delivery.[17] Tenecteplase has a weight-based dosing regimen and cannot be mixed with dextrose in the IV line. After administration of TNKase, a heparin infusion is required to prevent reoc-

clusion of the coronary artery. Other drugs in this category are also used (Table 12-3).

Intracoronary Thrombolytics

Although thrombolysis will open a coronary artery filled with fresh clot, subsequent cardiac interventions, such as angioplasty or placement of a stent, are often required to prevent reocclusion. Therefore many cardiologists prefer to take the patient undergoing MI directly to the cardiac catheterization laboratory, visualize the blocked coronary artery directly under fluoroscopy, and administer thrombolytics as needed. The most common IC fibrinolytics are t-PA and r-PA (Table 12-3).

The benefit of thrombolytic therapy correlates with the degree of restoration of normal blood flow in the infarct-related artery. Coronary artery patency is defined by angiographic perfusion grades developed by the Thrombolysis In Myocardial Infarction (TIMI) Study Group in 1985 (Box 12-3).[18] Achievement of TIMI grade 3 flow is associated with the best long-term survival.[19] Restoration of

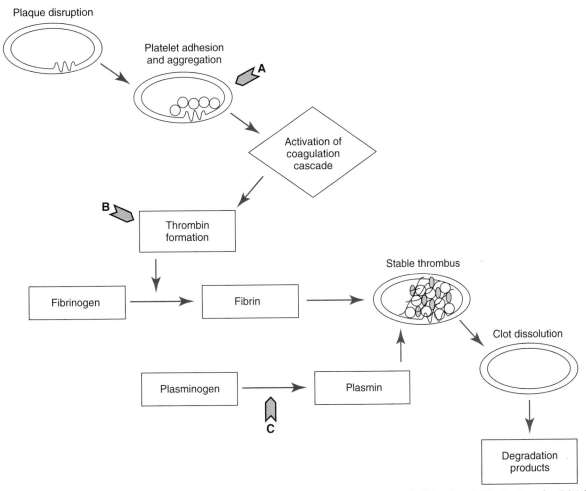

Figure 12-7   Thrombus formation and site of action of medications used in treatment of acute myocardial infarction. *A*, Site of action of antiplatelet agents such as aspirin and glycoprotein IIb/IIIa inhibitors. *B*, Heparin bonds with antithrombin III and thrombin to create an inactive complex. *C*, Thrombolytic agents convert plasminogen to plasmin, an enzyme responsible for degradation of fibrin clots.

Table **12-3** Thrombolytic Agents in Acute Myocardial Infarction

Drug	Dosage (IV)	Actions	Special Considerations
CLOT SPECIFIC			
t-PA (alteplase)	100 mg over 90 min with first 15 mg as bolus	Binds to fibrin at clot; promotes activation of plasminogen to plasmin	Short half-life, so heparin usually given with t-PA as bolus, followed by infusion Aspirin begun with t-PA administration and continued daily
r-PA (reteplase)	10 units as bolus, repeated in 30 min	Binds to fibrin at clot; promotes activation of plasminogen to plasmin	Heparin started with r-PA administration and continued for 24 hr Aspirin begun with r-PA administration and continued daily
TNKase (tenecteplase)	30-50 mg based on body weight, as single bolus	Binds to fibrin at clot; promotes activation of plasminogen to plasmin	Heparin started with TNKase administration Aspirin begun with TNKase administration and continued daily
NON–CLOT SPECIFIC			
SK (streptokinase)	1.5 million units over 60 min	Catalyzes conversion of plasminogen to plasmin, causing lysis of fibrin Has systemic lytic effects	May cause allergic reactions and hypotension Heparin may be administered IV or SQ Aspirin begun with SK administration and continued daily
APSAC (anistreplase)	30 units via slow bolus over 2-5 min	Molecular combination of SK and plasminogen with actions similar to SK. Has systemic lytic effects	May cause allergic reactions and hypotension Long half-life, so heparin usually started 4-6 hours after APSAC Aspirin begun with APSAC administration and continued daily

APSAC, Anisoylated plasminogen-streptokinase activator complex; r-PA, recombinant plasminogen activator; t-PA, tissue plasminogen activator; SK, Streptokinase; IV, intravenous; SQ, subcutaneous; mg, milligrams; min, minutes.

normal blood flow within 90 minutes of treatment results in improved left ventricular function and reduced mortality.[12,14] Because arterial reocclusion remains an ongoing concern, the combination of antiplatelet agents, such as glycoprotein (GP) IIb/IIIa receptor antagonists in conjunction with fibrinolytic agents is being actively studied.[20] The advantage to using both an antiplatelet and a fibrinolytic in combination is that the agents act on different parts of the coagulation cascade (Figure 12-7).

Nursing Management

Nursing priorities for management of the patient receiving thrombolytic therapy focus on (1) identifying candidates for reperfusion therapy, (2) monitoring for signs of bleeding, (3) observing for signs of reperfusion, and (4) providing patient education.

Identifying Candidates for Reperfusion Therapy

Nursing management of the patient undergoing thrombolytic therapy begins with identification of eligible candidates. In many institutions, checklists are used to facilitate rapid triage of patients who are candidates for thrombolytics. The nurse prepares the patient for thrombolytic (fibrinolytic) therapy by starting peripheral IV lines, drawing baseline laboratory values, obtaining vital signs, ensuring that diagnostic 12-lead ECG and chest radiography are performed, and asking about allergies and relevant medical history.

Monitoring for Signs of Bleeding

The most common complication related to thrombolysis is bleeding, not only as a result of the fibrinolytic therapy itself but also because the patients routinely receive postprocedure anticoagulation via a heparin drip to minimize the possibility of rethrombosis. Many patients also receive IV antiplatelet therapy (GP IIb/IIIa antagonists). Therefore the nurse continually monitors for clinical manifestations of bleeding. Mild gingival bleeding and oozing around venipuncture sites are common and are not a cause of concern. The monitoring is for any alteration in level of consciousness that might indicate an intracranial bleed and the infrequent but serious risk of internal bleeding that creates hemodynamic instability or requires a blood transfusion. At this point the physician is notified, all anticoagulant therapies are discontinued, and volume expanders or coagulation factors or both are administered.

In addition to accurate assessment of the patient for evidence of bleeding, nursing priorities include preventive measures to minimize the potential for bleeding. For example, patient handling is limited, injections are avoided, and manual pressure is applied to ensure hemostasis at venous and arterial puncture sites. Any IV lines must be placed before administering thrombolytic therapy, and a heparin lock can be very useful for obtaining laboratory specimens during treatment.

Observing for Evidence of Reperfusion

Reperfusion of a previously occluded coronary artery serves as a catalyst for the following clinical events:

1. Coronary artery can be seen to open when viewed under fluoroscopy in the cardiac catheterization laboratory.
2. Ischemic chest pain ceases abruptly as blood flow is restored.
3. Reperfusion dysrhythmias occur.
4. ST segment normalizes.
5. Creatine kinase (CK) washout is evident on laboratory analysis.

Reperfusion Dysrhythmias. A reliable indicator of reperfusion is the appearance of various "reperfusion" dysrhythmias. Premature ventricular contractions (PVC), bradycardias, heart block, idioventricular rhythms, VT, and rarely VF may occur. These dysrhythmias are probably caused by restored blood flow to ischemic tissue. Generally, reperfusion dysrhythmias are self-limiting, and aggressive drug or defibrillation therapy is not required. Vigilant monitoring of the patient's ECG is essential, however, because a stable condition may deteriorate rapidly, and emergency ACLS treatment must be available.

ST-Segment Normalization. Another noninvasive marker of recanalization is the rapid resolution of the previously elevated ST segments, which indicates restoration of blood flow to previously ischemic myocardial tissue. For this reason a monitoring lead should be chosen that clearly demonstrates ST elevation before initiation of therapy.[21]

Creatine Kinase Washout. Serum CK concentration rises rapidly and markedly after reperfusion of the ischemic myocardium. This phenomenon is termed *washout* because it is thought to result from the rapid release of CK, an enzyme released by damaged myocardial cells, into the circulation after restoration of blood flow to previously unperfused areas of the heart.

Providing Patient Education

Education for the patient receiving thrombolytic therapy includes information regarding the actions of thrombolytic agents, with emphasis on precautions to minimize bleeding. For example, the patient is cautioned against vigorous tooth brushing and asked to refrain from using straight-edge razors while receiving anticoagulant or antiplatelet agents. In addition, information is provided for follow-up cardiac assessment to evaluate the CAD and prevent further acute MI.

CATHETER INTERVENTIONS FOR CORONARY ARTERY DISEASE

Percutaneous catheter interventions (PCIs) are increasingly the first-line treatment for symptomatic CAD.

Indications

The eligibility criteria for PCIs include patients with symptomatic single-vessel and multivessel atherosclerotic disease, provided the plaque can be accessed by a catheter. For post-surgical patients with an occluded saphenous vein or internal mammary artery graft, PCI technology can open the vessel without resorting to more surgery. The major exclusions are heavily calcified vessels and diffuse disease in coronary arteries too small to be reached by a PCI catheter.

PCI Procedure

PCI is performed in the cardiac catheterization laboratory under fluoroscopy. Introducers or "sheaths" are inserted percutaneously into the femoral artery and vein. The venous sheath can be accessed to perform a right-sided heart catheterization with a pulmonary artery catheter or to insert a pacing catheter, or both. The arterial sheath is used to access the coronary arteries for the interventional procedure. The patient is systemically anticoagulated to prevent clots from forming on or in any of the catheters. A special guiding catheter designed to engage the coronary arteries is inserted through the arterial sheath and advanced retrograde through the aorta (against the normal flow of blood). Nitroglycerin or calcium channel blockers may be administered during the procedure to prevent coronary artery spasm and maximize coronary vasodilation. A guidewire is then advanced down the coronary artery and negotiated across the occluding atheroma. A specialized cardiac catheter is subsequently advanced over the guidewire and positioned across the atherosclerotic lesion (atheroma).

Several different types of PCI procedures are available. The most frequently used catheter procedures include percutaneous transluminal coronary angioplasty (PTCA), atherectomy, and stent insertion.

Percutaneous Transluminal Coronary Angioplasty

PTCA, also known as *balloon angioplasty*, involves use of a balloon-tipped catheter that, when advanced through an atherosclerotic lesion, can be inflated intermittently to dilate the stenotic area and improve blood flow through the vessel (Figure 12-8). The high balloon inflation pressure stretches the vessel wall, fractures the plaque, and enlarges the vessel lumen. A successful PTCA reduces the stenosis to less than 50% of the vessel lumen diameter. However, many interventional cardiologists aim to decrease the stenosis to less than 30% of the diameter to ensure an optimal result,[22] because restenosis within the first year after angioplasty occurs in more than one third of patients. This long-term complication is not caused by thrombus but rather by platelet-mediated intimal hyperplasia. Restenosis is diagnosed when patients experience a recurrence of anginal symptoms.[23]

Atherectomy

Atherectomy is the excision and removal of the atherosclerotic plaque by cutting, shaving, or grinding, using specialized coronary catheters. These devices use different mechanisms and may offer special advantages for different types of lesions. The current trend is to use a "lesion-specific" approach in the selection of a device for catheter intervention.[24,25]

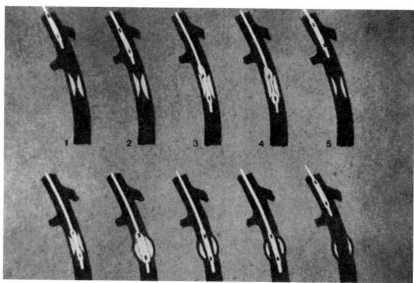

Figure 12-8 Balloon compression of atherosclerotic lesion. (From Kinney M et al: *Comprehensive cardiac care*, ed 8, St Louis, 1996, Mosby.)

Coronary Stents

A *stent* is a self-expanding or balloon-expandable tube (Figure 12-9). The stent is introduced into the coronary artery over a guidewire, usually in a vessel area that has been previously dilated with angioplasty or had plaque removed by atherectomy to debulk the atheroma. The expansion/debulking is performed before stent insertion to obtain a larger vascular lumen diameter. More than 65 stents are now approved for routine use.[19] Stents are employed in 80% of PCIs because they dramatically reduce the number of abrupt vessel closures within the first 24 hours, post-procedure.[26,27] In addition, some cardiologists are using intravascular ultrasound to evaluate the vessel lumen diameter after stent deployment.[28]

Medical Management

Physician responsibilities include management of the patient both in the cardiac catheterization laboratory and after the patient has transferred to the critical care unit. Primary interventions are to prescribe anticoagulant and antiplatelet drugs to prevent coronary artery reocclusion and to be aware of the potential for other complications.

Acute Arterial Reocclusion

Medications are administered to create an anticoagulant state that will prevent clots forming in the newly opened vessel. The mainstay of treatment has always been a heparin drip titrated to therapeutic activated partial thromboplastin time (aPTT) or activated coagulation time (ACT). A patient may also receive one of the GP IIb/IIIa inhibitor drugs as an IV infusion; these agents block the enzyme GP IIb/IIIa, which is essential for platelet aggregation. This category of drugs includes *abciximab* (ReoPro), *eptifibatide* (Integrilin), and *tirofiban* (Aggrastat)[29] (Table 12-4).

After the first 24 hours, oral antiplatelet therapy is routinely prescribed, with agents such as ticlopidine (Ticlid) or clopidogrel (Plavix) given for 2 to 4 weeks and aspirin indefinitely.[30,31] Conventional medications for treatment of CAD, such as nitroglycerin and calcium channel blockers, may also be prescribed.

Hemostatic Devices

Hemostatic devices address the problem of achieving hemostasis at the femoral access site after PCI sheath removal. The two principal methods are a percutaneous suture-mediated device or a collagen plug; at times, both are used together. One *percutaneous suture-mediated device*, the Perclose Prostar XL,[32] is inserted into the femoral artery in the same position as a conventional introducer sheath. The device contains needles and sutures that are used to suture the artery closed after PCI. At the end of the procedure, the artery is sutured closed with the device, which is immediately removed by the cardiologist, and the sutures are knotted firmly.

VasoSeal and Angioseal are vascular hemostatic devices that use a *collagen plug*. The collagen is injected through a preloaded syringe system into the supraarterial space to promote hemostasis at the arterial puncture site.[32,33] Gentle pressure is maintained over the puncture site for

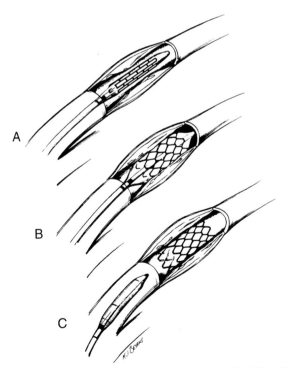

A. Stent is crimped onto balloon catheter for placement.
B. Stent is expanded against vessel wall.
C. Stent is supporting the vessel wall. Balloon catheter is withdrawn from coronary artery.

Figure 12-9   Intracoronary stent. (From Bevans M, McLimore E: *J Cardiovasc Nurs* 7(1): 34, 1992.)

Table 12-4 Glycoprotein (GP) IIb/IIIa Inhibitors in PCI for CAD

Drug	Indications/Dose	Comments
Abciximab (Reopro)	ACS: 0.25 mg/kg IVP, then 10 mcg/min until PCI. PCI: 0.25 mg/kg IVP, then 0.125 mcg/kg/min for 12 hours.	Used concomitantly with heparin and aspirin. May alter platelet function for up to 48 hours after infusion.
Eptifibatide (Integrilin)	ACS: IV bolus of 180 mcg/kg followed by infusion of 2 mcg/kg/min for up to 72 hours; if patient undergoes PCI, dose decreased to 0.5 mcg/kg/min and continued for 24 hours after procedure, for total of 96 hours PCI: 135 mcg/kg IVP, followed by infusion of 0.5 mcg/kg/min for 24 hours.	Concomitant heparin and aspirin may be administered. Platelet function returns to baseline in 6-8 hours. Contraindicated in patients with significant renal dysfunction.
Tirofiban (Aggrastat)	ACS (with or without PCI): 0.4 mcg/kg/min for 30 min, then continued at 0.1 mcg/kg/min for 48-108 hours post-ACS or for patients undergoing PCI	Administered in combination with heparin for patients having PCI. Platelet function returns to baseline in 4-8 hours. Dosage should be reduced in patients with severe renal dysfunction.

PCI, Percutaneous catheter intervention; *CAD*, coronary artery disease; *ACS*, acute coronary syndrome; *IVP*, intravenous push; *mg*, milligrams; *mcg*, micrograms; *min*, minutes; *kg*, kilograms.

approximately 5 minutes, until hemostasis is achieved. Such devices reduce bleeding complications, increase time to ambulation, and shorten time to discharge after PCI.[33]

Complications

Serious complications can result from PCI that necessitate emergency intervention. Persistent coronary artery spasm, coronary artery dissection, and acute coronary thrombosis can result in abrupt vessel closure within the first 24 hours. Other possible complications immediately after PCI include bleeding and hematoma formation at the site of vascular cannulation, compromised blood flow to the involved extremity, allergic reaction to radiopaque contrast dye, dysrhythmias, and *vasovagal response* (hypotension, bradycardia, diaphoresis) during manipulation or removal of introducer sheaths. If complications arise, most patients are returned promptly to the cardiac catheterization laboratory so that the artery may be visualized under fluoroscopy. Currently the majority of dissections and abrupt vessel closures are effectively treated with stent placement. For very-high-risk interventions, surgical backup support, although infrequently required, is recommended.[11]

Nursing Management

Nursing management of the patient after PCI incorporates a variety of nursing diagnoses (Box 12-4). **Nursing priorities are directed toward (1) monitoring for recurrent chest pain, (2) managing the vascular access site, (3) assessing for bleeding, and (4) providing patient education.**

Monitoring for Recurrent Chest Pain

It is essential that the nurse observe the patient for recurrent angina, a clinical indication of myocardial ischemia. Ischemic chest pain may be accompanied by elevated ST

nursing diagnosis priorities Box 12-4

Post-PTCA, Coronary Atherectomy, and Stent
- Ineffective Cardiopulmonary Tissue Perfusion related to acute myocardial ischemia
- Ineffective Altered Peripheral Tissue Perfusion related to decreased peripheral blood flow
- Activity Intolerance related to prolonged immobility or deconditioning
- Acute Pain related to transmission and perception of cutaneous, visceral, muscular, or ischemic impulses
- Anxiety related to threat to biologic, psychologic, and/or social integrity
- Deficient Knowledge: Discharge Regimen related to lack of previous exposure to information

PTCA, Percutaneous transluminal coronary angioplasty.

segments on the bedside monitor or the 12-lead ECG. Angina during interventional cardiology procedures is an expected occurrence at the time of balloon inflation or manipulation within the coronary artery. Intraprocedural angina is caused by the temporary interruption of blood flow through the involved artery, which should subside with balloon deflation and subsequent IV nitroglycerin administration. Angina after a coronary procedure may be a result of transient coronary vasospasm, or it may signal a more serious complication. In either case the nurse must act quickly to assess for manifestations of myocardial ischemia and initiate clinical interventions as indicated. The physician usually prescribes IV nitroglycerin titrated to alleviate chest pain. Continued angina despite maximal vasodilator therapy generally rules out transient coronary vasospasm as the source of ischemic pain, and a new evaluation in the cardiac catheterization laboratory must be considered to rule out an acute occlusion.

Managing Vascular Access Site

The patient is transferred to the coronary care or PCI unit after the procedure for nursing care and observation. The arterial and venous sheaths may be still present or may have been removed at the conclusion of the procedure.

Sheath Management. When a sheath remains in place after PCI, vigilant nursing assessment of the puncture site is essential. Bleeding or hematoma at the sheath insertion site may result from the effects of heparin or GP IIb/IIIa inhibitor infusion.[34] The nurse observes the patient for bleeding or swelling at the puncture site and frequently assesses adequacy of circulation to the involved extremity. The patient is instructed to keep the involved leg straight and not to elevate the head of the bed any more than 30 degrees while the sheath is in place to prevent dislodgement. The nurse also assesses the patient for back pain, which may indicate retroperitoneal bleeding from the internal lumen of the arterial puncture site.

Sheath Removal. After sheath removal, direct pressure is applied to the puncture site for 15 to 30 minutes; a sandbag may be ordered if direct pressure is inadequate for hemostasis. For stents or atherectomy, which require a larger sheath size, a C-clamp or femoral compression device may be used to apply continued pressure for 1 to 2 hours to ensure adequate hemostasis.

Patients usually are allowed to resume ambulation 2 to 8 hours after sheath removal depending on institution and protocol. Excessive bleeding or hematoma formation can become a serious problem because, if excessive, it may result in hypotension or compromised blood flow to the involved extremity.[35]

Palpating Peripheral Pulses. Pulses are usually monitored every 15 minutes for the first 1 to 2 hours immediately after the procedure, then hourly with vital signs until the sheaths are removed. After sheath removal, pulses are again monitored at 15-minute intervals for a brief period.

If the patient does not have sheaths because a hemostatic device was used at the end of the PCI, the nurse is still responsible for assessing the puncture site, peripheral distal pulses, and color/warmth of the extremity. The advantage to these devices is that they greatly shorten the patient's period of enforced bed rest and permit much earlier ambulation.

Assessing for Bleeding

The major complication of both heparin and the GP IIb/IIIa inhibitors is bleeding, and nursing management requires careful assessment of all potential bleeding sites, especially at the femoral sheath site. Extra precautions are used to immobilize the sheath insertion site, examples include these "precautions" are sometimes, but not always used or required a sheet tuck to the affected leg or a leg restraint.[35]

Providing Patient Education

Typically, patients undergoing elective angioplasty, atherectomy, or stent procedures are hospitalized for under 24 hours. All patients require education about their medication regimen and CAD risk-factor modification. Because of the abbreviated hospital stay, the nurse often can do little more than identify the offending risk factors and initiate basic instruction. Patients are referred to a local cardiac rehabilitation center for more extensive teaching and follow-up to facilitate understanding and compliance with risk factor modification.

Another important point of instruction concerns the discharge medications. Patients are discharged home on a regimen of antiplatelet drugs (e.g., clopidogrel, aspirin), as well as a nitrate (e.g., isosorbide) to promote vasodilation.[31] In addition, if the patient has coronary artery vasospasm, calcium channel blockers are prescribed. It is essential that the patient clearly understands the rationale for therapy and potential side effects of each drug. Patients must be provided with written information and an emergency telephone number to call if problems occur.

In all aspects of patient care management after PCI, health care professionals work as a team with the goal of providing the best possible outcome for each patient[19] (Box 12-5).

CARDIAC SURGERY

The nursing management of the patient undergoing cardiac surgery is demanding yet exciting work that requires the talents of an experienced team of critical care nurses. This section discusses the basic cardiac surgical procedures and highlights the key points of postoperative management.

Coronary Artery Bypass Surgery

Results of three major randomized trials support the view that *coronary artery bypass grafting* (CABG) to revascularize ischemic myocardium affords dramatic improvement of symptoms and quality of life.[36] Myocardial revascularization uses a conduit (vein or artery) to bypass an occluded coronary artery. Currently, the two most common conduits are the *saphenous vein graft* (SVG) and the *internal mammary artery* (IMA). The SVG is taken from the leg and anastomosed from the aorta beyond the coronary blockage (Figure 12-10). The IMA remains attached at the origin to the subclavian artery while the other end is anastomosed distal to the blocked coronary artery[36] (Figure 12-11).

Valvular Surgery

Symptomatic aortic valve disease is surgically managed by *aortic valve replacement* (AVR). Mitral valve disease can be

---

Box 12-5 COLLABORATIVE Management

Percutaneous Catheter Intervention (PCI)

1. Identify and treat potential complications related to PCI early (e.g., vasospasm, reocclusion).
2. Prevent complications related to vascular access site (e.g., hematoma, compromised circulation to extremity).
3. Provide effective patient education and follow-up to facilitate necessary lifestyle changes.

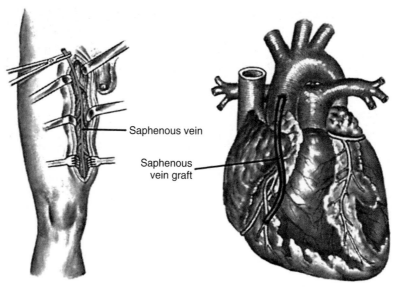

Figure 12-10 Saphenous vein graft.

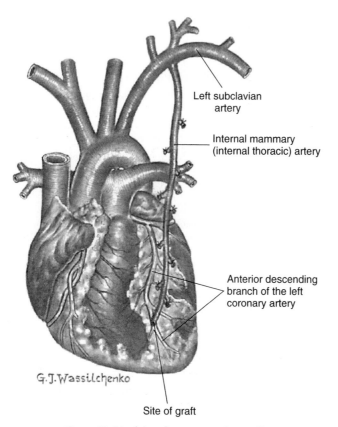

G.J.Wassilchenko

Figure 12-11 Internal mammary artery graft.

repaired by valve commissurotomy, valve repair, or valve replacement. *Commissurotomy* is performed for mitral stenosis and involves incising fused leaflets to increase valve mobility. Valve reconstruction or repair can sometimes be performed for mitral regurgitation.[37] If reconstruction of the valve is not possible, *mitral valve replacement* (MVR) is performed.

Mechanical versus Tissue Valves

The two categories of replacement valves are mechanical valves and biologic or tissue valves. *Mechanical* valves are made from combinations of metal alloys, pyrolite carbon, polyester (Dacron), and Teflon and have rigid occluding devices. The construction renders these valves highly durable, but all patients with mechanical valves require anticoagulation to reduce the incidence of thromboembolism. *Biologic* or *tissue* valves are constructed from animal or human cardiac tissue and have flexible occluding mechanisms (Figure 12-12). Because of their low thrombogenicity, tissue valves offer the patient freedom from therapeutic anticoagulation, but durability is limited to about 10 years.

Cardiopulmonary Bypass

Cardiopulmonary bypass (CPB) is a mechanical means of circulating and oxygenating a patient's blood while diverting most of the circulation from the heart and lungs during cardiac surgical procedures. Numerous clinical sequelae can result from CPB (Table 12-5). Knowledge of these physiologic effects allows the nurse to anticipate problems and intervene effectively in the recovery period.[38,39]

Minimally Invasive Cardiac Surgery

New techniques have recently been developed to address some of the problems associated with traditional cardiac procedures. These procedures are individualized for each patient. Small thoracotomy incisions may be used instead of a median sternotomy. Visualization of the coronary arteries or valves is through a thoracoscope instead of the open chest, and specially designed instruments are used to perform the CABG or valve surgery.[40] These procedures may be performed without CPB ("beating heart surgery") or may employ a modified form of CPB.

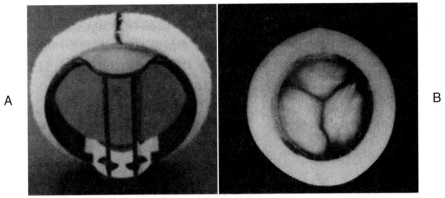

Figure 12-12   Prosthetic valves. **A,** St. Jude Medical mechanical heart valve, a mechanical central flow disk. **B,** Hancock II porcine aortic valve. Flexible Derlin stent and sewing ring are covered in polyester (Dacron) cloth. (**A** courtesy St Jude Medical, 1993, St Paul, Minn; **B** from Eagle K et al: *The practice of cardiology*, ed 2, Boston, 1989, Little, Brown.)

Table 12-5   Physiologic Effects of Cardiopulmonary Bypass (CPB)

Effect	Causes
Intravascular fluid deficit (hypotension)	Third spacing Postoperative diuresis Sudden vasodilation (drugs, rewarming)
Third spacing (weight gain, edema)	Decreased plasma protein concentration Increased capillary permeability
Myocardial depression (decreased cardiac output)	Hypothermia Increased systemic vascular resistance Prolonged CPB pump run Preexisting heart disease Inadequate myocardial protection
Coagulopathy (bleeding)	Systemic heparinization Mechanical trauma to platelets Depressed release of clotting factors from liver as a result of hypothermia
Pulmonary dysfunction (decreased lung mechanics and impaired gas exchange)	Decreased surfactant production Pulmonary microemboli Interstitial fluid accumulation in lungs
Hemolysis (hemoglobinuria)	Red blood cells damaged in pump circuit
Hyperglycemia (rise in serum glucose)	Decreased insulin release Stimulation of glycogenolysis
Hypokalemia (low serum potassium)	Intracellular shifts during CPB
Hypomagnesemia (low serum magnesium)	Postoperative diuresis secondary to hemodilution
Neurologic dysfunction (decreased level of consciousness, motor/sensory deficits)	Inadequate cerebral perfusion Microemboli to brain (air, plaque fragments, fat globules)
Hypertension (transient rise in blood pressure)	Catecholamine release and systemic hypothermia causing vasoconstriction

Postoperative Nursing Management

Nursing management of the patient after cardiac surgery incorporates a variety of nursing diagnoses (Box 12-6). **Nursing priorities are directed toward (1) normalizing cardiac output, (2) managing complications of blood loss, (3) promoting early extubation, (4) assessing for neurologic complications, (5) preventing infection, (6) pre-** serving renal function, and (7) providing patient educa-tion.

Normalizing Cardiac Output

Using standardized protocols, the nurse actively intervenes to normalize CO by optimizing the patient's heart rate (HR), preload, afterload, and contractility.

Heart Rate. In the presence of low CO, the HR can be appropriately regulated by means of temporary pacing or drug therapy. Temporary epicardial pacing usually is instituted when HR of the adult patient who has had cardiac surgery drops to less than 80 beats/min. In the case of tachycardia, IV β-blockers (e.g., esmolol) or calcium channel blockers (e.g., diltiazem) may be used in the acute postoperative period to slow supraventricular rhythms with a ventricular response that exceeds 110 beats/min. Because ventricular ectopy can result from hypokalemia, serum potassium levels are maintained in the high-normal range (4.5 mEq/L). Maintaining serum magnesium in a therapeutic range (2.0 mEq/L) has also been shown to reduce the incidence of dysrhythmias in the postoperative period.[41]

Atrial fibrillation occurs in a third of patients after cardiac surgery, with a peak occurrence in the first 2 to 3 days postoperatively. This rhythm may induce hemodynamic compromise, prolongs hospitalization, and increases the patient's risk of stroke.[42] Prophylactic administration of antidysrhythmic agents such as β-blockers has been shown to decrease the incidence of atrial fibrillation and its clinical sequelae.[43]

Preload. In most patients, reduced preload is the cause of low postoperative CO. If a pulmonary artery catheter has been inserted during surgery, monitoring pulmonary artery occlusion pressure (PAOP) or "wedge pressure" can provide a more accurate guide to left ventricular preload than monitoring central venous pressure (CVP) alone. To enhance preload, volume may be administered in the form of crystalloid, colloid, or packed red blood cells (RBC). The greatest hemodynamic stability in cardiac surgery patients may be achieved when filling pressures (pulmonary artery diastolic pressure [PADP] or PAOP [wedge pressure]) are maintained at higher ranges from 15 to 20 millimeters of mercury (mm Hg) (normal 5 to 12 mm Hg).

Afterload. Partly as a result of the peripheral vasoconstrictive effects of hypothermia, many patients who have had cardiac surgery demonstrate postoperative hypertension and elevated systemic vascular resistance (SVR). Although transient, postoperative hypertension can precipitate or exacerbate bleeding from the mediastinal chest tubes. In addition, the high SVR (afterload) can increase left ventricular workload. Therefore vasodilator therapy with intravenous sodium nitroprusside (Nipride) often is used to reduce afterload, control hypertension, and improve CO.

Contractility. If these adjustments in HR, preload, and afterload fail to produce significant improvement in CO, contractility can be enhanced with positive inotropic drug support or intra-aortic balloon pumping to augment circulation.

Controlling Bleeding Complications

Postoperative bleeding from the mediastinal chest tubes may be caused by inadequate hemostasis, disruption of suture lines, or coagulopathy associated with CPB or hypothermia. If bleeding in excess of 150 milliliters per hour (ml/hr) occurs early in the postoperative period, clotting factors (fresh-frozen plasma, fibrinogen, platelets) and additional protamine (used to reverse the effects of heparin) may be administered, along with prompt blood replacement. In some institutions, autotransfusion devices, which facilitate the collection and reinfusion of mediastinal blood drainage, may be used to replace RBC loss.[44]

Cardiac Tamponade. Cardiac tamponade may occur postoperatively if blood accumulates in the mediastinal space, impairing the heart's ability to pump. Signs of tamponade include elevated and equalized filling pressures (CVP, PADP, PAOP), decreased CO, decreased blood pressure (BP), jugular venous distention (JVD), pulsus paradoxus, muffled heart sounds, sudden cessation of chest tube drainage, and a widened cardiac silhouette on chest radiograph. Interventions for tamponade may include emergency sternotomy in the intensive care unit or a return to the operating room for surgical evacuation of the clot.

Temperature Regulation. Hypothermia can contribute to depressed myocardial contractility and bleeding in the patient who has had cardiac surgery. Patients are rewarmed using heated air or water blankets until the body temperature reaches 98.6° F (37.0° C).[45]

Promoting Early Extubation

Protocols that facilitate early extubation (within the first 4 to 8 hours) are now routine in most cardiovascular critical care units.[46] Early extubation requires a multidisciplinary approach that incorporates anesthesiologists, surgeons, nurses, and respiratory therapists.[47] Potential candidates are identified preoperatively so that the anesthetic regimen can be modified to support early extubation. One approach is to use short-acting anesthetic agents such as propofol (Diprivan) at the end of the surgery and minimize the use of narcotics. Another option is to administer neostigmine and glycopyrrolate at the end of the surgery to reverse the neuromuscular blockade used during the procedure. After extubation, supplemental oxygen is administered, and patients are medicated for incisional pain to facilitate adequate coughing and deep breathing.

Assessing for Neurologic Complications

The transient neurologic dysfunction observed in patients who have undergone cardiac surgery probably is attributable to the CPB pump run (see Table 12-5). The term *postcardiotomy delirium* is used to describe this postoperative syndrome, which initially may be seen as only a mild impairment of orientation but may progress to agitation, hallucinations, and paranoid delusions.[48] Treatment of delirium requires medications such as benzodiazepines or haloperidol (Haldol). Environmental modifications, such as noise reduction, restoring normal day/night lighting patterns, and placing familiar objects at the bedside, may help to calm and reorient the patient. Liberalizing visitation polices to allow family members a prolonged presence at the bedside is also recommended. Nursing management is organized to maximize optimal sleep patterns whenever possible.

Preventing Infection

Postoperative fever is fairly common after CPB. However, persistent temperature elevation to more than 101° F (38.3° C) must be investigated. Sternal wound infections and infective endocarditis are the most devastating infectious complications, but leg wound infection, pneumonia, and urinary tract infection also can occur. Infection rates are greater in diabetic patients. Maintaining a normal blood glucose level between 80 and 110 milligrams per deciliter (mg/dl) in the perioperative and postoperative period through a continuous insulin infusion decreases the incidence of wound infection, sepsis, and multisystem organ dysfunction.[49]

Preserving Renal Function

Hemolysis caused by trauma to RBCs in the extracorporeal circuit results in hemoglobinuria, which can damage renal tubules. Therefore small amounts of furosemide (Lasix) usually are given to promote urine flow if output is less than 30 ml/hour or is pink tinged.

Providing Patient Education

In addition to information on the procedure, post-CABG surgery education includes risk factor management for the prevention of atherosclerosis. Patients who have undergone valve surgery require information on the need for antibiotic prophylaxis before invasive procedures and specifics pertaining to their anticoagulation regimen if they have received a mechanical valve.

In all aspects of patient care management after cardiac surgery, health care professionals work as a team with the goal of providing the best possible outcome for each patient[36,37] (Box 12-7).

MECHANICAL CIRCULATORY ASSIST DEVICES: IABP

Mechanical circulatory assist devices are used in the treatment of heart failure when conventional pharmacologic therapy has proved ineffective. The primary goals of mechanical assist devices are to decrease myocardial workload and maintain adequate perfusion to vital organs. If the cardiac failure is reversible, a short duration of ventricular assistance is used to allow the myocardium time to recover. If the condition is irreversible, a mechanical assist device may be used as a bridge to transplant for qualified candidates.

The *intraaortic balloon pump* (IABP) is a widely used temporary mechanical circulatory assist device for supporting the failing heart and circulation. Therapeutic effects are based on the hemodynamic principles of diastolic augmentation and afterload reduction.

The most common type of intraaortic balloon (IAB) catheter is a sausage-shaped polyurethane balloon of 40-ml volume that is positioned in the descending thoracic aorta just below the takeoff of the left subclavian artery. The balloon catheter is attached to a bedside pumping console and is synchronized to the patient's cardiac cycle and movement of the aortic valve. The IAB inflates during diastole after the aortic valve has closed and deflates just before systole when the aortic valve is open (Figure 12-13). The properly timed IABP will decrease resistance to left ventricular ejection, decrease afterload, facilitate ventricular emptying, reduce myocardial oxygen demand, and increase CO. The overall physiologic effect of IABP therapy is an improvement in the balance between myocardial oxygen supply and demand.[50] Contraindications to balloon pumping include aortic aneurysm, aortic valve insufficiency, and severe peripheral vascular disease.

Box 12-7 COLLABORATIVE Management

Cardiac Surgery

1. Optimize cardiac function by manipulation of heart rate, preload, afterload, and contractility.
2. Identify and treat surgical complications early (e.g., bleeding, cardiac tamponade).
3. Prevent complications (e.g., infection, renal failure, postcardiotomy delirium).

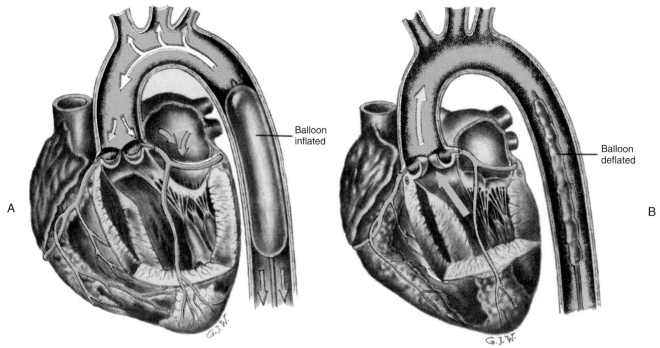

Figure 12-13 Mechanisms of action of intraaortic balloon pump (IABP). **A,** Diastolic balloon inflation augments coronary blood flow. **B,** Systolic balloon deflation decreases afterload.

IABP Insertion

The IAB catheter may be inserted in the cardiac catheterization laboratory, operating room, or critical care unit. The IAB catheter is inserted percutaneously through the femoral artery and advanced to the correct position in the descending thoracic aorta. The physician may insert the IAB catheter through a femoral introducer sheath or directly into the femoral artery to minimize vessel occlusion. After insertion the IAB catheter is attached to the pump console, filled with the prescribed volume of helium, and pumping is initiated.

Nursing Management

Nursing priorities related to managing the patient receiving IABP therapy focus on (1) preventing dysrhythmias, (2) monitoring for complications, and (3) weaning the patient from the IABP safely.

Preventing Dysrhythmias

The ECG and arterial pressure tracing are constantly monitored to verify the timing and effect of balloon counterpulsations (see Figure 12-13). For counterpulsation to occur, the pump must receive a trigger signal to identify the beginning of a new cardiac cycle. The trigger can be the R wave of the ECG, the upstroke of the arterial pressure waveform, or a pacemaker spike.[50] Dysrhythmias can adversely affect the timing of IAB catheter inflation and deflation, and there-

fore rhythm disturbances must be detected and treated promptly. Mean arterial pressure (MAP) is ideally maintained at about 80 mm Hg with adequate pumping.

Monitoring for Complications

Peripheral Circulation. The most common complication of IABP is lower extremity ischemia secondary to occlusion of the femoral artery. The vessel is blocked either by the catheter or by emboli from thrombus formation on the IAB.[51] Consequently, the presence and quality of peripheral pulses distal to the catheter insertion site are assessed frequently, along with color, temperature, and capillary refill of the involved extremity. Doppler localization of peripheral pulses may be required if pulses are difficult to palpate on the cannulated extremity. Signs of diminished perfusion must be reported immediately.[52]

Balloon Integrity. A potential complication of IAB therapy is perforation from a tear in the balloon. Perforation occurs because of the repeated contact of the balloon membrane with calcified plaque in the aorta as the balloon inflates and deflates. The patient is monitored for evidence of IAB leak, such as a gas leak alarm from the pump console and the presence of blood in tubing. If a balloon leak is detected, pumping is stopped and the physician immediately notified so that the IAB can be removed. If not promptly removed, or if pumping is attempted after the perforation, the IAB may become entrapped as the blood hardens within the catheter, creating a mass. In this event the balloon must be surgically removed.[52]

Balloon Catheter Position. The IAB catheter must be maintained in proper position to optimize its effectiveness and minimize complications. If the IAB catheter migrates proximally, it will occlude the left subclavian artery, or if it moves distally, it will occlude the renal arteries and compromise circulation to the kidneys. Therefore careful assessment of the left radial pulse and urine output is essential. Measures to prevent accidental displacement of the IAB catheter include ensuring that the patient observes complete bed rest, with the head of the bed elevated no more than 30 degrees, and avoids any flexion of the involved hip. "Log rolling," in which the patient is moved from side to side every 2 hours, is used to maintain skin integrity and to prevent pulmonary atelectasis.

Bleeding. Thrombocytopenia (low platelet count) may occur as a result of mechanical destruction of the platelets by the IAB pumping action. Platelet counts are closely monitored, and the patient is observed for evidence of bleeding. Because infection of the insertion site is a potential complication, the IAB catheter dressing is changed in accordance with the hospital policy for other invasive lines.

Weaning the IABP

Weaning the patient from the IABP is considered when hemodynamic stability has been achieved with no, or only minimal, pharmacologic support. One weaning procedure involves slowly decreasing the pumping frequency from every beat to every second or third beat, as tolerated. Decreasing IAB catheter volume is another method of weaning.[53] To prevent thrombus formation on the balloon surface; the IABP *must* remain at a minimal pumping ratio (or volume) until its removal. Dependence on the IABP for more than 48 hours suggests severe cardiac dysfunction and is usually associated with a poor prognosis.[53]

CARDIOVASCULAR DRUGS

Multiple medications are used in the treatment of critically ill cardiovascular patients. Intravenous medications are used for the acute rather than the chronic management of cardiovascular conditions. Safety issues must be considered regarding medication administration (see Box 10-7).

Nursing priorities are directed toward (1) **ensuring the medications are administered safely,** (2) **monitoring the patient's response to the medications,** and (3) **maintaining surveillance for adverse drug reactions.**

Antidysrhythmic Drugs

Antidysrhythmic drugs comprise a diverse category of pharmacologic agents used to terminate or prevent an array of abnormal cardiac rhythms. These drugs usually are classified according to their primary effect on the action potential of cardiac cells (Table 12-6). Classification of newer agents becomes more difficult because some of these agents have characteristics of more than one class and others have no characteristics of the current system.

Class I Drugs

Class I antidysrhythmic agents are *sodium channel blockers* that decrease the influx of sodium ions through "fast" channels during ventricular depolarization. Class I drugs exert their antidysrhythmic effect because they prolong the absolute (effective) refractory period, which decreases the

Table **12-6**	Classification of Antidysrhythmic Agents	
Class	**Action**	**Drugs**
I	Blocks sodium channels ("stabilizes" cell membrane)	
IA	Blocks sodium channels and delays repolarization, lengthening duration of action potential	Quinidine Procainamide Disopyramide
IB	Blocks sodium channels and accelerates repolarization, shortening duration of action potential	Lidocaine Mexiletine Tocainide
IC	Blocks sodium channels and slows conduction through His-Purkinje system, prolonging QRS duration	Flecainide Encainide Propafenone
II	Blocks β-adrenergic receptors	Esmolol Metoprolol Propranolol
III	Slows repolarization and prolongs duration of action potential	Amiodarone Ibutilide Sotalol
IV	Blocks calcium channels	Diltiazem Verapamil

risk of premature impulses from ectopic foci. In addition, these agents slow the rate of spontaneous depolarizations of pacemaker cells during the resting phase. Class I drugs are further subdivided into categories A, B, and C.[54]

Class IA antidysrhythmics, including *quinidine, procainamide,* and *disopyramide,* may result in measurable increases in the QRS duration and the QT interval. All class IA agents may depress myocardial contractility, with disopyramide having the most potent negative inotropic effect.[55] *Class IB* antidysrhythmics, including *lidocaine, mexiletine,* and *tocainide,* have only a moderate effect on sodium channels and actually shorten the action potential duration. *Class IC* drugs, including *encainide, flecainide,* and *propafenone,* are the most potent sodium channel blockers. Class IC drugs increase both the PR and the QRS intervals. Because the Cardiac Arrhythmia Suppression Trial (CAST) results indicated that treatment with encainide and flecainide is associated with increased mortality, these agents are infrequently used in clinical practice.[56]

Class II Drugs

Class II drugs are adrenergic blockers; the β-adrenergic blocking agents are known as β-*blockers.* These agents inhibit dysrhythmias mediated by the sympathetic nervous system by competing with endogenous catecholamines for available receptor sites. Knowledge of the effects of adrenergic receptor stimulation allows for anticipation of the therapeutic responses brought about by β-blockade (Table 12-7). The drugs *esmolol, metoprolol,* and *propranolol* are available as IV agents for the treatment of acute dysrhythmias. Of these, esmolol (Brevibloc) offers significant advantages for the critically ill patient because of its short half-life (approximately 9 minutes). Esmolol is used in the treatment of supraventricular tachycardias (SVT, e.g., atrial fibrillation/flutter).

Class III Drugs

Class III antidysrhythmics, including *amiodarone, ibutilide,* and *sotalol,* greatly slow ventricular repolarization, increasing the effective refractory period and the action potential duration. Although their effect on the action potential is similar, class III drugs differ greatly in their mechanism of action and their side effects. IV amiodarone is used as a first-line medication for VT in the ACLS algorithm for management of ventricular dysrhythmias. Amiodarone is also used with increasing frequency for atrial dysrhythmias.[57] Ibutilide (Corvert) is a short-term antidysrhythmic used for the rapid conversion of acute atrial fibrillation/flutter to sinus rhythm. Ibutilide is administered as a 10-minute infusion in a carefully monitored clinical setting. The most serious side effect of ibutilide is the potential for life-threatening dysrhythmias, especially torsades de pointes.[58] Sotalol is approved only for oral use.

Class IV Drugs

Class IV agents are *calcium channel blockers* that inhibit the influx of calcium through slow calcium channels during the plateau phase. This effect occurs primarily in the sinus and AV nodes and the atrial tissue. *Verapamil,* the first drug in this category available as an IV antidysrhythmic, depresses sinus and AV node conduction and is effective in terminating SVT caused by AV nodal reentry. *Diltiazem* (Cardizem) is also available in IV form and is highly effective in treating supraventricular dysrhythmias, with fewer hypotensive side effects.

Unclassified Antidysrhythmics

Adenosine. Adenosine (Adenocard) is an antidysrhythmic agent that remains unclassified under the current system. Adenosine occurs endogenously in the body as a building block of adenosine triphosphate (ATP). Given in IV boluses, adenosine slows conduction through the AV node, causing transient AV block. It is used clinically to convert SVT and to facilitate differential diagnosis of rapid dysrhythmias. Because of its short half-life, adenosine is administered intravenously as a rapid bolus, followed by a saline flush. The bolus is delivered as centrally as possible so that the drug reaches the heart before it is metabolized.[3] Side effects are transient because adenosine is rapidly taken up by the cells and is cleared from the body in 10 seconds.

Magnesium. Magnesium is also unclassified under the present system. Although its action as an antidysrhythmic agent is not entirely understood, clinical studies suggest that magnesium may reduce the incidence of both ventricular and supraventricular dysrhythmias in selected patient populations. Magnesium is the treatment of choice for torsades de

Table **12-7** Effects of Adrenergic Receptors

Receptor	Location	Response to Stimulation
α	Vessels of skin, muscles, kidneys, and intestines	Vasoconstriction of peripheral arterioles
β₁	Cardiac tissue	Increased heart rate
		Increased conduction
		Increased contractility
β₂	Vascular and bronchial smooth muscle	Vasodilation of peripheral arterioles
		Bronchodilation

pointes. For emergency treatment of torsades de pointes, 1 to 2 grams of magnesium may be administered rapidly over 1 to 2 minutes. For patients with confirmed hypomagnesemia by laboratory test, magnesium replacement is generally 1 gram IV (diluted) over 30 minutes.

Side Effects

Antidysrhythmic drugs carry the risk of serious side effects, some of which may be life threatening. The most severe complication is a *prodysrhythmic* effect, which may result in worsening of the underlying rhythm disturbance, occurrence of a new dysrhythmia, or development of a bradydysrhythmia. Torsades de pointes is a life-threatening prodysrhythmia caused by class IA agents.[54] The development of a prodysrhythmia is unpredictable, so the nurse plays an important role in evaluating ECG changes, monitoring drug levels, and assessing patient symptoms. Antidysrhythmic agents may also alter the amount of energy required for defibrillation and pacing. For example, increases in an antidysrhythmic dose may increase the amount of pacemaker output (mA) required to depolarize the myocardium.

Vasoactive Drugs
Inotropic Drugs

Critically ill patients with compromised cardiac function often require the use of medications to enhance myocardial contractility (*positive inotropes*). Clinically available inotropes include cardiac glycosides, sympathomimetics, and phosphodiesterase inhibitors. These agents increase myocardial contractility, resulting in improved CO, more complete emptying of the ventricles, and decreased filling pressures.

Cardiac Glycosides. Cardiac glycosides include *digitalis* and its derivatives (*digoxin*). Although these drugs have been used for centuries, their slow onset of action and risk of toxicity make them more appropriate for the management of chronic heart failure. Because digoxin causes a slowing of the sinus rate and a decrease in AV conduction, it may be administered intravenously in the acute care setting to control supraventricular dysrhythmias.

Sympathomimetics. Sympathomimetic agents stimulate adrenergic receptors, thereby simulating the effects of sympathetic nerve stimulation (Table 12-8). Included in this category are naturally occurring catecholamines (epinephrine, dopamine, norepinephrine), as well as synthetic catecholamines (dobutamine, isoproterenol). The cardiovascular effects of these drugs, which vary according to their selectivity for specific receptor sites, are often dose dependent as well.

Dopamine. Dopamine (Intropin) is one of the most widely used drugs in the critical care setting. It is a chemical precursor of norepinephrine that, in addition to both α-and β-receptor stimulation, can activate *dopaminergic* receptors in the renal and mesenteric blood vessels. The actions of dopamine are entirely dose related.[3]

Low-dose dopamine at less than 3 micrograms per kilogram of body weight per minute (mcg/kg/min) is used to stimulate renal perfusion and increase renal output.

Inotropic-dose dopamine (3 to 10 mcg/kg/min) is designed to enhance myocardial contraction and improve CO via cardiac β_1-adrenergic receptor stimulation.

High-dose or *vasopressor-dose* dopamine (greater than 10 mcg/kg/min) stimulates peripheral α-receptors in the

---

Table 12-8   Physiologic Effects of Sympathomimetic Agents

Drug	Dose	Receptor Activated*				Cardiovascular Effects		
		α	β_1	β_2	Dopa	CO	HR	SVR
Dobutamine	<5†	0	↑↑↑	↑	0	↑↑	↑	0/↓
	5-20	0	↑↑↑	↑↑	0	↑↑↑	↑↑	↓
	>20	0	↑↑↑	↑↑	0	↑↑↑	↑↑↑	↓↓
Dopamine	<3†	0	↑	↑	↑↑↑	0/↑	0/↑	0
	3-10	↑	↑↑↑	↑	↑↑↑	↑↑↑	↑	↑
	11-20	↑↑↑	↑↑↑	↑	↑↑	↑↑	↑↑	↑↑↑
	>20	↑↑↑↑	↑↑	↑	↑	↑	↑	↑↑↑↑
Epinephrine	<2‡	0	↑	↑↑	0	0/↑	0/↑	↓
	2-8	↑↑	↑↑↑	↑↑	0	↑↑↑	↑	↑
	9-20	↑↑↑	↑↑	↑↑	0	↑↑	↑↑	↑↑
Isoproterenol	1-7‡	0	↑↑↑	↑↑↑	0	↑↑↑	↑↑↑	↓↓↓
Norepinephrine	<2‡	↑↑↑	↑↑	0	0	↑	0/↓	↑↑↑
	2-16	↑↑↑↑	↑↑	0	0	↓	↓	↑↑↑↑
Phenylephrine	10-100‡	↑↑↑↑	0	0	0	0/↓	↓	↑↑↑

*See Table 12-7 for actions of receptors.
†Micrograms per kilogram body weight per minute (mcg/kg/min).
‡Micrograms per minute (mcg/min).
Dopa, Dopaminergic; *CO*, cardiac output; *HR*, heart rate; *SVR*, systemic vascular resistance; 0, no effect; ↑, increased; ↓, decreased (number of arrows indicates degree of effect, e.g., ↑ = mild effect and ↑↑↑↑ = strong effect).

vasculature to vasoconstrict the systemic arterial bed and raise BP in shock states. As with other vasopressors, dopamine must never be administered at high dose to hypovolemic patients; volume deficits must always be corrected first (Table 12-8).

Dobutamine. Dobutamine (Dobutrex), a synthetic catecholamine with predominantly β_1-adrenergic effects, increases myocardial contractility. It also produces some β_2-adrenergic stimulation, resulting in a mild peripheral vasodilation. Dobutamine is useful in the treatment of heart failure, especially in patients who benefit from the combination of inotropic stimulation and vasodilator therapy. The dosage range is wide, with a range of 2.5 to 20 mcg/kg/min, titrated on the basis of hemodynamic parameters.

Epinephrine. Epinephrine (Adrenalin) is produced by the adrenal gland as part of the body's response to stress. This agent has the ability to stimulate both α- and β-receptors, depending on the dose administered (see Table 12-8). In the critical care unit epinephrine is used to stimulate the cardiac β_1-adrenergic receptors to increase CO, and simultaneously activate peripheral α-receptors to vasoconstrict the arterial blood vessels. As the dosage is increased SVR and BP will rise. The impact on CO depends on the heart's ability to pump against the increased afterload. Epinephrine accelerates the sinus rate and may precipitate ventricular dysrhythmias in the ischemic heart.

Norepinephrine. Norepinephrine (Levophed) is able to stimulate α- and β_1-receptors. At low infusion rates, β_1-receptors are activated to produce increased contractility. At higher doses the α-receptors cause marked vasoconstriction. Clinically, norepinephrine is used most often as a vasopressor to elevate BP in shock states.

Vasopressin. Vasopressin, also known as *antidiuretic hormone* (ADH), has been used to treat a variety of clinical conditions. Recently this agent has become popular in the critical care setting for its vasoconstrictive effects. At higher doses, vasopressin directly stimulates contraction of vascular smooth muscle, resulting in vasoconstriction of capillaries and small arterioles. A one-time dose of 40 units intravenously is now recommended in the ACLS guidelines as first-line drug therapy for VF or pulseless VT that is refractory to initial defibrillation.[3] Continuous infusions of 0.01 units per minute (units/min) up to 0.1 units/min have been used in the treatment of vasodilatory shock in patients with refractory hypotension following CPB.[59] Patients must be monitored for side effects such as heart failure (due to the antidiuretic effects) and myocardial ischemia. Vasopressin should be infused through a central line to avoid the risk of peripheral extravasation and resultant tissue necrosis.[59]

Phosphodiesterase Inhibitors. Phosphodiesterase inhibitors represent a group of inotropic agents that are also potent vasodilators. Drugs in this classification inhibit the enzyme *phosphodiesterase*, resulting in increased levels of cyclic adenosine monophosphate (cAMP) and intracellular calcium. *Milrinone* (Primacor) is used to increase CO as a result of increased contractility (inotropic effect) and decreased

afterload (vasodilative effect). Filling pressures tend to decrease, whereas HR and BP remain fairly constant. Milrinone causes thrombocytopenia in some patients, so platelet levels must be monitored. It also can induce ventricular dysrhythmias (VT, premature ventricular complexes) in a significant number of patients.[60]

Vasodilator Drugs

Vasodilators are pharmacologic agents that improve cardiac performance by various degrees of arterial or venous dilation, or both. The goal of continuous IV vasodilator therapy may be a reduction of preload or afterload, or both. Afterload reduction is accomplished by vasodilation of arterial vessels. This decreases resistance to left ventricular ejection and may improve CO without increasing myocardial oxygen demands. Reduction of preload is accomplished by dilating venous vessels to increase capacitance (Table 12-9).

Nitric Oxide Smooth Muscle Relaxants

Direct-acting vasodilators include sodium nitroprusside and nitroglycerin via continuous infusion. These drugs stimulate nitric oxide within the vascular smooth muscle, resulting in decreased peripheral vascular resistance. Hypotension may occur as a result of peripheral vasodilation, and headaches may be caused by cerebral vasodilation. Compensatory mechanisms in response to the drop in BP may include reflex tachycardia and activation of the renin-angiotensin-aldosterone system, with resultant sodium and water retention.

Sodium Nitroprusside. Sodium nitroprusside (Nipride) is a potent, rapidly acting venous and arterial vasodilator, particularly suitable for rapid reduction of BP in hypertensive emergencies and perioperatively. Sodium nitoprusside also is effective for afterload reduction in heart failure and after cardiac surgery. Dosage is titrated to maintain a prescribed target BP and SVR. The patient should have a functioning arterial line inserted because of the risk of hypotension secondary to the extremely short half-life (seconds). Sodium nitroprusside is administered by continuous IV infusion, usually 0.25 to 6.0 mcg/kg/min. Prolonged administration can result in thiocyanate toxicity, manifested by nausea, confusion, and tinnitus.[61] This serious side effect limits long-term use at upper dose ranges.

Nitroglycerin. Intravenous nitroglycerin (Tridil) causes both arterial and venous vasodilation, but its venous effect is more pronounced. Nitroglycerin is used in the critical care setting for the treatment of acute heart failure because it reduces cardiac filling pressures, relieves pulmonary congestion, and decreases cardiac workload and oxygen consumption. In addition, nitroglycerin dilates the coronary arteries and is a useful adjunct in the treatment of unstable angina and acute MI. The initial dosage is 10 mcg/min, and the infusion is titrated upward to achieve the desired clinical effect: a reduction or elimination of chest pain, decreased PAOP, or decreased BP. Nitroglycerin also is administered prophylactically to prevent coronary vasospasm after coronary angioplasty, atherectomy, stent insertion, or throm-

| Table **12-9** | Characteristics of Common Vasodilators |

Class/Drug	Dosage	Preload Effects	Afterload Effects	Side Effects
DIRECT SMOOTH MUSCLE RELAXANTS				
Sodium nitroprusside (Nipride)	0.25-6.0 mcg/kg/min IV infusion	Moderate	Strong	Hypotension, thiocyanate toxicity, reflex tachycardia
Nitroglycerin (Tridil)	5.0-300 mcg/min IV infusion	Strong	Mild	Headache, reflex tachycardia, hypotension
CALCIUM CHANNEL BLOCKERS				
Nicardipine (Cardene)	5.0 mg/hour IV, titrated to 15 mg/hr	None	Strong	Hypotension, headache, reflex tachycardia
Nifedipine (Procardia)	10-20/TID mg PO; also available as extended release 30, 60, or 90 mg once per day P.	None	Strong	Hypotension, headache, reflex tachycardia
ANGIOTENSIN-CONVERTING ENZYME (ACE) INHIBITORS				
Captopril (Capoten)	6.25-100 mg PO every 8-12 hrs	Moderate	Moderate	Hypotension, chronic cough, neutropenia
Enalapril (Vasotec)	0.625 mg IV over 5 min, then every 6 hrs	Moderate	Moderate	Hypotension, elevation of liver enzymes
α-ADRENERGIC BLOCKERS				
Labetalol (Normodyne)	20-80 mg IV bolus every 10 min, then 1.0-2.0 mg/min infusion	Moderate	Moderate	Orthostatic hypotension, bronchospasm, atrioventricular (AV) block
Phentolamine (Regitine)	1.0-2.0 mg/min infusion	Moderate	Moderate	Hypotension, tachycardia

IV, Intravenous(ly); *PO*, by mouth; *mcg*, micrograms, *mg*, milligrams; *TID*, 3 times per day.

bolytic therapy. The most common side effects include hypotension, flushing, and headache.

Calcium Channel Blockers

Calcium channel blockers are a chemically diverse group of drugs with different pharmacologic effects.

Nifedipine and Nicardipine. The "pine"-suffix calcium channel blockers are used primarily as arterial vasodilators. Nifedipine (Procardia) and nicardipine (Cardene) are dihydropyridines and are used in the critical care setting to treat hypertension. These drugs reduce the influx of calcium in the arterial resistance vessels; both coronary and peripheral arteries are affected. Side effects of nifedipine and nicardipine are related to vasodilation and include hypotension, reflex tachycardia, flushing, headache, and ankle edema.

Verapamil and Diltiazem. Verapamil (Calan, Isoptin) and diltiazem (Cardizem) are part of another group of calcium channel blockers with different functions. These drugs dilate coronary arteries but have less effect on the peripheral vasculature. Verapamil and diltiazem are used in the treatment of angina, especially with a vasospastic component, and as antidysrhythmics in the treatment of SVT.

ACE Inhibitors

Angiotensin-converting enzyme (ACE) inhibitors produce vasodilation by blocking the conversion of angiotensin I to

angiotensin II. Because angiotensin is a potent vasoconstrictor, limiting its production decreases peripheral vascular resistance. In contrast to the direct vasodilators and nifedipine, ACE inhibitors do not cause reflex tachycardia or induce sodium and water retention. However, these drugs may cause a profound fall in BP, especially in hypovolemic patients. BP must be monitored carefully, especially during initiation of therapy.

Captopril and Enalapril. The drugs Captopril (Capoten) and enalapril (Vasotec) are used for symptoms of heart failure to decrease SVR (afterload) and PAOP (preload). Captopril is available in an oral form only but has a relatively rapid onset of action (approximately 1 hour). Enalapril is available in an IV form and may be used to decrease afterload in more emergent situations.

B-Type Natriuretic Peptide

Nesiritide (Natrecor) is a new vasodilator used in the treatment of acute heart failure. This agent is a recombinant form of human brain natriuretic peptide (BNP), the hormone released by cardiac cells in response to ventricular distention. The primary effects of nesiritide include decreasing filling pressures (PAOP, CVP), reducing vascular resistance (SVR, PVR), and increasing urine output. Compared with traditional vasodilator therapy for acute heart failure, nesiritide reportedly is as effective as nitroglycerin with fewer side effects (e.g., headache).[62] The recommended dose is an IV bolus of 2.0 mcg/kg, followed by continuous infusion of 0.01 mcg/kg/min. The primary side effect is hypotension. If this occurs, nesiritide may need to be discontinued for a time and then restarted at a lower dose after the patient has been stabilized.[62]

α-Adrenergic Blockers

Peripheral adrenergic blockers inhibit α-receptors in the peripheral vasculature, resulting in vasodilation. Orthostatic hypotension is a common side effect and may result in syncope. Long-term therapy also may be complicated by fluid and water retention.

Labetalol. Labetalol (Normodyne) combines both α- and β-blockade. It is used in the treatment of acute stroke, hypertensive emergencies and acute aortic dissection.[63]

Phentolamine. Phentolamine (Regitine) is a peripheral α-adrenergic blocker that causes decreased afterload through arterial vasodilation. Phentolamine is given as a continuous infusion at 1 to 2 mg/min and is titrated to achieve the required reduction in BP and SVR. Phentolamine is the drug of choice in the treatment of pheochromocytoma.[61] It is also used to treat the extravasation of dopamine. If this occurs, 5 to 10 mg is diluted in 10 ml of normal saline and administered intradermally into the infiltrated area.

Dopamine Receptor Agonists. *Fenoldopam* (Corlopam) is the first of a new class of vasodilators called selective, specific dopamine DA_1-receptor agonists.[64] Fenoldopam is a potent vasodilator that affects both peripheral, renal, and mesenteric arteries. It is administered via continuous IV infusion beginning at 0.1 mcg/kg/min and titrated up to the desired BP effect with a maximum recommended dosage of 0.5 mcg/kg/min.[64] It can be administered as an alternative to sodium nitroprusside or other antihypertensives in the treatment of hypertensive emergencies. Fenoldopam can also be used safely for patients with renal dysfunction or those at high risk for renal insufficiency after cardiac catheterization, cardiac surgery or PCI.[64] At lower doses (0.05 mcg/kg/min) fenoldopam may renal pefusion effects similar to low-renal-dose dopamine.

REFERENCES

1. Dhala A et al: Ventricular arrhythmias, electrophysiologic studies, and devices, *Crit Care Nurs Clin North Am* 11(3):375, 1999.
2. Baas LS, Beery TA, Hickey CS: Care and safety of pacemaker electrodes in intensive care and telemetry nursing units, *Am J Crit Care* 6(4):302, 1997.
3. American Heart Association: ECG guidelines. Part 6. Advanced cardiovascular life support, *Circulation* 102:I-136, 2000.
4. Carroll KC et al: Risks associated with removal of ventricular epicardial pacing wires after cardiac surgery, *Am J Crit Care* 7(6):444, 1998.
5. Bernstein AD et al: The NASPE/BPEG generic pacemaker code for antibradycardia and adaptive rate pacing and antitachyarrhythmia devices, *Pacing Clin Electrophysiol* 10:794, 1987.
6. Gregoratos G et al: ACC/AHA guidelines for implantation of cardiac pacemakers and antiarrhythmia devices, *Circulation* 97(13):1325, 1998.
7. Porterfield LM, Morton PG, Butze E: The evolution of internal defibrillators, *Crit Care Nurs Clin North Am* 11(3):303, 1999.
8. Hans-Joachim T et al: Single chamber vs dual chamber implantable defibrillators: indications and clinical results, *Am J Cardiol* 83(5B):8D, 1999.
9. Hein JJ et al: Atrioverter: an implantable device for the treatment of atrial fibrillation, *Circulation* 98:1651, 1998.
10. Knight L et al: Caring for patients with third-generation implantable cardioverter defibrillators: from decision to implant to patients' return home, *Crit Care Nurse* 17(5):46, 1997.
11. Ryan TJ et al: 1999 update: ACC/AHA guidelines for the management of patients with acute myocardial infarction, *J Am Coll Cardiol* 34(3):890, 1999.
12. White HD, Vande Werf F: Thrombolysis for acute myocardial infarction, *Circulation* 97:1632, 1998.
13. Casey K, Bedker DL, Roussel-McElmeel PL: Myocardial infarction: review of clinical trials and treatment strategies, *Crit Care Nurse* 18(2):39, 1998.
14. Gylys K, Gold M: Acute coronary syndromes: new developments in pharmacological treatment stategies, *Crit Care Nurse Suppl* 20(2):3, 2000.
15. Kline-Rogers E, Martin JS, Smith DD: New era of reperfusion in acute myocardial infarction, *Crit Care Nurse* 19(1):21, 1999.
16. A comparison of reteplase with alteplase for acute myocardial infarction. GUSTO III trial, *N Engl J Med* 337(16):1118, 1997.
17. Single-bolus tenecteplase compared with front-loaded alteplase in acute myocardial infarction: the ASSENT-2 double-blind randomised trial, *Lancet* 354(9180):716, 1999.
18. TIMI Study Group: The Thrombolysis In Myocardial Infarction (TIMI) Trial: Phase I findings, *N Engl J Med* 312:932, 1985.
19. Smith SC Jr: ACC/AHA guidelines for percutaneous coronary intervention (revision of the 1993 PTCA guidelines). American College of Cardiology/American Heart Association Task Force on Practice Guidelines, *Circulation* 103(24):3019, 2001.
20. Dracup KA, Cannon CP: Combination treatment strategies for the management of acute myocardial infarction: new directions with current therapies, *Crit Care Nurse Suppl*, April 1999, p 3.
21. Drew BJ, Krucoff MW: Multilead ST-segment monitoring in patients with acute coronary syndromes: a consensus statement for healthcare professionals, *Am J Crit Care* 8(6):372, 1999.
22. Senerchia CC: Highlights from the past decade of interventional device research, *Crit Care Nurs Clin North Am* 11(3):311, 1999.
23. Kuntz RE, Baim DS: Prevention of coronary restenosis: the evolving evidence base for radiation therapy, *Circulation* 101(18):2130, 2000.
24. Williams DO, Fahrenbach MC: Directional coronary atherectomy: but wait, there's more, *Circulation* 97:309, 1998.
25. Thorbs N et al: Coronary rotational atherectomy: a nursing perspective, *Crit Care Nurse* 20(2):77, 2000.
26. Jacobs AK: Coronary stents—have they fulfilled their promise? *N Engl J Med* 341(26):2005, 1999.
27. Carozza JP: In-stent restenosis: should an old device be used to treat a new problem? *J Am Coll Cardiol* 35(6):1577, 2000.
28. Lau KY et al: Frequency of ischemia during intracoronary ultrasound in women with and without coronary artery disease, *Crit Care Nurse* 19(5):44, 1999.
29. Dangas G, Colombo A: Platelet glycoprotein IIb/IIIa antagonists in percutaneous coronary revascularization, *Am Heart J* 138(1):S16, 1999.
30. Holmes DR et al: Coronary artery stents. ACC Expert Consensus Document, *J Am Coll Cardiol* 32(5):1471, 1998.
31. Quinn MJ, Fitzgerald DJ: Ticlodipine and clopidogrel, *Circulation* 100:1667, 1999.

32. Hamel WJ: Suppose a Perclose, *Prog Cardiovasc Nurs* 14(4): 136-142, 1999.

33. Schickel SI et al: Achieving femoral artery hemostasis after cardiac catheterization: a comparison of methods, *Am J Crit Care* 8(6):406, 1999.

34. Lincoff AM et al: Complementary clinical benefits of coronary artery stenting and blockade of platelet glycoprotein IIb/IIIa receptors, *N Engl J Med* 341(5):319, 1999.

35. Juran NB et al: Nursing interventions to decrease bleeding at the femoral access site after percutaneous coronary intervention, *Am J Crit Care* 8(5):303, 1999.

36. Eagle KA et al: ACC/AHA guidelines for coronary artery bypass graft surgery, *Circulation* 100(13):1464, 1999.

37. Bonow RO et al: ACC/AHA guidelines for the management of patients with valvular heart disease, *Circulation* 98(18):1949, 1998.

38. Seifert PC: Advances in myocardial protection, *J Cardiovasc Nurs* 12(3):29, 1998.

39. Jacquet LM et al: Randomized trial of intermittent antegrade warm versus cold crystalloid cardioplegia, *Ann Thorac Surg* 67(2):471, 1999.

40. Fitzgerald CA: Minimally invasive cardiac valve surgery, *Crit Care Nurs Q* 21(1):41, 1998.

41. Berger AK et al: Does adjunctive magnesium prevent atrial fibrillation following coronary artery bypass surgery? *Circulation* 94(suppl I):170, 1996.

42. Kern LS: Management of postoperative atrial fibrillation, *J Cardiovasc Nurs* 12(3):57, 1998.

43. Balser JR: Perioperative management of dysrhythmias, *Prob Anesth* 10:197, 1998.

44. Ley SJ: Intraoperative and postoperative blood salvage, *AACN Clin Issues Crit Care Nurs* 7(2):238, 1996.

45. Sanford MM: Rewarming cardiac surgical patients: warm water vs warm air, *Am J Crit Care* 6(1):39, 1997.

46. Goodwin MJ et al: Early extubation and early activity after open heart surgery, *Crit Care Nurse* 19(5):18, 1999.

47. Sakallaris BR et al: Same day transfer of patients to the cardiac telemetry unit after surgery: the Rapid After Bypass Back Into Telemetry (RABBIT) Program, *Crit Care Nurse* 20(2):50, 2000.

48. Segatore M, Dutkiewicz M, Adams D: The delirious cardiac surgical patient: theoretical aspects and principles of management, *J Cardiovasc Nurs* 12(4):32, 1998.

49. van den Berghe G et al: Intensive insulin therapy in critically ill patients, *N Engl J Med* 345(19):1359, 2001.

50. Cadwell CA, Quaal SJ: Intra-aortic balloon counterpulsation timing, *Am J Crit Care* 5(4):254, 1996.

51. Cook L et al: Intra-aortic balloon pump complications: a five-year retrospective study of 283 patients, *Heart Lung* 28(3):195, 1999.

52. Stavarski DH: Complications of intra-aortic balloon pumping: preventable or not preventable, *Crit Care Nurs Clin North Am* 8(4):409, 1996.

53. Krau SD: Successfully weaning the intra-aortic balloon pump patient: an algorithm, *DCCN* 18(3):2, 1999.

54. Kayser SR: Antiarrhythmic drug therapy. Part I. General principles of drug selection, *Prog Cardiovasc Nurs* 11(2):33, 1996.

55. Wooten JM, Earnest J, Reyes J: Review of common adverse effects of selected antiarrhythmic drugs, *Crit Care Nurs Q* 22(4):23, 2000.

56. Kayser SR: Antiarrhythmic drug therapy. Part II. Specific drugs, *Prog Cardiovasc Nurs* 11(3):33, 1996.

57. Futterman LG, Lemberg L: Amiodarone: a late comer, *Am J Crit Care* 6(3):233, 1997.

58. Ellenbogen KA et al: Efficacy of intravenous ibutilide for rapid termination of atrial fibrillation and flutter: a dose response study, *J Am Coll Cardiol* 28:130, 1996.

59. Albright TN, Zimmerman MA, Selzman CH: Vasopressin in the cardiac surgery intensive care unit, *Am J Crit Care* 11(4):326, 2002.

60. Albert NM: Advanced systolic heart failure: emerging pathophysiology and current management, *Prog Cardiovasc Nurs* 13(3):14, 1998.

61. Bisognano JD, Weder AB: Effective treatment of severe hypertension, *Prog Cardiovasc Nurs* 14(4):150, 1999.

62. Intravenous nesiritide vs nitroglycerin for treatment of decompensated congestive heart failure: a randomized controlled trial. VMAC study, *JAMA* 287:1531, 2002.

63. Harrington, C: Managing hypertension in patients with stroke: Are you prepared for Labatelol infusion? *Crit Care Nurse* 23(3):30, 2003.

64. Thompson EJ, King SL: Acetylcysteine and Fenoldopam: promising new approaches for preventing effects of contrast nephrotoxicity, *Crit Care Nurse* 23(3):39, 2003.

UNIT FOUR

PULMONARY ALTERATIONS

KATHLEEN M. STACY
JEANNE M. MAIDEN

13

Pulmonary Assessment and Diagnostic Procedures

Objectives

- Identify the components of a pulmonary history.
- Describe inspection, palpation, percussion, and auscultation of the patient with pulmonary alterations or dysfunction.
- Outline the steps in analyzing an arterial blood gas value.
- Identify key diagnostic procedures used in assessment of the patient with pulmonary dysfunction.
- Discuss the nursing management of a patient undergoing a pulmonary diagnostic procedure.
- Describe the use of pulse oximetry for bedside monitoring.

evolve Be sure to check out the free exercises on-line at *http://evolve.elsevier.com/Urden/priorities/*

Assessment of the patient with pulmonary alterations or dysfunction is a systematic process that incorporates the patient history and physical examination. The purpose of the assessment is (1) to recognize changes in the patient's pulmonary status that would necessitate nursing or medical intervention and (2) to determine the ways in which the patient's pulmonary dysfunction is interfering with self-care activities.[1] To complete the assessment, the patient's laboratory studies and diagnostic tests must be reviewed. This chapter focuses on priority clinical assessments, laboratory studies, and diagnostic tests for the critically ill patient with pulmonary dysfunction.

HISTORY

The initial presentation of the patient with pulmonary alterations determines the rapidity and direction of the interview. For a patient in acute respiratory distress, the history is curtailed to just a few questions about the patient's chief complaint and precipitating events. For a patient in no obvious distress, the history focuses on (1) reviewing the present illness, (2) determining the general respiratory status, (3) determining the general health status, and (4) evaluating lifestyle factors in relation to the pulmonary dysfunction[2,3] (Box 13-1).

A description of the patient's current symptoms is also obtained. Common pulmonary symptoms include dyspnea, cough, wheezing, edema, palpitations, fatigue, chest pain,[4] hemoptysis, and sputum production.[5] Information is elicited regarding the location, onset, duration, characteristics, setting, aggravating and alleviating factors, associated symptoms,[4] and efforts to treat the symptoms.[6] If the cough is productive, the patient is asked questions about the color, amount, odor, and consistency of the sputum.[7]

CLINICAL ASSESSMENT
Inspection

Nursing priorities for inspection of the patient with pulmonary dysfunction focus on (1) **observing the tongue and sublingual area,** (2) **assessing the chest wall configuration,** and (3) **evaluating respiratory effort.** If possible, the patient is positioned upright, with the arms resting at the sides.[3]

Observing Tongue and Sublingual Area

The patient's tongue and sublingual area are observed for a blue, gray, or dark-purple tint or discoloration, indicative of central cyanosis. *Central cyanosis* is a sign of hypoxemia, or inadequate oxygenation of the blood, and is considered life threatening. The fingers and toes may also appear discolored, indicative of peripheral cyanosis.[8]

Assessing Chest Wall Configuration

The size and shape of the patient's chest wall are assessed for an increase in the anteroposterior (AP) diameter and for structural deviations. Normally the ratio of AP diameter to lateral diameter ranges from 1:2 to 5:7.[1,9,10] An increase in the AP diameter suggests chronic obstructive pulmonary disease (COPD).[1] The shape of the chest is inspected for any structural deviations. In *pectus excavatum* (funnel chest) the sternum and lower ribs are displaced posteriorly, creating a funnel or pit-shaped depression in the chest. This causes a decrease in the AP diameter of the chest and may interfere with respiratory function. In *pectus carinatum* (pigeon breast) the sternum projects forward, causing an increase in the AP diameter of the chest. A *barrel chest* also results in increased AP diameter of the chest and is characterized by displacement of the sternum forward and the ribs outward. Spinal deformities such as kyphosis, lordosis, and scoliosis may also be present and may interfere with respiratory function.[9-11]

Evaluating Respiratory Effort

The patient's respiratory effort is evaluated for rate, rhythm, symmetry, and quality of ventilatory movements.[1] Normal breathing at rest is effortless and regular and occurs at a rate of 12 to 20 breaths/min.[3] Common patterns in patients with pulmonary dysfunction are *tachypnea*, manifested by increased rate and decreased depth of ventilation, and *hyperventilation*, manifested by increased rate and depth of ventilation. Patients with COPD often experience *air trapping*, or obstructive breathing. As the patient breathes, air becomes trapped in the lungs, and ventilations become progressively shallower until the patient actively and forcefully exhales.[12]

Box **13-1**	Pulmonary History Questions

PRESENT ILLNESS

What brought you to the hospital?
What were the precipitating events?
When did the problem start?

RESPIRATORY STATUS

Do you currently have a chronic lung disease, such as asthma, bronchitis, or emphysema?
Do you have a history of any lung disease, such as chronic respiratory infections or tuberculosis?
Have you had any chest surgery?

GENERAL HEALTH STATUS

Do you have any other chronic disease or illness?
Do you have a history of any other disease, illness, or surgery?
Are you currently taking any medications, prescription or nonprescription?

LIFESTYLE

Do you smoke, or have you smoked in the past?
Have you been exposed to secondhand smoke?
Have you ever been exposed to lung irritants or cancer-causing agents, such as asbestos, chemicals, fumes, beryllium, coal or stone quarry dust, or Agent Orange?

Additional Assessment Areas

Other areas assessed are patient position, use of accessory muscles, presence of intercostal retractions, unequal movement of the chest wall, flaring of nares, and pausing midsentence to take a breath.[1,10] The presence of other iatrogenic devices, such as chest tubes, central venous lines, artificial airways, and nasogastric tubes, may affect assessment findings and should be noted.

Palpation

Nursing priorities for palpation of the patient with pulmonary dysfunction focus on (1) **confirming tracheal position**, (2) **assessing respiratory excursion**, and (3) **evaluating tactile fremitus**. In addition, the thorax is assessed for any areas of tenderness, lumps, or bony deformities. The anterior, posterior, and lateral areas of the chest are evaluated systematically.[9,11]

Confirming Tracheal Position

The patient's tracheal position is confirmed at midline. Tracheal position is assessed by placing the fingers in the suprasternal notch and moving upward.[12] Deviation of the trachea to either side can indicate pneumothorax, unilateral pneumonia, diffuse pulmonary fibrosis, a large pleural effusion, or severe atelectasis. With atelectasis the trachea shifts to the same side as the problem, and with pneumothorax the trachea shifts to the opposite side of the problem.[11]

Assessing Respiratory Excursion

The patient's respiratory excursion is assessed for the degree and symmetry of movement. Respiratory excursion is evaluated by placing the hands on the anterolateral chest with the thumbs extended along the costal margin, pointing to the xiphoid process, or by placing the hands on the posterolateral chest with the thumbs on either side of the spine at the level of the tenth rib. The patient is instructed to take a few normal breaths, then a few deep breaths. Chest movement is assessed for equality, which signifies symmetry of thoracic expansion.[3,10,11] Asymmetry is an abnormal finding that can occur with pneumothorax, pneumonia, or other disorders that interfere with lung inflation. The degree of chest movement is felt to ascertain the extent of lung expansion. The thumbs should separate 3 to 5 cm during deep inspiration.[11] Lung expansion of the hyperinflated chest is less than that of the normal chest.[4,9]

Evaluating Tactile Fremitus

Assessment of tactile fremitus is performed to identify, describe, and localize any areas of increased or decreased fremitus. *Fremitus* refers to the palpable vibrations felt through the chest wall when the patient speaks. It is assessed by placing the palmar surface of the hands against opposite sides of the chest wall and having the patient repeat the word "ninety-nine." The hands are moved systematically around the thorax until the anterior, posterior, and both lateral areas have been assessed.[10,11] Fremitus varies from patient to patient and depends on the pitch and intensity of the voice. Fremitus is described as normal, decreased, or increased. With *normal* fremitus, vibrations can be felt over the trachea but are barely palpable over the periphery. With *decreased* fremitus, there is interference with the transmission of vibrations, as with pleural effusion, pneumothorax, bronchial obstruction, pleural thickening, and emphysema. With *increased* fremitus, there is an increase in the transmission of vibrations, as with pneumonia, lung cancer, and pulmonary fibrosis.[3]

Percussion

Nursing priorities for percussion of the patient with pulmonary dysfunction focus on (1) **evaluating the underlying lung structure** and (2) **assessing diaphragmatic excursion**. Although infrequently used, percussion is useful for confirming suspected abnormalities.

Evaluating Underlying Lung Structure

The patient's underlying lung structure is evaluated to estimate the amounts of air, liquid, or solid material present. The middle finger of the nondominant hand is placed on the chest wall. The distal portion, between the last joint and the nailbed, is then struck with the middle finger of the dominant hand. The hands are moved side-to-side, systematically around the thorax, to compare similar areas, until the anterior, posterior, and both lateral areas have been assessed. Five different tones can be elicited: resonance, hyperresonance, tympany, dullness, and flatness. These tones are distinguished by differences in intensity, pitch, duration, and quality[1,9,12] (Table 13-1).

Assessing Diaphragmatic Excursion

Diaphragmatic excursion is assessed by measuring the difference in the level of the diaphragm on inspiration and expiration. The patient is instructed to inhale and hold the breath. The posterior chest is percussed downward, over the intercostal spaces, until the dull sound produced by the diaphragm is heard. The spot is marked. The patient is then instructed to take a few breaths in and out, exhale completely, and then hold the breath. The posterior chest is percussed again, and the new area of dullness over the diaphragm is then located and marked. The difference between the two spots is noted and measured. Normal diaphragmatic excursion is 3 to 5 cm[9,11] and is *decreased* in ascites, pregnancy, hepatomegaly, and emphysema and *increased* in pleural effusion or disorders that elevate the diaphragm (e.g., atelectasis, paralysis).[4]

Auscultation

Nursing priorities for auscultation of the patient with pulmonary dysfunction focus on (1) **evaluating normal breath sounds**, (2) **identifying abnormal breath sounds**, **and** (3) **assessing voice sounds**. Auscultation requires a

Table **13-1** Percussion Tones: Description and Associated Conditions

Tone	Intensity	Pitch	Duration	Quality	Conditions
Resonance	Loud	Low	Long	Hollow	Normal lung Bronchitis
Hyperresonance	Very loud	Very low	Long	Booming	Asthma Emphysema Pneumothorax
Tympany	Loud	Musical	Medium	Drumlike	Large pneumothorax Emphysematous blebs
Dullness	Medium	Medium to high	Medium	Thudlike	Atelectasis Pleural effusion Pulmonary edema Pneumonia Lung mass
Flatness	Soft	High	Short	Extremely dull	Massive atelectasis Pneumonectomy

quiet environment, proper positioning of the patient, and a bare chest.[13] Breath sounds are best heard with the patient in the upright position.[5]

Evaluating Normal Breath Sounds

The patient's breath sounds are auscultated to evaluate the quality of air movement through the pulmonary system and to identify the presence of abnormal sounds. The diaphragm of the stethoscope is placed against the chest wall, and the patient is instructed to breathe in and out slowly with the mouth open. Both inspiratory and expiratory phases are assessed. Auscultation is done in a systematic sequence: side to side, top to bottom, posteriorly, laterally, and anteriorly[5,9,11] (Figure 13-1).

Normal breath sounds are different, depending on their location, and are classified in three categories: bronchial, bronchovesicular, and vesicular[3,9,12,13] (Table 13-2).

Identifying Abnormal Breath Sounds

Abnormal breath sounds are identified once the normal breath sounds have been clearly delineated. The three categories are absent or diminished, displaced bronchial, and adventitious breath sounds (Table 13-3). *Absent* or *diminished* breath sounds indicate little or no airflow to a particular portion of the lung (either a small segment or an entire lung). *Displaced bronchial* breath sounds are normal bronchial sounds heard in the peripheral lung fields instead of over the trachea and usually indicate fluid or exudate in the alveoli. *Adventitious* breath sounds are extra or added sounds heard in addition to the other sounds and are classified as crackles, rhonchi, wheezes, and pleural friction rubs.[3,7,13]

Crackles (also called *rales*) are short, discrete, popping or crackling sounds produced by fluid in the small airways or alveoli or by the snapping open of collapsed airways during inspiration. They are mainly heard on inspiration and are usually unchanged with coughing.[11] Crackles can be further classified as fine, medium, or coarse, depending on pitch.[13] *Rhonchi* are coarse, rumbling, low-pitched sounds produced by airflow over secretions in the larger airways or by narrowing of the large airways. They are mainly heard on expiration and are usually changed with coughing.[11] Rhonchi can further be classified as bubbling, gurgling, or sonorous, depending on the characteristics of the sound.[13] *Wheezes* are high-pitched, squeaking, whistling sounds produced by airflow through narrowed small airways. They are mainly heard on expiration but may be heard throughout the ventilatory cycle.[11] Depending on their severity, wheezes can be further classified as mild, moderate, or severe.[13] *Pleural friction rubs* are creaking, leathery, loud, dry, coarse sounds produced by irritated pleural surfaces rubbing together. They are usually heard best in the lower anterolateral chest area during the latter portion of inspiration and the beginning of expiration. Friction rubs are caused by inflammation of the pleura.[3,7,10,11]

Assessing Voice Sounds

Assessment of the patient's voice sounds is particularly useful in detecting lung consolidation or lung compression. Three abnormal voice sounds are bronchophony, whispering pectoriloquy, and egophony.

Bronchophony. The spoken voice is heard on auscultation with higher intensity and clarity than usual. Normally the spoken word is muffled when heard through the stethoscope. Bronchophony is assessed by placing the diaphragm of the stethoscope against the posterior side of the patient's chest and instructing the patient to say "ninety-nine." Bronchophony is present when the sound heard is clear, distinct, and loud.

Whispering Pectoriloquy. This abnormal sound is defined as unusually clear transmission of the whispered voice on auscultation. Normally the whispered word is unin-

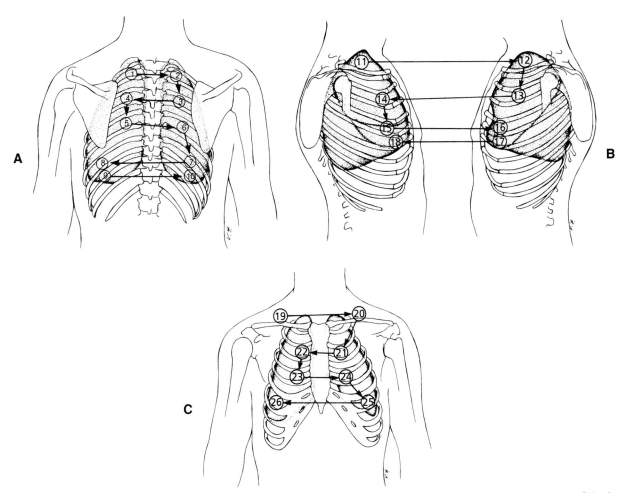

Figure 13-1 Auscultation sequence. **A**, Posterior. **B**, Lateral. **C**, Anterior. (From Perry AG, Potter PA: *Clinical nursing skills and techniques*, ed 5, St Louis, 2002, Mosby.)

Table **13-2**	Characteristics of Normal Breath Sounds
Sound	**Characteristics**
Vesicular	Heard over most of lung field; low pitch; soft, short exhalation and long inhalation
Bronchovesicular	Heard over main bronchus area and upper right posterior lung field; medium pitch; exhalation equals inhalation
Bronchial	Heard only over trachea; high pitch; loud and long exhalation

Modified from Thompson JM et al: *Mosby's clinical nursing*, ed 5, St Louis, 2002, Mosby.

telligible when heard through the stethoscope. Whispered pectoriloquy is assessed by placing the stethoscope against the posterior side of the patient's chest and instructing the patient to whisper "one, two, three." Whispering pectoriloquy is present when the sound heard is clear and distinct.

Egophony. The voice sounds increase in intensity and develop a nasal bleating quality on auscultation. Egophony is assessed by placing the stethoscope against the posterior side of the patient's chest and instructing the patient to say "e-e-e." Egophony is present when the "e" sound changes to an "a" sound.[11,13]

LABORATORY STUDIES
Arterial Blood Gases

Interpretation of arterial blood gas (ABG) levels can be difficult, especially if the health care professional is under pressure to do it quickly and accurately. One method to help ensure accuracy when analyzing ABG levels is to follow the same steps of interpretation that ask specific questions (Box 13-2).

Five-Step ABG Interpretation

Step 1: PaO_2 and Hypoxemia. The PaO_2 is a measure of partial pressure (tension) of oxygen dissolved in arterial blood plasma, reported in millimeters of mercury (mm Hg). PaO_2 reflects 3% of total oxygen in the blood.[14]

Table **13-3**   Abnormal Breath Sounds and Associated Conditions

Sound	Description	Conditions
Absent breath sounds	No airflow to particular portion of lung	Pneumothorax Pneumonectomy Emphysematous blebs Pleural effusion Lung mass Massive atelectasis Complete airway obstruction
Diminished breath sounds	Little airflow to particular portion of lung	Emphysema Pleural effusion Pleurisy Atelectasis Pulmonary fibrosis
Displaced bronchial sounds	Bronchial sounds heard in peripheral lung fields	Atelectasis with secretions Lung mass with exudate Pneumonia Pleural effusion Pulmonary edema
Crackles (rales)	Short, discrete, popping or crackling sounds	Pulmonary edema Pneumonia Pulmonary fibrosis Atelectasis Bronchiectasis
Rhonchi	Coarse, rumbling, low-pitched sounds	Pneumonia Asthma Bronchitis Bronchospasm
Wheezes	High-pitched, squeaking, whistling sounds	Asthma Bronchospasm
Pleural friction rubs	Creaking, leathery, loud, dry, coarse sounds	Pleural effusion Pleurisy

Box **13-2**   **Steps for Interpretation of Arterial Blood Gas (ABG) Values**

STEP 1

Look at arterial oxygen tension (PaO_2) and answer the following:
- Does the PaO_2 show hypoxemia?

STEP 2

Look at the pH and answer the following:
- Is the pH on the acid or alkaline side of 7.40?

STEP 3

Look at arterial carbon dioxide tension ($PaCO_2$) and answer the following:
- Does the $PaCO_2$ show respiratory acidosis, respiratory alkalosis, or normalcy?

STEP 4

Look at bicarbonate (HCO_3^-) and answer the following:
- Does the HCO_3^- show metabolic acidosis, alkalosis, or normalcy?

STEP 5

Look back at the pH and answer the following:
- Does the pH show a compensated or an uncompensated condition?

The normal range in PaO_2 for persons breathing room air at sea level is 80 to 100 mm Hg. However, the normal range is age dependent in two groups: infants and persons 60 years and older. The normal PaO_2 for infants breathing room air is 40 to 70 mm Hg.[15] The normal PaO_2 for persons 60 years and older decreases with age as changes occur in the ventilation/perfusion (V/Q) matching in the aging lung.[14] The correct PaO_2 for older persons can be ascertained as follows: 80 mm Hg (lowest normal value) minus 1 mm Hg for every year that a person is over age 60. Using this formula, a 65-year-old individual can have PaO_2 as low as 75 mm Hg (80 mm Hg – 5 mm Hg = 75 mm Hg) and still be within the normal range. An acceptable range for an 80-year-old person is 60 mm Hg (80 mm Hg – 20 mm Hg = 60 mm Hg). At any age, PaO_2 less than 40 mm Hg represents a life-threatening situation that requires immediate action.[14] In addition, PaO_2 less than the predicted lowest value indicates hypoxemia, which means that a lower-than-normal amount of oxygen is dissolved in plasma.

Step 2: Acid/Alkaline pH. The pH is the hydrogen ion (H^+) concentration of plasma. Calculation of pH is accomplished by using partial pressure of carbon dioxide ($PaCO_2$) and plasma bicarbonate (HCO_3^-).[15]

The normal pH of arterial blood is 7.35 to 7.45, with a mean of 7.40. If less than 7.40, pH is on the acid side of the mean. A pH less than 7.35 is known as *acidemia*, and the condition is *acidosis*. If greater than 7.40, pH is on the alkaline side of the mean. A pH greater than 7.45 is known as *alkalemia*, and the condition is *alkalosis*.[14,16]

Step 3: $Paco_2$ and Respiratory Acidosis/Alkalosis. The $Paco_2$ is a measure (mm Hg) of the partial pressure (tension) of carbon dioxide dissolved in arterial blood plasma. $Paco_2$ is the acid-base component that reflects the effectiveness of ventilation in relation to the metabolic rate.[15-17] In other words, $Paco_2$ indicates whether the patient can ventilate well enough to rid the body of the CO_2 produced as a consequence of metabolism.

The normal range for $Paco_2$ is 35 to 45 mm Hg. This range does not change as a person ages. $Paco_2$ greater than 45 mm Hg defines *respiratory acidosis*, which is caused by alveolar hypoventilation. Hypoventilation can result from COPD, oversedation, head trauma, anesthesia, drug overdose, neuromuscular disease, or hypoventilation with mechanical ventilation.[15-17] $Paco_2$ less than 35 mm Hg defines *respiratory alkalosis*, which is caused by alveolar hyperventilation. Hyperventilation can result from hypoxia, anxiety, pulmonary embolism, pregnancy, and hyperventilation with mechanical ventilation or may be a compensatory mechanism to metabolic acidosis.[15,17]

Step 4: Bicarbonate and Metabolic Acidosis/Alkalosis. Bicarbonate (HCO_3^-) is the acid-base component that reflects kidney function and is reduced or increased in the plasma by renal mechanisms. The normal range is 22 to 26 mEq/L.[17] HCO_3^- less than 22 mEq/L defines *metabolic acidosis*, which can result from ketoacidosis, lactic acidosis, renal failure, or diarrhea. The cumulative effect is a gain of acids or a loss of base. HCO_3^- greater than 26 mEq/L defines *metabolic alkalosis*, which can result from fluid loss from the upper gastrointestinal tract (vomiting or nasogastric suction), diuretic therapy, severe hypokalemia, alkali administration, or steroid therapy.[15]

Step 5: pH and Compensated/Uncompensated Conditions. If pH is abnormal (less than 7.35 or greater than 7.45), $Paco_2$ or HCO_3^- (or both) will also be abnormal. This is an *uncompensated* condition because there has not been enough time for the body to return the pH to normal range (Box 13-3). If pH is within normal limits and both $Paco_2$ and HCO_3^- are abnormal, the condition is *compensated* because there has been enough time for the body to restore the pH to normal range (Box 13-4). Differentiating the primary disorder from the compensatory response can be difficult. The primary disorder is the abnormality that caused the pH level to shift initially and thus is defined by the side of 7.40 on which the pH value lies. *Partial compensation* may also be present, as evidenced by abnormal pH, $Paco_2$, and HCO_3^-, which indicate the body is attempting to return the pH to normal range.[16,17]

Specific changes in the acid-base components accompany the various acid-base disorders[15] (Table 13-4). Other

---

Box 13-3 | ABG Values: Uncompensated Conditions

EXAMPLE 1

Pao_2	90 mm Hg
pH	7.25
$Paco_2$	50 mm Hg
HCO_3^-	22 mEq/L

Interpretation: Uncompensated respiratory acidosis

EXAMPLE 2

Pao_2	90 mm Hg
pH	7.25
$Paco_2$	40 mm Hg
HCO_3^-	17 mEq/L

Interpretation: Uncompensated metabolic acidosis

Box 13-4 | ABG Values: Compensated Conditions

EXAMPLE 1

Pao_2	90 mm Hg
pH	7.37
$Paco_2$	60 mm Hg
HCO_3^-	38 mEq/L

Interpretation: Compensated respiratory acidosis with metabolic alkalosis. (The acidosis is considered the main disorder and the alkalosis the compensatory response because the pH is on the acid side of 7.40.)

EXAMPLE 2

Pao_2	90 mm Hg
pH	7.42
$Paco_2$	48 mm Hg
HCO_3^-	35 mEq/L

Interpretation: Compensated metabolic alkalosis with respiratory acidosis. (The alkalosis is considered the main disorder and the acidosis the compensatory response because the pH is on the alkaline side of 7.40.)

---

factors must be considered when reviewing a patient's ABGs, including oxygen saturation, oxygen content, expected Pao_2, and base excess/deficit.

Oxygen Saturation

Oxygen (O_2) saturation is a measure of the amount of oxygen bound to hemoglobin (Hgb) compared with the maximal capability of Hgb for binding O_2. Oxygen saturation can be assessed as a component of ABG measurement (Sao_2) or can be measured noninvasively using a pulse oximeter (Spo_2).[14] O_2 saturation is reported as a percentage or as a decimal, with normal being greater than 95% on room air. Normally, the saturation level cannot reach 100% (on room air) because of the physiologic shunting.[14,18] When supplemental oxygen is administered, however, O_2 saturation may approach 100% so closely that it is reported as 100%.

Table **13-4**	Arterial Blood Gas (ABG) Values in Respiratory/Metabolic Disorders		
Disorder	pH	$Paco_2$ (mm Hg)	HCO_3^- (mEq/L)
RESPIRATORY ACIDOSIS			
Uncompensated	<7.35	>45	22-26
Partially compensated	<7.35	>45	26
Compensated	7.35-7.39	>45	26
RESPIRATORY ALKALOSIS			
Uncompensated	>7.45	<35	22-26
Partially compensated	>7.45	<35	22
Compensated	7.41-7.45	<35	22
METABOLIC ACIDOSIS			
Uncompensated	<7.35	35-45	22
Partially compensated	<7.35	<35	22
Compensated	7.35-7.39	35	22
METABOLIC ALKALOSIS			
Uncompensated	>7.45	35-45	26
Partially compensated	>7.45	45	26
Compensated	7.41-7.45	45	26
COMBINED RESPIRATORY/METABOLIC ACIDOSIS			
	<7.35	45	22
COMBINED RESPIRATORY/METABOLIC ALKALOSIS			
	>7.45	35	26

Pao_2, Arterial oxygen partial pressure (tension); HCO_3^-, bicarbonate.

Proper evaluation of the oxygen saturation level is vital. For example, an Sao_2 of 97% means that 97% of the available Hgb is bound with oxygen. The word "available" is essential to evaluating the Sao_2 level because Hgb level is not always within normal limits, and O_2 can bind only with what is available. A 97% saturation level associated with 10 g of Hgb does not deliver as much O_2 to the tissues as does a 97% saturation associated with 15 g of Hgb. Thus assessing only the Sao_2 level and finding it within normal limits must not lead to the conclusion that the patient's oxygenation status is normal. Hgb level must also be evaluated before a decision on oxygenation status can be made.[14,19]

Oxygen Content

Oxygen content (Cao_2) is a measure of the total amount of oxygen carried in the blood, including the amount dissolved in plasma (measured by Pao_2) and the amount bound to Hgb (measured by Sao_2). Cao_2 is reported in milliliters of oxygen carried per 100 ml of blood. The normal value is 20 ml O_2/100 ml blood. To calculate Cao_2, the Pao_2, Sao_2, and Hgb values are used (see Appendix). A change in any of these parameters will affect Cao_2.[14,19]

Expected Arterial Oxygen Tension

When a patient receives supplemental oxygen, Pao_2 is expected to rise. Knowing the level to which the Pao_2 should rise in normal subjects on a given fraction of inspired oxygen (Fio_2) and comparing that with the level to which the Pao_2 actually does rise in patients with pulmonary disease illustrates how well the lung is functioning. Calculating the expected Pao_2 is accomplished by multiplying the Fio_2 value by 5. Thus the expected Pao_2 with Fio_2 of 30% is at least 150 mm Hg (30 × 5), whereas the expected Pao_2 with Fio_2 of 50% is 250 mm Hg (50 × 5).[20] These expected Pao_2 values represent the oxygen level achievable with healthy lungs. Pulmonary disease can radically decrease the expected Pao_2 level. It is impossible to apply the "Fio_2 value × 5" rule to achieve the expected Pao_2 value when the patient is on a system that delivers oxygen by liters per minute (L/min)[14] (Table 13-5).

Intrapulmonary Shunting and Oxygen Tension Indices

Measuring the degree of intrapulmonary shunting that occurs in a patient at any one time, using the classic shunt equation and oxygen tension indices, can assess the efficiency of oxygenation. Intrapulmonary shunting, also called *shunt effect*, *low ventilation/perfusion*, *venous admixture*, and "wasted blood flow," refers to venous blood that flows to the lungs without being oxygenated because of nonfunctioning alveoli.[14,16,21] The classic *shunt equation* (Qs/Qt) refers to

Table **13-5**	Guideline Values for Estimating Fio_2 with Low-Flow O_2 Devices*	
100% O_2 Flow Rate (L/mim)		Fio_2 (%)
NASAL CANNULA OR CATHETER		
1		24
2		28
3		32
4		36
5		40
6		44
OXYGEN MASK		
5-6		40
6-7		50
7-8		60
MASK WITH RESERVOIR BAG		
6		60
7		70
8		80
9		90
10		99+

From Scanlon CL, Wilkins RL, Stoller JK: *Egan's fundamentals of respiratory care*, ed 7, St Louis, 1999, Mosby.
*Normal ventilatory pattern assumed.
Fio_2, Fraction of inspired oxygen.

the portion of cardiac output not exchanging with alveolar blood divided by the total cardiac output. *Direct* determination of intrapulmonary shunting requires use of the shunt equation, which is both invasive and cumbersome (see Appendix). A shunt greater than 10% is considered abnormal and indicative of a shunt-producing disorder.[14]

Intrapulmonary shunting often is *estimated* by using the oxygen tension indices. One advantage to these methods is the ease of performance, although they have been found to be unreliable in critically ill patients.[16] An estimate of intrapulmonary shunting can be determined by computing the difference between the alveolar and arterial oxygen concentrations. Normally, alveolar and arterial P_{O_2} values are approximately equal.[19] Unequal values indicate that venous blood is passing malfunctioning alveoli and returning unoxygenated to the left side of the heart.[20] The most common P_{O_2} indices used to estimate intrapulmonary shunting are Pa_{O_2}/Fi_{O_2} ratio, Pa_{O_2}/PA_{O_2} ratio, and the A-a gradient (see Appendix).

Pa_{O_2}/Fi_{O_2} Ratio

The Pa_{O_2}/Fi_{O_2} ratio is clinically the easiest formula to calculate because it does not call for the computation of the alveolar P_{O_2}. Normally, the Pa_{O_2}/Fi_{O_2} ratio is greater than 286; the lower the value, the worse the lung function.[19,22]

Pa_{O_2}/PA_{O_2} Ratio

The arterial/alveolar oxygen tension ratio (Pa_{O_2}/PA_{O_2}) is normally greater than 60%. The disadvantage to using this formula is that PA_{O_2} must be calculated, but the advantage is that the value is unaffected by changes in Fi_{O_2} as long as the underlying lung condition is stable.[19,22]

Alveolar-Arterial Gradient

The alveolar-arterial pressure gradient, $P(A\text{-}a)_{O_2}$, is normally less than 20 mm Hg on room air for patients less than age 61 years. This estimate of intrapulmonary shunting is the least reliable clinically but is frequently used in clinical decision making. One of the major disadvantages to using this formula is that the value is greatly influenced by the amount of oxygen the patient is receiving.[16]

Dead Space Equation

The efficiency of ventilation can be measured using the clinical dead space (Vd/Vt) equation (see Appendix). The formula measures the fraction of tidal volume not participating in gas exchange. Dead space greater than 0.6 indicates a dead space–producing disorder and is considered abnormal. The major limitations to using this formula are that it requires the measurement of exhaled CO_2 to complete and that the work of breathing by patients must remain stable during the collection.[22]

Sputum Studies

Careful analysis of sputum specimens is crucial for the rapid identification and treatment of pulmonary infections. The most difficult aspect of sputum examination is proper collection of the specimen. In general, collection of a good sputum sample requires a conscious, cooperative, sufficiently hydrated patient.[23] When the patient has difficulty producing sputum, heated nebulized saline may help to loosen secretions for expectoration.[24] Chest physiotherapy combined with nebulization can improve the success rate. Collection of a sputum specimen is best done in the morning because there is a greater volume of secretions as a result of nighttime pooling.[25]

Many critically ill patients cannot cough effectively, which requires sputum collection by other methods, including tracheobronchial aspiration, transtracheal aspiration, and fiberoptic bronchoscopy with a protected brush catheter. Because each method has its own benefits and risks, the patient's clinical condition determines the appropriate technique.[16]

Many critically ill patients have endotracheal or tracheostomy tubes already in place. Collecting sputum specimens from these patients requires special attention to technique (Box 13-5). Deep specimens are obtained to avoid collecting specimens that contain resident upper airway flora that may have migrated down the tube. Colonization of the lower airways with upper airway flora can occur within 48 hours of intubation.[26]

Once obtained, the sputum specimen is examined for volume, physical properties, mucopurulence, and color. Microscopic examination is then done to identify the source of the specimen. If a bacterial infection is suspected, Gram stain followed by culture and sensitivity (C&S) is performed.[16]

DIAGNOSTIC PROCEDURES

The various diagnostic procedures used to evaluate the patient with pulmonary dysfunction are presented in Table 13-6.

Box 13-5 **Procedure for Collection of Tracheal/Endotracheal Specimen**

1. Clear the endotracheal or tracheostomy tube of all local secretions, avoiding deep airway penetration.
2. Attach a sputum trap to a sterile suction catheter and advance the catheter into the trachea while trying to avoid contact with the endotracheal tube or tracheostomy tube.
3. After the catheter is fully advanced, apply suction until secretions return to the sputum trap. When enough secretions are collected, discontinue suctioning and remove the catheter.
4. Do not apply suction while the catheter is being withdrawn because this can contaminate the sample with sputum from the upper airway. Do not flush the catheter with sterile water because this dilutes the sample.
5. If the catheter becomes plugged with secretions, place it in a sterile container and send it to the laboratory. The specimen must be transported immediately or refrigerated if a delay is necessary.

Table 13-6 Pulmonary Diagnostic Procedures

Procedure	Evaluation	Comments
Bronchography	Detects obstruction or malformation of tracheobronchial tree.	Patient ingests radiopaque substance, then radiographs are taken. Inquire about possibility of pregnancy.
Chest radiography	Detects lung pathology (e.g., pneumonia, pulmonary edema, atelectasis, tuberculosis). Determines size and location of lung lesions and tumors. Verifies placement of endotracheal tube, central venous catheters, and chest tubes.	Noninvasive test with minimal radiation exposure. Inquire about possibility of pregnancy. PA and lateral films most common, but in critical care areas, AP portable films often necessary because patient cannot be transported. Lateral decubitus films aid in identification of pleural effusion.
Exercise testing	Identify early disability. Differentiate between cardiac and pulmonary disease.	Monitor for changes in SpO_2 during exercise. Monitor closely for exercise-induced hypotension and ventricular dysrhythmias.
Laryngoscopy, bronchoscopy, mediastinoscopy	Obtain cytology specimen or biopsy. Identify tumors, obstructions, secretions, and foreign bodies in tracheobronchial tree. Locate a bleeding site. May be used therapeutically to remove secretions, foreign bodies, other contaminants.	Patient is sedated before procedure, usually with a benzodiazepine (e.g., diazepam, midazolam). Monitor patient for subcutaneous emphysema after study; indicates tracheal or bronchial tear. Monitor for hemoptysis; some blood in sputum is normal after biopsy, but frank hemoptysis requires immediate attention.
Lung biopsy	Obtain specimen for cytologic evaluation.	*Transthoracic needle biopsy* performed under fluoroscopy; inquire about possibility of pregnancy. *Open lung biopsy* requires thoracotomy.
Magnetic resonance imaging (MRI)	Distinguishes tumors from other structures (e.g., tumor, pleural thickening, fibrosis).	Noninvasive test. Contraindicated for patients with pacemakers or implanted metallic devices.
Pulmonary angiography	Detects changes in lung tissue (e.g., masses). Diagnoses abnormalities in pulmonary vasculature, including thrombi and emboli. Identifies congenital abnormalities of circulation.	Invasive test. Inquire about possibility of pregnancy. Contrast media injected into pulmonary artery; ensure adequate hydration after study. Monitor arterial puncture point for hematoma and hemorrhage.
Pulmonary function tests (PFTs; see Table 13-7) • Spirometry • Ventilatory mechanics • Flow-volume loop • Diffusing capacity	Measure lung volumes, capacities, and flow rates. RV, FRC, and TLC require nitrogen washout technique. Identify features of restrictive or obstructive lung disease. Evaluate responsiveness to bronchodilator. Aids in evaluation of surgical risk.	Noninvasive studies. Frequently repeated after bronchodilator therapy.
Sleep studies	Documents a disability or cause of dyspnea. Diagnose and differentiate between *obstructive, central,* and *cardiac* sleep apnea.	Restrict caffeine before testing. Usually done during normal sleep hours.
Thoracentesis (may include pleural biopsy)	Obtain pleural fluid/tissue specimen. May be used therapeutically to remove pleural fluid.	Monitor patient for indications of pneumothorax. Monitor for leakage from puncture point. X-ray films are taken at different angles.
Thoracic computed tomography (CT)	Defines lesions, masses, cavities, or shadows seen on normal chest radiograph. Evaluates tracheal and bronchial narrowing. Aids in planning radiation therapy.	
Ultrasonography	Evaluates pleural disease. Visualizes diaphragm and detects disease around diaphragm (e.g., subphrenic hematoma, abscess).	Noninvasive test.
Ventilation scan Lung perfusion scan V/Q scan	Diagnoses ventilation and perfusion abnormalities (e.g., emphysema, pulmonary emboli).	Invasive test: radioisotope ingested and injected intravascularly. Inquire about possibility of pregnancy. Assure that amount of radioactive material is minimal.

PA, Posteroanterior; *AP*, anteroposterior; SpO_2, oxygen saturation; *V/Q*, ventilation/perfusion ratio.

Volume	Definition	Normal Value
LUNG VOLUMES AND CAPACITIES		
Tidal volume (Vt, V_T, V_T)	Volume of air moved in/out of lungs with each normal breath.	7 ml/kg ($\approx$500 ml)
Inspiratory reserve volume (IRV)	Volume of air that can be maximally inspired above normal inspiratory level.	3000 ml
Expiratory reserve volume (ERV)	Volume of air that can be maximally exhaled beyond normal expiratory level.	1000 ml
Residual volume (RV)	Volume of air remaining in lungs at end of a maximal expiration.	1000 ml
Inspiratory capacity (IC)	Vt + IRC; volume of air that can be maximally inspired from a normal expiratory level.	3500 ml
Functional residual capacity (FRC)	RV + ERV; volume of air remaining in lungs at end of a normal expiration.	2000 ml
Vital capacity (VC)	Vt + IRC + ERV; volume of air that can be maximally expired after a maximal inspiration.	4500 ml
Total lung capacity (TLC)	Vt + IRC + ERV+ RV; volume of air that lungs can hold with maximal inspiration.	5500-6000 ml
Respiratory rate or frequency (f)	Number of breaths per minute.	12-20
Minute ventilation (VE)	Vt × f; volume of air expired per minute.	5-10 L
Dead space (Vd)	Vd/Vt = $Paco_2$ − $Petco_2/Paco_2$*	<0.4
Alveolar ventilation (VA)	Vt − Vd; volume of tidal air involved in alveolar gas exchange.	350 ml
Forced vital capacity (FVC)	Volume of air in a forceful maximal expiration.	Same as VC: 4500 ml
Forced expiratory volume (FEV)	Volume of air exhaled in prescribed period. FEV_1 in 1 second; FEV_3 in 3 seconds.	FEV_1: >75% VC FEV_3: >95% VC

From Dennison RD: *Pass CCRN!*, ed 2, St. Louis, 2000, Mosby.
*See Appendix; volume or percentage of Vt that does not participate in gas exchange; includes volume of air in conducting pathways (anatomic dead space) plus volume of alveolar air not involved in gas exchange due to pathology (alveolar dead space); Vd/Vt >0.6 is usually an indication for mechanical ventilation.

Nursing Management

The nursing management of a patient undergoing a diagnostic procedure involves a variety of interventions. **Nursing priorities are directed toward (1) preparing the patient psychologically and physically for the procedure, (2) monitoring the patient's responses to the procedure, and (3) assessing the patient after the procedure.**

Preparing the patient includes teaching the patient about the procedure, answering any questions, and transporting and/or positioning the patient for the procedure. In addition to vital signs, monitoring the patient's responses to the procedure includes observing for signs of pain, anxiety, or respiratory decompensation (Box 13-6). Assessing the patient after the procedure includes observing for complications of the procedure and medicating the patient for any postprocedural discomfort. **Any evidence of respiratory distress should be immediately reported to the physician, and emergency measures to maintain breathing must be initiated.**

BEDSIDE MONITORING: PULSE OXIMETRY

Bedside pulmonary function tests (PFTs) are designed to quantify respiratory function and are an essential component of a thorough pulmonary evaluation. Measurement of lung volumes and capacities provides valuable information on the origin of a pulmonary disease process (Table 13-7).

Pulse oximetry is a noninvasive method for monitoring oxygen saturation (SpO_2). It is indicated in any situation that requires continuous observation of the patient's oxygenation status. The pulse oximeter consists of a microprocessor and a probe that attaches to the patient (finger, ear, toe, or nose). Two light-emitting diodes transmit red and infrared light wavelengths through the pulsating vascular bed to a photodetector on the other side. The photodetector converts the light signals into an electrical signal, which is then sent to the microprocessor, which converts the signal to a digital reading. The pulse oximeter is considered very accurate, within ±2% at SpO_2 greater than 70%.[27]

Nursing Management

Nursing priorities in pulse oximetry monitoring are directed toward minimizing the physiologic and technical factors that can limit the monitoring system.

Minimizing Physiologic Limitations

Physiologic limitations include elevated levels of abnormal hemoglobin, presence of vascular dyes, and poor tissue perfusion. The pulse oximeter cannot differentiate between normal and abnormal Hgb. Elevated levels of abnormal Hgb falsely elevate SpO_2. Vascular dyes (e.g., methylene blue, indigo carmine, indocyanine green, fluorescein) also interfere with pulse oximetry and can lead to falsely low readings. Poor tissue perfusion to the area with the probe leads to loss of pulsatile flow and signal failure.[27]

Minimizing Technical Limitations

Technical limitations include bright lights, excessive motion, and incorrect probe placement. Bright lights may interfere with the photodetector and cause inaccurate results. The probe must be covered to limit optical interference. Excessive motion can mimic arterial pulsations and can lead to false readings. Incorrect placement of the probe can lead to inaccurate results because part of the light can reach the photodetector without having passed through blood (*optical shunting*). Interventions to limit these problems include (1) using the proper probe in the appropriate spot (e.g., not using a finger probe on the ear), (2) applying the probe according to the directions, and (3) ensuring that the area being monitored has adequate perfusion.[27]

Box **13-6**	Clinical Manifestations of Respiratory Decompensation

INADEQUATE AIRWAY

Stridor
Noisy respirations
Supraclavicular and intercostal retractions
Flaring of nares
Labored breathing with use of accessory muscles

INADEQUATE VENTILATION

Absence of air exchange at nose and mouth (breathlessness)
Minimal/absent chest wall motion
Manifestations of obstructed airway
Central cyanosis
Decreased or absent breath sounds (bilateral, unilateral)
Restlessness, anxiety, confusion
Paradoxical motion involving significant portion of chest wall
Decreased Pao_2, increased $Paco_2$, decreased pH

INADEQUATE GAS EXCHANGE

Tachypnea
Decreased Pao_2
Increased dead space
Central cyanosis
Chest infiltrates on radiographic evaluation

REFERENCES

1. Rokosky JS: Assessment of the individual with altered respiratory function, *Nurs Clin North Am* 16:195, 1981.
2. Gehring PE: Physical assessment begins with a history, *RN* 54(11):26, 1991.
3. Brenner M, Welliver J: Pulmonary and acid-base assessment, *Nurs Clin North Am* 25:761, 1990.
4. Dettenmeier PA: *Pulmonary nursing care*, St Louis, 1992, Mosby.
5. Wilkins RL, Stoller J: Bedside assessment of the patient. In Scanlan CL, Wilkins RL, Stoller JK, editors: *Egan's fundamentals of respiratory care*, ed 7, St Louis, 1999, Mosby.
6. Wilson SF, Thompson JM: *Respiratory disorders*, St Louis, 1990, Mosby.

7. Stiesmeyer JK: A four-step approach to pulmonary assessment, *Am J Nurs* 93(8):22, 1993.

8. Carpenter KD: A comprehensive review of cyanosis, *Crit Care Nurs* 13(4):66, 1993.

9. King C: Examining the thorax and respiratory system, *RN* 45 (8):55, 1982.

10. Kuhn KW, McGovern M: Respiratory assessment of the elderly, *J Gerontol Nurs* 18(5):40, 1992.

11. Barkauskas V et al: *Health and physical assessment*, ed 2, St Louis, 1998, Mosby.

12. Seidel HM et al: *Mosby's guide to physical examination*, ed 4, St Louis, 1999, Mosby.

13. Boyda EK et al: *Pulmonary auscultation*, St Paul, Minn, 1987, 3M Health Care Group.

14. Davoric C, Franklin CM: *Handbook of hemodynamic monitoring*, Philadelphia, 1999 Saunders.

15. Porth CM: *Pathophysiology concepts of altered health states*, Philadelphia, ed 5, 1998, Lippincott-Raven.

16. Grif-Alspach J: *American Association of Critical-Care Nurses core curriculum for critical care nursing*, ed 5, Philadelphia, 1998, Saunders.

17. Tasota FJ, Wesmiller SW: Balancing act: keeping the blood pH in equilibrium, *Nursing 98* 28(12):34, 1998.

18. Jensen LA, Onyskiw JE, Prasad NG: Meta-analysis of arterial oxygen saturation monitoring by pulse oximetry in adults, *Heart Lung* 27:387, 1998.

19. Schallom L, Ahrens T: Clinical application: using oxygenation profiles to manage patients, *Crit Care Nurs Clin North Am* 11:437, 1999.

20. Shapiro BA, Peruzzi WT, Kozelowski-Templin R: *Clinical application of blood gases*, ed 5, St Louis, 1994, Mosby.

21. Misasi RS, Keyes J: Matching and mismatching ventilation and perfusion in the lung, *Crit Care Nurse* 16(3):23, 1996.

22. Ahrens T, Beattie S, Nienhaus T: Experimental therapies to support the failing lung, *AACN Clin Issues Adv Pract Acute Crit Care* 7:507, 1996.

23. Gilman G, Branson RD: Humidification for patients with artificial airways: more on the HME-booster, *Respir Care* 44:430, 1999.

24. Willams RL, Dexter JR: *Respiratory disease—a case study approach to patient care*, Philadelphia, 1998, Davis.

25. Scanlon CL, Wilkins RL, Stoller JK: *Egan's fundamentals of respiratory care*, ed 7, St Louis, 1999, Mosby.

26. Grap MJ, Munro CL: Ventilator-associated pneumonia: clinical significance and implications for nursing, *Heart Lung*, 26: 419, 1997.

27. St. John RE, Thomson PD: Noninvasive respiratory monitoring, *Crit Care Nurs Clin North Am* 11:423, 1999

14

Pulmonary
Disorders

Objectives

- Describe the etiology and pathophysiology of selected pulmonary disorders.
- Identify the clinical manifestations of selected pulmonary disorders.
- Explain the treatment of selected pulmonary disorders.
- Discuss the nursing priorities for managing the patient with selected pulmonary disorders.

evolve Be sure to check out the free exercises on-line at *http://evolve.elsevier.com/Urden/priorities/*

Understanding the pathology of a disease, areas of assessment on which to focus, and usual medical management allows the critical care nurse to anticipate and plan nursing interventions more accurately. This chapter discusses common pulmonary disorders seen in the critical care environment.

ACUTE RESPIRATORY FAILURE

Acute respiratory failure (ARF) is a clinical condition in which the pulmonary system fails to maintain adequate gas exchange.[1] ARF is one of the most common problems seen in critical care,[2] with a survival rate of about 55%.[3] ARF can be classified as *hypoxemic normocapnic* respiratory failure (type I) or *hypoxemic hypercapnic* respiratory failure (type II), depending on the patient's arterial blood gas (ABG) measurements. In *type I* respiratory failure the patient presents with low arterial oxygen tension (PaO_2) and normal arterial carbon dioxide tension ($PaCO_2$), whereas in *type II* respiratory failure, PaO_2 is low and $PaCO_2$ is high.[4]

Etiology

ARF results from a deficiency in pulmonary system performance.[1,4] ARF usually occurs secondary to another disorder that has altered the normal function of the pulmonary system in such a way as to decrease the ventilatory drive, decrease muscle strength, decrease chest wall elasticity, decrease the lung's capacity for gas exchange, increase airway resistance, or increase metabolic oxygen requirements.[5]

The etiologies of ARF may be classified as extrapulmonary or intrapulmonary, depending on the component of the respiratory system that is affected. *Extrapulmonary* causes include disorders that affect the brain, spinal cord, neuromuscular system, thorax, pleura, and upper airways. *Intrapulmonary* causes include disorders that affect the lower airways and alveoli, pulmonary circulation, and alveolar-capillary membrane[6] (Table 14-1).

Pathophysiology

Hypoxemia is the result of impaired gas exchange and is the hallmark of ARF. Hypercapnia may be present, depending on the underlying cause of the problem. The mains causes of hypoxemia are alveolar hypoventilation, ventilation/perfusion (V/Q) mismatching, and intrapulmonary shunting.[7] Type I respiratory failure usually results from V/Q mismatching and intrapulmonary shunting, whereas type II usually results from alveolar hypoventilation, which may or may not be accompanied by V/Q mismatching and intrapulmonary shunting.[1]

Alveolar Hypoventilation

Alveolar hypoventilation occurs when the amount of oxygen being brought into the alveoli is insufficient to meet the metabolic needs of the body.[6] This may result from increasing metabolic oxygen needs or decreasing ventilation.[5] Hypoxemia caused by alveolar hypoventilation is associated

Table **14-1**	Etiologies of Acute Respiratory Failure
Affected Area	**Disorders**[*]
EXTRAPULMONARY	
Brain	Drug overdose
	Central alveolar hypoventilation syndrome
	Brain trauma or lesion
	Postoperative anesthesia depression
Spinal cord	Guillain-Barré syndrome
	Poliomyelitis
	Amyotrophic lateral sclerosis
	Spinal cord trauma or lesion
Neuromuscular system	Myasthenia gravis
	Multiple sclerosis
	Neuromuscular blocking agents
	Organophosphate poisoning
	Muscular dystrophy
Thorax	Massive obesity
	Chest trauma
Pleura	Pleural effusion
	Pneumothorax
Upper airways	Sleep apnea
	Tracheal obstruction
	Epiglottitis
INTRAPULMONARY	
Lower airways and alveoli	Chronic obstructive pulmonary disease
	Asthma
	Bronchiolitis
	Cystic fibrosis
	Pneumonia
Pulmonary circulation	Pulmonary emboli
Alveolar-capillary membrane	Pulmonary edema
	Acute respiratory distress syndrome
	Inhalation of toxic gases
	Near-drowning

[*]Not an inclusive list.

with hypercapnia and usually results from extrapulmonary disorders.[1,7]

Ventilation/Perfusion Mismatching

V/Q mismatching occurs when ventilation and blood flow are mismatched in various regions of the lung in excess of what is normal. Blood passes through alveoli that are underventilated for the given amount of perfusion, leaving these areas with a lower-than-normal amount of oxygen. V/Q mismatching is the most common cause of hypoxemia and usually results from partially collapsed alveoli or aveoli partially filled with fluid.[6-8]

Intrapulmonary Shunting

The extreme form of V/Q mismatching, intrapulmonary shunting, occurs when blood reaches the arterial system without participating in gas exchange. The mixing of unoxygenated (shunted) blood and oxygenated blood lowers the average level of oxygen present in the blood. Intrapulmonary shunting occurs when blood passes through a portion of a lung that is not ventilated. This may be the result of (1) alveolar collapse secondary to atelectasis or (2) alveolar flooding with pus, blood, or fluid.[6]

Complications

If allowed to progress, hypoxemia can result in oxygen deficit at the cellular level. As the tissue demands for oxygen continue and the supply diminishes, an oxygen supply/demand imbalance occurs and tissue hypoxia develops. Decreased oxygen to the cells contributes to impaired tissue perfusion and development of lactic acidosis and multiple organ dysfunction syndrome.[8]

Assessment and Diagnosis

The patient with ARF may experience a variety of clinical manifestations, depending on the underlying cause and the extent of tissue hypoxia. The clinical manifestations typically seen in the patient with ARF are usually associated with development of hypoxemia, hypercapnia, and acidosis.[9] Because these are so varied, clinical symptoms are not considered reliable in predicting the degree of hypoxemia or hypercapnia[8] or the severity of ARF.[2]

Diagnosing and following the course of respiratory failure are best accomplished by arterial ABG analysis to determine $PaCO_2$, PaO_2, and blood pH levels. ARF is generally accepted as being present when the PaO_2 is less than 60 mm Hg or the $PaCO_2$ is greater than 50 mm Hg.[1] In patients with chronically elevated $PaCO_2$ levels, these criteria must be broadened to include a pH less than 7.35.[2,5]

Medical Management

Medical management of the patient with ARF is aimed at treating the underlying cause, promoting adequate gas exchange, correcting acidosis, initiating nutrition support, and preventing complications.[5] Medical interventions to promote gas exchange are aimed at improving oxygenation and ventilation.

Oxygenation

Interventions to improve oxygenation include supplemental oxygen (O_2) and positive airway pressure. O_2 therapy is used to correct hypoxemia, and although the absolute level of hypoxemia varies in each patient, most treatment approaches maintain arterial hemoglobin O_2 saturation (SaO_2) at greater than 90%,[10] supplying tissue needs but not producing hypercapnia or oxygen toxicity.[5] Supplemental O_2 administration is effective in treating hypoxemia related to alveolar hypoventilation and V/Q mismatching. When

intrapulmonary shunting exists, supplemental O_2 alone is ineffective.[11] In this situation, positive pressure is necessary to open collapsed alveoli and facilitate their participation in gas exchange. Positive pressure may be delivered noninvasively via a mask[2,12] or invasively via endotracheal tube (ETT) or tracheostomy.[2]

Ventilation

Interventions to improve ventilation include the use of noninvasive and invasive mechanical ventilation. Depending on the underlying cause and the severity of the ARF, the patient may be initially treated with noninvasive ventilation.[12] However, patients with pH less than 7.25 at initial presentation may be more likely to need invasive mechanical ventilation.[13] The selection of ventilatory mode and settings depends on the patient's underlying condition, severity of respiratory failure, and body size.[10] The patient is usually started on volume ventilation in the assist/control mode. In the patient with chronic hypercapnia the settings should be adjusted to keep ABG values within the parameters that the patient should maintain after extubation.[14]

Pharmacology

Medications to facilitate removal of secretions and dilate airways may also be of benefit in the treatment of the patient with ARF. Mucolytics are administered to help liquefy secretions, which facilitates their removal. Bronchodilators, such as xanthines, β_2-agonists, and anticholinergic agents, aid in smooth muscle relaxation and are of particular benefit to patients with airflow limitations. Steroids also are often administered to decrease airway inflammation and enhance the effects of the β_2-agonists.[1,5,15]

Sedation is necessary in many patients to assist with maintaining adequate ventilation. Sedation may be used to comfort the patient and decrease the work of breathing, particularly if the patient is fighting the ventilator. Analgesics should be administered for pain control.[12] In some patients, sedation does not decrease spontaneous respiratory efforts enough to allow adequate ventilation. Neuromuscular paralysis may be necessary to facilitate optimal ventilation. Paralysis also may be necessary to decrease O_2 consumption in the severely compromised patient.[16]

Acidosis

Acidosis may occur in the patient for a number of reasons. Hypoxemia causes impaired tissue perfusion, which leads to the production of lactic acid and the development of metabolic acidosis. Impaired ventilation leads to the accumulation of carbon dioxide (CO_2) and the development of respiratory acidosis. Once the patient is adequately oxygenated and ventilated, the acidosis should correct itself. The use of sodium bicarbonate to correct the acidosis has been shown to be of minimal benefit to the patient,[17] although it may still be used if the acidosis persists or is severe (pH less than 7.2).[5]

Nutrition Support

The initiation of nutrition support is of utmost importance in the management of the patient with ARF. The goals of nutrition support are to meet the overall nutritional needs of the patient while avoiding overfeeding in order to prevent nutrition delivery–related complications and to improve patient outcomes.[18] Failure to provide the patient with adequate nutrition support results in the development of malnutrition. Both malnutrition and overfeeding can interfere with the performance of the pulmonary system, perpetuating ARF. *Malnutrition* decreases the patient's ventilatory drive and muscle strength, whereas *overfeeding* increases CO_2 production, which then increases the patient's ventilatory demand, resulting in respiratory muscle fatigue.[19]

The *enteral* route is the preferred method of nutrition administration. If a patient cannot tolerate enteral feedings or cannot receive enough nutrients enterally, the patient will be started on parenteral nutrition. Because the parenteral route is associated with a higher rate of complications, the goal is to switch to enteral feedings as soon as the patient can tolerate them.[18,19] Nutrition support should be initiated before the third day of mechanical ventilation for the well-nourished patient and within 24 hours for the malnourished patient.[18]

Complications

The ARF patient may experience a number of complications, including ischemic-anoxic encephalophathy,[20] cardiac dysrhythmias,[21] venous thromboembolism,[22] and gastrointestinal (GI) bleeding.[23] *Ischemic-anoxic encephalopathy* results from hypoxemia, hypercapnia, and acidosis.[20] *Dysrhythmias* are precipitated by hypoxemia, acidosis, electrolyte imbalances, and the administration of β_2-agonists and xanthines.[21] Maintaining oxygenation, normalizing electrolytes, and monitoring drug levels help to prevent and treat encephalopathy and dysrhythmias.[20,21] *Venous thromboembolism* (VTE) is precipitated by venous stasis resulting from immobility and can be prevented through the use of graduated compression stockings and low-dose unfractionated heparin or low-molecular-weight (LMW) heparin.[22] GI bleeding can be prevented through the use of histamine (H_2) antagonists, cytoprotective agents, or gastric proton pump inhibitors.[23] In addition, the patient is at risk for the complications associated with an artificial airway, mechanical ventilation, enteral or parenteral nutrition, and peripheral arterial cannulation.

Nursing Management

Nursing management of the patient with ARF incorporates a variety of nursing diagnoses (Box 14-1). Nursing care is directed by the specific etiology of the respiratory failure, although some common interventions are used. **Nursing priorities are directed toward (1) optimizing oxygenation and ventilation, (2) providing comfort and emotional support, (3) maintaining surveillance for complications, and (4) providing patient education.**

Optimizing Oxygenation and Ventilation

Positioning. Positioning of the patient with ARF depends on the type of lung injury and the underlying cause of hypoxemia. For those patients with V/Q mismatching, positioning is used to facilitate better matching of ventilation with perfusion to optimize gas exchange.[24] Because gravity normally facilitates preferential ventilation and perfusion to the dependent areas of the lungs, the best gas exchange would take place in the dependent areas of the lungs.[11] Thus the goal of positioning is to place the least affected area of the patient's lung in the most dependent position. Patients with unilateral lung disease should be positioned with the healthy lung in a *dependent* position.[24,25] Patients with diffuse lung disease may benefit from being positioned with the right lung down, because it is larger and more vascular than the left lung.[25,26] For those patients with alveolar hypoventilation, the goal of positioning is to facilitate ventilation. These patients benefit from *nonrecumbent* positions, such as sitting or a semierect position.[27]

Preventing Desaturation. A number of activities can prevent desaturation, including (1) performing procedures only as needed, (2) hyperoxygenating the patient before suctioning, (3) providing adequate rest and recovery time between various procedures, and (4) minimizing O_2 consumption. Interventions to minimize O_2 consumption include limiting the patient's physical activity, administering sedation to control anxiety, and providing measures to control fever. The patient should be continuously monitored with a pulse oximeter to warn of signs of desaturation.

Promoting Secretion Clearance. Interventions to promote secretion clearance include providing adequate systemic hydration, humidifying supplemental O_2, coughing, and suctioning. Postural drainage and chest percussion and vibration have been found to be of little benefit in the critically ill patient.[28,29]

To facilitate deep breathing, the patient's thorax should be maintained in alignment and the head of the bed elevated at least 30 degrees. This position best accommodates diaphragmatic descent and intercostal muscle action. In addition, semirecumbency has been shown to decrease the risk of aspiration and inhibit the development of nosocomial pneumonia.[30] Frequent repositioning (at least every 2 hours) or continuous lateral rotation therapy is essential because it results in a change in ventilatory pattern and V/Q matching.

Once the patient is extubated, deep breathing and incentive spirometry should be started as soon as possible. *Deep breathing* involves having the patient take a deep breath and hold it for approximately 3 seconds or longer. *Incentive spirometry* involves having the patient take at least 10 deep, effective breaths per hour using an incentive spirometer. These actions help to prevent atelectasis and to reexpand any collapsed lung tissue. The chest should be auscultated during inflation to ensure that all dependent parts of the lung are well ventilated and to help the patient understand the depth of breath necessary for optimal effect. Coughing should be avoided unless secretions are present because it promotes collapse of the smaller airways.

Providing Patient Education

Early in the patient's hospital stay, the patient and family should be taught about ARF, its etiologies, and its treatment. As the patient moves toward discharge, teaching should focus on the interventions necessary for preventing the recurrence of the precipitating disorder. The patient who smokes should be encouraged to stop smoking and be referred to a smoking cessation program. In addition, the importance of participating in a pulmonary rehabilitation program should be stressed.

Box 14-2 COLLABORATIVE Management

Acute Respiratory Failure

1. Identify and treat underlying cause.
2. Administer oxygen therapy.
3. Intubate patient.
4. Initiate mechanical ventilation.
5. Administer medications.
   - Mucolytics
   - Bronchodilators
   - Steriods
   - Sedatives
   - Analgesics
6. Position patient to optimize ventilation/perfusion matching.
7. Suction as needed.
8. Provide adequate rest and recovery time between various procedures.
9. Correct acidosis.
10. Initiate nutritional support.
11. Maintain surveillance for complications.
    - Encephalopathy
    - Cardiac dysrhythmias
    - Venous thromboembolism
    - Gastrointestinal bleeding
12. Provide comfort and emotional support.

Collaborative management of the patient with acute respiratory failure is outlined in Box 14-2.

ACUTE RESPIRATORY DISTRESS SYNDROME

Acute respiratory distress syndrome (ARDS), also and formerly called "adult" respiratory distress styndrome,[31] is the pulmonary manifestion of *multiple organ dysfunction syndrome*.[32] This syndrome is characterized by noncardiac pulmonary edema and disruption of the alveolar-capillary membrane[33] as a result of injury to the pulmonary vasculature or the airways.[34] Many diagnostic criteria have been used to identify ARDS, which has led to confusion, particularly among researchers. In an attempt to standardize the identification of this disorder, the American-European Consensus Committee on ARDS recommended the following criteria be used to diagnose ARDS:

- Acute in onset
- Ratio of partial pressure of oxygen (Pao_2) to fraction of inspired oxygen (Fio_2) less than or equal to 200 mm Hg, regardless of positive end-expiratory pressure (PEEP) level
- Bilateral infiltrates on chest radiography
- Pulmonary artery occlusion pressure (PAOP) of 18 mm Hg or less *or* no clinical evidence of left atrial hypertension.[31]

Etiology

The various clinical conditions associated with development of ARDS are categorized as direct or indirect, depending on the primary site of injury (Box 14-3).[31,33] In *direct* injuries the lung epithelium sustains a direct insult. In *indirect* injuries the insult occurs elsewhere in the body, and mediators are transmitted through the bloodstream to the lungs.[32] Sepsis, aspiration of gastric contents, diffuse pneumonia, and trauma are major risk factors for development of ARDS.[33]

Box 14-3 Risk Factors for Acute Respiratory Distress Syndrome (ARDS)

DIRECT INJURY

Aspiration
Near-drowning
Toxic inhalation
Pulmonary contusion
Pneumonia
Oxygen toxicity
Transthoracic radiation

INDIRECT INJURY

Sepsis
Nonthoracic trauma
Hypertransfusion
Cardiopulmonary bypass (CPB)
Severe pancreatitis
Embolism (air, fat, amniotic fluid)
Disseminated intravascular coagulation (DIC)
Shock states

Pathophysiology

The progression of ARDS can be described in three phases: exudative, proliferative, and fibrotic. ARDS is initiated with stimulation of the inflammatory-immune system as a result of direct or indirect injury (Figure 14-1). Inflammatory mediators are released from the site of injury, resulting in the activation and accumulation of the neutrophils, macrophages, and platelets in the pulmonary capillaries. These cellular mediators initiate the release of humoral mediators.[31,34-36]

Exudative Phase

Approximately 24 hours after the initial insult, the exudative phase ensues.[35,36] Once released, the humoral mediators damage the alveolar-capillary membranes, resulting in increased capillary membrane permeability. This leads to the leakage of fluid filled with protein, blood cells, fibrin, and activated cellular and humoral mediators into the pulmonary interstitium.[35,37] Damage to pulmonary capillaries also results in development of microthrombi and elevation of pulmonary artery pressures.[37] As fluid enters the pulmonary interstitium, the lymphatics are overwhelmed and

unable to drain all the accumulating fluid, resulting in the development of *interstitial* edema.[37] Fluid is then forced from the interstitial space into the alveoli, resulting in *alveolar* edema. Pulmonary interstitial edema also causes compression of the alveoli and small airways. Alveolar edema causes swelling of the type I alveolar epithelial cells and flooding of the alveoli. Protein and fibrin in the edema fluid precipitate the formation of hyaline membranes over the alveoli.[35,37]

Proliferative Phase

After 7 to 10 days the proliferative phase begins as disordered healing starts in the lungs.[38] Type II alveolar epithelial cells multiply and attempt to replace the damaged type I alveolar epithelial cells. Eventually the type II alveolar epithelial cells are also damaged, leading to impaired surfactant production. Injury to the alveolar epithelial cells and the loss of surfactant lead to alveoli collapse.[35,38] Hypoxemia occurs as a result of intrapulmonary shunting and V/Q mismatching secondary to compression, collapse, and flooding of the alveoli and small airways. Increased work of breathing occurs as a result of

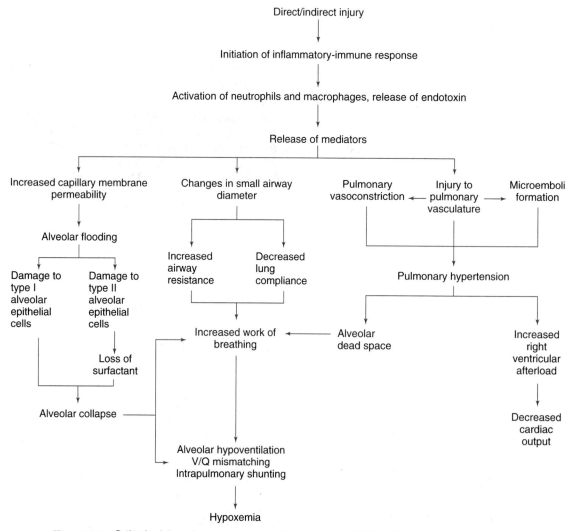

Figure 14-1   Pathophysiology of acute respiratory distress syndrome (ARDS). *V/Q*, Ventilation/perfusion ratio.

increased airway resistance, decreased functional residual capacity (FRC), and decreased lung compliance secondary to atelectasis and compression of the small airways.[35-37] Hypoxemia and the increased work of breathing lead to patient fatigue and the development of alveolar hypoventilation.[35,37] *Pulmonary hypertension* occurs as a result of damage to the pulmonary capillaries, microthrombi, and hypoxic vasoconstriction leading to the development of increased alveolar dead space and right ventricular afterload. Hypoxemia worsens as a result of alveolar hypoventilation and increased alveolar dead space. Right ventricular afterload increases and leads to right ventricular dysfunction and a decrease in cardiac output.[37] This phase of ARDS may last up to a month.[37]

Fibrotic Phase

After 2 to 3 weeks the fibrotic phase commences. Cellular granulation and collagen deposition occur within the alveolar-capillary membrane, resulting in the development of pulmonary fibrosis.[32,37] Structural and vascular remodeling take place as the alveoli become enlarged and irregularly shaped and the pulmonary capillaries become scarred and obliterated. This leads to further stiffening of the lungs, which increases pulmonary hypertension and worsens hypoxemia.[32,39]

Recovery occurs over several weeks, with resolution of the fibrosis and restoration of the alveolar-capillary membrane. Survival of ARDS is directly related to the absence of multiple organ dysfunction syndrome and sepsis.[3]

Assessment and Diagnosis

Initially the patient with ARDS may present with a variety of clinical manifestations, depending on the precipitating event. As the disorder progresses, the patient's signs and symptoms may be associated with the phase of ARDS the patient is experiencing (Table 14-2). During the *exudative* phase the patient presents with tachypnea, restlessness,

Table 14-2   ARDS Phases: Pathophysiology and Patient Examination

Pathophysiology	Physical Examination
EXUDATIVE PHASE	
Parenchymal surface hemorrhage	Restless, apprehensive, tachypneic
Interstitial or alveolar edema	Respiratory alkalosis
Compression of terminal bronchioles	Pao_2 normal
Destruction of type 1 alveolar cells	CXR: normal
	Chest examination: moderate use of accessory muscles; lungs clear
	Elevated PA pressures
	Normal or low PAOP
PROLIFERATIVE PHASE	
Destruction of type 2 alveolar cells	Elevated PA pressures
Gas exchange compromised	Increased workload on right ventricle
Increased peak inspiratory pressure	Increased use of accessory muscles
Decreased compliance (static and dynamic)	Fine crackles or rales
Refractory hypoxemia	Increasing agitation related to hypoxia
• Intraalveolar atelectasis	CXR: interstitial or alveolar infiltrates; elevated diaphragm
• Increased shunt fraction	Hyperventilation, hypercarbia
• Decreased diffusion	Decreased Svo_2
Decreased functional residual capacity	Widening alveolar-arterial gradient
	Increased work of breathing
FIBROTIC PHASE	
Interstitial fibrosis	Worsening hypercarbia and hypoxemia
Increased dead space ventilation	Lactic acidosis (related to aerobic metabolism)
Alteration in perfusion	Increased heart rate
	Decreased blood pressure
	Change in skin temperature and color
	Decreased capillary filling
End-organ dysfunction	*Brain*: Changes in mentation, agitation, hallucinations
	Heart: Decreased CO → angina, congestive heart failure, papillary muscle dysfunction, arrhythmias, and myocardial infarction
	Renal: Decreased urine output and GFR
	Skin: Mottled, ischemic
	Liver: Elevated AST, bilirubin, alkaline phosphatase, and PT/PTT; decreased albumin

From Phillips JK: *Crit Care Clin North Am* 11:233, 1999.
ARDS, Acute respiratory distress syndrome; *Pao_2*, arterial oxygen tension; *CXR*, chest radiograph; *PA*, pulmonary artery; *PAOP*, pulmonary arterial occlusion pressure; *Svo_2*, mixed-venous oxygen saturation; *CO*, cardiac output; *GFR*, glomerular filtration rate; *AST*, serum aspartate transaminase (GOT, glutamic-oxaloacetic transaminase); *PT*, prothrombin time; *PTT*, partial thromboplastin time.

apprehension, and moderate increase in accessory muscle use. During the *proliferative* phase the patient's signs and symptoms progress to agitation, dyspnea, fatigue, excessive accessory muscle use, and fine crackles as respiratory failure develops.[35]

ABG analysis reveals a low PaO_2, despite increases in supplemental O_2 administration (refractory hypoxemia).[35] Initially the $PaCO_2$ is low as a result of hyperventilation but eventually increases as the patient fatigues. The pH is high initially but decreases as respiratory acidosis develops.[35,36]

Initially the chest x-ray film may be normal because changes in the lungs do not become evident for up to 24 hours. As the pulmonary edema becomes apparent, diffuse, patchy interstitial and alveolar infiltrates appear. This progresses to multifocal consolidation of the lungs, which appears as a "white out" on the chest radiograph.[36]

Medical Management

Medical management of the patient with ARDS involves a multifaceted approach. This strategy includes treating the underlying cause, promoting gas exchange, supporting tissue oxygenation, and preventing complications.[32,39] Given the severity of hypoxemia, the patient is intubated and mechanically ventilated to facilitate adequate gas exchange.[40]

Oxygen Therapy

Oxygen is administered at the lowest level possible to support tissue oxygenation. Continued exposure to high O_2 levels can lead to oxygen toxicity, which further perpetuates the entire process. The goal of O_2 therapy is to maintain SaO_2 at 90% or greater using the lowest O_2 level, preferably less than 0.65.[39]

Positive End-Expiratory Pressure

Because the hypoxemia that develops with ARDS is often refractory or unresponsive to oxygen therapy, it is necessary to facilitate oxygenation with PEEP. The purpose of using PEEP in the patient with ARDS is to improve oxygenation while reducing FiO_2 to less toxic levels.[39] PEEP has several positive effects on the lungs, including opening collapsed alveoli, stabilizing flooded alveoli, and increasing FRC. Thus PEEP decreases intrapulmonary shunting and increases compliance.[35] PEEP also has several negative effects, including (1) decreasing cardiac output (CO) as a result of decreasing venous return secondary to increased intrathoracic pressure[35] and (2) volutrauma as a result of gas escaping into the surrounding spaces secondary to alveolar rupture.[32] The amount of PEEP a patient requires is determined by evaluating both SaO_2 and CO. In most cases a PEEP of 10 to 15 cm H_2O is adequate.[39] If too high, PEEP can result in overdistention of the alveoli, which can impede pulmonary capillary blood flow, decrease surfactant production, and worsen intrapulmonary shunting.[38] If too low, PEEP allows the alveoli to collapse during expiration, damaging them further.[41]

Ventilation

Traditionally the patient with ARDS was ventilated with a mode of volume ventilation such as assist/control ventilation (A/CV) or synchronized intermittent mandatory ventilation (SIMV), with tidal volumes adjusted to deliver 10 to 15 ml/kg. Current research now indicates that this approach may have actually led to further lung injury. It is now known that repeated opening and closing of the alveoli causes injury to the lung units (*atelectrauma*), resulting in inhibited surfactant production, and increased inflammation (*biotrauma*), resulting in the release of mediators and an increase in pulmonary capillary membrane permeability.[32] In addition, overdistention of the alveoli (*volutrauma*) leads to excessive alveolar wall stress and damage to the alveolar-capillary membrane, resulting in air escaping into the surrounding spaces.[32,42] Thus several different approaches have been developed to facilitate the mechanical ventilation of the patient with ARDS.

Permissive Hypercapnia. The permissive hypercapnia approach to mechanical ventilation uses smaller tidal volumes (5 to 8 ml/kg) to ventilate the patient, in an attempt to limit the effects of volutrauma, in conjunction with normal respiratory rates, in an attempt to limit the effects of atelectrauma and biotrauma. Normally the patient's respiratory rate would have to be increased to compensate for the small tidal volume to maintain normocapnia. In ARDS, however, increasing the respiratory rate can lead to worsening alveolar damage and should be avoided. Thus the patient's CO_2 level is allowed to rise, and the patient becomes hypercapnic. As a general rule, the patient's $PaCO_2$ should not rise faster than 10 mm Hg per hour and overall should not exceed 80 to 100 mg Hg. Because of the negative cardiopulmonary effects of severe acidosis, the arterial pH is generally maintained at 7.20 or greater. To maintain the pH, the patient is given intravenous sodium bicarbonate, or the respiratory rate and tidal volume are increased.[40,42,43] Permissive hypercapnia is contraindicated in patients with increased intracranial pressure, pulmonary hypertension, seizures, and cardiac failure.[38]

Pressure Control Ventilation. In pressure control ventilation (PCV) mode, each breath is delivered or augmented with a preset amount of inspiratory pressure as opposed to tidal volume, which is used in volume ventilation. Thus the actual tidal volume the patient receives varies from breath to breath. PCV is used to limit and control the amount of pressure in the lungs and decrease the incidence of volutrauma. The goal is to keep the patient's plateau pressure (end-inspiratory static pressure) less than 30 to 40 cm H_2O.[39] A known problem with PCV is that as the patient's lungs become stiffer, it becomes more and more difficult to maintain an adequate tidal volume, and severe hypercapnia may occur.[40]

Inverse Ratio Ventilation. Another alternative ventilatory mode used in managing the patient with ARDS is inverse ratio ventilation (IRV), either pressure controlled or volume controlled. IRV prolongs the inspiratory (I) time and shortens the expiratory (E) time, thus reversing the normal I/E ratio.[42] The goal of IRV is to maintain a more constant mean airway pressure throughout the ventilatory cycle, which helps keep alveoli open and participating in gas exchange. It also increases FRC and decreases the work of breathing. In addition, as the breath is delivered over a longer period, the peak inspiratory pressure in the lungs is decreased.[40] A major disadvantage to IRV is the development of auto-PEEP. As the expiratory phase of ventilation is shortened, air can become trapped in the lower airways, creating unintentional PEEP (auto-PEEP), which can cause hemodynamic compromise and worsening gas exchange. Patients on IRV usually require heavy sedation and neuromuscular blockade to prevent them from fighting the ventilator.[40]

Tissue Perfusion

Adequate tissue perfusion depends on an adequate supply of oxygen being transported to the tissues. An adequate CO and hemoglobin level is critical to oxygen transport. CO depends on heart rate, preload, afterload, and contractility. A variety of fluids and medications are used to manipulate this parameter. Newer approaches to fluid management include maintaining a very low intravascular volume (PAOP 5 to 8 mm Hg) with fluid restriction and diuretics while supporting CO with vasoactive and inotropic medications. The goal is to decrease the amount of fluid leakage into the lungs.[39]

Nursing Management

Nursing management of the patient with ARDS incorporates a variety of nursing diagnoses (Box 14-4). **Nursing priorities are directed toward (1) optimizing oxygenation and ventilation, (2) providing comfort and emotional support, and (3) maintaining surveillance for complications.**

Optimizing Oxygenation and Ventilation

Nursing interventions to optimize oxygenation and ventilation include positioning, preventing desaturation, and promoting secretion clearance (see Nursing Management of ARF).

Prone Positioning. A number of studies have shown that prone positioning for the patient with ARDS results in an improvement in oxygenation.[44] Although several theories propose how prone positioning improves oxygenation, the discovery that ARDS causes greater damage to the dependent areas of the lungs probably provides the best explanation. It was originally thought that ARDS was a diffuse homogenous disease that affected all areas of the lungs equally. It is now known that the dependent lung areas are more heavily damaged than the nondependent lung areas. Turning the patient prone improves perfusion to less damaged parts of lungs and improves V/Q matching and decreases intrapulmonary shunting.[26,40] Prone positioning appears to be more effective when initiated during the early phases of ARDS.[45]

Collaborative management of the patient with ARDS is outlined in Box 14-5.

PNEUMONIA

Pneumonia is an acute inflammation of the lung parenchyma that is caused by an infectious agent that can lead to alveolar consolidation. Pneumonia can be classified as

---

nursing diagnosis
priorities   Box **14-4**

Acute Respiratory Distress Syndrome (ARDS)

- Impaired Gas Exchange related to ventilation/perfusion mismatching or intrapulmonary shunting
- Decreased Cardiac Output related to alterations in preload
- Imbalanced Nutrition: Less than Body Requirements related to lack of exogenous nutrients or increased metabolic demand
- Anxiety related to threat to biologic, psychologic, and/or social integrity
- Compromised Family Coping related to critically ill family member

---

Box **14-5** COLLABORATIVE Management

Acute Respiratory Distress Syndrome (ARDS)

1. Administer oxygen therapy.
2. Intubate patient.
3. Initiate mechanical ventilation.
   - Permissive hypercapnia
   - Pressure control ventilation
   - Inverse ratio ventilation
4. Utilize positive end-expiratory pressure (PEEP).
5. Administer medications.
   - Bronchodilators
   - Sedatives
   - Analgesics
   - Neuromuscular blocking agents
6. Maximize cardiac output.
   - Preload
   - Afterload
   - Contractility
7. Position patient prone.
8. Suction as needed.
9. Provide adequate rest and recovery time between various procedures.
10. Initiate nutritional support.
11. Maintain surveillance for complications.
    - Encephalopathy
    - Cardiac dysrhythmias
    - Venous thromboembolism
    - Gastrointestinal bleeding
    - Atelectrauma
    - Biotrauma
    - Volutrauma
    - Oxygen toxicity
12. Provide comfort and emotional support.

community-acquired pneumonia (CAP) or hospital-acquired (nosocomial) pneumonia (HAP). CAP is acquired outside the hospital.[46,47] Severe CAP is pneumonia requiring admission to the intensive care unit and accounts for about 10% of all patients with pneumonia.[47] HAP, or *nosocomial pneumonia*, is acquired inside the hospital and is usually much more serious than CAP because many of the causative agents are resistant to conventional antibiotic therapy.[48,49] *Ventilator-associated pneumonia* (VAP) is a subgroup of HAP that refers to an infection developing during mechanical ventilation later than 48 hours after intubation. VAP has an average incidence of 20% to 25%.[49]

Etiology

The spectra of etiologic pathogens of pneumonia vary with the type of pneumonia, as do the risk factors for the disease.

Severe Community-Acquired Pneumonia

Pathogens that can cause severe CAP include *Streptococcus pneumoniae*, *Haemophilus influenzae*, *Moraxella catarrhalis*, *Legionella*, *Klebsiella pneumoniae*, *Staphylococcus aureus*, *Mycoplasma pneumoniae*, *Chlamydia pneumoniae*, and *Pseudomonas aeruginosa*.[46,47] A number of factors determine the severity of CAP. Bacterial factors include the size of the pathogen inoculum and virulence of the organism. Pulmonary factors include multilobar involvement, underlying lung disease, and pulmonary neoplasm. Systemic factors include advanced age, compromised host, and presence of congestive heart failure (CHF) or hepatic/renal insufficiency.[46]

Hospital-Acquired Pneumonia

Nosocomial pneumonia is usually caused by *P. aeruginosa* or *S. aureus* (two pathogens most frequently associated with VAP[48]), *K. pneumoniae*, *Escherichia coli*, *Serratia marcescens*, and *Enterobacter* species.[49] Risk factors are associated with the host, devices, and personnel or the procedure. Host-related factors include age greater than 65 years, underlying illness (e.g., chronic obstructive pulmonary disease [COPD], immunosuppression, diabetes), alcoholism, smoking, depressed consciousness, malnutrition, and thoracoabdominal surgery. Device-related factors include endotracheal intubation, mechanical ventilation, and gastric intubation with enteral feedings. Personnel/procedure-related factors include cross-contamination by hands, infected personnel, antibiotic therapy, histamine blockers, antacid therapy, and enteral feedings.[50]

Pathophysiology

Development of acute pneumonia implies a defect in host defenses, a particularly virulent organism, or an overwhelming inoculation event. A number of conditions predispose a patient to developing pneumonia, including depressed gag and cough reflexes, decreased ciliary activity, increased secretions, decreased lymphatic flow, atelectasis, fluid in the alveoli, immunologic defect, and impaired alveolar macrophages[51] (Table 14-3).

Bacterial invasion of the lower respiratory tract can occur by (1) inhalation of aerosolized infectious particles, (2) aspiration of organisms colonizing the oropharynx, (3) migration from adjacent sites or colonization, (4) direct inoculation of organisms into the lower airway, (5) spread of infection to the lungs from adjacent structures, (6) spread of infection to the lung through the blood, and (7) reactivation of latent infection (usually in the setting of immunosuppression). The most common mechanism appears to be aspiration of oropharyngeal organisms.[52]

Colonization of the patient's oropharynx with infectious organisms is a major contributor to the development of nosocomial pneumonia (Figure 14-2). Normally the oropharynx has a stable population of resident flora that may be anaerobic or aerobic. When stress occurs, as with illness, surgery, or

Table **14-3** Precipitating Conditions in Pneumonia	
Condition	**Etiologies**
Depressed epiglottal/cough reflexes	Unconsciousness, neurologic disease, tracheal/endotracheal tubes, anesthesia, aging
Decreased ciliary activity	Smoke inhalation, smoking history, oxygen toxicity, hypoventilation, intubation, viral infections, aging, COPD
Increased secretion	COPD, viral infections, bronchiectasis, general anesthesia, endotracheal intubation, smoking
Atelectasis	Trauma, foreign body obstruction, tumor, splinting, shallow ventilation, general anesthesia
Decreased lymphatic flow	Heart failure, tumor
Fluid in alveoli	Heart failure, aspiration, trauma
Abnormal phagocytosis and humoral activity	Neutropenia, immunocompetent disorders, chemotherapy
Impaired alveolar macrophages	Hypoxemia, metabolic acidosis, smoking history, hypoxia, alcohol use, viral infections, aging

COPD, Chronic obstructive pulmonary disease.

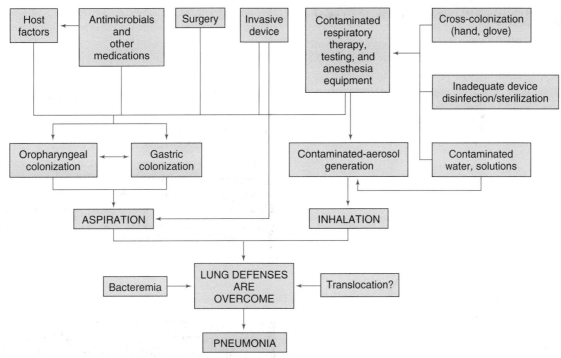

Figure 14-2   Pathophysiology of pneumonia. (From Tablan OC et al: *Am J Infect Contr* 22:247, 1994.)

infection, pathogenic organisms replace normal resident flora. Previous antibiotic therapy also affects the resident flora population, making replacement by pathologic organisms more likely. The pathogens are then able to invade the sterile lower respiratory tract. Disruption of the gag and cough reflexes, altered consciousness, abnormal swallowing, and artificial airways all predispose the patient to aspiration and colonization of the lungs and subsequent infection. Histamine blockers, antacids, and enteral feedings also contribute to this problem because they raise the pH of the stomach and promote bacterial overgrowth. The nasogastric tube then acts as a wick, facilitating the movement of bacteria from the stomach to the pharynx, where the bacteria can be aspirated.[48,53]

Infection results in pulmonary inflammation with or without significant exudates. Increased capillary permeability occurs with increased interstitial and alveolar fluid. V/Q mismatching and intrapulmonary shunting occur, resulting in hypoxemia as lung consolidation progresses. Untreated pneumonia can result in ARF and initiation of the inflammatory immune response. The patient may develop a pleural effusion, the result of the vascular response to inflammation, whereby capillary permeability is increased and fluid from the pulmonary capillaries diffuses into the pleural space.[51]

Assessment and Diagnosis

The clinical manifestations of pneumonia will vary with the offending pathogen. The patient may present with a variety of signs and symptoms, including dyspnea, fever, chills, cough (productive or nonproductive), purulent sputum, and crackles on auscultation.[47]

Chest radiography is used to evaluate the patient with suspected pneumonia. The diagnosis is established by the presence of a new pulmonary infiltrate. The radiographic pattern of the infiltrates will vary with the organism.[54] A sputum Gram stain and culture are done to facilitate the identification of the infectious pathogen. If the sputum culture fails to identify the offending organism, serology testing is conducted. Complete blood count with differential, chemistry panel, blood cultures, and ABGs are obtained.[55]

Medical Management

Medical management of the patient with pneumonia includes antibiotic therapy, oxygen therapy for hypoxemia, mechanical ventilation if ARF develops, fluid management for hydration, nutritional support, and treatment of associated medical problems and complications. For patients having difficulty mobilizing secretions, mucolytics and therapeutic bronchoscopy may be necessary.

Antibiotic Therapy

Although bacteria-specific antibiotic therapy is the goal, this may not always be possible because of difficulties in identifying the organism and the seriousness of the patient's condition. The time involved obtaining cultures should be balanced against the need to begin some treatment based on the patient's condition. Empiric therapy has become the accepted approach; choice of antibiotic treatment is based on the most likely etiologic organism while avoiding toxicity, superinfection, and unnecessary cost. If available, Gram stain results should be used to guide antibiotic choices. Antibiotics should be chosen that offer broad coverage of the usual pathogens in the hospital or community. Failure to respond to such therapy may indicate that the chosen antibiotic regimen does not appropriately cover all the etiologic pathogens or that a new source of infection has developed. Antibiotics are continued for 10 to 14 days.[47]

Independent Lung Ventilation

In patients with unilateral pneumonia or severely asymmetric pneumonia, this alternative mode of mechanical ventilation may be necessary to facilitate oxygenation. As the alveoli in the affected lung become flooded with pus, the lung becomes less compliant and difficult to ventilate. This results in a shifting of ventilation to the good lung without a concomitant shift in perfusion and thus an increase in V/Q mismatching. Independent lung ventilation (ILV) allows each lung to be ventilated separately, thus controlling the amount of flow, volume, and pressure each lung receives. A double-lumen ETT is inserted, and each lumen is usually attached to a separate mechanical ventilator. The ventilator settings are then customized to the needs of each lung to facilitate optimal oxygenation and ventilation.[56]

Nursing Management

Nursing management of the patient with pneumonia incorporates a variety of nursing diagnoses (Box 14-6). **Nursing priorities are directed toward (1) optimizing oxygenation and ventilation, (2) preventing the spread of infection, (3) providing comfort and emotional support, and (4) maintaining surveillance for complications.** In addition, the patient's response to the antibiotic therapy should be monitored for adverse effects.

Optimizing Oxygenation and Ventilation

Nursing interventions to optimize oxygenation and ventilation include positioning, preventing desaturation, and promoting secretion clearance (see Nursing Management of ARF).

Preventing Spread of Infection

Prevention should be directed at eradicating pathogens from the environment and interrupting the spread of organisms from person to person. Significant progress has been made in removing contaminants from the patient environment through proper disinfection of respiratory equipment and increased use of disposable supplies. Other possible environmental sources of pathogens include suctioning equipment and indwelling lines. These invasive tools must be given proper aseptic care.

Proper handwashing technique is the primary measure available to prevent the spread of bacteria from person to person. In addition, meticulous oral care, including suctioning of the secretions pooling above the cuff of the artificial airway, is critical to decreasing the bacterial colonization of the oropharynx.[50]

Collaborative management of the patient with pneumonia is outlined in Box 14-7.

ASPIRATION LUNG DISORDER

The presence of abnormal substances in the airways and alveoli as a result of aspiration is misleadingly called "aspiration pneumonia" because the aspiration of toxic substances into the lung may or may not involve an infection. *Aspiration lung disorder* is more accurate because injury to the lung can result from the chemical, mechanical, or bacterial characteristics of the aspirate.

Etiology

A number of factors have been identified that place the patient at risk for aspiration (Box 14-8). Gastric contents and oropharyngeal bacteria (see Pneumonia) are the most common aspirates of the critically ill patient.[57] The effects of gastric contents on the lungs will vary based on the pH of the liquid. If pH is less than 2.5, the patient will develop a severe chemical pneumonitis, resulting in hypoxemia.[58] If

---

nursing diagnosis priorities   Box **14-6**

Pneumonia
- Ineffective Airway Clearance related to excessive secretions or abnormal viscosity of mucus
- Impaired Gas Exchange related to ventilation/perfusion mismatching or intrapulmonary shunting
- Risk for Infection Risk Factor: invasive monitoring devices
- Powerlessness related to lack of control over current situation or disease progression

---

Box **14-7** COLLABORATIVE Management

Pneumonia
1. Administer oxygen therapy.
2. Initiate mechanical ventilation as required.
3. Administer medications.
   - Antibiotics
   - Mucolytics
   - Bronchodilators
4. Position patient to optimize ventilation/perfusion matching.
5. Suction as needed.
6. Provide adequate rest and recovery time between various procedures.
7. Maintain surveillance for complications.
   - Acute respiratory failure
8. Provide comfort and emotional support.

Altered level of consciousness
Depressed gag, cough, or swallowing reflex
Presence of feeding tubes (all types)
Presence of artificial airways
Ileus or gastric distention
History of gastrointestinal disorders
• Dysphagia
• Achalasia
• Gastroesophageal reflux disease
• Esophageal strictures

pH is greater than 2.5, the immediate damage to the lungs is reduced,[58] but the elevated pH may have promoted bacterial overgrowth of the stomach.[50] Once the bacteria-laden gastric contents are aspirated into the lungs, overwhelming bacterial pneumonia can develop.[48]

Pathophysiology

The type of lung injury that develops after aspiration is determined by such factors as quality of the aspirate and status of the patient's respiratory defense mechanisms.

Acid Liquid

Aspiration of acid (pH less than 2.5) liquid gastric contents results in the development of bronchospasm and atelectasis almost immediately. Over the next 4 hours, tracheal damage, bronchitis, bronchiolitis, alveolar-capillary breakdown, interstitial edema, and alveolar congestion and hemorrhage occur. Severe hypoxemia develops as a result of intrapulmonary shunting and V/Q mismatching. As the disorder progresses, necrotic debris and fibrin fill the alveoli, hyaline membranes form, and hypoxic vasoconstriction occurs, resulting in elevated pulmonary artery pressures.[58] The clinical course will follow one of three patterns: (1) rapid improvement in 1 week, (2) initial improvement followed by deterioration and development of ARDS or pneumonia, or (3) rapid death from progressive ARF.[57,58]

Acid Food Particles

Aspiration of acid nonobstructing food particles can produce the most severe pulmonary reaction because of extensive pulmonary damage. Severe hypoxemia, hypercapnia, and acidosis occur.[58]

Nonacid Liquid

Aspiration of nonacid (pH greater than 2.5) liquid gastric contents is similar to acid liquid aspiration initially, but with minimal structural damage. Intrapulmonary shunting and V/Q mismatching usually start to reverse within 4 hours, and hypoxemia clears within 24 hours.[57]

Nonacid Food Particles

Aspiration of nonacid nonobstructing food particles is similar to acid aspiration initially, with significant edema and hemorrhage occurring within 6 hours. After the initial reaction, the response changes to a foreign body–type reaction with granuloma formation around the food particles in 1 to 5 days. In addition to hypoxemia, hypercapnia and acidosis result from hypoventilation.[58]

Assessment and Diagnosis

The patient with aspiration lung disorder presents clinically with signs of acute respiratory distress, and gastric contents may be present in the oropharynx. The patient has shortness of breath, coughing, wheezing, cyanosis, and signs of hypoxemia. Tachypnea, tachycardia, hypotension, fever, and crackles also are present. Copious amounts of sputum are produced as alveolar edema develops.[57,58]

ABGs reflect severe hypoxemia. Chest radiograph changes appear 12 to 24 hours after the initial aspiration, with no pattern diagnostic of the event. Infiltrates will appear in a variety of distribution patterns depending on the position of the patient during aspiration and the volume of the aspirate. Established bacterial infection results in leukocytosis and positive sputum cultures.[57]

Medical Management

Management of the patient with aspiration lung disorder includes both emergency and follow-up treatment. When aspiration is witnessed, emergency treatment should be instituted to secure the airway and minimize pulmonary damage. The patient should be placed in a slight (6 to 8 inches head-down) Trendelenburg position and turned to the right lateral decubitus position to aid drainage and avoid involvement of other lung areas. Oropharyngeal suctioning should immediately follow.[59] Direct visualization by bronchoscopy is indicated to remove large particulate aspirate or to confirm an unwitnessed aspiration event. Bronchoalveolar lavage is not recommended because this practice disseminates the aspirate in lungs and increases damage. Prophylactic antibiotics are not recommended as well.[58]

After airway clearance, attention should be given to supporting oxygenation and hemodynamics. Hypoxemia should be corrected with supplemental O_2 or mechanical ventilation with PEEP, if necessary. Hemodynamic changes result from fluid shifts that can occur after massive aspirations, causing noncardiogenic pulmonary edema. Monitoring intravascular volume is essential, and judicious fluid replacement should maintain adequate urine output and vital signs.[57,58]

Nursing Management

Nursing management of the patient with aspiration lung disorder incorporates a variety of nursing diagnoses (Box 14-9). **Nursing priorities are directed toward (1) optimizing oxygenation and ventilation, (2) preventing further aspiration**

Aspiration Lung Disorder

- Impaired Gas Exchange related to ventilation/perfusion mismatching or intrapulmonary shunting
- Ineffective Airway Clearance related to excessive secretions or abnormal viscosity of mucus
- Risk for Aspiration
- Risk for Infection
- Ineffective Coping related to situational crisis and personal vulnerability

events, (3) **providing comfort and emotional support**, and (4) **maintaining surveillance for complications**.

Optimizing Oxygenation and Ventilation

Nursing interventions to optimize oxygenation and ventilation include positioning, preventing desaturation, and promoting secretion clearance (see Nursing Management of ARF).

Preventing Aspiration

One of the most important interventions for preventing aspiration is identifying the patient at risk for aspiration. Actions to prevent aspiration include confirming feeding tube placement, checking for signs and symptoms of feeding intolerance and aspiration of gastric contents into lungs, elevating the head of the bed at least 30 degrees or turning the patient on the right side if remaining flat is essential, ensuring proper inflation of artificial airway cuffs, and frequent suctioning of the oropharynx of an intubated patient to prevent secretions from pooling above the cuff of the tube.[60]

Collaborative management of the patient with aspiration lung disorder is outlined in Box 14-10.

PULMONARY EMBOLISM

A pulmonary embolism (PE) occurs when a clot (thrombotic emboli) or other matter (nonthrombotic emboli) lodges in the pulmonary arterial (PA) system, disrupting the blood flow to a region of the lungs. The majority of thrombotic emboli arise from the deep leg veins, particularly the iliac, femoral, and popliteal veins. Other sources include the right ventricle, upper extremities, and pelvic veins. Nonthrombotic emboli arise from fat, tumors, amniotic fluid, air, and foreign bodies.[61] This section focuses on thrombotic emboli.

Etiology

A number of predisposing factors and precipitating conditions put a patient at risk for developing a PE (Box 14-11).

Box **14-11** **Risk Factors for Pulmonary Thromboembolism**

PREDISPOSING FACTORS

Venous Stasis
Atrial fibrillation
Decreased cardiac output (CO)
Immobility

Injury to Vascular Endothelium
Local vessel injury
Infection
Incision
Atherosclerosis

Hypercoagulability
Polycythemia

PRECIPITATING CONDITIONS
Previous pulmonary embolism

Cardiovascular Disease
Congestive heart failure
Right ventricular infarction
Cardiomyopathy
Cor pulmonale

Surgery
Orthopedic
Vascular
Abdominal

Cancer
Ovarian
Pancreatic
Stomach
Extrahepatic bile duct system

Trauma (Injury or Burns)
Lower extremities
Pelvis
Hips

Gynecologic Status
Pregnancy
Postpartum
Oral contraceptives
Estrogen replacement therapy

Box **14-10** **COLLABORATIVE** Management

Aspiration Lung Disorder

1. Administer oxygen therapy.
2. Secure the patient's airway.
3. Place patient in slight Trendelenburg position.
4. Turn patient to right lateral decubitus position.
5. Suction patient's oropharyngeal area.
6. Initiate mechanical ventilation as required.
7. Maintain surveillance for complications.
   - Pneumonia
   - Acute respiratory failure
   - Acute respiratory distress syndrome
8. Provide comfort and emotional support.

Of the three predisposing factors—hypercoagulability, injury to vascular endothelium, and venous stasis (Virchow's triad)—venous stasis appears to be the most significant.[62]

Pathophysiology

A massive PE occurs with the blockage of a lobar or larger artery, resulting in occlusion of more than 40% of the pulmonary vascular bed. Blockage of the PA system has both pulmonary and hemodynamic consequences. Pulmonary effects include increased alveolar dead space, bronchoconstriction, and compensatory shunting. The hemodynamic effects include an increase in pulmonary vascular resistance (PVR) and right ventricular workload.[63]

Increased Dead Space

Alveolar dead space increases because an area of the lung is receiving ventilation without being perfused. The ventilation to this area is known as *wasted ventilation* because it does not participate in gas exchange. This effect leads to alveolar dead space ventilation and an increase in the work of breathing. To limit the amount of dead space ventilation, localized bronchoconstriction occurs.[61,63]

Bronchoconstriction

Bronchoconstriction develops as a result of alveolar hypocarbia, hypoxia, and the release of mediators. *Alveolar hypocarbia* results from decreased CO_2 in the affected area and leads to constriction of the local airways, increased airway resistance, and redistribution of ventilation to perfused areas of the lungs. A variety of mediators are released from the site of injury, either from the clot or the surrounding lung tissue, which further causes constriction of the airways.[61,63] Bronchoconstriction promotes the development of atelectasis.[61]

Compensatory Shunting

Compensatory shunting occurs as a result of the unaffected areas of the lungs having to accommodate the entire CO. This creates a situation in which perfusion exceeds ventilation and blood is returned to the left side of the heart without participating in gas exchange. This leads to the development of hypoxemia.[61,63]

Hemodynamic Consequences

The major hemodynamic consequence of a PE is the development of pulmonary hypertension, which is part of the effect of a mechanical obstruction when more than 50% of the vascular bed is occluded. In addition, the mediators released at the injury site and the development of hypoxia cause pulmonary vasoconstriction, which further exacerbates pulmonary hypertension. As PVR increases, so does the workload of the right ventricle, as reflected by a rise in PA pressures. Consequently, right ventricular failure occurs, which can lead to a decrease in left ventricular preload, CO, and blood pressure, leading to shock.[61,63]

Assessment and Diagnosis

The patient with PE may have various presenting symptoms; dyspnea, pleuritic chest pain, and cough are most common. Additional symptoms may include palpitations, apprehension, leg swelling, diaphoresis, hemoptysis, nonpleuritic chest pain, wheezing, and syncope. The most common physical signs include tachypnea, rales, and tachycardia. Additional signs may include increased pulmonic component of the second heart sound, fever, right ventricular lift, pleural friction rub, and cyanosis.[64]

Initial laboratory studies and diagnostic procedures may include ABG analysis, electrocardiogram (ECG), and chest radiography. ABGs may show low PaO_2 (hypoxemia), low $PaCO_2$ (hypocarbia), and high pH (respiratory alkalosis). Hypocarbia with resulting respiratory alkalosis is caused by tachypnea.[65] Common ECG findings include sinus tachycardia[65] and T-wave inversion in leads V_1 to V_4.[61] The classic findings of P pulmonale (S wave in lead I, Q wave with inverted T wave in lead III) are seen in fewer than 15% of the patients.[61] Chest x-ray findings vary from normal to abnormal and are of little value in confirming the presence of a PE. Abnormal findings include enlargement of the right descending pulmonary artery (Palla sign), a wedge-shaped density above the diaphragm (Hampton hump),[61] and the presence of atelectasis and small pleural effusions.[65]

Differentiating a PE from other illnesses can be difficult because many clinical manifestations of PE are found in other disorders.[65] Thus other tests may be necessary, including V/Q scan, pulmonary angiogram, and deep vein thrombosis (DVT) studies.[61,65] In patients with underlying pulmonary conditions that are likely to affect the results of a V/Q scan, spiral computed tomography (CT) may be substituted.[66] A definitive diagnosis of a PE requires confirmation by a high-probability V/Q scan, positive pulmonary angiogram, or strong clinical suspicion coupled with abnormal findings on lower extremity DVT studies.[65]

Medical Management

Medical management of the patient with PE involves both prevention and treatment strategies. Prevention strategies include the use of prophylactic anticoagulation with low-dose or adjusted-dose heparin, LMW heparin, and oral anticoagulants. The use of graduated compression stockings and intermittent pneumatic leg compression have also been demonstrated as effective methods of prophylaxis in low-risk patients.[67]

Treatment strategies include preventing the recurrence of a PE, administering thrombolytic therapy, reversing the effects of pulmonary hypertension, promoting gas exchange, and preventing complications. Medical interventions to promote gas exchange include supplemental O_2, intubation, and mechanical ventilation.

Interventions to prevent PE recurrence include administration of unfractionated or LMW heparin and warfarin (Coumadin) and interruption of the inferior vena cava (IVC). Heparin is administered to prevent further clots from forming and has no effect on the existing clot. The heparin should be adjusted to maintain the activated partial thromboplastin time (aPTT) in the range of 1.5 to 2.5 times control.[62,68] Warfarin should be started at the same time, and when the international normalized ratio (INR) reaches 3.0, the heparin should be discontinued. The patient should receive warfarin for 3 to 6 months. Interruption of the IVC is reserved for patients in whom anticoagulation is contraindicated. The procedure involves placement of a percutaneous venous filter (e.g., Greenfield filter) into the IVC, usually below the renal arteries. The filter prevents further thrombotic emboli from migrating into the lungs.[61,68]

Definitive actions are directed at treating the current PE and include the administration of thrombolytic agents. Measures to correct the hypoxemia include supplemental O_2 and intubation and mechanical ventilation.

The administration of thrombolytic agents in the treatment of PE has had limited success. Currently, thrombolytic therapy is reserved for the patient with a massive PE and concomitant hemodynamic instability, although that criterion is broadening. Either recombinant tissue-type plasminogen activator (rt-PA) or streptokinase may be used. The therapeutic window for using thrombolytic therapy is 14 days.[61,69]

To reverse the hemodynamic effects of pulmonary hypertension, additional measures may be taken. These include the administration of inotropic agents and fluid. Fluids should be administered to increase right ventricular preload, which would stretch the right ventricle and increase contractility, thus overcoming the elevated PA pressures. Inotropic agents also can be used to increase contractility to facilitate an increase in CO.[61]

Nursing Management

Prevention of PE should be a major nursing focus because most critically ill patients are at risk for PE. Nursing actions are aimed at preventing the development of DVT, which is a major complication of immobility and a leading cause of PE. These measures include the use of antiembolic and pneumatic compression stockings, elevation of the legs, active/passive range of motion (ROM) exercises, adequate hydration, and progressive ambulation. Patients at risk should be routinely assessed for signs of a DVT, specifically, deep calf pain (Homans sign), calf tenderness, or redness.[61]

Nursing management of the patient with a PE incorporates a variety of nursing diagnoses (Box 14-12). **Nursing priorities are directed toward (1) optimizing oxygenation and ventilation, (2) monitoring for bleeding, (3) providing comfort and emotional support, (4) maintaining surveillance for complications, and (5) providing patient education.**

Optimizing Oxygenation and Ventilation

Nursing interventions to optimize oxygenation and ventilation include positioning, preventing desaturation, and promoting secretion clearance (see Nursing Management of ARF).

Monitoring for Bleeding

The patient receiving anticoagulant or thrombolytic therapy should be observed for signs of bleeding. The patient's gums, skin, urine, stool, and emesis should be screened for signs of overt or covert bleeding. In addition, monitoring the patient's INR or aPTT is critical to managing the anticoagulation therapy.

Providing Patient Education

Early in the patient's hospital stay, the patient and family should be taught about PE and its causes and treatment. As the patient moves toward discharge, teaching should focus on the interventions necessary for preventing the recurrence of deep vein thrombosis and subsequent emboli, signs and symptoms of deep vein thrombosis and anticoagulant complications, and measures to prevent bleeding. The patient who smokes should be encouraged to stop smoking and should be referred to a smoking cessation program.

Collaborative management of the patient with PE is outlined in Box 14-13.

STATUS ASTHMATICUS

Asthma is a chronic obstructive pulmonary disease characterized by partially reversible airflow obstruction, airway inflammation, and airway hyperresponsiveness (AHR) to a variety of stimuli.[70] Status asthmaticus is a severe asthma attack that fails to respond to conventional therapy with bronchodilators, which may result in ARF.[71]

Etiology

The precipitating cause of the asthmatic attack is usually an upper respiratory infection, allergen exposure, or a reduction in antiinflammatory medications. Other factors include overreliance on bronchodilators, environmental pollutants, lack of access to health care, failure to identify worsening airflow obstruction, and noncompliance with the health care regimen.[72]

Pathophysiology

An asthma attack is initiated when exposure to an irritant or trigger occurs, resulting in the initiation of the inflammatory immune response in the airways. Bronchospasm occurs along with increased vascular permeability and increased mucus production. Mucosal edema and thick, tenacious mucus further increase airway responsiveness. The combination of bronchospasm, airway inflammation, and AHR results in narrowing of the airways and airflow obstruction.[70,71] These changes have significant effects on the pulmonary and cardiovascular systems.

Pulmonary Effects

As the diameter of the airways decreases, airway resistance increases, resulting in increased residual volume, hyperinflation of the lungs, increased work of breathing, and abnormal distribution of ventilation. V/Q mismatching occurs, which results in hypoxemia. Alveolar dead space increases with hypoxic vasoconstriction, resulting in hypercapnia.[70]

Cardiovascular Effects

Inspiratory muscle force increases in an attempt to ventilate the hyperinflated lungs, resulting in a significant increase in negative intrapleural pressure. This leads to an increase in venous return and pooling of blood in the right ventricle. The stretched right ventricle causes the intraventricular septum to shift, thereby impinging on the left ventricle. In addition, the left ventricle has to work harder to pump blood from the highly negative pressure in the thorax to elevated pressure in the systemic circulation. This leads to a decrease in CO and a fall in systolic blood pressure on inspiration (*pulsus paradoxus*).[72]

Assessment and Diagnosis

Initially the patient may present with a cough, wheezing, and dyspnea. As the attack continues, the patient develops tachypnea, tachycardia, diaphoresis, increased accessory muscle use, and pulsus paradoxus of 18 mm Hg or greater.

Decreased level of consciousness, inability to speak, significantly diminished or absent breath sounds, and inability to lie supine herald onset of ARF.[73]

Initial ABGs indicate hypocapnia and respiratory alkalosis caused by hyperventilation. As the attack continues and the patient starts to fatigue, hypoxemia and hypercapnia develop. Lactic acidosis may result from lactate overproduction by the respiratory muscles. The end result is the development of respiratory and metabolic acidosis.[71]

Deterioration of pulmonary function tests despite aggressive bronchodilator therapy is diagnostic of status asthmaticus and indicates the potential need for intubation. A peak expiratory flow rate (PEFR) less than 40% of predicted[71] or forced expiratory volume in 1 second (FEV$_1$) less than 20% of predicted[72] indicates severe airflow obstruction, and the need for intubation with mechanical ventilation may be imminent.

Medical Management

Medical management of the patient with status asthmaticus is directed toward supporting oxygenation and ventilation. Bronchodilators, corticosteroids, oxygen therapy, and intubation and mechanical ventilation are the mainstays of therapy.

Bronchodilators

Inhaled β$_2$-agonists and anticholinergics are the bronchodilators of choice for status asthmaticus. β$_2$-Agonists promote bronchodilation and can be administered by nebulizer or metered-dose inhaler (MDI). Larger and more frequent doses usually are given, and the drug is titrated to the patient's response. Anticholinergics that inhibit bronchoconstriction are not very effective alone, but in combination with β$_2$-agonists, anticholinergics have a synergistic effect and produce a greater improvement in airflow. The routine use of xanthines is not recommended in the treatment of status asthmaticus because xanthines have not been shown to have therapeutic benefit.[71-73]

Corticosteroids

In treatment of status asthmaticus, systemic corticosteroids have antiinflammatory effects that limit mucosal edema, decrease mucus production, and potentiate β$_2$-agonists. Inhaled corticosteroids should also be continued or started.[71-74] Corticosteroids usually take effect in 6 to 8 hours.[71]

Oxygen Therapy

Initial treatment of hypoxemia is with supplemental O$_2$. High-flow O$_2$ therapy is administered to maintain the patient's SaO$_2$ greater than 92%.[71]

Intubation and Mechanical Ventilation

Indications for mechanical ventilation include cardiac or respiratory arrest, disorientation, failure to respond to bronchodilator therapy, and exhaustion.[75,76] A large ETT

(8 mm) should be used to decrease airway resistance and to facilitate suctioning of secretions.[76] Ventilating the patient with status asthmaticus can be very difficult. High inflation pressures should be avoided because of the potential for volutrauma. PEEP is contraindicated because the patient is prone to developing air trapping. Patient-ventilator asynchrony also can be a major problem. Sedation and neuromuscular paralysis may be necessary to allow for adequate ventilation of the patient.

Nursing Management

Nursing management of the patient with status asthmaticus incorporates a variety of nursing diagnoses (Box 14-14). **Nursing priorities are directed toward (1) optimizing oxygenation and ventilation, (2) providing comfort and emotional support, (3) maintaining surveillance for complications, and (4) providing patient education.**

Optimizing Oxygenation and Ventilation

Nursing interventions to optimize oxygenation and ventilation include positioning, preventing desaturation, and promoting secretion clearance (see Nursing Management of ARF).

Providing Patient Education

Early in the patient's hospital stay, the patient and family should be taught about asthma and its triggers and treatment. As the patient moves toward discharge, teaching should focus on the interventions necessary for preventing the recurrence of status asthmaticus, early warning signs of worsening airflow obstruction, correct use of an inhaler and a peak flowmeter, measures to prevent pulmonary infections, and signs and symptoms of a pulmonary infection. The patient who smokes should be encouraged to stop smoking and should be referred to a smoking cessation program. The importance of participating in a pulmonary rehabilitation program should be stressed.

Collaborative management of the patient with status asthmaticus is outlined in Box 14-15.

nursing diagnosis priorities   Box **14-14**

Status Asthmaticus
- Impaired Gas Exchange related to alveolar hypoventilation
- Ineffective Breathing Pattern related to musculoskeletal fatigue or neuromuscular impairment
- Ineffective Airway Clearance related to excessive secretions or abnormal viscosity of mucus
- Anxiety related to threat to biologic, psychologic, and/or social integrity
- Deficient Knowledge: Discharge Regimen related to lack of previous exposure to information

Box **14-15** **COLLABORATIVE** Management

Status Asthmaticus
1. Administer oxygen therapy.
2. Intubate patient.
3. Initiate mechanical ventilation.
4. Administer medications.
   - Bronchodilators
   - Corticosteriods
   - Sedatives
5. Maintain surveillance for complications.
   - Acute respiratory failure
6. Provide comfort and emotional support.

THORACIC SURGERY

Thoracic surgery refers to a number of surgical procedures that involve opening the thoracic cavity (thoracotomy) and the organs of respiration. Indications for thoracic surgery range from tumors and abscesses to repair of the esophagus and thoracic vessels[77] (Table 14-4). This discussion focuses on the surgical procedures that involve removal of lung tissue.

Preoperative Care

Before surgery, complete evaluation of the patient is needed to determine the appropriateness of surgery as a treatment and to determine whether lung tissue can be removed without jeopardizing respiratory function. This is especially important when a lobectomy or pneumonectomy is being considered. When resection is undertaken for tumor treatment, preoperative care includes evaluation of the type and extent of tumor and the patient's physical condition.[78]

The evaluation of the patient's physical status should focus on the adequacy of cardiopulmonary function. The preoperative evaluation should include pulmonary function tests to determine the patient's ability to lose lung tissue. Cardiac function also should be evaluated. Uncontrolled dysrhythmias, acute myocardial infarction, severe CHF, and unstable angina are contraindications to surgery.[78]

Surgical Considerations

The type and location of surgery will dictate the surgical approach.[79] The most common approach is the posterolateral thoracotomy, which allows for exposure of both the lung and mediastinum. Other approaches include anterolateral thoracotomy, axillary incision, and median sternotomy.

Special care is taken to avoid drainage of blood or secretions into the unaffected lung during surgery because of the potential for hypoxemia and cardiac dysfunction. A double-lumen ETT is used during the surgery to protect the unaffected lung from secretions and necrotic tumor fragments. In addition, the deflated lung is suctioned and ventilated every 20 to 30 minutes during the procedure.

After pneumonectomy, on closure of the operative site, the mediastinal position requires evaluation using manometry

Table **14-4** Thoracic Surgical Procedures

Procedure	Definition	Indications
Segmental resection (segmentectomy)	Resection of bronchovascular segment of lung lobe	Small peripheral lesions Patients with borderline lung function who would not tolerate more extensive procedure
Wedge resection	Removal of small section of lung tissue	Small peripheral lesions (without lymph node involvement) Peripheral granulomas Pulmonary blebs
Lobectomy	Resection of one or more lobes of lung	Lesions confined to single lobe Pulmonary tuberculosis Bronchiectasis Lung abscesses or cysts Trauma
Pneumonectomy	Removal of entire lung with or without resection of mediastinal lymph nodes	Malignant lesions Unilateral tuberculosis Extensive unilateral bronchiectasis Multiple lung abscesses Massive hemoptysis Bronchopleural fistula
Bronchoplastic reconstruction (sleeve resection)	Resection of lung tissue and bronchus with end-to-end reanastomosis of bronchus	Small lesions involving carina or major bronchus without evidence of metastasis May be combined with lobectomy
Decortication	Removal of fibrous membrane from pleural surface of lung	Fibrothorax resulting from hemothorax or empyema
Bullectomy	Resection of large bullae	Severe emphysema with large bullae compressing surrounding tissue
Lung volume reduction surgery (reduction pneumoplasty, pneumectomy)	Resection of most damaged portions of lung tissue, allowing more normal chest wall configuration	Emphysema
Tracheal resection	Resection of portion of trachea with end-to-end reanastomosis of trachea	Tracheal stenosis Tumors Trauma
Thoracoscopy	Endoscopic procedure performed through small chest incisions	Evaluation of pulmonary, pleural, mediastinal, or pericardial conditions Biopsy of lung, pleural, or mediastinal lesions Recurrent spontaneous pneumothorax Evacuation of empyema, hemothorax, pleural effusion, or pericardial effusion Thymectomy Blebectomy/bullectomy Pleurodesis Sympathectomy Closure of bronchopleural fistula Lysis of adhesions

and chest radiography. With the patient in the supine position, pressure in the empty chest cavity should be −4 to −6 cm H_2O. When the pressure is abnormal, air or fluid can be added or withdrawn. If the abnormality is not corrected, a mediastinal shift can result in hemodynamic compromise and cardiac dysfunction. A chest radiograph shows the location of the mediastinum.[79]

Complications and Medical Management

Complications associated with lung resection include ARF, bronchopleural fistula, hemorrhage, cardiovascular disturbances, and mediastinal shift.

Acute Respiratory Failure

In the postoperative period, ARF may result from atelectasis or pneumonia. Atelectasis may result from anesthesia, the surgical procedure, immobilization, and pain. Treatment should correct the underlying problems and support gas exchange. Supplemental O_2 and mechanical ventilation with PEEP may be necessary.[80]

Bronchopleural Fistula

Development of a postoperative bronchopleural fistula is a major cause of mortality after a lung resection. A bronchopleural fistula develops when the suture line fails to secure occlusion of the bronchial stump and an opening develops. This can result from an imperfect stump closure, perforation of the stump (e.g., with a suction catheter), high pressure within the airways (e.g., caused by mechanical ventilation),[81] or infection.[82] During surgery, careful attention is given to isolating and closing the bronchus in an attempt to secure a lasting seal with subsequent stump healing.[79] In addition, early extubation is encouraged to eliminate the possibility of perforation of the stump and high airway pressures.[81] Clinical manifestations of a bronchopleural fistula include shortness of breath and coughing up serosanguineous sputum. Immediate surgery is usually necessary to close the stump to prevent flooding of the remaining lung with fluid from the residual space.[82] If this flooding occurs, the patient should be placed with the operative side down (remaining lung up), and a chest tube should be inserted to drain the residual space.

Hemorrhage

Hemorrhage is an early, life-threatening complication that can occur after a lung resection. Hemorrhage can result from bronchial or intercostal artery bleeding or disruption of a suture or clip around a pulmonary vessel.[81] Excessive chest tube drainage can signal excessive bleeding. During the immediate postoperative period, chest tube drainage should be measured every 15 minutes, decreasing this frequency as the patient stabilizes. If chest tube loss is greater than 100 ml/hour, fresh blood is noted, or if drainage suddenly increases, hemorrhage should be suspected.

Cardiovascular Disturbances

Cardiovascular complications after thoracic surgery include dysrhythmias and pulmonary edema. Resection of large lung areas or pneumonectomy may be followed by a rise in central venous pressure. With the loss of one lung, the right ventricle must empty its stroke volume into a vascular bed that has been reduced by 50%. A higher-pressure system is created, which increases right ventricular workload, precipitating right ventricular failure. Depending on previous heart function, acute decompensation of both ventricles can result. Measures are taken to support cardiac function and avoid intravascular volume excess, including optimizing preload, afterload, and contractility with vasoactive agents.[80,81]

Mediastinal Shift

The pneumonectomy patient also should be monitored for a shift in the mediastinum. The mediastinal position can be determined by palpating for tracheal deviation, palpating and auscultating the position of the apex of the heart, and obtaining a chest radiograph. Mediastinal shift should be corrected by injecting or withdrawing air or fluid.[82]

Postoperative Nursing Management

Nursing care of the patient who has had thoracic surgery incorporates a number of nursing diagnoses (Box 14-16). **Nursing priorities are directed toward** (1) **optimizing oxygenation and ventilation**, (2) **preventing atelectasis**, (3) **maintaining the chest tube system**, (4) **assisting the patient to return to an adequate activity level**, and (5) **maintaining surveillance for complications**.

Optimizing Oxygenation and Ventilation

Nursing interventions to optimize oxygenation and ventilation include positioning, preventing desaturation during procedures, and promoting secretion clearance.

Preventing Atelectasis

Nursing interventions to prevent atelectasis include proper patient positioning and early ambulation, deep-breathing

---

nursing diagnosis
priorities   Box **14-16**

Thoracic Surgery

- Ineffective Breathing Pattern related to decreased lung expansion
- Impaired Gas Exchange related to ventilation/perfusion mismatching or intrapulmonary shunting
- Impaired Gas Exchange related to alveolar hypoventilation
- Acute Pain related to transmission and perception of cutaneous, visceral, muscular, or ischemic impulses
- Disturbed Body Image related to actual change in body structure, function, or appearance
- Compromised Family Coping related to critically ill family member

exercises, incentive spirometry, and pain management. The goal is to promote maximal lung ventilation and prevent hypoventilation.

Patient Positioning and Early Ambulation. The nurse should consider the surgical incision site and the type of surgery when positioning the patient. After lobectomy the patient should be turned onto the nonoperative side to promote V/Q matching. When the good lung is dependent, blood flow is greater to the area with better ventilation, and V/Q matching is better. V/Q mismatching results when the affected lung is positioned down because of the increase in blood flow to an area with less ventilation. The patient should be turned frequently to promote secretion removal but should have the affected lung dependent as little as possible. The patient with pneumonectomy should be positioned supine or on the operative side during the initial period. Turning onto the operative side promotes splinting of the incision and facilitates deep-breathing exercises. Tilting the patient slightly toward the unaffected side is possible, but the surgeon should indicate when free side-to-side positioning is safe.[82]

When sitting at the bedside or ambulating, patients must be encouraged to keep the thorax in straight alignment while they breathe deeply. This position best accommodates diaphragmatic descent and intercostal muscle action. The sitting or standing position provides enhanced ventilation to areas of the lung that are dependent in the supine position, thus accommodating maximal inflation and promoting gas exchange. Ambulation is essential in restoring lung function and should be initiated as soon as possible.[83]

Deep Breathing and Incentive Spirometry. These interventions should be performed regularly by thoracotomy patients. Deep breathing involves taking a deep breath and holding it for approximately 3 seconds or longer. Incentive spirometry involves taking at least 10 deep, effective breaths per hour using a spirometer. These activities help reexpand collapsed lung tissue, promoting early resolution of the pneumothorax in patients with partial lung resections. The chest should be auscultated during inflation to ensure that all dependent parts of the lung are well ventilated and to help the patient understand the depth of breath necessary for optimal effect. Coughing, which should be encouraged only when secretions are present, assists in mobilizing secretions for removal.[83]

Pain Management. Pain can be a major problem after thoracic surgery. Pain can increase the workload of the heart, precipitate hypoventilation, and inhibit mobilization of secretions. Clinical manifestations of pain include tachypnea, tachycardia, elevated blood pressure, facial grimacing, splinting of the incision, hypoventilation, moaning, and restlessness. Several alternatives for pain management after thoracic surgery can be used. The two most common methods are systemic narcotic administration and epidural narcotic administration. Systemic narcotics can be administered intra-

venously, intramuscularly, or by patient-controlled analgesia (PCA). The patient should be assisted with splinting the incision with a pillow or blanket when deep breathing and coughing. Splinting stabilizes the area and reduces pain when moving, deep breathing, or coughing.[84]

Maintaining Chest Tube System

Chest tubes are placed after all thoracic surgery procedures (except pneumonectomy) to remove air and fluid. The drainage initially appears bloody, becoming serosanguineous and then serous over the first 2 to 3 postoperative days. Approximately 100 to 300 ml of drainage occurs during the first 2 hours postoperatively, decreasing to less than 50 ml/hour over the next several hours. Routine "milking," or stripping, of chest tubes is not recommended because excessive negative pressure can be generated in the chest. If blood clots are in the drainage tubing or an obstruction is present, the chest tubes may be carefully milked.

Air leaks should be evaluated during auscultation of the lungs. In the early phase an air leak is usually heard over the affected area because the pleura has not yet tightly sealed. As healing occurs, this leak should disappear. An increase in an air leak or appearance of a new air leak should prompt investigation of the chest drainage system to discover whether air is leaking into the system from outside or the leak is originating from the patient's incision. Increased air leaks not related to the thoracic drainage system may indicate disruption of sutures.

Assisting Return to Adequate Activity Level

Within a few days after surgery, ROM exercises for the shoulder on the operative side should be performed. The patient frequently splints the operative side and avoids shoulder movement because of pain. If immobility is allowed, stiffening of the shoulder joint can result. This "frozen shoulder" may require physical therapy and rehabilitation to regain satisfactory shoulder joint ROM.[79,82]

Usually on the day after surgery the patient is able to sit in a chair. Activity should be systematically increased, with attention to the patient's activity tolerance. With adequate pulmonary function before surgery and a surgical approach designed to preserve respiratory function, full return to previous activity levels is possible. This may take as long as 6 months to 1 year, depending on the tissue resected and the patient's general condition.

LONG-TERM MECHANICAL VENTILATOR DEPENDENCE

Long-term mechanical ventilator dependence (LTMVD) is a secondary disorder that occurs when a patient requires assisted ventilation for more than 3 days.[85] LTMVD results from complex medical problems that prevent the normal weaning process in a timely manner, resulting in ventilator dependence. *Ventilator dependence* can be described as a state in which the patient is mechanically ventilated longer than expected given the patient's underlying condition[86] and has usually failed at least one weaning attempt.[87]

Etiology and Pathophysiology

A wide variety of physiologic and psychologic factors contribute to the development of LTMVD. Physiologic factors include conditions that result in decreased gas exchange, increased ventilatory workload, increased ventilatory demand, decreased ventilatory drive, and increased respiratory muscle fatigue (Box 14-17).[87-91] Psychologic factors include conditions that result in loss of breathing pattern control, lack of motivation and confidence, and delirium (Box 14-18).[101] The development of LTMVD also is effected by the severity and duration of the patient's current illness and any underlying chronic health problems.[92]

Box 14-17 Physiologic Factors Contributing to Ventilator Dependence (LTMVD)

DECREASED GAS EXCHANGE
Ventilation/perfusion mismatching
Intrapulmonary shunting
Alveolar hypoventilation
Anemia
Acute heart failure

INCREASED VENTILATORY WORKLOAD
Decreased lung compliance
Increased airway resistance
Small endotracheal tube
Decreased ventilator sensitivity
Improper positioning
Abdominal distention
Dyspnea

INCREASED VENTILATORY DEMAND
Increased pulmonary dead space
Increased metabolic demands
Improper ventilator mode/settings
Metabolic acidosis
Overfeeding

DECREASED VENTILATORY DRIVE
Respiratory alkalosis
Metabolic alkalosis
Hypothyroidism
Sedatives
Malnutrition

INCREASED RESPIRATORY MUSCLE FATIGUE
Increased ventilatory workload
Increased ventilatory demand
Malnutrition
Hypokalemia
Hypomagnesemia
Hypophosphatemia
Hypothyroidism
Critical illness polyneuropathy
Inadequate muscle rest

Box 14-18 Psychologic Factors Contributing to Ventilator Dependence (LTMVD)

LOSS OF BREATHING PATTERN CONTROL
Anxiety
Fear
Dyspnea
Pain
Ventilator asynchrony
Lack of confidence in ability to breathe

LACK OF MOTIVATION AND CONFIDENCE
Inadequate trust in staff
Depersonalization
Hopelessness
Powerlessness
Depression
Inadequate communication

DELIRIUM
Sensory overload
Sensory deprivation
Sleep deprivation
Pain
Medications

Medical and Nursing Management

The goal of medical and nursing management of the patient with LTMVD is successful weaning. The Third National Study Group on Weaning From Mechanical Ventilation, sponsored by the American Association of Critical-Care Nurses, proposes the *weaning continuum model*, which divides weaning into three stages: preweaning, weaning process, and weaning outcome.[93] Nursing management of the LTMVD patient incorporates a variety of nursing diagnoses (Box 14-19).

Preweaning Stage

For the LTMVD patient the preweaning phase consists of resolving the precipitating event that necessitated ventilatory assistance and preventing the physiologic and psychologic factors that can interfere with weaning. Before any attempts at weaning, the patient should be assessed for weaning readiness, an approach determined, and a method selected.[85]

Weaning Preparedness. The patient should be physiologically and psychologically prepared to initiate the weaning process by addressing those factors that can interfere with weaning. Aggressive medical management should be initiated to prevent and treat V/Q mismatching, intrapulmonary shunting, anemia, cardiac failure, decreased lung compliance, increased airway resistance, acid-base disturbances, hypothyroidism, abdominal distention, and electrolyte imbalances. Interventions to decrease the work of breathing also should be implemented, such as replacing a small ETT with a larger tube or a tracheostomy, suctioning airway secretions, administering bronchodilators, optimizing the ventilator settings and trigger sensitivity, and positioning the patient in straight alignment with the head of the bed elevated at least 30 degrees. Enteral or parenteral nutrition should be started and the patient's nutritional state optimized. Physical therapy should be initiated for the patient with critical illness polyneuropathy because increased mobility facilitates weaning. A means of communication should be established with the patient. Sedatives can be administered to provide anxiety control, but the avoidance of respiratory depression is critical.[94]

Weaning Readiness. Methods for assessing weaning readiness have not been proved to be very accurate in predicting weaning success in the patient with LTMVD.[85,95] Left ventricular dysfunction, fluid imbalance, and nutritional deficiency may increase the duration of mechanical ventilation,[96] however, and the upward trending of the albumin level may be predictive of weaning success.[97] Any assessment of weaning readiness should incorporate the many variables affecting the patient's ability to wean.[98] Cardiac function, gas exchange, pulmonary mechanics, nutritional status, fluid-electrolyte balance, and motivation should all be considered when making the decision to wean. The assessment is ongoing to reflect the dynamic nature of the process.

Weaning Approach. Although weaning the patient requiring short-term mechanical ventilation is a relatively simple process usually accomplished with a nurse and respiratory therapist, weaning the patient with LTMVD is a much more complex process that usually requires a multidisciplinary team approach.[95] Teams who use a coordinated and collaborative approach to weaning have demonstrated improved patient outcomes and decreased weaning times.[95] The team should consist of a physician, nurse, respiratory therapist, dietitian, physical therapist, and a case manager,

clinical outcomes manager, or clinical nurse specialist. Additional members, if possible, should include an occupational therapist, speech therapist, discharge planner, and social worker. Together the team members should develop a comprehensive plan of care for the patient that is efficient, consistent, progressive, and cost-effective.[95]

Weaning Method. Weaning methods include the T-tube (T-piece) approach, constant positive airway pressure (CPAP), pressure support ventilation (PSV), and synchronized intermittent mandatory ventilation (SIMV). No method has consistently proved to be superior to the others,[85] although evidence supports the use of PSV for weaning over T-tube or SIMV weaning.[99] Often these weaning methods are used in combination, such as SIMV with PSV, CPAP with PSV, or SIMV with CPAP.[85]

Weaning Process Stage

For the long-term ventilator patient the weaning process phase consists of initiating the weaning method selected and minimizing the physiologic and psychologic factors that can interfere with weaning.[93] The patient must not become exhausted during this phase because exhaustion can cause a setback in the weaning process.[100] During this phase the patient is assessed for weaning progress and signs of weaning intolerance.[85]

Weaning Initiation. Weaning should be initiated in the morning when the patient is rested. Before starting the weaning process, the patient is provided with an explanation of how the process works, a description of the sensations to expect, and reassurances that the patient will be closely monitored and returned to the original ventilator mode and settings if any difficulty arises.[85] This information should be reinforced with each weaning attempt.

T-tube and CPAP weaning are accomplished by removing the patient from the ventilator and then fitting the patient with a T-tube or placing the patient on CPAP mode for a specified duration, known as a *weaning trial*, for a specified number of times per day. When the weaning trial is over, the patient is placed on the assist-control mode (continuous mandatory ventilation mode on the Puritan-Bennett 7200 ventilator) and allowed to rest to prevent respiratory muscle fatigue. Gradually the duration of time spent weaning is increased, as is the frequency, until the patient is able to breathe spontaneously for 24 hours. If PSV is used with CPAP, the PSV is initially set to provide the patient with an assisted tidal volume of 10 to 12 ml/kg, with gradual weaning until a level of 6 to 8 cm H_2O of pressure support is achieved. SIMV and PSV weaning are accomplished by gradually decreasing the number of breaths or the amount of pressure support by a specified amount until the patient is able to breathe spontaneously for 24 hours.[85,100]

Weaning Progress. Evaluation of progress when using a weaning method that gradually withdraws ventilatory support (e.g., SIMV, PSV) can be accomplished by measuring the percentage of the minute ventilation requirement provided by the ventilator. If the percentage steadily decreases, weaning is progressing. Evaluation when using a weaning method that removes ventilatory support (e.g., T-tube, CPAP) can be accomplished by measuring the amount of time the patient remains free from support. If the time steadily increases, weaning is progressing.[85]

Weaning Intolerance. Once the weaning process has begun, the patient should be continuously assessed for signs of intolerance. These signs indicate when to return the patient to the ventilator or to the previous ventilator settings. Common indicators include dyspnea, accessory muscle use, restlessness, anxiety, change in facial expression, changes in heart rate and blood pressure, rapid shallow breathing, and discomfort.[85,95]

Facilitative Therapies. When the patient is having difficulty, additional therapies may be needed to facilitate weaning, including ventilatory muscle training and biofeedback.[95] Inspiratory muscle training is used to enhance the strength and endurance of the respiratory muscles.[95,100] Biofeedback can be used to promote relaxation and assist in the management of dyspnea and anxiety.[95,101]

Weaning Outcome Stage

Weaning Completed. Weaning is deemed successful when a patient is able to breathe spontaneously for 24 hours without ventilatory support. At this time the patient may be extubated or decannulated, although this is not necessary for weaning to be considered successful.[86]

Incomplete Weaning. Weaning is deemed incomplete when a patient has reached a *plateau* (5 days at same ventilatory support level without change) in the weaning process despite managing the physiologic and psychologic factors that impede weaning. Thus the patient is *unable* to breathe spontaneously for 24 hours without full or partial ventilatory support. At this time the patient should be placed in a subacute ventilator facility or discharged home under ventilator support with home care nursing follow-up.[86,102]

REFERENCES

1. Christie HA, Goldstein LS: Respiratory failure and the need for ventilatory support. In Scanlan CL, Wilkins RL, Stoller JK, editors: *Egan's fundamentals of respiratory care*, ed 7, St Louis, 1999, Mosby.
2. Zuege DJ, Whitelaw WA: Management of acute respiratory failure in chronic obstructive pulmonary disease, *Curr Opin Pulm Med* 3:190, 1997.
3. Vasileyev S, Schaap RN, Mortensen JD: Hospital survival rates of patients with acute respiratory failure in modern respiratory intensive care units: an international, multicenter, prospective survey, *Chest* 107:1083, 1995.
4. Balk R, Bone RC: Classification of acute respiratory failure, *Med Clin North Am* 67:551, 1983.
5. Curtis JR, Hudson LD: Emergent assessment and management of acute respiratory failure in COPD, *Clin Chest Med* 15:481, 1994.
6. Raju P, Manthous CA: The pathogenesis of respiratory failure, *Respir Care Clin North Am* 6:195, 2000.
7. Green KE, Peters JI: Pathophysiology of acute respiratory failure, *Clin Chest Med* 15:1, 1994.
8. Misasi RS, Keyes JL: The pathophysiology of hypoxia, *Crit Care Nurse* 14(4):55, 1994.
9. Vaughan P: Acute respiratory failure in the patient with chronic obstructive lung disease, *Crit Care Nurse* 1(6):46, 1981.
10. Moore FA, Haenel JB: Ventilatory strategies for acute respiratory failure, *Am J Surg* 173:53-56, 1997.
11. Misasi RS, Keyes JL: Matching and mismatching ventilation and perfusion in the lung, *Crit Care Nurse* 16(3):23, 1996.
12. Peter JV, Moran JL, Phillips-Hughes J: Noninvasive ventilation in acute respiratory failure: a meta-analysis update, *Crit Care Med* 30:555, 2002.
13. Soo Hoo GW, Hakimian N, Santiago SM: Hypercapnic respiratory failure in COPD patients: response to therapy, *Chest* 117:169, 2000.
14. Seithi JM, Siegel MD: Mechanical ventilation in chronic obstructive lung disease, *Clin Chest Med* 21:799, 2000.
15. American Thoracic Society: Standards for the diagnosis and care of patients with chronic obstructive pulmonary disease, *Am J Respir Crit Care Med* 152:S77, 1995.
16. Shapiro BA et al: Practice parameters for sustained neuromuscular blockade in the adult critically ill patient: an executive summary. Society of Critical Care Medicine, *Crit Care Med* 23:1601, 1995.
17. Forsythe SM, Schmidt GA: Sodium bicarbonate for the treatment of lactic acidosis, *Chest* 117:260, 2000.
18. Parrish CR, Krenitsky J, McCray S: *Nutrition support for the mechanically ventilated patient*, Aliso Viejo, Calif, 1998, American Association of Critical-Care Nurses.
19. Chan S, McCowen KC, Blackburn GL: Nutrition management in the ICU, *Chest* 115:145, 1999.
20. Naik-Tolani S, Oropello JM, Benjamin E: Neurologic complications in the intensive care unit, *Clin Chest Med* 20:423, 1999.
21. Francis GS: Cardiac complications in the intensive care unit, *Clin Chest Med* 20:269, 1999.
22. Legere BM, Dweik RA, Arroliga AC: Venous thromboembolism in the intensive care unit, *Clin Chest Med* 20:367, 1999.
23. Liolios A, Oropello JM, Benjamin E: Gastrointestinal complications in the intensive care unit, *Clin Chest Med* 20:329, 1999.
24. Wong WP: Use of body positioning in the mechanically ventilated patient with acute respiratory failure: application of Sackett's rules of evidence, *Physiother Theory Pract* 15:25, 1999.
25. Force TR et al: Patient position and motion strategies, *Respir Care Clin North Am* 4:665, 1998.
26. Lasater-Erhand M: The effect of patient position on arterial saturation, *Crit Care Nurse* 15(5):31, 1995.
27. Cosenza JJ, Norton LC: Secretion clearance: state-of-the-art from a nursing perspective, *Crit Care Nurse* 6(4):23, 1986.
28. Kollef MH: Outcome research as a tool for defining the role of respiratory care practitioners in the intensive care unit setting, *New Horizons* 6:91, 1998.
29. Jones A, Rowe BH: Bronchopulmonary hygiene physical therapy in bronchietasis and chronic obstructive pulmonary disease: a systematic review, *Heart Lung* 29:125, 2000.
30. Cook DJ et al: Toward understanding evidence uptake: semirecumbency for pneumonia prevention, *Crit Care Med* 30:1472, 2002.
31. Bernard GR et al: The American-European Consensus Conference on ARDS: definitions, mechanisms, relevant outcomes, and clinical trial coordination, *Am J Respir Crit Care Med* 149:818, 1994.
32. Fein AM, Calalang-Colucci MG: Acute lung injury and acute respiratory distress syndrome in sepsis and septic shock, *Crit Care Clin* 16:289, 2000.
33. Brower RG et al: Treatment of ARDS, *Chest* 120:1347, 2001.
34. Lee WL, Downey GP: Neutrophil activation and acute lung injury, *Curr Opin Crit Care* 7:1, 2001.

35. Phillips JK: Management of patients with acute respiratory distress syndrome, *Crit Care Clin North Am* 11:233, 1999.

36. Van Soeren MH et al: Pathophysiology and implications for treatment of acute respiratory distress syndrome, *AACN Clin Issues* 11:179, 2000.

37. Tomashefski JF: Pulmonary pathology of acute respiratory distress syndrome, *Clin Chest Med* 21:435, 2001.

38. O'Connor MF, Hall JB: ARDS: current treatment and ventilator strategies, *Anesth Clin North Am* 16:155, 1998.

39. Artigas A et al: The American European Consensus Conference on ARDS. Part 2. Ventilatory, pharmacologic, supportive therapy, study design strategies, and issues related to recovery and remodeling, *Am J Respir Crit Care Med* 157:1332, 1998.

40. Hirvela ER: Advances in the management of acute respiratory distress syndrome: protective ventilation, *Arch Surg* 135:126, 2000.

41. Kacmarek RM: Strategies to optimize alveolar recruitment, *Curr Opin Crit Care* 7:15, 2001.

42. Luca B, Nicolo P, Fabio S: Permissive hypercapnia, *Curr Opin Crit Care* 7:34, 2001.

43. Bulger E et al: Current clinical options for the treatment and management of acute respiratory distress syndrome, *J Trauma* 48:562, 2000.

44. Curley MAQ: Prone positioning of patients with acute respiratory distress syndrome: a systematic review, *Am J Crit Care* 8:397, 1999.

45. Balas MC: Prone positioning of patients with acute respiratory distress syndrome: applying research to practice, *Crit Care Nurse* 20(1):24, 2000.

46. Cunha BA: Community-acquired pneumonia: diagnostic and therapeutic approach, *Med Clin North Am* 85:79, 2001.

47. Ewig S, Torres A: Severe community-acquired pneumonia, *Clin Chest Med* 20:575, 1999.

48. Torres A, El-Ebiary M, Rano A: Respiratory infectious complications in the intensive care unit, *Clin Chest Med* 20:287, 1999.

49. Cross JT, Campbell GD: Therapy of nosocomial pneumonia, *Med Clin North Am* 85:1583, 2001.

50. Harris JR, Miller TH: Preventing nosocomial pneumonia: evidence-based practice, *Crit Care Nurse* 20(1):51, 2000.

51. Nelson S et al: Pathophysiology of pneumonia, *Clin Chest Med* 16:1, 1995.

52. Longworth DL: Pulmonary infections. In Scanlan CL, Wilkins RL, Stoller JK, editors: *Egan's fundamentals of respiratory care*, ed 7, St Louis, 1999, Mosby.

53. Kollef MH: Epidemiology and risk factors for nosocomial pneumonia: emphasis on prevention, *Clin Chest Med* 20:653, 1999.

54. Ghariba AM, Stern EJ: Radiology of pneumonia, *Med Clin North Am* 85:1461, 2001.

55. Barlett JG et al: Community-acquired pneumonia in adults: guidelines for management, *Clin Infect Dis* 26:811, 1998.

56. Thomas AR, Bryce TL: Ventilation in the patient with unilateral lung disease, *Crit Care Clin* 14:743, 1998.

57. DePaso WJ: Aspiration pneumonia, *Clin Chest Med* 12:269, 1991.

58. Tietjen PA, Kaner RJ, Quinn CE: Aspiration emergencies, *Clin Chest Med* 15:117, 1994.

59. Chokshi S, Asper R, Khandheria B: Aspiration pneumonia: a review, *Am Fam Physician* 33:195, 1986.

60. Goodwin RS: Prevention of aspiration pneumonia: a research-based protocol, *Dimen Crit Care Nurs* 15(2):58, 1996.

61. Goldhaber SZ: Pulmonary embolism, *N Engl J Med* 339:93, 1998.

62. Legere BM, Dweik AR, Arroliga AC: Venous thromboembolism in the intensive care unit, *Clin Chest Med* 20:367, 1999.

63. Kelley MA, Abbuhl S: Massive pulmonary embolism, *Clin Chest Med* 15:547, 1994.

64. Lee LC, Shah K: Clinical manifestations of pulmonary embolism, *Emerg Med Clin North Am* 19:925, 2001.

65. Baker WF: Diagnosis of deep venous thrombosis and pulmonary embolism, *Med Clin North Am* 82:459, 1998.

66. Kline JA et al: New diagnostic tests for pulmonary embolism, *Ann Emerg Med* 35:168, 2000.

67. Hull RD, Pineo GF: Prophylaxis of deep vein thrombosis and pulmonary embolism, *Med Clin North Am* 82:477, 1998.

68. Edlow JA: Emergency department management of pulmonary embolism, *Emerg Med Clin North Am* 19:995, 2001.

69. Arcasoy SM, Kreit JW: Thrombolytic therapy of pulmonary embolism, *Chest* 115:1695, 1999.

70. McDowell KM: Pathophysiology of asthma, *Respir Care Clin N Am* 6:15, 2000.

71. Cohen NH, Eigen H, Shaughnessy TE: Status asthmaticus, *Crit Care Clin* 13:459, 1997.

72. Jagoda A et al: Refractory asthma. Part 1. Epidemiology, pathophysiology, pharmacologic interventions, *Ann Emerg Med* 29:262, 1997.

73. Burns SM, Lawson C: Pharmacological and ventilatory management of acute asthma exacerbations, *Crit Care Nurse* 19(4):39, 1999.

74. Jantz MA, Sahn SA: Corticosteriods in acute respiratory failure, *Am J Respir Crit Care Med* 160:1079, 1999.

75. Jagoda A et al: Refractory asthma. Part 2. Airway interventions and management, *Ann Emerg Med* 29:275, 1997.

76. Jain S, Hanania NA, Guntupalli KK: Ventilation of patients with asthma and obstructive lung disease, *Crit Care Clin* 14:685, 1998.

77. Litwack K: Practical points in the care of the thoracic surgery patient, *Post Anesth Nurs* 5:276, 1990.

78. Ferguson, MK: Preoperative assessment of pulmonary risk, *Chest* 115:S58, 1999.

79. Langston W: Surgical resection of lung cancer, *Nurs Clin North Am* 27:665, 1992.

80. Boysen PG: Perioperative management of the thoracotomy patient, *Clin Chest Med* 14:321, 1993.

81. Kopec SE: The postpneumonectomy state, *Chest* 114:1158, 1998.

82. Brenner Z, Addona C: Caring for the pneumonectomy patient: challenges and changes, *Crit Care Nurse* 15(5):65, 1995.

83. Brooks, JA: Postoperative nosocomial pneumonia: nurse-sensitive interventions, *AACN Clin Issues* 12:305, 2001.

84. Desai PM: Pain management and pulmonary dysfunction, *Crit Care Clin* 15:151, 1999.

85. Burns SM: *Weaning from long-term mechanical ventilation*, Aliso Viejo, Calif, 1998, American Association of Critical-Care Nurses.

86. Knebel AR et al: Weaning from mechanical ventilation: concept development, *Am J Crit Care Nurs* 3:416, 1994.

87. Pierson DJ: Long-term mechanical ventilation and weaning, *Respir Care* 40:289, 1995.

88. Vallverdú I, Mancebo J: Approach to patients who fail initial weaning trials, *Respir Care Clin N Am* 6:365, 2000.

89. MacIntyre NR: Respiratory factors in weaning from mechanical ventilatory support, *Respir Care* 40:244, 1995.

90. Pierson DJ: Nonrespiratory aspects of weaning from mechanical ventilation, *Respir Care* 40:263, 1995.

91. Hund EF et al: Critical illness polyneuropathy: clinical findings and outcomes of a frequent cause of neuromuscular weaning, *Crit Care Med* 24:1328, 1996.

92. MacIntyre NR: Psychological factors in weaning from mechanical ventilatory support, *Respir Care* 40:277, 1995.

93. Knebel AR et al: Weaning from mechanical ventilatory support: refinement of a model, *Am J Crit Care Nurs* 7:149, 1998.

94. Scheinhorn DJ, Chao DC, Stearn-Hassenpflug M: Approach to patients with long-term weaning failure, *Respir Care Clin N Am* 6:437, 2000.

95. Burns SM et al: Weaning from long-term mechanical ventilation, *Am J Crit Care* 4:4, 1995.

96. Clochesy JM: Weaning chronically critically ill adults from mechanical ventilatory support: a descriptive study, *Am J Crit Care* 4:93, 1995.

97. Sapijaszko MJA et al: Nonrespiratory predictor of mechanical ventilation dependency in intensive care unit patients, *Crit Care Med* 24:601, 1996.

98. Ingersoll GL et al: Measurement issues in mechanical ventilation weaning research, *Online J Knowledge Synthesis Nurs* 2(12):24, 1995.

99. Brochard L et al: Comparison of three methods of gradual withdrawal from ventilatory support during weaning from mechanical ventilation, *Am J Respir Crit Care Med* 150:898, 1994.

100. Brochard LJ, Lessard MR: Weaning from ventilatory support, *Clin Chest Med* 17:475, 1996.

101. Jacavone J, Young J: Use of pulmonary rehabilitation strategies to wean a difficult-to-wean patient: case study, *Crit Care Nurse* 18(6):29, 1998.

102. Gracey DR: Options for long-term ventilatory support, *Clin Chest Med* 18:563, 1997.

KATHLEEN M. STACY

15

Pulmonary Therapeutic Management

Objectives

- Describe nursing management of a patient receiving oxygen therapy.
- List the indications and complications of the different artificial airways.
- Outline the principles of airway management.
- Discuss the various modes of invasive and noninvasive mechanical ventilation.
- Describe the management of a patient receiving mechanical ventilation.

evolve Be sure to check out the free exercises on-line at *http://evolve.elsevier.com/Urden/priorities/*

A wide variety of therapeutic interventions are employed in the management of the patient with pulmonary dysfunction. This chapter focuses on the priority interventions used to manage pulmonary disorders in the critical care setting.

OXYGEN THERAPY

Normal cellular function depends on an adequate supply of oxygen being delivered to the cells to meet their metabolic needs. The goal of oxygen therapy is to provide a sufficient concentration of inspired oxygen to permit full use of the oxygen-carrying capacity of the arterial blood, thus ensuring adequate cellular oxygenation given an adequate cardiac output (CO) and hemoglobin (Hgb) concentration.[1,2]

Principles of Therapy

Oxygen (O_2) is an atmospheric gas that must also be considered a drug because, as with most other drugs, O_2 has both detrimental and beneficial effects. Oxygen is one of the most commonly used and misused drugs. As a drug, O_2 must be administered for good reason and in a proper, safe manner. Oxygen is generally ordered in liters per minute (L/min); as a concentration of O_2 expressed as a percent, such as 40%, or as a fraction of inspired O_2 (FIO_2), such as 0.4.

The primary indication for O_2 therapy is hypoxemia.[3] The amount of O_2 administered depends on the pathophysiologic mechanisms affecting the patient's oxygenation status. In most cases the amount required should provide arterial oxygen partial pressure (PaO_2) of greater than 60 mm Hg or arterial hemoglobin saturation (SaO_2) of greater than 90% during both rest and exercise.[2] The O_2 concentration delivered to an individual patient is a clinical judgment based on the many factors that influence O_2 transport (e.g., Hgb concentration, CO, PaO_2).[1,2]

Once O_2 therapy has begun, the patient is continuously assessed for level of oxygenation and associated factors. The patient's oxygenation status is evaluated several times daily until the desired O_2 level is reached and has stabilized. If the desired response to the O_2 amount delivered is not achieved, the oxygen supplementation is adjusted and the patient's condition reevaluated. It is important to use this dose-response method so that the lowest possible O_2 level is administered that will still achieve a satisfactory PaO_2 or SaO_2.[2,3]

Methods of Delivery

Oxygen therapy can be delivered by many different devices (Table 15-1). Common problems with these devices include system leaks and obstructions, device displacement, and skin irritation. These devices are classified as either low-flow, reservoir, or high-flow systems.[3]

Low-Flow Systems

A low-flow oxygen delivery system provides supplemental O_2 directly into the patient's airway at flows of 8 L/min or less. Because this flow is insufficient to meet the patient's inspiratory volume requirements, it results in a variable FIO_2 as the inspired O_2 is mixed with room air. The patient's ventilatory pattern also affects FIO_2 of a low-flow system. As the patient's ventilatory pattern changes, the inspired O_2 concentration varies because of differing amounts of room-air gas mixing with the constant O_2 flow. A nasal cannula is an example of a low-flow device.[3]

Reservoir Systems

A reservoir system incorporates some type of device to collect and store oxygen between breaths. When the patient's inspiratory flow exceeds the oxygen flow of the O_2 delivery system, the patient is able to draw from the O_2 reservoir to meet inspiratory volume needs. Thus there is less mixing of the inspired O_2 with room air. A reservoir O_2 delivery system can deliver a higher FIO_2 than a low-flow system. Examples of reservoir systems are simple face masks, partial rebreathing masks, and nonrebreathing masks.[3]

High-Flow Systems

With a high-flow system, the oxygen flows out of the device into the patient's airways in amounts sufficient to meet all inspiratory volume requirements. This type of system is not affected by the patient's ventilatory pattern. An air-entrainment mask is an example of a high-flow system.[1,3]

Complications

As with most drugs, oxygen has adverse effects and complications resulting from its use. The adage "if a little is good, a lot is better" does not apply to oxygen. The lung is designed to handle a concentration of 21% O_2, with some adaptability to higher concentrations, but adverse effects and oxygen toxicity can result if a high concentration is administered for too long.[4]

Oxygen Toxicity

The most detrimental effect of breathing a high O_2 concentration is the development of oxygen toxicity. Toxicity can occur in any patient breathing O_2 concentrations of greater than 50% for more than 24 hours. Patients most likely to develop oxygen toxicity are those who require intubation, mechanical ventilation, and high O_2 concentrations for extended periods.[1,3]

Hyperoxia, or the administration of higher-than-normal O_2 concentrations, produces an overabundance of O_2 free radicals. These radicals are responsible for the initial damage to the alveolar-capillary membrane. Oxygen free radicals are toxic metabolites of O_2 metabolism. Normally, enzymes neutralize the radicals, which prevents damage. During administration of high O_2 levels, the large number of O_2 free radicals produced exhausts the supply of neutralizing enzymes. Thus the lung parenchyma and vasculature are damaged, resulting in the initiation of acute respiratory distress syndrome (ARDS).[1,4]

Table 15-1 Oxygen (O₂) Therapy Systems

Device	O₂ Flow (L/min)	FiO₂ %	Stability	Advantages	Disadvantages	Best Use
LOW-FLOW SYSTEMS						
Nasal cannula	*Adults:* 0.25-8.0 *Infants:* 2.0 or less	22-45	Variable	Use in adults, children, infants; easy to apply; disposable, low cost; well tolerated	Unstable, easily dislodged; high flows uncomfortable; can cause dryness and bleeding; polyps, deviated septum may block flow	Stable patient needing low FiO₂; home care patient requiring long-term therapy
Nasal catheter	0.25-8.0	22-35	Variable	Use in adults, children, infants; good stability; disposable, low cost	Difficult to insert; high flows increase back pressure; needs regular changing; polyps, deviated septum may block insertion; may provoke gagging, air swallowing, and aspiration	Procedures in which cannula is difficult to use, such as bronchoscopy; long-term therapy for infants
Transtracheal catheter	0.25-4.0	22-35	Variable	Lower O₂ use/cost; eliminates nasal/skin irritation; improved compliance; increased exercise tolerance; increased mobility; enhanced image	High cost; surgical complications; infection; mucus plugging; lost tract	Home care or ambulatory patients who need increased mobility or do not accept nasal oxygen
RESERVOIR SYSTEM						
Reservoir cannula	0.25-4.0	22-35	Variable	Lower O₂ use/cost; increased mobility; less discomfort because of lower flows	Unattractive, cumbersome; poor compliance; must be regularly replaced; breathing pattern affects performance	Home care or ambulatory patients who need increased mobility
Simple mask	5-12	35-50	Variable	Use on adults, children, infants; quick, easy to apply; disposable, inexpensive	Uncomfortable; must be removed for eating; prevents radiant heat loss; blocks vomitus in unconscious patients	Emergencies, short-term therapy requiring moderate FiO₂

Continued

Table **15-1** Oxygen (O_2) Therapy Systems—cont'd

Device	O_2 Flow (L/min)	FIO_2 %	Stability	Advantages	Disadvantages	Best Use
Partial-rebreathing mask	6-10*	35-60	Variable	Same as simple mask; moderate to high FIO_2	Same as simple mask; potential suffocation hazard	Emergencies, short-term therapy requiring moderate to high FIO_2
Nonrebreathing mask	6-10*	55-70	Variable	Same as simple mask; high FIO_2	Same as simple mask; potential suffocation hazard	Emergencies, short-term therapy requiring high FIO_2
Nonrebreathing circuit (closed)	$3 \times VE^*$	21-100	Fixed	Full range of FIO_2	Potential suffocation hazard; requires 50 psi air/O_2; blender failure common	Patients requiring precise FIO_2 at any level (21%-100%)
HIGH-FLOW SYSTEM						
Air-entrainment mask (AEM)	Varies; >60 output	24-50	Fixed	Easy to apply; disposable, inexpensive; stable, precise FIO_2	Limited to adult use; uncomfortable, noisy; must be removed for eating; FIO_2 >0.40 not ensured; FIO_2 varies with back pressure	Unstable patients requiring precise, low FIO_2
Air-entrainment nebulizer	10-15 input At least 60 output	28-100	Fixed	Provides temperature control and extra humidification	FIO_2 <28% or >40% not ensured; FIO_2 varies with back pressure; high infection risk	Patients with artificial airways requiring low to moderate FIO_2

Modified from Scanlan CL, Wilkins RL, Stoller JK, editors: *Egan's fundamentals of respiratory care*, ed 7, St Louis, 1999, Mosby.
*Prevent bag collapse on inspiration.
FIO_2, Fraction of inspired oxygen; *VE*, minute ventilation; *psi*, pounds per square inch.

A number of clinical manifestations are associated with oxygen toxicity. The first symptom is substernal chest pain that is exacerbated by deep breathing. A dry cough and tracheal irritation follow. Eventually, definite pleuritic pain occurs on inhalation, followed by dyspnea. Upper airway changes may include a sensation of nasal stuffiness, sore throat, and eye and ear discomforts. Chest radiographs and pulmonary function tests show no abnormalities until symptoms are severe. Complete, rapid reversal of these symptoms occurs as soon as normal O_2 concentration returns.[4]

Carbon Dioxide Retention

In patients with severe chronic obstructive pulmonary disease (COPD), carbon dioxide (CO_2) retention may occur as a result of administering O_2 in higher concentrations. One theory for this phenomenon proposes that the normal stimulus to breathe (increasing CO_2 levels) is muted in patients with COPD, and decreasing O_2 levels become the stimulus to breathe. When O_2 is administered and hypoxemia corrected, the stimulus to breathe is abolished and hypoventilation develops, resulting in a further increase in arterial CO_2 partial pressure ($PaCO_2$).[3] Another theory is that O_2 administration abolishes the compensatory response of hypoxic pulmonary vasoconstriction. This results in an increase in perfusion of underventilated alveoli and development of dead space, producing ventilation/perfusion (V/Q) mismatching. As alveolar dead space increases, so does CO_2 retention.[3,5] In another theory the rise in CO_2 is related to the proportion of deoxygenated Hgb to oxygenated Hgb (Haldane effect). Because deoxygenated Hgb carries more CO_2 than oxygenated Hgb, when O_2 is administered, it increases the amount of oxygenated Hgb, which results in increased release of CO_2 at the lung level.[5] Because of the risk of CO_2 accumulation, all chronically hypercapnic patients require careful low-flow O_2 delivery.[3]

Absorption Atelectasis

Breathing high O_2 concentrations washes out the nitrogen that normally fills the alveoli and helps hold the alveoli open (residual volume). In absorption atelectasis, as oxygen replaces the nitrogen in the alveoli, the alveoli start to shrink and collapse because O_2 is absorbed into the bloodstream faster than it can be replaced in the alveoli, particularly in minimally ventilated lung areas.[1,3]

Nursing Management

Nursing priorities for the patient receiving oxygen focus on (1) ensuring the oxygen is being administered as ordered and (2) observing for complications of the therapy. Confirming that the O_2 therapy device is properly positioned and replacing it after removal is important. During meals an oxygen mask should be changed to a nasal cannula if the patient can tolerate one. The patient receiving O_2 therapy should also be transported with the oxygen. In addition, SaO_2 should be periodically monitored using a pulse oximeter.

ARTIFICIAL AIRWAYS

Pharyngeal Airways

Pharyngeal airways are used to maintain airway patency by keeping the tongue from obstructing the upper airway. The two types of pharyngeal airways are oropharyngeal and nasopharyngeal. Complications of these airways include trauma to the oral or nasal cavity, obstruction of the airway, laryngospasm, gagging, and vomiting.[6,7]

Oropharyngeal Airway

An oropharyngeal airway is made of plastic and is available in a variety of sizes. The proper size is selected by holding the airway against the side of the patient's face and ensuring it extends from the corner of the mouth to the angle of the jaw. If improperly sized, the artificial airway will occlude the airway. An oral airway is placed by inserting a tongue depressor into the patient's mouth to displace the tongue downward and then passing the airway into the patient's mouth, slipping it over the patient's tongue. When properly placed, the tip of the artificial airway lies above the epiglottis at the base of the tongue. The oropharyngeal airway should only be used in an unconscious patient who has an absent or diminished gag reflex.[6,7]

Nasopharyngeal Airway

A nasopharyngeal airway is usually made of plastic or rubber and also is available in a variety of sizes. The proper size is selected by holding the airway against the side of the patient's face and ensuring it extends from the tip of the nose to the earlobe. A nasal airway is placed by lubricating the tube and inserting it midline along the floor of the naris into the posterior pharynx. When properly placed, the tip of the artificial airway lies above the epiglottis at the base of the tongue.[6,7]

Endotracheal Tubes

An endotracheal tube (ETT) is the most common artificial airway for providing short-term airway management. Indications for endotracheal intubation include maintenance of airway patency, protection of the airway from aspiration, application of positive-pressure ventilation, facilitation of pulmonary toilet, and use of high O_2 concentrations.[8] An ETT may be placed using the orotracheal or nasotracheal route.[9,10] In most situations involving emergency placement, the orotracheal route is used because the approach is simpler and affords use of a larger-diameter ETT.[10-12] Nasotracheal intubation provides greater patient comfort over time and is preferred when the patient has a jaw fracture[9,11,13] (Table 15-2).

ETTs are sized according to the inner diameter of the tube and have a radiopaque marker that runs the length of the tube. On one end of the tube is a cuff that is inflated using the pilot balloon. Because of the high incidence of cuff-related problems, low-pressure high-volume cuffs are preferred. On the other end of the tube is a 15-mm adapter

Table **15-2** Advantages of Orotracheal, Nasotracheal, and Tracheostomy Tubes		
Orotracheal	**Nasotracheal**	**Tracheostomy**
Easier access	Easily secured and stabilized	Easily secured and stabilized
Avoids nasal and sinus complications	Reduced risk of unintentional extubation	Reduced risk of unintentional decannulation
Allows for larger-diameter tube, which facilitates: • Work of breathing • Suctioning • Fiberoptic bronchoscopy	Well tolerated by patient Enables swallowing, oral hygiene Facilitates communication Avoids need for bite block	Well tolerated by patient Enables swallowing, speech, oral hygiene Avoids upper airway complications Allows for larger-diameter tube, which facilitates: • Work of breathing • Suctioning • Fiberoptic bronchoscopy

that facilitates the connection of the tube to a manual resuscitation bag (MRB), T-tube, or ventilator[14] (Figure 15-1).

Intubation

Before intubation the necessary equipment is gathered and organized to facilitate the procedure. Readily available equipment should include (1) suction system with catheters and tonsil suction, (2) MRB with a mask connected to 100% O_2, (3) laryngoscope handle with assorted blades, (4) variety of ETT sizes, and (5) stylet. Before the procedure is initiated, all equipment is inspected to ensure it is in working order. The patient should be prepared for the procedure, if possible, with an intravenous (IV) catheter in place and should be monitored with a pulse oximeter. The patient is sedated before the procedure (as clinical condition allows), and a topical anesthetic is applied to facilitate placement of the tube. A paralytic agent may be necessary if the patient is extremely agitated.[7,11,12]

The procedure is initiated by positioning the patient with the neck flexed and head slightly extended in the "sniff" position. The oral cavity and pharynx are suctioned and dental devices removed. The patient is preoxygenated and ventilated using the MRB and mask with 100% O_2. Each intubation attempt is limited to 30 seconds. Once the ETT is inserted, the patient is assessed for bilateral breath sounds and chest movement. Absence of breath sounds indicates esophageal intubation, whereas breath sounds heard over only one side indicate mainstem intubation. A disposable end-tidal CO_2 detector is used to verify correct airway placement, after which the cuff of the tube is inflated and the tube secured. A chest radiograph is obtained to confirm placement. The ETT tip should be approximately 3 to 4 cm above the carina when the patient's head is in the neutral position. Once final adjustment of the position is complete, the level of insertion (marked in centimeters on the side of the tube) at the teeth is noted.[7,10,12]

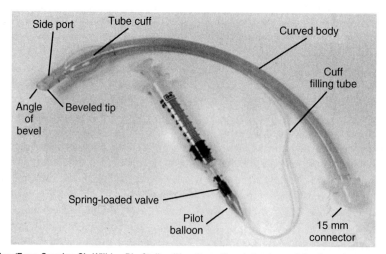

Figure 15-1 Endotracheal tube. (From Scanlan CL, Wilkins RL, Stoller JK, editors: *Egan's fundamentals of respiratory care*, ed 7, St Louis, 1999, Mosby.)

Complications

Potential complications during the intubation procedure include nasal and oral trauma, pharyngeal and hypopharyngeal trauma, vomiting with aspiration, and cardiac arrest.[15,16] Hypoxemia and hypercapnia may result in bradycardia, tachycardia, dysrhythmias, hypertension, and hypotension.[7,12] Complications while the ETT is in place include nasal and oral inflammation and ulceration, sinusitis and otitis, laryngeotracheal injuries, and tube obstruction or displacement. Complications that may occur days to weeks after ETT removal include laryngeal or tracheal stenosis and cricoid abscess (Table 15-3). Delayed complications usually require some form of surgical intervention to correct.[15]

Tracheostomy Tubes

A tracheostomy tube is the preferred method of airway maintenance in the patient requiring long-term intubation. Although no ideal time to perform the procedure has been identified, it is generally accepted that if the patient has been intubated or is anticipated to be intubated for more than 2 to 3 weeks, a tracheotomy should be performed.[16] A tracheotomy is also indicated in upper airway obstruction or trauma and in patients with neuromuscular diseases.[17]

A tracheostomy tube provides the best route for long-term airway maintenance because it avoids the oral, nasal, pharyngeal, and laryngeal complications associated with an ETT. Because the tracheostomy tube is shorter, of wider diameter, and less curved than an ETT, the resistance to airflow is less, and breathing is easier. Additional advantages of a tracheostomy tube include easier secretion removal, increased patient acceptance and comfort, the possibility of the patient being able to eat and talk, and the facilitation of ventilator weaning[11,16] (see Table 15-2).

Tracheostomy tubes are made of plastic or metal and may be single-lumen or double-lumen tubes. Single-lumen tubes consist of the tube and a built-in *cuff*, which is connected to a pilot balloon for inflation purposes, and an *obturator*, which is used during tube insertion. The double-lumen tubes consist of the tube with the attached cuff, the obturator, and an inner cannula that can be removed for cleaning and then reinserted or, if disposable, replaced by a new sterile inner cannula. The inner cannula can quickly be removed if it becomes obstructed, making the system safer for patients with significant secretion problems. Single-lumen tubes provide a larger inside diameter for airflow than double-lumen tubes, thus reducing airflow resistance and allowing the patient to ventilate through the tube with greater ease. Plastic tracheostomy tubes also have a 15-mm adapter on the end[18] (Figure 15-2).

Tracheotomy

A tracheostomy tube is inserted through an open or a percutaneous procedure. An open procedure is usually performed in the operating room, whereas a percutaneous procedure can be done at the patient's bedside.[17]

Complications

Complications that may occur during the tracheotomy procedure include misplacement of the tracheal tube, hemorrhage, laryngeal nerve injury, pneumothorax, pneumomediastinum, and cardiac arrest.[19] Potential complications while the tracheostomy tube is in place include stomal infection, hemorrhage, tracheomalacia, tracheoesophageal fistula, tracheoinnominate artery fistula, and tube obstruction or displacement. Complications that may occur days to weeks after tracheostomy tube removal include tracheal stenosis and a tracheocutaneous fistula. (Table 15-4). Delayed complications usually require some form of surgical intervention to correct.[15]

Nursing Management

The patient with an endotracheal or tracheostomy tube requires additional measures to address the effects associated with tube placement on the respiratory and other body systems.

Nursing priorities in the management of the patient with an artificial airway focus on (1) providing humidification, (2) monitoring cuff inflation and cuff pressure, (3) suctioning the airway and monitoring for complications, (4) facilitating communication, and (5) performing extubation and decannulation. Because the tube bypasses the upper airway system, warming and humidifying of air must be performed by external means. Because the cuff of the tube can cause damage to the walls of the trachea, proper cuff inflation and management is imperative. In addition, the normal defense mechanisms are impaired and secretions may accumulate; thus suctioning may be needed to promote secretion clearance. Because the tube does not allow airflow over the vocal cords, developing a method of communication is also very important. Lastly, observing the patient to ensure proper placement of the tube and patency of the airway is essential (Box 15-1).

Providing Humidification

Humidification of air normally is performed by the mucosal layer of the upper respiratory tract. When this area is bypassed, such as occurs with both endotracheal and tracheostomy tubes, or when supplemental O_2 is used, humidification by external means is necessary. Various humidification devices add water to inhaled gas to prevent drying and irritation of the respiratory tract, to prevent undue loss of body water, and to facilitate secretion removal.[20,21] The humidification device should provide inspired gas conditioned (heated) to body temperature and saturated with water vapor.[22]

Monitoring Cuff Inflation/Pressure

Because the cuff of the endotracheal or tracheostomy tube is a major source of the complications associated with artificial airways, proper cuff management is essential. To prevent the complications associated with cuff design, only low-pressure high-volume cuffed tubes are used in clinical practice.[14,23]

Table **15-3**   Prevention/Treatment of Endotracheal Tube (ETT) Complications

Complication	Causes	Prevention	Treatment
Tube obstruction	Patient biting tube Tube kinking during repositioning Cuff herniation Dried secretions, blood, or lubricant Tissue from tumor Trauma Foreign body	Place bite block. Sedate patient PRN. Suction PRN. Humidify inspired gases.	Replace tube.
Tube displacement	Movement of patient's head Movement of tube by tongue Traction on tube from ventilator tubing Self-extubation	Secure tube to upper lip. Restrain patient's hands. Sedate patient PRN. Ensure that only 2 inches of tube extends beyond lip. Support ventilator tubing.	Replace tube.
Sinusitis, nasal injury	Obstruction of paranasal sinus drainage Pressure necrosis of nares	Avoid nasal intubations. Cushion nares from ETT and tape/ties.	Remove all tubes from nasal passages. Administer antibiotics.
Tracheoesophageal fistula	Pressure necrosis of posterior tracheal wall, resulting from overinflated cuff and rigid nasogastric tube	Inflate cuff with minimal amount of air necessary. Monitor cuff pressures q8h.	Position cuff of ETT distal to fistula. Place gastrostomy tube for enteral feedings. Place esophageal tube for secretion clearance proximal to fistula.
Mucosal lesions	Pressure at tube and mucosal interface	Inflate cuff with minimal amount of air necessary. Monitor cuff pressures q8h. Use appropriate-size ETT.	May resolve spontaneously. Perform surgical intervention.
Laryngeal or tracheal stenosis	Injury to area from end of tube or cuff, resulting in scar tissue formation and airway narrowing	Inflate cuff with minimal amount of air necessary. Monitor cuff pressures q8h. Suction area above cuff frequently.	Perform tracheostomy. Place laryngeal stent. Perform surgical repair.
Cricoid abscess	Mucosal injury with bacterial invasion	Inflate cuff with minimal amount of air necessary. Monitor cuff pressures q8h. Suction area above cuff frequently.	Perform incision and drainage of area. Administer antibiotics.

PRN, As needed; *q8h,* every 8 hours.

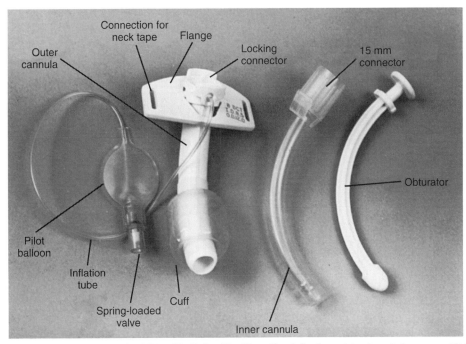

Figure 15-2   Tracheostomy tube. (From Scanlan CL, Wilkins RL, Stoller JK, editors: *Egan's fundamentals of respiratory care*, ed 7, St Louis, 1999, Mosby.)

Even with these tubes, cuff pressures can be generated that are high enough to lead to tracheal ischemia and injury. Both cuff inflation techniques and cuff pressure monitoring are critical components of the care of the patient with an artificial airway.[10,23]

Cuff Inflation Techniques. Two different cuff inflation techniques are currently used. The *minimal leak* (ML) technique consists of injecting air into the cuff until no leak is heard, then withdrawing the air until a small leak is heard on inspiration. Problems with ML technique include difficulty maintaining PEEP and aspiration around the cuff. The *minimal occlusion volume* (MOV) technique consists of injecting air into the cuff until no leak is heard at peak inspiration. The problem with MOV technique is that it generates higher cuff pressures than the ML technique. The choice of technique is determined by individual patient needs. If the patient needs a seal to provide adequate ventilation or is at high risk for aspiration, the MOV technique is used. If these are not concerns, usually the ML technique is used.[10,11,23]

Cuff Pressure Monitoring. Cuff pressures are monitored at least every shift with a cuff pressure manometer. Cuff pressures should be maintained at 20 to 25 mm Hg (24 to 30 cm H_2O) because greater pressures decrease blood flow to the capillaries in the tracheal wall and lesser pressures increase the risk of aspiration. Pressures greater than 22 mm Hg (30 cm H_2O) should be reported to the physician. In addition, cuffs are not routinely deflated because this increases the risk of aspiration.[10,23]

Foam Cuff Tracheostomy Tubes. One tracheostomy tube has a cuff made of foam that is self-inflating. The cuff is deflated during insertion, after which the pilot port is opened to atmospheric pressure (room air), and the cuff self-inflates. Once inflated, the foam cuff conforms to the size and shape of the patient's trachea, reducing pressure against the tracheal wall. The pilot port is left open to atmospheric pressure or is attached to the mechanical ventilator tubing, allowing the cuff to inflate and deflate with the cycling of the ventilator. Routine maintenance of a foam cuff tracheostomy tube includes aspirating the pilot port every 8 hours to measure cuff volume, to remove any condensation from the cuff area, and to assess the integrity of the cuff. Removal is accomplished by deflating the cuff, which can be complicated if the plastic sheath covering the foam is perforated. When perforation occurs, the foam may not be deflatable because the air cannot be totally aspirated.[24]

Suctioning the Airway

Suctioning is often required to maintain a patent airway in the patient with an endotracheal or tracheostomy tube. Suctioning is a sterile procedure that is performed only when required by the patient, not on a routine schedule.[10,23] Indications for suctioning include coughing, secretion in the airway, respiratory distress, presence of rhonchi on auscultation, increased peak airway pressures on the ventilator, and decreasing SaO_2 or PaO_2.[10] Complications associated with suctioning include hypoxemia, atelectasis, bronchospasm,

Table **15-4** Prevention/Treatment of Tracheostomy Tube Complications

Complication	Causes	Prevention	Treatment
Hemorrhage	Vessels opening after surgery Vessel erosion caused by tube	Use appropriate-size tube. Treat local infection. Suction gently. Humidify inspired gases. Position tracheal window not lower than third tracheal ring.	Pack lightly. Perform surgical intervention.
Wound infection	Colonization of stoma with hospital flora	Perform routine stoma care.	Remove tube, if necessary. Perform aggressive wound care and debridement. Administer antibiotics.
Subcutaneous emphysema	Positive-pressure ventilation Coughing against a tight, occlusive dressing or sutured or packed wound	Avoid suturing or packing wound closed around tube.	Remove any sutures or packing if present.
Tube obstruction	Dried blood or secretions False passage into soft tissues Opening of cannula positioned against tracheal wall Foreign body Tissue from tumor	Suction PRN. Humidify inspired gases. Use double-lumen tube. Position tube so that opening does not press against tracheal wall.	Remove/replace inner cannula. Replace tube.
Tube displacement	Patient movement Coughing Traction on ventilatory tubing	Tie tapes to allow only one finger width between tape and neck. Suture tube in place. Use tubes with adjustable neck plates for patients with short necks. Support ventilator tubing. Sedate patient PRN. Restrain patient PRN.	Cover stoma and manually ventilate patient by mouth. Replace tube.
Tracheal stenosis	Injury to area from end of tube or cuff, resulting in scar tissue formation and airway narrowing	Inflate cuff with minimal amount of air necessary. Monitor cuff pressures q8h.	Perform surgical repair.
Tracheoesophageal fistula	Pressure necrosis of posterior tracheal wall, resulting from overinflated cuff and rigid nasogastric tube	Inflate cuff with minimal amount of air necessary. Monitor cuff pressures q8h.	Perform surgical repair.
Tracheoinnominate artery fistula	Direct pressure from elbow of cannula against innominate artery Placement of tracheal stoma below fourth tracheal ring Downward migration of tracheal stoma, resulting from traction on tube High-lying innominate artery	Position tracheal window not lower than third tracheal ring.	Hyperinflate cuff to control bleeding. Remove tube and replace with endotracheal tube; apply digital pressure through stoma against sternum. Perform surgical repair
Tracheocutaneous fistula	Failure of stoma to close after removal of tube	—	Perform surgical repair.

PRN, As needed; q8h, every 8 hours.

Box **15-1**

Artificial Airways

Unintentional Extubation/Decannulation
- Open patient's airway with head-tilt/chin-lift maneuver.
- Maintain airway patency with oropharyngeal or nasopharyngeal airway.

Patient Not Breathing
- Manually ventilate patient with manual resuscitation bag (MRB) and face mask with 100% oxygen.
- If patient has tracheostomy, cover stoma to prevent air from escaping.

dysrhythmias, increased intracranial pressure (ICP), and airway trauma.[23]

Complications. Hypoxemia can result from disconnecting the O_2 source from the patient or removing the oxygen from the patient's airways when suction is applied. Atelectasis is thought to occur when the suction catheter is larger than one-half the ETT's diameter. Excessive negative pressure occurs when suction is applied, promoting collapse of the distal airways. Bronchospasm is the result of the stimulation of the airways with the suction catheter. Cardiac dysrhythmias, particularly bradycardias, are attributed to vagal stimulation. Airway trauma occurs with impaction of the catheter in the airways and when excessive negative pressure is applied to the catheter.[10,23]

Suctioning Protocol. Several practices in suctioning protocols are helpful in limiting the complications of suctioning. Hypoxemia can be minimized by giving the patient three hyperoxygenation breaths (breaths at 100% F_{IO_2}) with the ventilator before the procedure and again after each pass of the suction catheter.[10,25] If the patient exhibits signs of desaturation, hyperinflation (breaths at 150% tidal volume) should be added to the procedure.[10] Atelectasis can be avoided by using a suction catheter with an external diameter less than one-half the internal diameter of the ETT.[23] Using no more than 120 mm Hg of suction will decrease the chances of hypoxemia, atelectasis, and airway trauma.[10] Limiting the duration of each suction pass to 10 to 15 seconds[10] and the number of passes to three or less also will help minimize hypoxemia, airway trauma, and cardiac dysrhythmias.[26] The process of applying intermittent (instead of continuous) suction has not been shown to be of benefit.[27] In addition, instillation of normal saline to help remove secretions has no proven benefit[28] and may actually contribute to the development of hypoxemia[10,29] and lower airway colonization, resulting in nosocomial pneumonia.[10,30]

Closed Tracheal Suction System. One device to facilitate suctioning a patient on the ventilator is the closed tracheal suction system (CTSS). This device consists of a suction catheter in a plastic sleeve that attaches directly to the ventilator tubing. CTSS allows the patient to be suctioned while remaining on the ventilator. Advantages include maintenance of oxygenation and PEEP during suctioning, reduction of hypoxemia-related complications, and protection of staff members from the patient's secretions. CTSS is convenient to use, requiring only one person to perform the procedure.

Concerns related to CTSS include autocontamination, inadequate removal of secretions, and increased risk of unintentional extubation resulting from the extra weight of the system on the ventilator tubing. Autocontamination is not an issue if the catheter is cleaned properly after every use and is changed every 24 hours. Inadequate removal of secretions may or may not be a problem, and further investigation is required to settle this issue.[31]

Facilitating Communication

One of the major stressors for the patient with an artificial airway is impaired communication. This is related to the inability to speak, insufficient explanations from staff members, inadequate understanding, fear of being unable to communicate, and difficulty with communication methods.[32] Interventions to facilitate communication in the patient with an endotracheal or tracheostomy tube include (1) performing a complete assessment of the patient's ability to communicate, (2) teaching the patient how to communicate, (3) using a variety of methods to communicate, and (4) facilitating the patient's ability to communicate by providing the patients eye glasses or hearing aid.[33]

The use of verbal and nonverbal language and a variety of devices can assist the short-term and long-term ventilator-assisted patient. Nonverbal communication may include the use of sign language, gestures, lip reading, pointing, facial expressions, or eye blinking. Simple devices available include pencil and paper; Magic Slates; magnetic boards with plastic letters; picture, alphabet, or symbol boards; and flash cards. More sophisticated devices include typewriters, computers, talking tracheostomy and endotracheal tubes, and external hand-held vibrators. Regardless of the method selected, the patient must be taught how to use the device.[10,33]

Passy-Muir Valve. One of the newer devices used to assist the mechanically ventilated patient with a tracheostomy to speak is the Passy-Muir valve. This one-way valve opens on inhalation, allowing air to enter the lungs through the tracheostomy tube, and closes on exhalation, forcing air over the vocal cords and out the mouth, thus permitting the patient to speak. Before placing the valve on a tracheostomy tube, the cuff must be deflated to allow air to pass around the tube, and the tidal volume of the ventilator must be increased to compensate for the air leak. In addition to assisting the patient to communicate, the Passy-Muir valve can assist the ventilator-dependent patient with relearning normal breathing patterns. The valve is contraindicated in patients with laryngeal or pharyngeal dysfunction, excessive secretions, and poor lung compliance.[34]

Performing Extubation/Decannulation

Once the artificial airway is no longer needed, it is removed. *Extubation*, the process of removing an ETT, is a simple procedure that can be accomplished at the bedside.[10,11] Complications of extubation include sore throat, stridor, hoarseness, odynophagia, vocal cord immobility, pulmonary aspiration, and cough.[15] *Decannulation*, the process of removing a tracheostomy tube, is also a simple process that can be performed at the bedside. After the removal of the tracheostomy tube, the stoma is usually covered with a dry dressing, with the expectation that the stoma will close within several days.[10,11] Difficulty removing the tracheostomy tube as a result of a tight stoma is usually the only complication associated with decannulation.[15]

INVASIVE MECHANICAL VENTILATION
Indications

Mechanical ventilation is indicated for a variety of physiologic and clinical reasons. Physiologic objectives include supporting cardiopulmonary gas exchange (alveolar ventilation, arterial oxygenation), increasing lung volume (end-expiratory lung inflation, functional residual capacity), and reducing the work of breathing. Clinical objectives include reversing hypoxemia and acute respiratory acidosis, relieving respiratory distress, preventing or reversing atelectasis and respiratory muscle fatigue, permitting sedation and neuromuscular blockade, decreasing O_2 consumption, reducing ICP, and stabilizing the chest wall.[35]

Types of Ventilators

Two main ventilator types are currently available. *Negative-pressure* ventilators are applied externally to the patient and decrease the atmospheric pressure surrounding the thorax to initiate inspiration; these ventilators generally are not used in the critical care environment. *Positive-pressure* ventilators use a mechanical drive mechanism to force air into the patient's lungs through an endotracheal or tracheostomy tube.[33,37]

Ventilator Mechanics

The ventilator must complete four phases of ventilation to properly ventilate the patient: (1) change from exhalation to inspiration, (2) inspiration, (3) change from inspiration to exhalation, and (4) exhalation. The ventilator uses four different variables to begin, sustain, and terminate each of these phases. These variables are described in terms of *volume*, *pressure*, *flow*, and *time*.

Trigger. The trigger is the phase variable that initiates the change from exhalation to inspiration. Breaths may be pressure or flow triggered, based on the sensitivity setting of the ventilator and the patient's inspiratory effort or time triggered, based on the rate setting of the ventilator. A breath initiated by the patient is known as a *patient-triggered*

or *assisted* breath, whereas a breath initiated by the ventilator is known as a *machine-triggered* or *controlled* breath. A *time-triggered* breath is a machine-controlled breath in which the ventilator initiates a breath after a preset time has elapsed. It is controlled by the rate setting on the ventilator; thus a rate of 10 breaths/min yields one breath every 6 seconds. *Flow-triggered* or *pressure-triggered* breaths are patient-assisted breaths in which the patient initiates the breath by decreasing flow or decreasing pressure within the breathing circuit. Flow triggering, or *flow-by*, is controlled by adjusting the flow sensitivity setting of the ventilator, whereas pressure triggering is controlled by adjusting the pressure sensitivity setting. Many ventilators offer different trigger types in combination. Thus a breath may be both time-triggered and flow-triggered, depending on the patient's ability to interact with the ventilator and initiate a breath.

Limit. The limit, or *target*, is the variable that maintains inspiration. Inspiration can be pressure, flow, or volume limited. In a pressure-limited breath a preset pressure is attained and maintained during inspiration. In a flow-limited breath a preset flow is reached before the end of inspiration. In a volume-limited breath a preset volume is delivered during the inspiration. The limit variable only sustains inspiration and does not end inspiration.

Cycle. The cycle variable ends inspiration. The four classifications of positive-pressure ventilators are based on the cycle variable. *Volume-cycled* ventilators are designed to deliver a breath until a present volume is delivered. *Pressure-cycled* ventilators deliver a breath until a preset pressure is reached within the patient's airway. *Flow-cycled* ventilators deliver a breath until a preset inspiratory flow rate is achieved. *Time-cycled* ventilators deliver a breath over a preset interval.

Baseline. The baseline is the variable that is controlled during exhalation. Pressure is typically used to adjust baseline. The patient exhales to a certain baseline pressure that is set on the ventilator. Baseline may be set at zero, which is atmospheric pressure, or above atmospheric pressure, which is called *positive end-expiratory pressure* (PEEP).

Modes of Ventilation

The term *ventilator mode* refers to how the machine will ventilate the patient. Selection of a particular mode of ventilation determines how much the patient will participate in the ventilatory pattern. The choice depends on the patient's situation and the goals of treatment. The mode is determined by the combination of phase variables selected, with a variety of modes available[36-38] (Table 15-5). Many of these modes may be used in conjunction with each other. Because brands vary in their ability to perform certain functions, not all modes are available on all ventilators.[37]

Ventilator Settings

A variety of settings on the ventilator allow the ventilator parameters to be individualized to the patient and also allow selection of the desired ventilation mode (Table 15-6). In

Table 15-5   Modes of Mechanical Ventilation

Mode	Clinical Application	Nursing Implications
Control (volume or pressure) ventilation (CV) Delivers gas at preset rate and tidal volume or pressure (depending on selected cycling variable), regardless of patient's inspiratory efforts	Used as primary ventilatory mode in apneic patients	Used in patients unable to initiate a breath Spontaneously breathing patients must be sedated/paralyzed.
Assist/control (volume or pressure) ventilation (A/C) or continuous mandatory ventilation (CMV) Delivers gas at preset tidal volume or pressure (depending on selected cycling variable) in response to patient's inspiratory efforts and will initiate breath if patient fails to do so within preset time	Used as primary mode of ventilation in spontaneously breathing patients with weak respiratory muscles	Hyperventilation can occur in patients with increased respiratory rates. Sedation may be necessary to limit number of spontaneous breaths.
Synchronous intermittent mandatory (volume or pressure) ventilation (SIMV) Delivers gas at preset tidal volume or pressure (depending on selected cycling variable) and rate while allowing patient to breathe spontaneously; ventilator breaths are synchronized to patient's respiratory effort.	Used both as primary mode of ventilation in variety of clinical situations Used as weaning mode	May increase work of breathing and promote respiratory muscle fatigue
Positive end-expiratory pressure (PEEP) Positive pressure applied at end of expiration of ventilator breaths (used with CV, A/C, and SIMV) *Constant positive airway pressure (CPAP)* Positive pressure applied during spontaneous breaths	Used in patients with hypoxemia refractory to oxygen therapy Increase FRC and improve oxygenation by opening collapsed alveoli at end expiration	Side effects include decreased cardiac output, volutrauma, and increased intracranial pressure. No ventilator breaths are delivered in PEEP and CPAP mode unless used with CV, A/C, or SIMV.
Pressure support ventilation (PSV) Preset positive pressure used to augment patient's inspiratory efforts; patient controls rate, inspiratory flow, and tidal volume.	Used as primary mode of ventilation in patients with stable respiratory drive Used with SIMV to support spontaneous breaths Used as weaning mode in patients difficult to wean	Advantages include increased patient comfort, decreased work of breathing, decreased respiratory muscle fatigue, and promotion of respiratory muscle conditioning
Volume-assured pressure support ventilation (VAPSV)	Tidal volume is set to ensure patient receives minimum tidal volume with each pressure support breath.	
Independent lung ventilation (ILV) Each lung ventilated separately	Used in patients with unilateral lung disease, bronchopleural fistulas, and bilateral asymmetric lung disease	Requires double-lumen endotracheal tube, two ventilators, sedation, and/or pharmacologic paralysis
High-frequency ventilation (HFV) Delivers small volume of gas at rapid rate • HFPPV: 60–100 breaths/min • HFJV: 100–600 cycles/min • HFO: 900–3000 cycles/min	Used when conventional mechanical ventilation compromises hemodynamic stability Bronchopleural fistulas Short-term procedures Diseases with risk of volutrauma	Patients require sedation and/or pharmacologic paralysis. Inadequate humidification can compromise airway patency. Assessment of breath sounds is difficult.
Inverse ratio ventilation (IRV) Proportion of inspiratory to expiratory time is greater than 1:1; can be initiated using pressure-controlled breaths (PC-IRV) or volume-controlled breaths (VC-IRV)	Used in patients with hypoxemia refractory to PEEP Longer inspiratory time increases FRC and improves oxygenation by opening collapsed alveoli. Shorter expiratory time induces auto-PEEP that prevents alveoli from recollapsing.	Requires sedation and/or pharmacologic paralysis because of discomfort Increased intrathoracic pressure can result in excessive air trapping and decreased cardiac output.

FRC, Functional residual capacity; *HFPPV,* high-frequency positive-pressure ventilation; *HFJV,* high-frequency jet ventilation; *HFO,* high-frequency oscillation.

Table **15-6**	Ventilator Settings
Parameter	**Description**
Respiratory rate or frequency (f)	Number of breaths the ventilator delivers per minute Usual setting: 4-20 breaths/min
Tidal volume (Vt)	Volume of gas delivered during each ventilator breath Usual volume: 10 ml/kg
Oxygen concentration (FIO_2)	Fraction of inspired oxygen delivered Settings: 20%-100%; usually adjusted to maintain PaO_2 >60 mm Hg or SaO_2 >90%
Inspiration/expiration (I/E) ratio	Duration of inspiration to duration of expiration Usual setting: 1:2 to 1:1.5, unless IRV to be used
Flow rate	Speed with which tidal volume is delivered Usual setting: 40-100 L/min
Sensitivity (pressure/flow trigger)	Determines amount of effort that patient must generate to initiate a ventilator breath Pressure triggering: 0.5-1.5 cm H_2O below baseline Flow triggering: 1.0-3.0 L/min below baseline flow
Pressure limit	Regulates maximal pressure that ventilator can generate to deliver tidal volume When pressure limit reached, ventilator terminates the breath and spills undelivered volume into atmosphere. Usual setting: 10 cm H_2O above peak inspiratory pressure

PaO_2, Arterial oxygen tension; SaO_2, arterial hemoglobin oxygen saturation; *IRV*, inverse ratio ventilation.

addition, each ventilator has a patient-monitoring system that allows all aspects of the patient's ventilatory pattern to be assessed, monitored, and displayed.[37,39]

Complications

Some mechanical ventilation complications are preventable, whereas other complications can be minimized but cannot be eradicated. Physiologic complications include volutrauma, cardiovascular compromise, gastrointestinal (GI) disturbances, patient-ventilator dyssynchrony, and nosocomial pneumonia.

Volutrauma

Volutrauma, formerly known as *barotrauma*, results from alveolar overdistention secondary to mechanical ventilation. Overdistention may be related more to the volume of air in the lungs than to the pressure inside the lungs and thus is now called *volutrauma*. Regardless of the underlying cause, overdistention causes alveolar rupture and air leakage into the pulmonary interstitial space. Once in the space, the air travels out through the hilum and into the mediastinum (pneumomediastinum), pleural space (pneumothorax), subcutaneous tissues (subcutaneous emphysema), pericardium (pneumopericardium), peritoneum (pneumoperitoneum), and retroperitoneum (pneumoretroperitoneum). The resultant disorders vary from the fairly benign to the potentially lethal; the most lethal disorder is pneumothorax or pneumopericardium resulting in cardiac tamponade. Volutrauma occurs in 4% to 15% of all mechanically ventilated patients. Patients with ARDS, status asthmaticus, and aspiration pneumonitis are at a higher risk.[35,40,41]

Cardiovascular Compromise

Positive-pressure ventilation (PPV) increases intrathoracic pressure, which decreases venous return to the right side of the heart. Impaired venous return decreases preload, which results in a decrease in CO.[35,40,41] As a secondary consequence, hepatic and renal dysfunction may occur. In addition, PPV impairs cerebral venous return. In patients with impaired autoregulation, PPV can result in increased ICP.[40]

Gastrointestinal Disturbances

GI disturbances also may result from PPV. Gastric distention occurs when air leaks around the endotracheal or tracheostomy tube cuff and overcomes the resistance of the lower esophageal sphincter.[37,40] Vomiting may result from pharyngeal stimulation from the artificial airway. These problems can be prevented by inserting a nasogastric tube and ensuring appropriate cuff inflation.[37,40] Hypomotility and constipation may result from immobility and administration of paralytic agents, analgesics, and sedatives.[35]

Patient-Ventilator Dyssynchrony

Because the normal ventilatory pattern is usually initiated by the establishment of negative pressure within the chest, the application of positive pressure can lead to patient difficulties in breathing on the ventilator. To achieve optimal ventilatory assistance, the patient should breathe in synchrony with the machine. The selected mode of ventilation, the settings, and the type of ventilatory circuitry used can also increase the work of breathing and lead to the patient breathing out of synchrony with the ventilator.

Patient-ventilatory dyssynchrony can result in decreased effectiveness of mechanical ventilation, development of auto-PEEP, and psychologic distress in the patient. Patients who are not breathing in synchrony with the ventilator appear to be fighting or "bucking" the ventilator. To minimize this problem, the ventilator is adjusted to work with the patient and accommodate the patient's spontaneous breathing pattern. If this is not possible, the patient may need to be sedated or pharmacologically paralyzed.[35,37,40]

Nosocomial Pneumonia

Nosocomial pneumonia may develop after placement of an artificial airway because the tube bypasses or impairs many of the lung's normal defense mechanisms. Once an artificial airway is placed, contamination of the lower airways follows within 24 hours from factors that directly and indirectly promote airway colonization. Respiratory therapy devices such as ventilators, nebulizers, and intermittent positive-pressure breathing machines also increase the risk of pneumonia. The severity of the patient's illness, presence of acute lung injury, and malnutrition significantly increase the likelihood of infection. Therapeutic measures such as nasogastric tubes, antacids, and histamine inhibitors also facilitate development of pneumonia. Nasogastric tubes promote aspiration by acting as a wick for stomach contents, whereas antacids and histamine inhibitors increase the pH level of the stomach, promoting growth of bacteria that can then be aspirated.[40,42]

Weaning

Weaning is the gradual withdrawal of the mechanical ventilator and the reestablishment of spontaneous breathing. Weaning should begin only after the original process requiring ventilator support for the patient has been corrected and patient stability achieved. Other factors to consider when weaning are length of time on ventilator, sleep deprivation, and nutritional status. Major factors that affect the patient's ability to wean include the lungs' ability to participate in ventilation and respiration, cardiovascular performance, and psychologic readiness.[43] This discussion focuses on weaning the patient from short-term (3 days or less) mechanical ventilation. Managing the patient requiring long-term mechanical ventilation is discussed in Chapter 14.

Readiness to Wean

Once the decision is made to wean the patient, the patient is assessed for readiness to wean. Evaluation includes level of consciousness, physiologic and hemodynamic stability, adequacy of oxygenation and ventilation, spontaneous breathing capability, and respiratory rate and pattern. Pulmonary mechanics also may be measured. Two strong predictors for weaning readiness are vital capacity (VC) greater than 15 ml/kg and negative inspiratory pressure (NIP) of −30 cm H_2O or less.[44]

Once readiness to wean has been established, the patient is prepared for the weaning trial. The patient is positioned upright to facilitate breathing and suctioned to ensure airway patency. The process is explained, and the patient is reassured and offered diversional activities. The patient is assessed immediately before the start of the trial and frequently during the weaning period for signs of weaning intolerance[43-45] (Box 15-2).

Weaning Methods

A number of methods can be used to wean a patient from the ventilator. The method selected depends on the patient, pulmonary status, and length of time on the ventilator. The three main methods for weaning are (1) T-tube (T-piece) trials, (2) synchronized intermittent mandatory ventilation (SIMV), and (3) pressure support ventilation (PSV).[35,43,44]

T-Piece. T-piece weaning trials consist of alternating periods of ventilatory support, usually on assist/control (A/C) or continuous mandatory ventilation (CMV), with periods of spontaneous breathing. The trial is initiated by removing the patient from the ventilator and having the patient breathe spontaneously on a T-piece O_2 delivery system. After a set time the patient is placed back on the ventilator. The goal is to progressively increase the duration of time spent off the ventilator. During the weaning process the patient is observed closely for respiratory muscle fatigue.[35,37,45] Continuous positive airway pressure (CPAP) may be added to prevent atelectasis and improve oxygenation.[37]

Synchronized Intermittent Mandatory Ventilation. The goal of SIMV weaning is the gradual transition from ventilatory support to spontaneous breathing. The transition is initiated by placing the ventilator in the SIMV mode and slowly decreasing the rate until zero (or close to zero) is

---

Box 15-2	Weaning Intolerance Indicators

- Decrease in level of consciousness
- Systolic blood pressure increased or decreased by 20 mm Hg
- Diastolic blood pressure greater than 100 mm Hg
- Heart rate increased by 20 beats/min
- Premature ventricular contractions greater than 6/min, couplets, or runs of ventricular tachycardia
- Changes in ST segment (usually elevation)
- Respiratory rate greater than 30 breaths/min or less than 10 breaths/min
- Respiratory rate increased by 10 breaths/min
- Spontaneous tidal volume less than 250 ml
- $Paco_2$ increased by 5 to 8 mm Hg and/or pH less than 7.30
- Spo_2 less than 90%
- Use of accessory muscles of ventilation
- Complaints of dyspnea, fatigue, or pain
- Paradoxical chest wall motion
- Diaphoresis

Table **15-7** Troubleshooting Ventilator Alarms

Problem	Causes	Interventions
Low exhaled tidal volume (Vt)	Altered settings	Check settings.
	Conditions that trigger high-pressure or low-pressure alarm	Evaluate patient; check respiratory rate.
	Patient stops spontaneous respirations	Check connections for leaks.
	Leak in system preventing Vt delivery	Suction patient's airway.
	Cuff insufficiently inflated	Check cuff pressure.
	Leak through chest tube	Calibrate spirometer.
	Airway secretions	
	Decreased lung compliance	
	Disconnected/malfunctioning spirometer	
Low inspiratory pressure	Altered settings	Reset alarm.
	Unattached tubing or leak around ETT	Reconnect tubing.
	ETT displaced into pharynx or esophagus	Modify cuff pressures.
	Poor cuff inflation or leak	Tighten humidifier.
	Tracheoesophageal fistula	Check chest tube.
	Too low peak flow; low Vt	Adjust peak flow to meet or exceed patient demand; correct for patient's Vt.
	Decreased airway resistance from decreased secretions or relief of bronchospasm	Reposition/change ETT.
	Increased lung compliance from decreased atelectasis	
	Reduction in pulmonary edema	
	Resolution of ARDS	
	Change in position	
Low exhaled minute volume	Altered settings	Check settings.
	Leak in system	Assess patient's respiratory rate, work of breathing, and mental status.
	Airway secretions	Evaluate system for leaks.
	Decreased lung compliance	Suction airway.
	Malfunctioning spirometer	Assess patient for changes in disease state.
	Decreased patient-triggered respiratory rate from drugs, sleep, hypocapnia, alkalosis, fatigue, change in neurologic status	Calibrate spirometer.
Low PEEP/CPAP	Altered settings	Check settings and correct.
	Leak in system	Observe for leaks in system.
	Increased patient inspiratory flow	If unable to correct problem, increase PEEP setting.
	Decreased ventilator expiratory flow	

Parameter	Cause	Action
High respiratory rate	Increased metabolic demand Drug administration Hypoxia, hypercapnia, acidosis, shock Pain, fear, anxiety	Evaluate ABGs. Assess patient. Calm and reassure patient.
High pressure limit	Improper alarm setting Airway obstruction from patient "fighting ventilator" (holding breath as ventilator delivers Vt) Patient circuit collapse Tubing kinked ETT in right mainstem bronchus or against carina Cuff herniation Increased airway resistance from bronchospasm, airway secretions, plugs, or coughing Water from humidifier in ventilator tubing Decreased lung compliance from tension pneumothorax Change in patient position ARDS, pulmonary edema, atelectasis, pneumonia, abdominal distention	Reset alarms. Clear obstruction from tubing. Unkink tubing; reposition patient off tubing. Empty water from tubing. Check breath sounds. Reassure patient; sedate if necessary. Check ABGs for hypoxemia. Observe for abdominal distention that would put pressure on diaphragm. Check cuff pressures. Obtain chest radiograph and evaluate for ETT position, pneumothorax, and pneumonia; reposition ETT. Administer bronchodilators.
Low-pressure oxygen inlet	Improper oxygen alarm setting Oxygen not connected to ventilator Dirty oxygen intake filter	Correct alarm setting. Reconnect/connect oxygen line to 50-psi source. Clean/replace oxygen filter.
I/E ratio	Inspiratory longer than expiratory time Use of inspiratory phase that is too long, with fast rate Peak flow setting too low while rate too high Machine too sensitive	Change inspiratory time, or adjust peak flow. Check inspiratory phase, or hold. Check machine sensitivity.
Temperature	Sensor malfunction Overheating from too low or no gas flow Sensor picking up outside airflow (from heaters, open doors/windows, air conditioners) Improper water levels	Test/replace sensor. Check gas flow. Protect sensor from outside source that would interfere with readings. Check water levels.

PEEP, Positive end-expiratory pressure; *CPAP*, continuous positive airway pressure; *I/E*, inspiration/expiration; *ETT*, endotracheal tube; *ARDS*, acute respiratory distress syndrome; *ABGs*, arterial blood gases; *psi*, pounds per square inch.

reached. The rate is usually decreased one to three breaths at a time, and an arterial blood gas (ABG) sample is usually obtained 30 minutes later. This method of weaning can increase the work of breathing, and thus the patient must be closely monitored for signs of respiratory muscle fatigue.[35,37,43,45]

Pressure Support Ventilation. PSV weaning consists of placing the patient on the pressure support mode and setting the pressure support at a level that facilitates the patient's achieving a spontaneous tidal volume of 10 to 12 ml/kg. PSV augments the patient's spontaneous breaths with a positive-pressure "boost" during inspiration. During the weaning process the level of pressure support is gradually decreased in increments of 3 to 6 cm H_2O while maintaining tidal volume of 10 to 15 ml/kg, until a level of 5 cm H_2O is achieved. If the patient is able to maintain adequate spontaneous respirations at this level, extubation is considered. PSV also can be used with SIMV weaning to help overcome the resistance in the ventilator system.[37,43,45]

Nursing Management

Nursing priorities for the patient with invasive mechanical ventilation focus on monitoring the patient for both patient-related and ventilator-related complications. Monitoring should include a total patient assessment, with particular emphasis on the pulmonary system, placement of the ETT, and observation for subcutaneous emphysema and synchrony with the ventilator. Assessment of the ventilator includes a review of all the ventilator settings and alarms (Table 15-7). In addition, peak inspiratory pressure, exhaled tidal volume, and ABGs are monitored and safety issues addressed (Box 15-3).

Bedside evaluation of vital capacity, minute ventilation, ABG values, and other pulmonary function tests may be warranted, according to the patient's condition. The use of pulse oximetry can facilitate continuous, noninvasive

assessment of oxygenation. Static and dynamic compliance should also be monitored to assess for changes in lung compliance (see Appendix).

NONINVASIVE MECHANICAL VENTILATION

Noninvasive mechanical ventilation is a relatively new method of ventilation that uses a mask instead of an ETT to administer PPV. Advantages of PPV include decreased frequency of nosocomial pneumonia, increased comfort, and the noninvasive nature of the procedure, which allows easy application and removal. PPV is indicated in both type I and type II acute respiratory failure and when intubation is not an option. Contraindications to noninvasive mechanical ventilation include hemodynamic instability, dysrhythmias, apnea, uncooperativeness, intolerance of the mask, and the inability to maintain a patent airway, clear secretions, and properly fit the mask.[46]

Noninvasive mechanical ventilation can be applied using a nasal or facial mask and ventilator or a BiPAP (Respironics) machine (Figure 15-3). This mode of therapy uses a combination of PSV (ventilator) or inspiratory positive airway pressure (IPAP) (BiPAP) and PEEP (ventilator) or expiratory positive airway pressure (EPAP) (BiPAP) to assist the spontaneously breathing patient with ventilation. On inspiration, the patient receives PSV or IPAP to increase tidal volume and minute ventilation, which results in increased alveolar ventilation, decreased $PaCO_2$ level, relief of dyspnea, and reduced accessory muscle use. On expiration the patient receives PEEP or EPAP to increase functional residual capacity, which results in an increased PaO_2 level. Humidified supplemental O_2 is administered to maintain a clinically acceptable PaO_2 level, and timed breaths may be added if necessary.[47]

Nursing Management

Nursing priorities for the patient with noninvasive mechanical ventilation focus on monitoring the patient for both patient-related and ventilator-related complications. As with invasive mechanical ventilation, the patient must be closely monitored while receiving noninvasive mechanical ventilation. Respiratory rate, accessory muscle use, and oxygenation status are continually assessed to ensure the patient is tolerating this method of ventilation. Continued pulse oximetry with a set alarm parameter is initiated.[47]

The key to ensuring adequate ventilatory support is a properly fitted mask. Either a nasal mask or a full-face mask may be used, depending on the patient. A properly fitted mask minimizes air leakage and discomfort for the patient. Transparent dressings placed over the pressure points of the face help minimize air leakage and prevent facial skin necrosis from the mask.[38] The BiPAP machine is able to compensate for air leaks.[47]

The patient is positioned with the head of the bed elevated at 45 degrees to minimize the risk of aspiration and facilitate breathing. *Insufflation* of the stomach is a compli-

---

patient safety _____ Box **15-3**

Invasive Mechanical Ventilation

Ventilator System Maintenance

- Maintain a functional manual resuscitation bag (MRB) connected to oxygen at the bedside.
- Ensure that ventilator tubing is free of water.
- Positioning ventilator tubing to avoid kinking.
- Maintain patency of ventilator tubing and connections.
- Change ventilator tubing per hospital policy.
- Monitor temperature of inspired air.

Ventilator Malfunction

- Remove patient from ventilator and ventilate manually with MRB.
- Ensure that alarms are sufficiently audible with respect to distance and competing noise in unit.

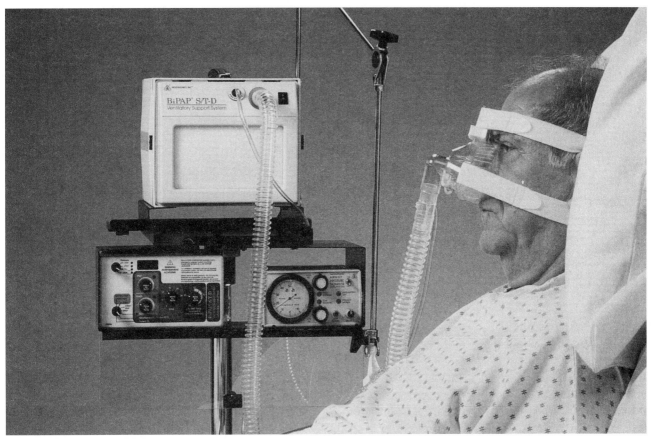

Figure 15-3   Noninvasive mechanical ventilation. (Courtesy Respironics, Murrysville, Pa.)

cation of this mode of therapy and places the patient at risk for aspiration. Thus the patient is closely monitored for gastric distention, and a nasogastric tube is placed for decompression as necessary.[38] Often patients are very anxious and have high levels of dyspnea before the initiation of noninvasive mechanical ventilation. Once adequate ventilation has been established, anxiety and dyspnea are usually sufficiently relieved. Heavy sedation should be avoided, but if needed, it would constitute the need for intubation and invasive mechanical ventilation. Spending 30 minutes with the patient after the initiation of noninvasive ventilation is important because the patient needs reassurance and must learn how to breathe on the machine[47] (Box 15-4).

---

patient safety   Box **15-4**

Noninvasive Mechanical Ventilation

- **Never restrain a patient requiring noninvasive mechanical ventilation with a full-face mask**.
- Patient must be able to remove the mask in the event that mask becomes displaced or patient vomits.
- A displaced mask can force the patient's bottom jaw inward and occlude the patient's airway.

REFERENCES

1. O'Connor BS, Vender JS: Oxygen therapy, *Crit Care Clin* 11:67, 1995.
2. Owens MW et al: Respiratory care modalities. In Bone RC, editor: *Pulmonary and critical care medicine*, St Louis, 1998, Mosby.
3. Scanlan CL, Heuer A: Medical gas therapy. In Scanlan CL, Wilkins RL, Stoller JK, editors: *Egan's fundamentals of respiratory care*, ed 7, St Louis, 1999, Mosby.
4. Carraway MS, Piantadosi CA: Oxygen toxicity, *Respir Care Clin N Am* 5:265, 1999.
5. Hanson CW et al: Causes of hypercarbia with oxygen therapy in patients with chronic obstructive pulmonary disease, *Crit Care Med* 24:23, 1996.
6. Marshak AB, Scanlan CL: Emergency life support. In Scanlan CL, Wilkins RL, Stoller JK, editors: *Egan's fundamentals of respiratory care*, ed 7, St Louis, 1999, Mosby.
7. Levitan R, Ochroch EA: Airway management and direct laryngoscopy: a review and update, *Crit Care Clin* 16:373, 2000.
8. Hess DR: Indications for translaryngeal intubation, *Respir Care* 44:604, 1999.
9. Rodricks MB, Deutschman CS: Emergent airway management: indications and methods in the face of confounding conditions, *Crit Care Clin* 16:389, 2000.
10. Henneman E, Ellstrom K, St. John RE: *Airway management*, Aliso Viejo, Calif, 1999, American Association of Critical-Care Nurses.
11. Scanlan C, Simmons K: Airway management. In Scanlan CL, Wilkins RL, Stoller JK, editors: *Egan's fundamentals of respiratory care*, ed 7, St Louis, 1999, Mosby.

12. Hurford WE: Orotracheal intubation outside the operating room: anatomic considerations and techniques, *Respir Care* 44:615, 1999.

13. Hurford WE: Nasotracheal intubation, *Respir Care* 44:643, 1999.

14. Colice GL: Technical standards for tracheal tubes, *Clin Chest Med* 12:433, 1991.

15. Stauffer JL: Complications of endotracheal intubation and tracheotomy, *Respir Care* 44:824, 1999.

16. Heffner JE: Tracheotomy: indications and timing, *Respir Care* 44:807, 1999.

17. Pryor JP, Reilly PM, Shapiro MB: Surgical airway management in the intensive care unit, *Crit Care Clin* 16:473, 2000.

18. Weilitz PB, Dettenmeier PA: Back to basics: test your knowledge of tracheostomy tubes, *Am J Nurs* 94(2):46, 1994.

19. Reibel J: Tracheotomy/tracheostomy, *Respir Care* 44:820, 1999.

20. Branson RD: Humidification for patients with artificial airways, *Respir Care* 44:630, 1999.

21. Fink J, Scanlon CL: Humidity and bland aerosol therapy. In Scanlan CL, Wilkins RL, Stoller JK, editors: *Egan's fundamentals of respiratory care*, ed 7, St Louis, 1999, Mosby.

22. Peterson BD: Heated humidifiers: structure and function, *Respir Care Clin N Am* 4:243, 1998.

23. Hess DR: Managing the artificial airway, *Respir Care* 44:759, 1999.

24. Bivona: *Fome-Cuf users manual*, Gary, Ind, 1991, Bivona.

25. Grap MJ et al: Endotracheal suctioning: ventilator vs. manual delivery of hyperoxygenation breaths, *Am J Crit Care* 5:192, 1996.

26. Stone KS: Ventilator versus manual resuscitation bag as the method of delivering hyperoxygenation before endotracheal suctioning, *AACN Clin Issues Crit Care Nurs* 1:289, 1990.

27. Czarnik RE et al: Deferential effects of continuous versus intermittent suction on tracheal tissue, *Heart Lung* 20:144, 1991.

28. Raymond SJ: Normal saline instillation before suctioning: helpful or harmful? A review of the literature, *Am J Crit Care* 4:267, 1995.

29. Kinloch D: Instillation of normal saline during endotracheal suctioning: effects on mixed venous oxygen saturation, *Am J Crit Care* 8:231, 1999.

30. Hagler DA, Traver GA: Endotracheal saline and suction catheters: sources of lower airway contamination, *Am J Crit Care* 3:444, 1994.

31. Johnson KL et al: Closed versus open endotracheal suctioning: costs and physiologic consequences, *Crit Care Med* 22:658,1994.

32. Jablonski RS: The experience of being mechanically ventilated, *Qual Health Res* 4:186, 1994.

33. Williams ML: An algorithm for selecting a communication technique with intubated patients, *Dimens Crit Care Nurs* 11:222, 1992.

34. Bell SD: Use of Passy-Muir tracheostomy speaking valve in mechanically ventilated neurological patients, *Crit Care Nurse* 16(1):63, 1996.

35. American College of Chest Physicians: ACCP consensus conference: mechanical ventilation, *Chest* 194:1833, 1993.

36. Chatburn RL, Scanlan CL: Ventilator modes and functions. In Scanlan CL, Wilkins RL, Stoller JK, editors: *Egan's fundamentals of respiratory care*, ed 7, St Louis, 1999, Mosby.

37. Pilbeam SP: *Mechanical ventilation: physiological and clinical applications*, ed 3, St Louis, 1998, Mosby.

38. Pierce LNB: *Traditional and nontraditional modes of mechanical ventilation*, Aliso Viejo, Calif, 1998, American Association of Critical-Care Nurses.

39. Hicks GH, Scanlan CL: Initiating and adjusting ventilatory support. In Scanlan CL, Wilkins RL, Stoller JK, editors: *Egan's fundamentals of respiratory care*, ed 7, St Louis, 1999, Mosby.

40. Mutlu GM, Factor P: Complications of mechanical ventilation, *Respir Care Clin N Am* 6:213, 2000.

41. Sandur S, Stoller JK: Pulmonary complications of mechanical ventilation, *Clin Chest Med* 20:223, 1999.

42. Ahmed QA, Niederman MS: Respiratory infection in the chronically critically ill patient: ventilator-associated pneumonia and tracheobronchitis, *Clin Chest Med* 22:71, 2001.

43. Chao DC, Scheinhorn DJ: Weaning from mechanical ventilation, *Crit Care Clin* 14:799, 1998.

44. Hannemann SK: *Weaning from short-term mechanical ventilation*, Aliso Viejo, Calif, 1998. American Association of Critical-Care Nurses.

45. Shelledy DC: Discontinuing ventilatory support. In Scanlan CL, Wilkins RL, Stoller JK, editors: *Egan's fundamentals of respiratory care*, ed 7, St Louis, 1999, Mosby.

46. Mehta S, Hill NS: Noninvasive ventilation, *Am J Respir Crit Care Med* 163:540, 2001.

47. Abou-Shola N, Meduri GU: Noninvasive mechanical ventilation in patients with acute respiratory failure, *Crit Care Med* 24:705, 1996.

UNIT FIVE

NEUROLOGIC ALTERATIONS

BEVERLY CARLSON

16

Neurologic Assessment and Diagnostic Procedures

Objectives

- Identify the components of a neurologic history.
- Describe the five components of the neurologic assessment.
- Discuss the neurologic changes associated with intracranial hypertension.
- Identify key diagnostic procedures used in assessment of the patient with neurologic dysfunction.
- Discuss the nursing management of a patient undergoing a neurologic diagnostic procedure.

Assessment of the critically ill patient with neurologic dysfunction includes a review of the patient's health history, a thorough physical examination, and an analysis of the patient's laboratory data. Numerous invasive and noninvasive diagnostic procedures may also be performed to assist in the identification of the patient's disorder. This chapter focuses on priority clinical assessments, laboratory studies, and diagnostic procedures for the critically ill patient with a neurologic dysfunction.

CLINICAL ASSESSMENT

A thorough clinical assessment of the patient with neurologic dysfunction is imperative for the early identification and treatment of neurologic disorders. Once completed, the assessment serves as the foundation for developing the management plan for the patient. The assessment process can be brief or may involve a detailed history and examination, depending on the nature and immediacy of the patient's situation.

HISTORY

Neurologic assessment encompasses a variety of applications and a multitude of techniques. The factor common to all neurologic assessments is the need to obtain a comprehensive history of events preceding hospitalization. An adequate neurologic history includes information about clinical manifestations, associated complaints, precipitating factors, progression, and familial occurrences. If the patient is incapable of providing this information, family members or significant others should be contacted as soon as possible. When someone other than the patient is the source of the history, the individual should have daily contact with the patient. Frequently, valuable information is gained, which directs the caregiver to focus on certain aspects of the patient's clinical assessment.[1]

PHYSICAL EXAMINATION

Five major components make up the neurologic examination of the critically ill patient. **Nursing assessment priorities focus on evaluating (1) level of consciousness, (2) motor function, (3) pupillary function, (4) respiratory function**, and (5) **vital signs**. Until all five components have been assessed, a complete neurologic examination has not been performed.[1]

Level of Consciousness

Assessment of the level of consciousness (LOC) is the most important aspect of the neurologic examination. In most situations, a patient's LOC deteriorates before any other neurologic changes are noted. These deteriorations often are subtle and must be monitored carefully. **Nursing priorities in assessment of level of consciousness focus on (1) evaluating arousal or alertness** and (2) **appraising content of consciousness or awareness**. Universally accepted definitions for various LOCs do not exist. Although vague, specific categories are often used to describe the patient's LOC[1-3] (Box 16-1).

Evaluating Arousal

Assessment of the arousal component of consciousness is an evaluation of the reticular activating system and its connection with the thalamus and the cerebral cortex. Arousal is the lowest level of consciousness, and observation centers on the patient's ability to respond appropriately to verbal or noxious stimuli. To stimulate the patient, the nurse should begin with verbal stimuli in a normal tone. If the patient does not respond, the nurse should increase the stimuli by using a shouting level with the patient. If the patient still does not respond, the nurse should further increase the stimuli by shaking the patient. Noxious stimuli should follow if previous attempts to arouse the patient are unsuccessful. *Central stimulation* should be used to assess arousal (Box 16-2).

Box 16-1	Categories of Consciousness
Alert	Patient responds immediately to minimal external stimuli.
Lethargic	State of drowsiness or inaction in which patient needs increased stimulus to be awakened, but is still easily arousable.
	Verbal, mental, and motor responses are slow and sluggish.
Obtunded	Very drowsy when not stimulated; follows simple commands when stimulated.
	Dull indifference to external stimuli; response is minimally maintained.
Stuporous	Minimal spontaneous movement; arousable only by vigorous and continuous external stimuli.
	Motor responses to tactile stimuli are appropriate; verbal responses are minimal and incomprehensible.
Comatose	Vigorous stimulation fails to produce any voluntary neural response.
	Both arousal and awareness are absent.
	No verbal responses; motor responses may be purposeful withdrawal to pain (light coma), nonpurposeful, or absent (deep coma).

Box 16-2	Stimulation Techniques in Patient Arousal

CENTRAL STIMULATION
- *Trapezius pinch*: Squeeze trapezius muscle between thumb and first two fingers.
- *Sternal rub*: Apply firm pressure to sternum with knuckles, using a rubbing motion.

PERIPHERAL STIMULATION
- *Nailbed pressure*: Apply firm pressure, using object such as a pen, to nailbed.
- *Pinching of inner aspect of arm/leg*: Firmly pinch small portion of patient's tissue on sensitive inner aspect of arm or leg.

Appraising Awareness

Content of consciousness is a higher-level brain function and involves assessment of the patient's orientation to person, place, and time. Assessment of content of consciousness requires the patient to give appropriate answers to a variety of questions. Changes in the patient's answers that indicate increasing degrees of confusion and disorientation may be the first sign of neurologic deterioration.[1,3]

Glasgow Coma Scale

The most widely recognized LOC assessment tool is the Glasgow Coma Scale (GCS).[4] This scored scale is based on evaluation of three categories: eye opening, verbal response, and best motor response (Table 16-1). The best possible score is 15, and the lowest GCS score is 3. Generally a score of 7 or less indicates coma. Originally the scoring system was developed to assist in general communication concerning the severity of neurologic injury. Recent testing of GCS revealed a moderate to high agreement rating among both physicians and nurses.[5,6]

Several points are important when GCS is used for serial assessment. It provides data about LOC only and never should be considered a complete neurologic examination. GCS is not a sensitive tool for evaluation of an altered sensorium and does not account for possible aphasia. GCS is also a poor indicator of lateralization of neurologic deterioration.[6] *Lateralization* involves decreasing motor response on one side or unilateral changes in pupillary reaction.

② Motor Function

Nursing priorities in assessment of motor function focus on (1) evaluating muscle size and tone and (2) estimating muscle strength. Each side should be assessed individually and then compared together.[1,7]

Evaluating Muscle Size and Tone

Initially the muscles should be inspected for size and shape. The presence of atrophy or hypertrophy is noted. Muscle tone is assessed by evaluating the opposition to passive movement. The patient is instructed to relax the extremity while the nurse performs passive range of motion and evaluates the degree of resistance. Muscle tone is appraised for signs of flaccidity (no resistance), hypotonia (little resistance), hypertonia (increased resistance), spasticity, or rigidity.[7]

Estimating Muscle Strength

Having the patient perform a number of movements against resistance assesses muscle strength. The strength of the movement is then graded on a six-point scale (Box 16-3). Asking the patient to grasp, squeeze, and release the nurse's index and middle fingers tests the upper extremities. If weakness or asymmetry is suspected, the patient is instructed to extend both arms with the palms turned upward and hold that position with the eyes closed. If the patient has a weaker side, that arm will drift downward and pronate. The lower extremities are tested by asking the patient to push and pull the feet against resistance.[8]

Abnormal Motor Responses

If the patient is incapable of comprehending and following a simple command, noxious stimuli are required to determine motor responses. The stimulus is applied to each extremity separately to allow evaluation of individual extremity function. *Peripheral stimulation* is used to assess motor function.[9] Motor responses elicited by noxious stimuli are interpreted

---

Table 16-1   Glasgow Coma Scale

Category	Score	Response
Eye opening	4	Spontaneous—eyes open spontaneously without stimulation.
	3	To speech—eyes open with verbal stimulation but not necessarily to command.
	2	To pain—eyes open with noxious stimuli.
	1	None—no eye opening regardless of stimulation.
Verbal response	5	Oriented—accurate information about person, place, time, reason for hospitalization, and personal data.
	4	Confused—answers not appropriate to question, but use of language is correct.
	3	Inappropriate words—disorganized, random speech, no sustained conversation.
	2	Incomprehensible sounds—moans, groans, and incomprehensible mumbles.
	1	None—no verbalization despite stimulation.
Best motor response	6	Obeys commands—performs simple tasks on command; able to repeat performance.
	5	Localizes to pain—organized attempt to localize and remove painful stimuli.
	4	Withdraws from pain—withdraws extremity from source of painful stimuli.
	3	Abnormal flexion—decorticate posturing spontaneously or in response to noxious stimuli.
	2	Extension—decerebrate posturing spontaneously or in response to noxious stimuli.
	1	None—no response to noxious stimuli; flaccid.

Box **16-3** | Muscle Strength Grading Scale

0—No movement or muscle contraction
1—Trace contraction
2—Active movement with gravity eliminated
3—Active movement against gravity
4—Active movement with some resistance
5—Active movement with full resistance

differently than those elicited by voluntary demonstration[8] (Box 16-4 and Figure 16-1).

Pupillary Function

Nursing priorities in assessment of pupillary function focus on (1) estimating pupil size and shape, (2) evaluating pupillary reaction to light, and (3) assessing eye movements.

Pupillary function is an extension of the autonomic nervous system. Parasympathetic control of the pupil occurs through innervation of the oculomotor nerve, or third cranial nerve (CN III), which exits from the brain stem in the midbrain area. When the parasympathetic fibers are stimulated, the pupil constricts. Sympathetic control originates in the hypothalamus and travels down the entire length of the brain stem. When the sympathetic fibers are stimulated, the pupil dilates. Pupillary changes provide a valuable tool to assessment because of pathway location. The oculomotor nerve lies at the junction of the midbrain and the tentorial notch. Any increase of pressure that exerts force down through the tentorial notch compresses CN III. Oculomotor nerve compression results in a dilated, nonreactive pupil. Sympathetic pathway disruption occurs with brain stem involvement. Loss of sympathetic control leads to pinpoint, nonreactive pupils.

Box **16-4** | Classification of Abnormal Motor Function

Spontaneous	Occurs without regard to external stimuli and may not occur by request.
Withdrawal	Occurs when the extremity receiving the painful stimulus flexes normally in an attempt to avoid the noxious stimulus.
Localization	Occurs when the extremity opposite the extremity receiving pain crosses midline of the body in an attempt to remove the noxious stimulus from the affected limb.
Decortication	Abnormal flexion response that may occur spontaneously or in response to noxious stimuli (Figure 16-1, *A* and *C*).
Decerebration	Abnormal extension response that may occur spontaneously or in response to noxious stimuli (Figure 16-1, *B* and *C*).
Flaccid	No response to painful stimuli.

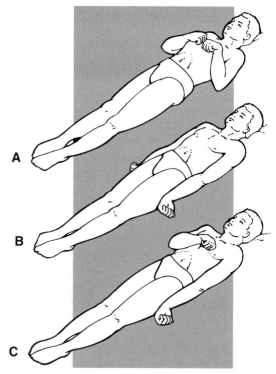

Figure 16-1 Abnormal motor responses. **A,** Decorticate posturing. **B,** Decerebrate posturing. **C,** Decorticate posturing on right side and decerebrate posturing on left side of body.

Control of eye movements occurs with interaction of three cranial nerves: oculomotor (CN III), trochlear (CN IV), and abducens (CN VI). The pathways for these cranial nerves provide integrated function through the internuclear pathway of the medial longitudinal fasciculus (MLF) located in the brain stem. The MLF provides coordination of eye movements with the vestibular (CN VIII) nerve and the reticular formation.[1,3]

Estimating Pupil Size and Shape

Pupil size should be documented in millimeters with the use of a pupil gauge to reduce the subjectivity of description. Although most people have pupils of equal size, a discrepancy up to 1 mm between the two pupils is normal. Inequality of pupils is known as *anisocoria* and occurs in 16% to 17% of the population.[10] Change or inequality in pupil size, especially in patients who previously have not shown this discrepancy, is a significant neurologic sign. It may indicate impending danger of herniation and should be reported immediately. With the location of CN III at the notch of the tentorium, pupil size and reactivity play a key role in the physical assessment of intracranial pressure (ICP) changes and herniation syndromes. In addition to CN III compression, changes in pupil size occur for other reasons. Large pupils may result from the instillation of cycloplegic agents, such as atropine or scopolamine, or may indicate extreme stress. Extremely small pupils may indicate narcotic overdose, lower brain stem compression, or bilateral damage to the pons.[10]

Pupil shape also is noted in the assessment of pupils. Although the pupil is normally round, an irregularly shaped or oval pupil may be noted in patients with elevated ICP. An oval pupil can indicate the initial stages of CN III compression.[2] An oval pupil typically is associated with elevated ICP of 18 to 35 mm Hg.[11]

Evaluating Pupillary Reaction to Light

The pupillary light reflex depends on both optic nerve (CN II) and CN III function. The technique for evaluation of the pupillary light response involves use of a narrow-beamed bright light shone into the pupil from the outer canthus of the eye. If the light is shone directly onto the pupil, glare or reflection of the light may prevent proper visualization. Pupillary reaction to light is identified as brisk, sluggish, or nonreactive (fixed). Each pupil should be evaluated for both direct light response and consensual response.

The *consensual* pupillary response is constriction in response to a light shone into the opposite eye. This reflex occurs as a result of crossing of nerve fibers at the optic chiasm. Evaluation of consensual response is necessary to rule out optic nerve dysfunction as a cause for lack of a direct light reflex. Because CN II is the afferent pathway for the light reflex, shining a light into a blind eye will produce neither a direct light response in that eye nor a consensual response in the opposite eye. A consensual response in the blind eye produced by shining a light into the opposite eye demonstrates an intact oculomotor nerve. CN III compression associated with transtentorial herniation will affect both the direct light response and the consensual response in the affected pupil.[1,10]

Assessing Eye Movements

In the conscious patient, function of the three cranial nerves of the eye and their MLF innervation can be assessed by asking the patient to follow a finger through the full range of eye motion. If the eyes move together into all six fields, extraocular movements are intact.[1]

In the unconscious patient, assessment of ocular function and innervation of the MLF is performed by eliciting the *doll's eye reflex*. If the patient is unconscious as a result of trauma, the nurse must ascertain the absence of cervical injury before performing this examination. To assess the oculocephalic reflex, the nurse holds the patient's eyelids open and briskly turns the head to one side while observing the eye movements, then briskly turns the head to the other side and observes. If the eyes deviate to the opposite direction in which the head is turned, "doll's eyes" are present, and the oculocephalic reflex arc is intact (Figure 16-2, A). If the oculocephalic reflex arc is not intact, the reflex is absent (Figure 16-2, C). This lack of response, in which the eyes remain midline and move with the head, indicates significant brain stem injury. The reflex may also be absent

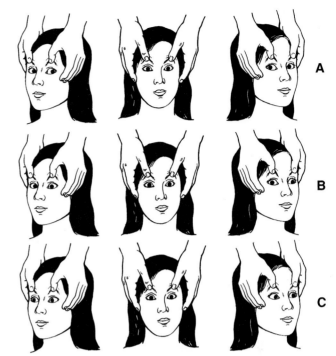

Figure 16-2   Oculocephalic (doll's eye) reflex. **A**, Normal. **B**, Abnormal. **C**, Absent.

in severe metabolic coma. An abnormal oculocephalic reflex is present when the eyes rove or move in opposite directions from each other (Figure 16-2, B). Abnormal oculocephalic reflex indicates some degree of brain stem injury.[1,3]

Respiratory Function

Nursing priorities in assessment of respiratory function focus on (1) observing respiratory pattern and (2) evaluating airway status. The activity of respiration is a highly integrated function that receives input from the cerebrum, brain stem, and metabolic mechanisms. A close correlation exists in clinical assessment among altered LOC, level of brain or brain stem injury, and respiratory pattern noted. Under the influence of the cerebral cortex and the diencephalon, three brain stem centers control respiration. The lowest center, the *medullary* respiratory center, sends impulses through the vagus nerve to innervate muscles of inspiration and expiration. The *apneustic* and *pneumotaxic* centers of the pons are responsible for the length of inspiration and expiration and the underlying respiratory rate.[1,3]

Observing Respiratory Pattern

Changes in respiratory patterns assist in identifying the level of brain stem dysfunction or injury (Table 16-2). Evaluation of respiratory pattern must also include evaluation of the effectiveness of gas exchange in maintaining adequate oxygen and carbon dioxide (CO_2) levels. Hypoventilation is not uncommon in the patient with an altered LOC.

Table 16-2 Respiratory Patterns in Neurologic Dysfunction

Pattern	Description	Significance
Cheyne-Stokes	Rhythmic crescendo and decrescendo of rate and depth of respiration; includes brief periods of apnea	Usually seen with bilateral deep cerebral lesions or some cerebellar lesions
Central neurogenic hyperventilation	Very deep, very rapid respirations with no apneic periods	Usually seen with lesions of midbrain and upper pons
Apneustic	Prolonged inspiratory and/or expiratory pause of 2 to 3 seconds	Usually seen in lesions of middle to lower pons
Cluster breathing	Clusters of irregular, gasping respirations separated by long periods of apnea	Usually seen in lesions of lower pons or upper medulla
Ataxic respirations	Irregular, random pattern of deep and shallow respirations with irregular apneic periods	Usually seen in lesions of medulla

Alterations in oxygenation or CO_2 levels can result in further neurologic dysfunction. ICP increases with hypoxemia or hypercapnia.[1]

Evaluating Airway Status

Assessment of the respiratory function in a patient with neurologic deficit must include assessment of airway maintenance and secretion control. Cough, gag, and swallow reflexes responsible for protection of the airway may be absent or diminished.[1]

Vital Signs

Nursing priorities in assessment of vital signs focus on (1) evaluating blood pressure and (2) monitoring heart rate and rhythm. As a result of the brain and brain stem influences on cardiac, respiratory, and body temperature functions, changes in vital signs can indicate deterioration in neurologic status.

Evaluating Blood Pressure

A common manifestation of intracranial injury is systemic hypertension. Cerebral autoregulation, responsible for the control of cerebral blood flow (CBF), frequently is lost with any type of intracranial injury. After cerebral injury the body often is in a hyperdynamic state (increased heart rate, blood pressure, and cardiac output) as part of a compensatory response. With the loss of autoregulation, as blood pressure increases, CBF and cerebral blood volume increase, and therefore ICP increases. Control of systemic hypertension is necessary to stop this cycle. However, caution must be exercised. The mean arterial pressure must be maintained at a level sufficient to produce adequate CBF in the presence of elevated ICP. Attention must also be paid to the pulse pressure because widening of this value may occur in the late stages of intracranial hypertension.

Monitoring Heart Rate and Rhythm

The medulla and the vagus nerve provide parasympathetic control to the heart. When stimulated, this lower brain stem system produces bradycardia. Sympathetic stimulation increases the rate and contractility. Various intracranial pathologies and abrupt ICP changes can produce cardiac dysrhythmias, such as bradycardia, premature ventricular contractions (PVCs), atrioventricular (AV) block, or ventricular fibrillation and myocardial damage.[12]

Cushing's Triad

Cushing's triad is a set of three clinical manifestations—bradycardia, systolic hypertension, and widening pulse pressure—related to pressure on the medullary area of the brain stem. These signs often occur in response to intracranial hypertension or a herniation syndrome. The appearance of Cushing's triad is a late finding that may be absent in neurologic deterioration. Attention should be paid to alteration in each component of the triad and intervention initiated accordingly.[3]

NEUROLOGIC CHANGES ASSOCIATED WITH INTRACRANIAL HYPERTENSION

Assessment of the patient for signs of increasing ICP is an important responsibility of the critical care nurse. Increasing ICP can be identified by changes in level of consciousness, pupillary reaction, motor response, vital signs, and respiratory patterns (Figure 16-3).

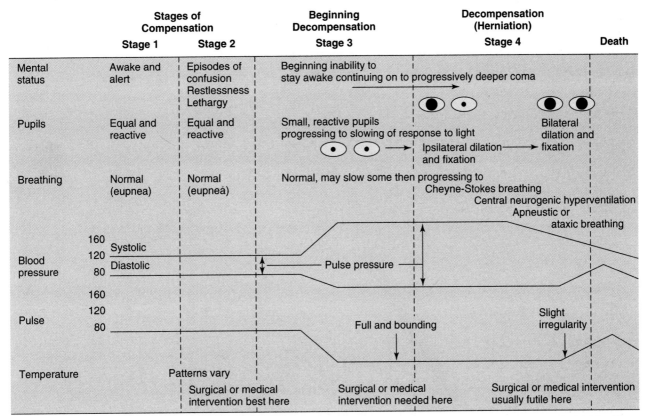

Figure 16-3   Clinical correlates of compensated and decompensated phases of intracranial hypertension. (From Beare PG, Myers JL: *Adult health nursing*, ed 3, St Louis, 1998, Mosby.)

LABORATORY STUDIES

The major laboratory study performed in the patient with neurologic dysfunction is cerebrospinal fluid (CSF) analysis obtained through lumbar puncture or ventriculostomy[1] (Table 16-3).

DIAGNOSTIC PROCEDURES

A variety of diagnostic procedures are used to evaluate the patient with neurologic dysfunction[1,13,14] (Table 16-4).

Nursing Management

The nursing management of a patient undergoing a diagnostic procedure involves a variety of interventions. **Nursing priorities are directed toward (1) preparing the patient** **psychologically and physically for the procedure, (2) monitoring the patient's responses to the procedure, and (3) assessing the patient after the procedure.**

Preparing the patient includes teaching the patient about the procedure, answering any questions, and transporting and positioning the patient for the procedure. Monitoring the patient's responses to the procedure includes observing the patient for signs of pain, anxiety, or hemorrhage and monitoring vital signs. Assessing the patient after the procedure includes observing for complications and medicating the patient for discomfort. Any evidence of increasing ICP should be immediately reported to the physician, and emergency measures to maintain circulation must be initiated.

Table **16-3**   Cerebrospinal Fluid (CSF) Analysis

Parameter	Normal	Abnormal	Possible Causes
Pressure (initial readings)	75-180 mm H₂O (5-15 mm Hg)	<60 mm	Faulty needle placement Dehydration Spinal block along subarachnoid space
		>200 mm	Block of foramen magnum Muscle tension Abdominal compression Brain tumor Subdural hematoma Brain abscess Brain cyst Cerebral edema (any cause) Hydrocephalus
Color	Clear, colorless	Cloudy	Increased cell count microorganisms
		Yellow	Xanthochromic (RBC pigments) High protein content
		Smoky	Presence of RBCs
Red blood cells (RBCs)	None	Blood-tinged Grossly bloody	Traumatic tap Traumatic tap Subarachnoid hemorrhage
White blood cells (WBCs)	0-6 mm³	>10 mm³ (WBC counts range from below 100 to many thousands depending on causative factor; all are abnormal findings.)	Occurs in many conditions Bacterial/viral infection of meninges Neurosyphilis Tuberculous meningitis Metastatic neoplastic lesions Parasitic infections Acute demyelinating diseases After introduction of air or blood into subarachnoid space
Protein*	15-45 mg/100 ml (dl) (1% of serum protein)	<10 mg/dl >60 mg/dl	Little clinical significance Occurs in many conditions Complete spinal block Guillain-Barré syndrome Carcinomatosis of meninges Tumors close to pial or ependymal surfaces or in cerebellopontine angle Acute and chronic meningitis Meningeal hemorrhage Demyelinating disorders Degenerative diseases
Glucose	50-75 mg/dl (approximately 60% of blood glucose level)	<40 mg/dl	Acute bacterial meningitis Tuberculous meningitis Meningeal carcinomatosis Diabetes
		>100 mg/dl	
Chloride	700-750 mg/100 ml; 125 mM	<625 mg/dl	Hypochloremia Tuberculous meningitis
		>800 mg/dl	Not of neurologic significance; correlated with blood levels of chloride

From Rudy E: *Advanced neurological and neurosurgical nursing*, ed 4, St Louis, 1984, Mosby.
*Protein level will be increased if CSF contains blood.

Table 16-4 Neurologic Diagnostic Procedures

Procedure	Purposes	Comments
Angiography	Visualizes extracranial and intracranial vasculature Identifies aneurysm, AV malformation, vasospasm, vascular tumors	Contraindicated if patient has bleeding disorder or is receiving anticoagulants. May cause local hematoma, vasospasm, vessel occlusion, allergic reaction to contrast media, transient or permanent neurologic dysfunction. *Before test:* ● Keep patient NPO for 4 hours and provide sedation before study. ● Check for allergy to iodine. *After test:* ● Ensure hydration (contrast medium used). ● Maintain bed rest for 8-12 hours. ● Monitor arterial puncture point for hemorrhage or hematoma. ● Assess neurovascular status of affected limb. ● Monitor for indications of systemic emboli.
Cisternogram	Views CSF flow Identifies hydrocephalus Evaluates CSF leakage through dural tear Evaluates abnormality of structures at base of brain and upper cervical cord region	Contraindicated in intracranial hypertension.
Computed tomography (CT)	Views intracranial structures: size, shape, location, shifts Differentiates among tumors, hemorrhage, and infarction Identifies hydrocephalus, cerebral edema, infectious processes, trauma, aneurysm, hematoma, AV malformation, and cerebral atrophy	Patient must be cooperative. Contrast media may be used. ● Check for allergy to iodine or seafood before study. ● Patient is NPO for 4-8 hours before study. ● Sedation may be given. ● Monitor for signs of allergic reaction. ● Encourage fluids.
Digital subtraction angiography (DSA): brain, spine	Visualizes vasculature, especially carotid and larger cerebral arteries Evaluates occlusive vascular disease Identifies tumors, aneurysms, AV malformations and vascular abnormalities	May be done intravenous (IV) or intraarterial. ● IV: less invasive with fewer complications than cerebral angiography. ● Intraarterial: care as for angiography. Contrast media is used. ● Check for allergy to iodine or seafood before study. ● Patient is NPO for 4-8 hours before study. ● Monitor for signs of allergic reaction. ● Encourage fluids.
Electroencephalography (EEG)	Differentiates epilepsy from mass lesion Detects focus of seizure activity Evaluates drug intoxication Evaluates cerebral blood flow Localizes tumor, abscess, and other mass lesions May be used in designation of brain death	Stimulants, anticonvulsants, tranquilizers, and antidepressants may be withheld for 24-48 hours before study. Hair is shampooed before and after study.

AV, Arteriovenous; *NPO,* nothing by mouth; *CSF,* cerebrospinal fluid.

Continued

Table **16-4** Neurologic Diagnostic Procedures—cont'd

Procedure	Purposes	Comments
Electromyography (EMG); nerve conduction velocity studies	Detects muscle disease Identifies peripheral neuropathies and nerve compression Identifies nerve regeneration and muscle recovery	Patient must be cooperative. Contraindicated in patients on anticoagulants, with bleeding disorders, or with skin infection. May be uncomfortable for patient.
Electronystagmography (ENG)	Detects nystagmus, which may aid in identification of cerebellar or vestibular problem	Hair is shampooed before and after study.
Evoked-potential studies (EPS)	Evaluate brain's electrical potentials (responses) to external stimuli; evaluate sensory and somatosensory neurologic pathways Identifies neuromuscular disease, cerebrovascular disease, spinal cord injury, head injury, peripheral nerve disease, tumors Determines prognosis in severe head injury Contributes to diagnosis of multiple sclerosis, brain stem injury	
Isotope ventriculography	Visualizes CSF circulation system	No CSF withdrawn. May cause meningeal irritation and aseptic meningitis.
Lumbar puncture (LP) or cisternal puncture	Obtains CSF for analysis Measures CSF opening pressure (about equivalent to intracranial pressure for most patients if done recumbent and no blockage is present)	Cisternal puncture is higher risk but may be used if there is scar tissue, which prevents LP. Patient must be cooperative. Contraindicated in patients with intracranial hypertension because herniation may occur. Contraindicated in bleeding disorders and in patients receiving anticoagulants. Patient kept flat for 4-8 hours to prevent headache. May cause headache, low back pain, meningitis, abscess, CSF leak, puncture of spinal cord.
Magnetic resonance angiography (MRA)	As for CT except better visualization of vasculature Identifies aneurysms, AV malformations, and vasospasm Identifies large vein patency and venous sinuses	Patient must be cooperative. Cannot be performed in patient receiving mechanical ventilation. Contraindicated in patients with implanted metallic devices, including pacemakers. Tends to overestimate degree of stenosis.
Magnetic resonance imaging (MRI)	As for CT except better visualization of vasculature Identifies vascular lesions, tissue abnormalities, cerebral hemorrhage, cerebral infarction, epileptic foci, and multiple sclerosis Identifies brain stem abnormalities Identifies type, location, and extent of brain injury	More sensitive than CT scan, especially for posterior fossa. Patient must be cooperative. Cannot be performed in patient receiving mechanical ventilation. Contraindicated in patients with implanted metallic devices, including pacemakers.
Myelography	Visualization of spinal subarachnoid space Detects spinal cord lesions and cord/nerve root compression Detects pressure on spinal nerve roots	If done with oil-based iophendylate (Pantopaque): • Patient must lie flat for 4-8 hours after study. • May cause headache, nerve root irritation, allergic reaction, and adhesive arachnoiditis. If done with water-soluble metrizamide (Amipaque): • Patient should have head of bed elevated.

- May cause headache, nausea, vomiting, back and neck ache, chest pain, seizures, hallucinations, speech disorders, dysrhythmias, and allergic reaction.
Encourage fluids with either type of dye.

Test	Purpose	Nursing considerations
Nerve conduction velocity studies	Identifies peripheral neuropathies and nerve compression	Needle electrodes are used.
Oculoplethysmography (OPG)	Indirectly measures ocular artery pressure Reflects adequacy of cerebrovascular blood flow in the carotid artery	Contraindicated in patients who have undergone eye surgery within last 6 months, who have had lens implants or cataracts, or who have had retinal detachment. May cause conjunctival hemorrhage, corneal abrasions, and transient photophobia.
Pneumoencephalography	Visualizes ventricular system and subarachnoid space Identifies intracranial tumors Identifies cerebral atrophy	Care as for LP. Contraindicated in patients with intracranial hypertension. May cause headache, nausea, vomiting, autonomic dysfunction, herniation, subdural hematoma, air embolus, and seizures. Patient kept flat for 12-24 hours after study.
Positron emission tomography (PET) Single-proton emission computed tomography (SPECT)	Evaluates oxygen and glucose metabolism Evaluates cerebral blood flow Identifies cerebral ischemia, injuries, epilepsy, and Alzheimer's disease	Patient must be cooperative. Contraindicated in pregnant patients.
Radioisotope brain scan	Identifies tumors, cerebrovascular disease, cerebral infarction, trauma, infectious processes, and seizures	Generally, has been replaced by CT scan. Reassure patient that amount of radioactive material is minimal. Patient must be cooperative. Contraindicated in pregnant patients.
Regional cerebral blood flow (xenon-133 [^{133}Xe] inhalation)	Evaluates blood flow to the cerebral cortex Identifies cerebrovascular disease Detects regions of increased or decreased perfusion Determines presence of collateral blood flow Evaluates cerebral vasospasm	Reassure patient that amount of radioactive material is minimal. Contraindicated in pregnant patients.
Skull radiography	Detects skull fracture, facial fracture, tumor, bone erosion, cranial anomalies, air-fluid level in sinuses, abnormal intracranial calcification, and radiopaque foreign bodies	Linear and basal fractures are frequently missed by routine x-ray films. Contraindicated in pregnant patients.
Somnography	Records EEG during sleep Evaluates sleep and sleep disorders	
Spinal cord angiography	Differentiates among spinal AV malformation, angioma, tumor, and ischemia	As for angiography. May cause thrombosis of spinal vessels; allergy to contrast agent may occur.
Spinal radiography	Detects vertebral dislocation or fracture, degenerative disease, tumor, bone erosion, and calcification Identifies structural spinal deficits and rules out associated cervical spinal injuries	Care must be taken to prevent fracture displacement and spinal cord injury. C1-C2 view best via open mouth. C6-C7 view best with arms pulled down. Contraindicated in pregnant patients.
Suboccipital puncture	Obtains CSF for analysis Measures CSF pressure Useful when LP contraindicated	May cause trauma to the medulla.

C1-C2, first to second cervical vertebrae area.

Continued

Table 16-4 Neurologic Diagnostic Procedures—cont'd

Procedure	Purposes	Comments
Transcranial Doppler imaging	Measures blood flow velocity through the cerebral arteries Identifies cerebral vasospasm, emboli, vascular stenosis, and brain death	
Ventriculography	Obtains CSF for analysis Measures CSF pressure Used especially when intracranial hypertension contraindicates LP	May cause meningeal irritation, seizures, herniation, and intracerebral/intraventricular hemorrhage.

From Dennison RD: *Pass CCRN!*, ed 2, St Louis, 2000, Mosby.
CSF, cerebrospinal fluid.

REFERENCES

1. Barker E: *Neuroscience nursing: a spectrum of care*, ed 2, St Louis, 2002, Mosby.
2. Hickey JV: *The clinical practice of neurological and neurosurgical nursing*, ed 4, Philadelphia, 1997, Lippincott.
3. Goetz CG, Pappert EJ: *Textbook of clinical neurology*, Philadelphia, 1999, Saunders.
4. Teasdale G, Jennett W: Assessment of coma and impaired consciousness: a practical scale, *Lancet* 2:81, 1974.
5. Juarez VJ, Lyons M: Interrater reliability of the Glasgow Coma Scale, *J Neurosci Nurs* 27:283, 1995.
6. Fischer J, Mathieson C: The history of the Glasgow Coma Scale: implications for practice, *Crit Care Nurs Q* 23(4):52, 2001.
7. Barnwell P: Assessing motor and sensory function: a focused survey, *Aust Emerg Nurs J* 2(3):16, 1999.
8. O'Hanlon-Nichols T: Neurologic assessment, *Am J Nurs* 99(6):44, 1999.
9. Lower J: Rapid neuro assessment, *Am J Nurs* 92(6):38, 1992.
10. Bishop BS: Pathologic pupillary signs: self-learning module. Part 1, *Crit Care Nurs* 11(6):59, 1991.
11. Marshall LF et al: The oval pupil: clinical significance and relationship to intracranial hypertension, *J Neurosurg* 58:566, 1983.
12. Keller C, Williams A: Cardiac dysrhythmias associated with central nervous system dysfunction, *J Neurosci Nurs* 25:349, 1993.
13. Shpritz DW: Neurodiagnostic studies, *Nurs Clin North Am* 34:593, 1999.
14. Bradley WG et al: *Neurology in clinical practice*, ed 3, Boston, 2000, Butterworth Heinemann.

BEVERLY CARLSON

Neurologic Disorders

Objectives

- Describe the etiology and pathophysiology of neurologic disorders seen in critical care.
- Identify the clinical manifestations of the selected neurologic disorders.
- Explain the treatment of the selected neurologic disorders.
- Discuss the nursing priorities for managing a patient with neurologic dysfunction.

evolve Be sure to check out the free exercises on-line at *http://evolve.elsevier.com/Urden/priorities/*

An understanding of the pathology of a disease or condition, the areas of assessment on which to focus, and the usual medical management allows the critical care nurse to anticipate and plan nursing interventions more accurately. Although a wide array of neurologic disorders exists, only a few routinely require care in the critical care environment.

COMA

Coma is a state of unconsciousness in which both wakefulness and awareness are lacking. The patient cannot be aroused and demonstrates no purposeful response to the environment.[1] As with consciousness, the state of coma comprises a continuum of many levels. The patient in a *light coma* demonstrates purposeful withdrawal in response to noxious stimuli. The patient in *deep coma* lacks any response, even to noxious stimuli. Levels of coma between these two extremes are difficult to differentiate clearly.

Epidemiology and Etiology

The state of coma is a symptom rather than a disease; coma results from an underlying process. As with any other life-threatening condition, however, coma requires identification and therapeutic management even when the cause cannot be determined or treated.

The incidence of coma is difficult to ascertain. Because a variety of both neurologic and nonneurologic conditions can produce coma, this state of unconsciousness is unfortunately very common in critical care. Of the survivors of severe head injury, 59% experience a period of coma;[2] 10% of patients with head injury remain in coma.[3]

The causes of coma can be divided into the general categories of (1) structural neurologic lesions and (2) metabolic and toxic conditions (Box 17-1) and (3) psychiatric disorders (not discussed here). *Structural lesions* that can result in coma include vascular lesions, trauma, brain tumors, and brain abscesses.[4] Metabolic and diffuse brain dysfunction accounts for more than half of all cases of coma.[5] *Metabolic and toxic conditions* that can result in coma include cardiopulmonary decompensation, poisoning, alcohol, hypertensive encephalopathy, meningitis, encephalitis, postconvulsive states, and other metabolic conditions.

Pathophysiology

Consciousness involves both *arousal* (wakefulness) and *awareness*; neither of these functions is present in the patient in coma. Ascending fibers of the reticular activating system (RAS) in the pons, hypothalamus, and thalamus maintain arousal as an autonomic function. Neurons in the cerebral cortex are responsible for awareness. Diffuse dysfunction of both cerebral hemispheres and diffuse or focal RAS dysfunction is necessary to produce coma.[6] Small focal lesions in the posterior hypothalamic and midbrain regions can also produce coma, whereas unilateral cerebral lesions usually do not unless they increase intracranial pressure (ICP). Alterations in cerebral function that also can produce coma include ischemia, hypoxia, infection, metabolic imbalance, toxic exposure, and structural disruption.

The pathophysiologic continuum of coma is comparable to the stages of anesthesia. Slight or moderate cortical depression produces clouding of consciousness, impairment of contact with the environment, loss of discrimination, and euphoria. In complete cortical suppression, motor and reflex functions are controlled solely by subcortical structures. Midbrain depression produces a loss of reflex response and a loss of several visceral functions. Finally, brain stem depression results in gradual abolition of respiratory and circulatory control.

Box 17-1   Causes of Coma

STRUCTURAL LESIONS	
Subarachnoid hemorrhage	Hypercapnia
Intracerebral hemorrhage	Hypoglycemia/hyperglycemia
Subdural hematoma	Electrolyte imbalance (sodium, calcium, magnesium, phosphorus)
Epidural hematoma	Water imbalance
Thrombotic or embolic brain infarction	Acidosis/alkalosis
Brain tumor	Hypothyroidism (myxedema)
Brain abscess	Addisonian crisis
Trauma	Thiamine deficiency (Wernicke encephalopathy)
	Sepsis
METABOLIC AND TOXIC CONDITIONS	Poisoning (lead, mushroom, cyanide, methanol, carbon monoxide)
Meningitis	Drug overdose
Encephalitis	Lactic acidosis
Alcohol	Hypertensive encephalopathy
Hepatic failure	Hypothermia/hyperthermia
Renal failure (uremia)	Postictal state
Cardiac failure	
Ischemia, hypoxemia, anoxia	

Assessment and Diagnosis

Diagnosis of the coma state is a clinical diagnosis, readily established by assessment of the level of consciousness (LOC). Determining the full nature and cause of coma, however, requires a thorough history and physical examination. A past medical history is essential because events immediately preceding the change in LOC can often provide valuable clues as to the origin of the coma. When limited information is available and the coma is profound, the response of the patient to emergency treatment may provide clues to the underlying diagnosis. The patient who becomes responsive with the administration of naloxone, for example, can be presumed to have ingested some type of opiate.

Detailed serial neurologic examinations are essential for all patients in coma. Assessment of motor function, pupillary responses, and respiratory pattern provides valuable diagnostic information.[5] Pupillary light responses are often the key to differentiating between structural and metabolic causes of coma because these responses are usually intact in metabolic-induced coma, with the exceptions of anoxic encephalopathy, barbiturate intoxication, and hypothermia.[1,5] Focal or asymmetric motor deficits usually indicate structural lesions (Table 17-1).

Structural causes of coma are usually readily apparent with computed tomography (CT) or magnetic resonance imaging (MRI). Lumbar puncture (LP), unless contraindicated by signs of increased ICP, facilitates the analysis of cerebrospinal fluid (CSF) pressure and content. CT scanning to identify patients at high risk for brain herniation must always precede LP. The risk of herniation with LP in the patient with increased ICP is estimated at 1% to 12%.[5]

Laboratory studies are also used to identify metabolic or endocrine abnormalities. Occasionally, the cause of coma is never clearly determined.

Medical Management

The goal of medical management of the patient in a coma is identification and treatment of the underlying cause of coma. Initial medical management includes emergency measures to support vital functions and prevent further neurologic deterioration. Protection of the airway and ventilatory assistance are often needed. Administration of thiamine (at least 100 mg), glucose, and a narcotic antagonist is suggested whenever the cause of coma is not immediately known.[1,5,7] Thiamine is administered before glucose because the coma produced by thiamine deficiency, Wernicke's encephalopathy, can be precipitated by a glucose load.[5] The cervical neck is stabilized until traumatic injury is ruled out.

The patient who remains in coma after emergency treatment requires supportive measures to maintain physiologic body functions and prevent complications. Continued airway protection and nutritional support are essential. Fluid and electrolyte management is often complex because of alterations in the neurohormonal system. Anticonvulsant therapy may be necessary to prevent further ischemic damage to the brain.

Prognosis

The health care team and the patient's family jointly make decisions regarding the level of medical management to be provided. Family members require informational support in

Table 17-1 Clinical Manifestations of Metabolically/Structurally Induced Comas

Manifestation	Metabolically Induced Coma	Structurally Induced Coma
Blink to threat (CNs II, VII)	Equal	Asymmetric
Ocular discs (CN II)	Flat, good pulsation	Papilledema
Extraocular movement (CNs III, IV, VI)	Roving eye movements. Normal doll's eye reflex and caloric tests	Gaze paresis, CN III palsy, MLF syndrome (internuclear ophthalmoplegia)
Pupils (CNs II, III)	Equal and reactive. May be large (atropine), pinpoint (opiates), or midposition and fixed (glutethimide [Doriden])	Asymmetric/nonreactive. May be midposition (midbrain injury), pinpoint (pons injury), or large (tectal injury)
Corneal reflex (CNs V, VIII)	Symmetric response	Asymmetric response
Grimace to pain (CN VII)	Symmetric response	Asymmetric response
Motor function movement	Symmetric	Asymmetric
Motor tone	Symmetric	Paratonic, spastic, flaccid, especially if asymmetric
Posture	Symmetric	Decorticate, especially if symmetric. Decerebrate, especially if asymmetric
Deep tendon reflexes	Symmetric	Asymmetric
Babinski sign	Absent or symmetric response	Present
Sensation	Symmetric	Asymmetric

CN, Cranial nerve; MLF, medial longitudinal fasciculus.

terms of probable cause of the coma and prognosis for recovery of both consciousness and function. Prognosis depends on the cause of the coma and the length of time unconsciousness persists. Sixty percent of patients in nontraumatic coma persisting for 6 or more hours die; 12% remain in a vegetative state. Only 3% of patients in coma for longer than 1 week recover.[7] Patients in nontraumatic coma persisting for more than 1 month are unlikely ever to regain consciousness.[5] As a general rule, *metabolic* coma has a better prognosis than coma caused by a structural lesion, and *traumatic* coma generally has a better outcome than nontraumatic coma.[7]

Much research has been directed toward identifying prognostic indicators for the patient in a coma after a cardiopulmonary arrest. As with all types of coma, the best prognosis is associated with early arousal. The comatose patient who responds to pain with reflex posturing (decorticate or decerebrate) in 1 to 3 hours after arrest has a 20% to 30% chance of survival with a good outcome. In one study the presence of speech at 24 hours after arrest predicted complete neurologic recovery.[8] Survival is unlikely in the coma patient who has absent pupillary light reflexes for more than 6 hours after cardiopulmonary resuscitation.[9]

Although these statistics are helpful in guiding decision making, outcome for an individual cannot be predicted with 100% accuracy, regardless of the cause or duration of coma.[5]

Nursing Management

Nursing management of the patient in a coma incorporates a variety of nursing diagnoses (Box 17-2) and is directed by the specific etiology of the coma, although some common interventions are used. Most important, the patient in a coma is totally dependent on the health care team. **Nursing priorities are directed toward (1) assessing for changes in neurologic status and clues to the origin of the coma, (2) supporting all body functions, (3) maintaining surveillance for complications, (4) providing comfort and emotional support, and (5) initiating rehabilitation measures.** The two key nursing interventions addressed here are eye care and coma stimulation therapy.

nursing diagnosis
priorities   Box **17-2**

Coma

- Decreased Intracranial Adaptive Capacity related to failure of normal intracranial compensatory mechanisms
- Ineffective Airway Clearance related to excessive secretions or abnormal viscosity of mucus
- Ineffective Breathing Pattern related to decreased lung expansion
- Imbalanced Nutrition Less than Body Requirments related to lack of exogenous nutrients or increased metabolic demand
- Risk for Aspiration
- Compromised Family Coping related to critically ill family member

Eye Care

The blink reflex is often diminished or absent in the comatose patient. The eyelids may be flaccid and dependent on body positioning to remain in a closed position, and edema may prevent complete closure. Loss of these protective mechanisms results in drying and ulceration of the cornea, which can lead to permanent scarring and blindness.

Two common interventions to protect the eyes are instilling saline or methylcellulose lubricating drops and taping the eyelids in the shut position. Evidence suggests that an alternative technique may be more effective in preventing corneal epithelial breakdown. In addition to instilling saline drops every 2 hours, a polyethylene film is taped over the eyes, extending beyond the orbits and eyebrows. The film creates a moisture chamber around the cornea and assists in keeping the eyes moist and in the closed position.[10] This technique also prevents damage to the eyes resulting from tape or gauze placed directly on the delicate eyelid skin.

Coma Stimulation Therapy

Coma stimulation has been used in rehabilitation settings for many years and is based on the belief that structured brain stimulation fosters brain recovery.[2,3,11-13] The purpose of coma stimulation is to stimulate the RAS and increase the patient's level of alertness. Preliminary research suggests that coma stimulation therapy may reduce the duration of coma and enhance functional recovery.[11,13-16] Based on the belief that maximal reorganization of the brain takes place in the early weeks after an insult, coma stimulation therapy must begin in the critical care unit to increase the potential for maximal recovery.

The methods used in coma stimulation therapy result in anticipated neurologic responses (Boxes 17-3 and 17-4). Recently, electrical stimulation of the right median nerve was used effectively to improve coma scores of comatose closed head–injured patients.[14] Simple auditory and tactile stimulation are used most often in the critical care environment. Stimuli must be meaningful rather than random. Taped voices of family and friends talking to the patient have been found to be particularly effective.[12]

The family must be included in all aspects of planning and implementing the coma stimulation program. Some experts advocate bombarding the patient with stimuli up to 16 hours a day, whereas others support providing stimulation every hour. In the critical care unit, a program consisting of a single-stimulation activity, lasting no more than 10 to 30 minutes per session, two to four times a day, allows time for necessary patient care activities and rest periods.[4] Family visits and nursing activities augment this program with additional auditory and tactile stimulation. Medical stability, including normal ICP and hemodynamic values, is required before initiation of coma stimulation, and the therapy is usually not started until the second week after neurologic insult. Research has demonstrated that various auditory stimuli produce no untoward physiologic effects,[17] including no

| Box 17-3 | Sensory Stimuli Used in Coma Stimulation Therapy |

AUDITORY	VISUAL	OLFACTORY	GUSTATORY	TACTILE	KINESTHETIC
Verbal orientation	Photographs	Vinegar	Mouthwash swabs	Hand holding	Turning
Music	Penlight	Spices	Lemon juice	Rubbing lotion	Range of motion
Bells	Familiar objects	Perfume	Sweet or salty solutions	Heat/cold	Chair
Clapping	Faces	Potpourri		Cotton balls	Tilt table
Tuning fork	Flashcards	Orange/lemon peel		Rough surfaces	
				Familiar objects	

From Sosnowski C, Ustik M: *J Neurosci Nurs* 26:336, 1994.

| Box 17-4 | Responses to Stimulation |

AUDITORY	VISUAL	OLFACTORY	GUSTATORY	TACTILE	KINESTHETIC
Startle reaction	Eye blink	Grimacing	Grimacing	Localization	Spasticity of joints
Visual tracking toward sound	Visual tracking	Tearing	Spitting	Withdrawal	Assisted range of motion
Follows commands		Head turning	Swallowing	Posturing	Follows commands

From Sosnowski C, Ustik M: *J Neurosci Nurs* 26:336, 1994.

significant change in ICP or cerebral perfusion pressure (CPP).[18] However, any increase in ICP, development of seizure activity, or sustained increase in blood pressure, heart rate, or respiratory rate is considered unfavorable and reason to terminate or revise the stimulation program.[3]

Collaborative management of the patient in a coma is outlined in Box 17-5.

STROKE

Stroke is a descriptive term for the onset of acute neurologic deficit persisting for more than 24 hours and caused by the interruption of blood flow to the brain. Stroke, or *cerebrovascular accident* (CVA), is the third leading cause of death in

| Box 17-5 COLLABORATIVE Management |

Coma

1. Identify and treat underlying cause.
2. Protect airway.
3. Provide ventilatory assistance as required.
4. Support circulation as required.
5. Initiate nutritional support.
6. Provide eye care.
7. Implement a coma stimulation program.
8. Maintain surveillance for complications.
   - Infections
   - Metabolic alterations
   - Cardiac dysrhythmias
   - Temperature alterations
9. Provide comfort and emotional support.
10. Design and implement appropriate rehabilitation program.

the United States, after heart disease and cancer. The number of stroke survivors currently in the United States is estimated at 4 million.[19] Morbidity associated with stroke is the leading cause of adult disability, and 29% of all strokes are recurrent.[20] The 1997 estimated annual cost for care and loss of productivity associated with stroke was $41 billion.[21]

The national concern for the incidence and effects of stroke is illustrated by the inclusion of emergent stroke care in the American Heart Association guidelines for basic and advanced life support. Major public education programs, stroke appraisal screening programs, development of stroke centers, and algorithms for stroke management are based on the success these same approaches have had with coronary artery disease.

Ischemic Stroke

Epidemiology and Etiology

Ischemic stroke results from low cerebral blood flow (CBF), usually caused by occlusion of a blood vessel. The occlusion can be thrombotic or embolic. Hypoperfusion resulting from hypotension also produces ischemic stroke. Eighty percent of all strokes are ischemic in nature.[22] The 30-day survival after ischemic stroke is approximately 67% to 85%.

Strokes are preventable. Most *thrombotic* strokes result from accumulation of atherosclerotic plaque in the vessel lumen, especially at bifurcations, or curves, of the vessel. The pathogenesis of cerebrovascular disease is the same as for coronary vasculature. The greatest risk factor for ischemic stroke is *hypertension*. Other risk factors are diabetes, elevated blood lipids, carotid artery disease, alcohol consumption, and smoking.[23] Common sites of atherosclerotic plaque are the bifurcation of the common carotid artery, the origins of the middle and anterior cerebral arteries, and the origins of the vertebral arteries.[22] Ischemic strokes secondary to vertebral artery dissection have been reported after chiropractic manipulation of the cervical spine.[24]

Embolic stroke occurs when an embolus from the heart or lower circulation travels distally and lodges in a small vessel, resulting in loss of blood supply. At least 30% of ischemic strokes are attributed to a cardioembolic phenomenon.[22] The presence of valvular heart disease triples the risk for stroke.[25] Other risk factors include atrial fibrillation, myocardial infarction, ventricular aneurysm, and cardiomyopathy. Embolic strokes also arise from atherosclerosis of the ascending aorta.[26] Recent research has linked chronic inflammation, evidenced by elevated serum C-reactive protein,[23,27] and chronic periodontitis with significantly increased risk for stroke.[28]

Pathophysiology

Ischemic stroke is a cerebral hemodynamic insult. When CBF is reduced to a level insufficient to maintain neuronal viability, ischemic injury occurs. In focal stroke an area of marginally perfused tissue, the *ischemic penumbra*, surrounds a core of ischemic cells.[29] Sustained anoxic insult initiates a chain of events producing brain infarction. Irreversible neuronal injury soon follows. If infarction occurs, the affected brain tissue eventually softens and liquefies.

The phenomenon of a focal ischemic stroke is identical to that associated with myocardial infarction; thus "brain attack" is used in public education strategies. Often a history of transient ischemic attacks (TIAs), brief episodes of neurologic symptoms, or reversible ischemic neurologic deficit (RIND), which last less than 24 hours, offers a warning that stroke is likely to occur. Sudden onset indicates embolism as the final insult to flow.[22] The size of the stroke depends on the size and location of the occluded vessel and the availability of collateral blood flow. Global ischemia results when severe hypotension or cardiopulmonary arrest produces a transient drop in blood flow to all areas of the brain.[30]

Cerebral edema sufficient to produce clinical deterioration develops in 10% to 20% of patients with ischemic stroke and can result in intracranial hypertension. The edema results from a loss of normal metabolic function of the cells and peaks at 3 to 5 days. This process is usually the cause of death during the first week after a stroke.[30] Secondary hemorrhage at the site of the stroke lesion, known as *hemorrhagic conversion*, and seizures are the two other major acute neurologic complications of ischemic stroke.[22] Mortality in the first 20 days after ischemic stroke ranges from 8% to 30%.

Assessment and Diagnosis

The characteristic sign of an ischemic stroke is the sudden onset of focal neurologic signs persisting for more than 24 hours. These signs usually occur in combination.

Hemiparesis, aphasia, and hemianopia are common neurologic symptoms associated with ischemic stroke (Box 17-6). Changes in LOC usually occur only with brain stem or cerebellar involvement, seizure, hypoxia, hemorrhage, or elevated ICP. These changes may be exhibited as stupor, coma, confusion, and agitation.[31] The reported frequency of seizures in patients with ischemic stroke is variable, ranging from 5% to 20%. If seizures occur, they are usually seen within 24 hours of insult.[32]

Confirmation of the diagnosis of ischemic stroke is the first step in the emergent evaluation of these patients. Differentiation from intracranial hemorrhage is vital, with noncontrast CT scanning the method of choice and considered the most important initial diagnostic study. In addition to excluding intracranial hemorrhage, CT can also assist in identifying early neurologic complications and the etiology of the insult. MRI will demonstrate actual infarction of cerebral tissue earlier than a CT but is less useful in the emergent differential diagnosis. Because of the strong correlation between acute ischemic stroke and heart disease, 12-lead electrocardiogram (ECG), chest radiograph, and continuous cardiac monitoring are suggested to detect a cardiac etiology or coexisting condition. Echocardiography is valuable in identifying a cardioembolic phenomenon when a sufficient index of suspicion warrants.[33] Laboratory evaluation of hematologic function, electrolyte and glucose levels, and renal and hepatic function is also recommended. Arterial

---

Box **17-6**	Neurologic Abnormalities in Acute Ischemic Strokes

LEFT (DOMINANT) HEMISPHERE

Aphasia; right hemiparesis, right-sided sensory loss, right visual field defect, poor right conjugate gaze; dysarthria; difficulty in reading, writing, or calculating

RIGHT (NONDOMINANT) HEMISPHERE

Neglect of left visual space, left visual field defect, left hemiparesis, left-sided sensory loss, poor left conjugate gaze, extinction of left-sided stimuli; dysarthria; spatial disorientation

BRAIN STEM/CEREBELLUM/POSTERIOR HEMISPHERE

Motor or sensory loss in all four limbs, crossed signs, limb or gait ataxia, dysarthria, dysconjugate gaze, nystagmus, amnesia, bilateral visual field defects

SMALL SUBCORTICAL HEMISPHERE OR BRAIN STEM
Pure Motor Stroke

Weakness of face and limbs on side of body without abnormalities of higher brain function, sensation, or vision

Pure Sensory Stroke

Decreased sensation of face and limbs on one side of body without abnormalities of higher brain function, motor function, or vision

From Adams HP et al: *Circulation* 90:1588, 1994.

blood gas (ABG) analysis is performed if hypoxia is suspected, and an electroencephalogram (EEG) is obtained if seizures are suspected. LP is performed only if subarachnoid hemorrhage is suspected and the CT scan is negative.[34]

Medical Management

Major changes have taken place in the medical management of ischemic stroke since 1996. Based on results of the National Institute of Neurologic Disorders and Stroke (NINDS) rt-PA Stroke Study, thrombolytic therapy with intravenous (IV) recombinant tissue plasminogen activator (rt-PA) is now recommended within 3 hours of onset of ischemic stroke.[35] Contraindications to thrombolysis are listed in Box 17-7.[36] Confirmation of diagnosis with CT must be accomplished before rt-PA administration. The recommended dose of rt-PA is 0.9 mg/kg, up to a maximum dose of 90 mg. Ten percent of the total dose is administered as an initial IV bolus over 1 minute, and the remaining 90% is administered by IV infusion over 60 minutes.[37]

The desired result of thrombolytic therapy is to dissolve the clot and reperfuse the ischemic brain. The goal is to reverse or minimize the effects of stroke. The major risk and complication of rt-PA therapy is bleeding, especially intracranial hemorrhage. Unlike thrombolytic protocols for acute myocardial infarction, subsequent therapy with anticoagulant or antiplatelet agents is *not* recommended after rt-PA administration in ischemic stroke. Persons receiving thrombolytic therapy for stroke should not receive aspirin, heparin, warfarin, ticlopidine, or other antithrombotic or antiplatelet aggregating drug for at least 24 hours after treatment.[38]

Recent studies have demonstrated that these guidelines are safe for use in routine clinical practice.[39] The major barrier to effective application of thrombolytic therapy for ischemic stroke is prehospital and in-hospital delays. This therapeutic breakthrough dictates that all involved in the acute care of the ischemic patient must be prepared for rapid evaluation of the stroke patient and for rapid, knowledgeable institution of guideline protocols.[40]

Other emergent care of the patient with ischemic stroke must include airway protection and ventilatory assistance to maintain adequate tissue oxygenation.[34] Hypertension often is present in the early period as a compensatory response and in most cases must not be lowered. For the patient who has not received thrombolytic therapy, antihypertensive therapy is considered only if the mean blood pressure (BP) is greater than 130 mm Hg or the systolic BP is greater than 220 mm Hg.[41] Criteria differ for the patient who has received rt-PA. The BP for these patients is kept below 180/105 mm Hg to prevent intracranial hemorrhage. IV labetalol or sodium nitroprusside is used to achieve BP control.[42] Body temperature and glucose levels also must be normalized.[30]

Medical management also must include the identification and treatment of acute complications, such as cerebral edema or seizure activity. Prophylaxis for these complications is not recommended. Surgical decompression is recommended if a large cerebellar infarction compresses the brain stem.[34]

Additional therapies, both preventive and therapeutic, under investigation include emergent carotid endarterectomy, embolectomy or angioplasty; hemodilution of the blood; and administration of cytoprotective agents such as steroids, barbiturates, nimodipine, naloxone, glutamate antagonists, and monoclonal antibodies. These therapies are not recommended at this time for routine use because of insufficient evidence.[29,41]

Subarachnoid Hemorrhage
Epidemiology and Etiology

Subarachnoid hemorrhage (SAH) is bleeding into the subarachnoid space, usually caused by rupture of a cerebral aneurysm or arteriovenous malformation (AVM). SAH accounts for 6% to 7% of all strokes, with nontraumatic SAH affecting more than 30,000 Americans each year. The incidence of SAH is greater in women and increases with age. Overall mortality is 25%, with most patients dying on the first day after insult. The rate of significant morbidity approximates 50% of all survivors.[43] Unfortunately, no appreciable decrease in the incidence of SAH has occurred over time. Approximately 2 million people in the United States are believed to have an unruptured cerebral aneurysm, the congenital anomaly responsible for most cases of SAH. The risk for rupture is 1% to 2% annually. The known risk factors for SAH include hypertension, smoking, alcohol use, and stimulant use.[43] As in ischemic stroke, the single most important risk factor is hypertension.

| Box **17-7** | Exclusion Criteria for Intravenous rt-PA Therapy for Acute Ischemic Stroke |

1. Evidence of intracranial hemorrhage on pretreatment evaluation.
2. Suspicion of subarachnoid hemorrhage.
3. Recent (within 3 months) intracranial or intraspinal surgery, serious head trauma, or previous stroke.
4. History of intracranial hemorrhage.
5. Uncontrolled hypertension at time of treatment (e.g., >185 mm Hg systolic or >110 mm Hg diastolic).
6. Seizure at the onset of stroke.
7. Active internal bleeding.
8. Intracranial neoplasm, arteriovenous malformation, or aneurysm.
9. Known bleeding diathesis, including but not limited to:
   - Current use of oral anticoagulants (e.g., warfarin) or INR >1.7 or PT >15 seconds.
   - Administration of heparin within 48 hours preceding onset of stroke, with elevated aPTT at presentation.
   - Platelet count <100,000/mm^3.

rt-PA, Recombinant tissue plasminogen activator; *INR*, international normalized ratio; *PT*, prothrombin time; *aPTT*, activated partial thromboplastin time.

Causes of SAH include cerebral aneurysms, AVMs, hypertensive intracerebral hemorrhages, and bleeding from a cerebral tumor. Cerebral aneurysm rupture accounts for approximately 75% of all cases of spontaneous SAH.[1] An aneurysm is an outpouching of the wall of a blood vessel that results from weakening of the wall of the vessel. Ninety percent of aneurysms are congenital and of unknown cause. The other 10% may result from traumatic injury (that stretches and tears the muscular middle layer of an arterial vessel), from infectious material (most often from infectious vegetation on valves in the left side of the heart after bacterial endocarditis) that lodges against a vessel wall and erodes the muscular layer, or from undetermined causes. Multiple aneurysms occur in 20% to 25% of patients and often are bilateral, occurring in the same location on both sides of the cerebrovascular system. An individual can live a full life span with an unruptured cerebral aneurysm. Aneurysm rupture usually occurs during the fifth and sixth decades of life.[1]

AVM rupture is responsible for less than 10% of all SAHs.[1] An AVM is a tangled mass of arterial and venous blood vessels that shunt blood directly from the arterial side into the venous side, bypassing the capillary system. They may be small focal lesions or large diffuse lesions that occupy almost an entire hemisphere. AVMs are always congenital, although the exact embryonic cause for these malformations is unknown. AVMs also occur in the spinal cord and renal, gastrointestinal, and integumentary systems. Small superficial AVMs are seen as port-wine stains of the skin. In contrast to the middle-aged population with SAH from aneurysm, SAH from an AVM usually occurs in the second to fourth decades of life.[1]

Pathophysiology

The pathophysiology of the two most common causes of SAH is distinctly different.

Cerebral Aneurysm. As the individual with a congenital cerebral aneurysm matures, blood pressure rises and more stress is placed on the poorly developed and thin vessel wall. Ballooning out of the vessel occurs, giving the aneurysm a berrylike appearance. Most cerebral aneurysms are saccular or berrylike with a stem or neck. Aneurysms are usually small, 2 to 7 mm in diameter, and often occur at the base of the brain on the circle of Willis (Figure 17-1). Most cerebral aneurysms occur at the bifurcation of blood vessels.[31]

The aneurysm becomes clinically significant when the vessel wall becomes so thin that it ruptures, sending arterial blood at a high pressure into the subarachnoid space. For a brief moment after the aneurysm ruptures, ICP is believed to approach mean arterial pressure, and cerebral perfusion falls. In other cases the unruptured aneurysm expands and places pressure on surrounding structures. This is particularly true with posterior communicating artery aneurysms because they put pressure on the oculomotor nerve (CN III), causing ipsilateral pupil dilation and ptosis.[31]

Arteriovenous Malformation. The pathophysiologic features of an AVM are related to the size and location of the malformation. One or more cerebral arteries, known as *feeders*, supply an AVM. These feeder arteries tend to enlarge over time and increase the volume of blood shunted through the malformation, as well as increase the overall mass effect. Large, dilated, tortuous draining veins also develop as a result of increasing arterial blood flow being delivered at a higher than normal pressure. Normal vascular flow has

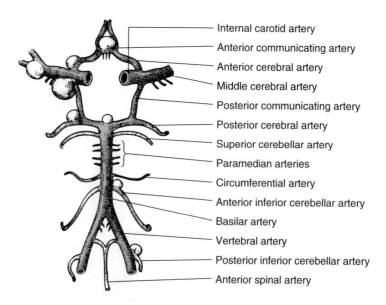

- Internal carotid artery
- Anterior communicating artery
- Anterior cerebral artery
- Middle cerebral artery
- Posterior communicating artery
- Posterior cerebral artery
- Superior cerebellar artery
- Paramedian arteries
- Circumferential artery
- Anterior inferior cerebellar artery
- Basilar artery
- Vertebral artery
- Posterior inferior cerebellar artery
- Anterior spinal artery

Figure 17-1   Common sites of berry aneurysms. Size of aneurysm in drawing is proportional to the frequency of occurrence at the various sites. (From Wyngaarden JB, Smith LH, editors: *Cecil's textbook of medicine*, ed 16, Philadelphia, 1982, Saunders.)

rial pressure of 70 to 80 mm Hg, mean arteriole pres-
 to 45 mm Hg, and mean capillary pressure that
35 to 10 mm Hg as it connects with the venous
 this capillary bridge allows blood with a mean
35 to 45 mm Hg to flow into the venous system.
vein has no muscular layer as does an artery, the
e extremely engorged and rupture easily. Cerebral
 may be present in the patient with an AVM as a
onic ischemia from shunting of blood through the
AVM and away from normal cerebral circulation.[31]

Assessment and Diagnosis

The patient with an SAH characteristically has an abrupt
onset of pain, described as the "worst headache of my life." A
brief loss of consciousness, nausea, vomiting, focal neurologic deficits, and a stiff neck may accompany the headache.
The SAH may result in coma or death.

Patient history may reveal one or more incidents of sudden onset of headache with vomiting in the weeks preceding
a major SAH. These are "warning leaks" of an aneurysm in
which small amounts of blood ooze from the aneurysm into
the subarachnoid space. The presence of blood is an irritant
to the meninges, particularly the arachnoid membrane. This
irritation causes headache, stiff neck, and photophobia.
These small "warning leaks" seldom are detected because
the condition is not severe enough for the patient to seek
medical attention. If a neurologic deficit, such as third cranial nerve palsy, develops before aneurysm rupture, medical
intervention is sought, and the aneurysm may be surgically
secured before the devastation of a rupture can occur.
Symptoms of an unruptured AVM—headaches with dizziness or syncope or fleeting neurologic deficits—also may be
found in the history.[31]

Diagnosis of SAH is based on clinical presentation, CT
scan, and LP. Noncontrast CT is the cornerstone of definitive SAH diagnosis.[43,44] In 92% of cases, CT scan can
demonstrate a clot in the subarachnoid space, if performed
within 24 hours of the onset of the hemorrhage. On the basis
of the appearance and the location of the SAH, diagnosis of
cause—aneurysm or AVM—may be made from the CT scan.
MRI is relatively insensitive for detecting blood in the subarachnoid space.

If the initial CT scan is negative, LP is performed to
obtain CSF for analysis. CSF after SAH is bloody in appearance, with a red blood cell count greater than 1000/mm[3]. If
LP is performed more than 5 days after the SAH, CSF fluid is
xanthochromic (dark amber) because the blood products
have broken down. Cloudy CSF usually indicates an infectious process such as bacterial meningitis, not SAH.[31]

Once the SAH has been documented, cerebral angiography is necessary to identify the exact cause of the SAH. If a
cerebral aneurysm rupture is the cause, angiography is also
essential for identifying the exact location of the aneurysm
in preparation for surgery. Once located, the aneurysm is
graded using the Hunt and Hess classification scale, which

categorizes the patient based on the severity of the neurologic deficits associated with the hemorrhage (Box 17-8).[45]
If AVM rupture is the cause, angiography is necessary to
identify the feeding arteries and draining veins of the
malformation.

Medical Management

SAH is a medical emergency, and time is of the essence.
Preservation of neurologic function is the goal. Initial treatment must always support vital functions. Airway management and ventilatory assistance may be necessary. Early
diagnosis is also essential. A ventriculostomy is performed to
control ICP if the patient's LOC is depressed.[43]

Evidence suggests that only 19% of the deaths attributable to aneurysmal SAH are related to the direct effects of the
initial hemorrhage.[46] Research has shown that rebleeding
accounts for 22% of deaths from aneurysmal SAH, cerebral
vasospasm for 23%, and nonneurologic medical complications for 23%.[46] Principal nonneurologic causes of death are
systemic inflammatory response syndrome (SIRS) and secondary organ dysfunction.[47] Once initial intervention has
provided necessary support for vital physiologic functions,
medical management of acute SAH is aimed primarily
toward the prevention and treatment of the complications
of SAH that can produce further neurologic damage and
death.

Rebleeding. Rebleeding is the occurrence of a second
SAH in an unsecured aneurysm or less often an AVM.[5] The
incidence of rebleeding with conservative therapy is 20% to
30% in the first month, with the highest occurrence on the
first day after initial hemorrhage.[43] Mortality from aneurysmal rebleeding is 48% to 78%.[48]

Historically, conservative measures to prevent rebleeding have included BP control and SAH precautions (see
Nursing Management of stroke). An elevation in BP is a

Box **17-8**	Classification of Subarachnoid Hemorrhage
Grade I	Asymptomatic or minimal headache Slight nuchal rigidity
Grade II	Moderate to severe headache Nuchal rigidity No neurologic deficit other than cranial nerve palsy
Grade III	Drowsiness Confusion Mild focal deficit
Grade IV	Stupor Moderate to severe hemiparesis Possible early decerebrate rigidity Vegetative disturbances
Grade V	Deep coma Decerebrate rigidity Moribund appearance

normal compensatory response to maintain adequate cerebral perfusion after a neurologic insult. In the belief that hypertension contributes to rebleeding, the agent nitroprusside, metoprolol, or hydralazine is often used to maintain a systolic BP no greater than 150 mm Hg. Individualized guidelines must be determined based on clinical condition and preexisting values of the patient. Evidence suggests that rebleeding is associated more with variations in BP than with absolute values, and that BP control does not lower the incidence of rebleeding.[43] Prophylactic anticonvulsant therapy is recommended to prevent seizures.[22,43]

Surgical Aneurysm Clipping. Definitive treatment for the prevention of rebleeding is surgical clipping with complete obliteration of the aneurysm. Timing of the surgery is a key medical management issue. Since the introduction of microsurgery and improved surgical techniques, patients usually are taken to the operating room within the first 48 hours after rupture. This early surgical intervention to secure the aneurysm eliminates the risk of rebleeding and allows more aggressive therapy in the postoperative period for the treatment of vasospasm. Early surgery also allows the neurosurgeon to flush out the excess blood and clots from the basal cisterns (reservoir of CSF around the base of the brain and circle of Willis) to reduce the risk of vasospasm. Early surgery is recommended for patients with grade I or II SAH and some patients with grade III. In patients with grade III SAH the initial hemorrhage did not produce significant neurologic deficit, but the risk of rebleeding, with tragically high mortality, is present until the aneurysm is secured. Because of the patient's clinical condition and the technical difficulty of the surgery, early surgical repair of the aneurysm is not always possible. Early surgery continues to be controversial for patients with grade IV or V SAH and patients with vasospasm. However, recent studies have not supported the fear of worse ischemic sequelae with early surgery in these patients.[48] Careful consideration of the patient's clinical situation is necessary in determining the optimal time for surgery.

The surgical procedure involves a craniotomy to expose and isolate the area of aneurysm. A clip is placed over the neck of the aneurysm to eliminate the area of weakness (Figure 17-2). This technically difficult procedure requires an experienced neurosurgeon. Early in surgery the clot may break away from the aneurysm as it is surgically exposed. Extensive hemorrhage into the craniotomy site results, and cessation of the hemorrhage often causes increased neurologic deficits. Deficits also may occur as a result of surgical manipulation to gain access to the site of the aneurysm.[31]

Surgical AVM Excision. Management of AVM traditionally has involved surgical excision or conservative management of such symptoms as seizures and headache. The decision for surgical excision depends on the location and size of the AVM. Some malformations are located so deep in the cerebral structures (thalamus or midbrain) that attempts to remove the AVM would cause severe neurologic deficits.

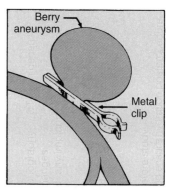

Figure 17-2 Clipping of aneurysm. (From Chipps EM, Clanin NJ, Campbell VG: *Neurologic disorders*, St Louis, 1992, Mosby.)

History of a previous hemorrhage and the patient's age and overall condition are also taken into account when making the decision regarding surgical intervention.

Surgical excision of large AVMs includes the risk of reperfusion bleeding. As feeding arteries of the AVM are clamped off, the arterial blood that usually flowed into the AVM is now diverted into the surrounding circulation. In many cases the surrounding tissue has been in a state of chronic ischemia, and the arterial vessels feeding these areas are maximally dilated. As arterial blood begins to flow at a higher volume and pressure into these dilated arteries, seeping of blood from the vessels may occur. Evidence of reperfusion bleeding in the operating room is an indication that no more arterial blood can be diverted from the AVM without risk of serious intracerebral hemorrhage. In the postoperative phase, low BP is maintained to prevent further reperfusion bleeding. In large AVMs, two to four stages of surgery may be required over 6 to 12 months.[31]

Embolization. Embolization is used to secure a cerebral aneurysm or AVM that is surgically inaccessible because of size, location, or medical instability of the patient. Embolization involves several new interventional neuroradiology techniques. All the techniques use a percutaneous transfemoral approach in a manner similar to an angiogram. Under fluoroscopy the catheter is threaded up to the internal carotid artery. Special microcatheters are then manipulated into the area of the vascular anomaly, and embolic materials are placed endovascularly. Three different embolization techniques are used, depending on the underlying pathologic derangement.[31]

The first type of embolization is used to embolize an AVM. Small silastic beads or glue is slowly introduced into the vessels feeding the AVM. Blood flow then carries the material to the site, and embolization is achieved. This procedure may be used in combination with surgery. One to three sessions of embolization of the feeding vessels are performed to reduce the size of the lesion before a craniotomy is performed for total excision. The primary risk is lodging of the embolic substance in a vessel that feeds normal tissue, which creates an embolic stroke with immediate onset of neurologic symptoms.

The second type of embolization involves placement of one or more detachable balloons into an aneurysmal sac or AVM. A liquid polymerizing agent is used to inflate the balloon. The material then solidifies. The third technique involves placement of one or more detachable platinum coils into an aneurysm to produce an endovascular thrombus. The advantage of this technique is that an electric current creates positive charging of the coil, which induces electrothrombosis. The most common complication of these two techniques is the development of distal ischemia resulting from emboli. Again, the onset of neurologic symptoms is immediate. Other risks include subtotal occlusion, intraprocedural rupture of the vasculature, and death.[31]

Cerebral Vasospasm. The presence or absence of cerebral vasospasm significantly affects the outcome of aneurysmal SAH. This complication does not occur with SAH resulting from AVM rupture. Cerebral vasospasm is a narrowing of the lumen of the cerebral arteries, possibly in response to subarachnoid blood clots coating the outer surface of the blood vessels. Because aneurysms occur at the circle of Willis, the major vessels responsible for feeding the cerebral circulation are affected by vasospasm. Depending on the arterial vessels involved in the vasospasm reaction, decreased arterial flow occurs in large areas of the cerebral hemispheres.[31]

An estimated 50% of all SAH patients develop vasospasm, which is demonstrable by angiography. Of these patients, 32% develop symptomatic vasospasm, resulting in ischemic stroke and/or death for 15% to 20% despite the use of maximal therapy.[43] The onset of vasospasm is usually 4 to 12 days after the initial hemorrhage.[49]

A variety of therapies have been evaluated in an attempt to reverse or overcome cerebral vasospasm. Research centers are evaluating such diverse therapies as barbiturate coma[50] and intraventricular sodium nitroprusside.[51] To date, three treatments are often used: induced hypertensive hypervolemic hemodilution therapy, oral nimodipine, and transluminal cerebral angioplasty.

Hypertensive Hypervolemic Hemodilution Therapy. HHH therapy involves increasing the patient's BP and cardiac output (CO) with vasoactive medications and diluting the patient's blood with fluid and volume expanders. Systolic BP is maintained between 150 and 160 mm Hg. The increase in volume and pressure forces blood through the vasospastic area at higher pressures. Hemodilution facilitates flow through the area by reducing blood viscosity. In many anecdotal reports, neurologic deficits improved as systolic BP increased from 130 mm Hg to between 150 and 160 mm Hg.[49] The Stroke Council of the American Heart Association has recommended HHH therapy for prevention and treatment of vasospasm.[43]

The obvious deterrent to use of induced hypertension is the risk of rebleeding in an unsecured aneurysm. Surgical clipping of the aneurysm before HHH therapy is preferred.

Cerebral edema, elevated ICP, cardiac failure, and electrolyte imbalance are also risks of HHH therapy. Careful monitoring of the patient's neurologic status, hemodynamic parameters, ICP, and serum electrolytes is necessary.[43]

Oral Nimodipine. Oral nimodipine is strongly recommended to reduce the poor outcomes associated with vasospasm. The exact nature of the effect of nimodipine is not clear, but its use has demonstrated consistently positive effects on outcome without any demonstrable effect on the incidence or severity of vasospasm.[49] Nimodipine is administered by mouth or nasogastric tube (NGT) prophylactically in all patients with SAH. Nimodipine may produce hypotension, especially when administered concurrently with other antihypertensive agents. Nimodipine is not effective if administered sublingually. To administer nimodipine via NGT, the soft capsule is punctured at both ends and the contents are withdrawn and administered through the tube, followed by flushing.[31]

Transluminal Cerebral Angioplasty. Transluminal cerebral angioplasty is used when pharmacologic management of cerebral vasospasm has failed. It is performed only when CT or MRI provides evidence that infarction has not yet occurred. An interventional neuroradiologist performs the procedure, and the patient is under local, general, or neuroleptic analgesia. The technique of cerebral angioplasty is very similar to that used in the coronary vasculature. Risks include intimal perforation or rupture, cerebral artery thrombosis or embolism, recurrence of stenosis, and severe diffuse vasospasm unresponsive to therapy. Hemorrhage at the femoral site also may occur. Transluminal cerebral angioplasty is recommended when conventional therapy is unsuccessful.[43,49]

Hyponatremia. Hyponatremia develops in 10% to 43% of patients with SAH, usually occurring about the same time as vasospasm, several days after initial hemorrhage. Strong evidence indicates that the use of fluid restriction to treat hyponatremia is associated with poor outcome in the SAH patient. The Stroke Council has strongly recommended that fluid restriction not be used in this instance and instead recommends sodium replenishment with isotonic fluids.[43]

Hydrocephalus. Development of hydrocephalus is a late complication common after SAH. Blood that has circulated in the subarachnoid space and has been absorbed by the arachnoid villi may obstruct the villi and reduce the rate of CSF absorption. Over time, increasing volumes of CSF in the intracranial space produce communicating hydrocephalus. Treatment consists of placing a drain to remove CSF. This can be accomplished temporarily by inserting a ventriculostomy or permanently by placing a ventriculoperitoneal shunt.[31]

Intracerebral Hemorrhage
Epidemiology and Etiology.

Intracerebral hemorrhage (ICH) is bleeding directly into cerebral tissue. ICH destroys cerebral tissue, causes cerebral edema, and increases ICP. The source of intracerebral bleeding is usually a small artery, but it can result also from rupture of an AVM or aneurysm. The most important cause of spontaneous ICH is hypertension, so this section concentrates on spontaneous hypertensive ICH.[52]

Spontaneous ICH is more than twice as common as SAH. The likeliness of death or disability is higher with ICH than with either ischemic stroke or SAH.[52,53] Mortality for hemorrhagic stroke is 35% to 52% within 1 month; half these deaths occur in the first 48 hours.[53] The key risk factors for ICH are age and hypertension. ICH occurs more often in men than in women and more often in nonwhite populations.[52,53]

ICH is most often caused by hypertensive rupture of a cerebral vessel, resulting from a long-standing history of hypertension. Anticoagulation or thrombolytic therapy; coagulation disorders; drug abuse; and hemorrhage into cerebral infarct or brain tumors are other possible causes of spontaneous ICH.[53] Many patients develop headache and neurologic symptoms after straining to have a bowel movement. Often on questioning, the patient with a hypertensive hemorrhage admits to having discontinued antihypertensive medication 2 to 3 weeks before the hemorrhage.

Pathophysiology

The pathophysiology of ICH is caused by continued elevated BP exerting force against smaller arterial vessels that have become damaged from arteriosclerotic changes. Eventually these arteries break, and blood bursts from the vessels into the surrounding cerebral tissue, creating a hematoma. ICP rises precipitously in response to the increase in overall intracranial volume.[31]

Assessment and Diagnosis.

Initial assessment usually reveals a critically ill patient who often is unconscious and requires ventilatory support. History from a relative or significant other describes a sudden onset of focal deficit often accompanied by severe headache, nausea, vomiting, and rapid neurologic deterioration. Approximately 50% of patients sustain early loss of consciousness, a key differential feature from ischemic stroke.[52,53] More than half of patients with ICH present with a smooth progression of neurologic symptoms, an uncommon finding in either ischemic stroke or SAH.[53] One third of patients have maximal symptoms at onset. Vital signs usually reveal a severely elevated BP (200/100 to 250/150 mm Hg). Signs of increased ICP are often present by the time the patient arrives in the emergency department. Diagnosis is established easily with CT. Angiography is recommended only in patients considered surgical candidates without a clear cause of hemorrhage.[52,53]

Medical Management

ICH is a medical emergency. Initial management requires attention to airway, breathing, and circulation. Intubation is usually necessary. Blood pressure management must be based on individual factors. Reduction in BP is usually necessary to decrease ongoing bleeding, but lowering BP too much or too rapidly may compromise CPP, especially in the patient with elevated ICP. National guidelines recommend keeping the *mean* arterial pressure (MAP) below 130 mm Hg in patients with a history of hypertension and below 110 mm Hg after surgical treatment for ICH.[53] Vasopressor therapy after fluid replacement is recommended if systolic BP falls below 90 mm Hg.[52,53]

Increased ICP is common with ICH and is a major contributor to mortality. Recommended management includes mannitol when indicated, hyperventilation, and neuromuscular blockade with sedation. Steroids are avoided. CPP must be kept greater than 70 mm Hg.[52,53]

The goal for fluid management is euvolemia with a recommended pulmonary arterial occlusion pressure (PAOP) of 10 to 14 mm Hg. Body temperature is kept at less than 38.5° C using acetaminophen or cooling blankets. Short-acting benzodiazepines or propofol is recommended to treat agitation or hyperactivity. Pneumatic compression devices are used to decrease risk of pulmonary embolism. Prophylactic antiepileptic therapy may be used.

The benefit of surgical treatment of spontaneous ICH is unclear. Recommendations for surgical removal of the clot depend on the size and location of the hematoma, the patient's ICP, and other neurologic symptoms. Medical treatment is recommended if the hemorrhage is small (less than 10 cm³) or neurologic deficit is minimal. Likewise, surgery offers no improvement in outcome for patients with a Glasgow Coma Scale (GCS) score of 4 or less. Surgical evacuation of the clot is recommended for patients with cerebellar hemorrhage greater than 3 cm with neurologic deterioration or hydrocephalus with brain stem compression and for young patients with moderate or large lobar hemorrhage with clinical deterioration.[52,53] Numerous techniques are being investigated to lessen the risk of brain damage associated with craniotomy for ICH.

Nursing Management

Nursing management of the patient with stroke incorporates a variety of nursing diagnoses (Box 17-9). **Nursing priorities are directed toward (1) performing frequent neurologic and hemodynamic assessments, (2) maintaining surveillance for complications, and (3) providing patient education.**

Performing Frequent Assessments

The goal of frequent assessments is early recognition of neurologic and hemodynamic deterioration. Close monitoring of the patient's neurologic signs and vital signs is essential and requires almost continuous observation. Automatic noninvasive devices such as BP cuff and pulse oximeter are helpful. Seizure activity must be identified and treated immediately. All personnel working with the patient must be aware of the desired hemodynamic and neurologic parameters set by the physician and understand that the physician must be notified at the first sign of change.

Stroke

- Decreased Intracranial Adaptive Capacity related to failure of normal intracranial compensatory mechanisms
- Ineffective Cerebral Tissue Perfusion related to vasospasm or hemorrhage
- Unilateral Neglect related to perceptual disruption
- Impaired Verbal Communication related to cerebral speech center injury
- Impaired Swallowing related to neuromuscular impairment, fatigue, and limited awareness
- Disturbed Body Image related to actual change in body structure, function, or appearance
- Deficient Knowledge: Discharge Regimen related to lack of previous exposure to information

Maintaining Surveillance for Complications. The patient with stroke should be monitored closely for signs of bleeding, vasospasm, and increased ICP. Other complications of stroke include aspiration, malnutrition, pneumonia, deep vein thrombosis, pulmonary embolism, decubitus ulcers, contractures, and joint abnormalities.[31] Nursing measures to prevent these complications are well known.

Additional complications that may be seen in the patient with stroke are related to the area of the brain that has been damaged. Damage to the temporoparietal area can create a variety of disturbances that affect the patient's ability to interpret sensory information. Damage to the *dominant* hemisphere (usually left) produces problems with speech and language and abstract and analytical skills. Damage to the *nondominant* hemisphere (usually right) produces problems with spatial relationships. The resulting deficits include agnosia, apraxia, and visual field defects. Perceptual deficits are not as readily noticeable as motor deficits but may be more debilitating and can lead to the inability to perform skilled or purposeful tasks. The patient also may develop impaired swallowing.[31]

Bleeding and Vasospasm. In the patient with cerebral aneurysm, sudden onset of or an increase in headache, nausea and vomiting, increased BP, and changes in respiration herald the onset of rebleeding. The first indication of vasospasm is usually the appearance of new focal or global neurologic deficits. SAH precautions must be implemented to prevent any stress or straining that could precipitate rebleeding. Precautions include BP control, bed rest, dark quiet environment, and stool softeners. Short-acting analgesics and sedatives are used to relieve pain and anxiety. The patient must be kept calm. Limb restraints cause straining and must be avoided. If restraint is necessary, only a vest or jacket type of restraint is used. The head of the bed should be elevated to 35 to 45 degrees at all times. The patient is taught to avoid any activities that create the Valsalva maneuver, such as pushing with the legs to move up in bed, straining for a bowel movement, or holding the breath during procedures or discomfort. Deep vein thrombosis precautions are routinely implemented. Collaboration with the

patient and family is used to establish a visitation plan to meet patient and family needs. Often, family members at the bedside can assist the patient to remain calm.[31]

Increased Intracranial Pressure. Of the numerous signs and symptoms of increased ICP, change in LOC is the most sensitive indicator. Others include unequal pupil size, decreased pupillary response to light, headache, projectile vomiting, altered breathing patterns, Cushing's triad (bradycardia, systolic hypertension, bradypnea), diminished brain stem reflexes, papilledema, and abnormal extension (decerebrate posturing) or flexion (decorticate posturing).[31]

Impaired Swallowing. Normal swallowing occurs in four phases that are controlled by the cranial nerves. Damage to the brain, brain stem, or cranial nerves can result in a variety of swallowing deficits that can place the patient at risk for aspiration. The stroke patient is observed for signs of dysphagia, including drooling; difficulty handling oral secretions; absence of gag, cough, or swallowing reflex; moist, gurgling voice quality; decreased mouth and tongue movements; and presence of dysarthria. A speech therapy consult is initiated if any of these signs are present, and the patient must not be orally fed. In the absence of these warning signs, the patient may be fed, as ordered by the physician, although the patient must be continually monitored for signs of aspiration.[31]

Providing Patient Education

Rehabilitation starts in the critical care area, with a multidisciplinary team designing and implementing an individualized plan for maximizing the patient's potential for neurologic rehabilitation. Early in the patient's hospital stay, the patient and family must be taught about stroke, its etiologies, and its treatment. As the patient moves toward discharge, teaching focuses on the interventions necessary for preventing the recurrence of the event and on maximizing the patient's rehabilitation potential. The patient's family must be encouraged to participate in the patient's care; learn how to feed, dress, and bathe the patient; and learn some basic rehabilitation techniques. In addition, the importance of participating in a neurologic rehabilitation program or support group must be stressed.

Collaborative management of the patient with a stroke is outlined in Box 17-10.

GUILLAIN-BARRÉ SYNDROME

Guillain-Barré syndrome (GBS), once thought to be a single entity characterized by inflammatory peripheral neuropathy, is now understood to be a combination of clinical features with varying forms of presentation and multiple pathologic processes.[54-58] Most patients with GBS do not require admission to a critical care unit. However, the prototype of GBS, known as *acute inflammatory demyelinating polyradiculoneuropathy* (AIDP), involves a rapidly progressive, ascending peripheral nerve dysfunction leading to paralysis that may produce respiratory failure. Because of the need for ventilatory support, AIDP is one of the few peripheral neurologic diseases that necessitates a critical care environment. In this discussion, all references to GBS pertain to the AIDP prototype.

Box 17-10 COLLABORATIVE Management

Stroke

1. Differentiate the cause of the stroke.
   - Ischemic
   - Subarachnoid hemorrhage
     - Cerebral aneurysm
     - Arteriovenous malformation (AVM)
   - Intracerebral bleed
2. Implement treatment dependent on cause of bleed.
   - Ischemic
     - Thrombolytic therapy
     - Blood pressure control
   - Subarachnoid hemorrhage
     - Surgical aneurysm clipping or AVM excision
     - Embolization
   - Intracerebral bleed
     - Blood pressure control
3. Protect patient's airway.
4. Provide ventilatory assistance as required.
5. Perform frequent neurologic assessments.
6. Maintain surveillance for complications.
   - Cerebral edema
   - Cerebral ischemia/vasospasm
   - Rebleeding
   - Impaired swallowing
   - Neurologic deficits
7. Provide comfort and emotional support.
8. Design and implement appropriate rehabilitation program.
9. Educate patient and family.

Epidemiology and Etiology

The annual incidence of GBS is 1.6 to 1.9 per 100,000 persons. It occurs more often in males and is the most frequently acquired demyelinating neuropathy. Occasionally, clusters of cases are reported, such as occurred following the 1977 swine flu vaccinations.[59]

The precise cause of GBS remains unknown, but the syndrome involves an immune-mediated response involving both cell-mediated immunity and development of immunoglobulin G (IgG) antibodies. Most patients report a viral infection 1 to 3 weeks before onset of clinical manifestations, usually involving the upper respiratory tract. Other antecedent causes, or triggering events, associated with GBS include other viral infections (influenza; cytomegalovirus, hepatitis, Epstein-Barr virus, human immunodeficiency virus), bacterial infections (gastrointestinal *Campylobacter jejuni* and *Mycoplasma pneumoniae*), vaccines (rabies, tetanus, influenza), lymphoma, surgery, and trauma.[54,55,57,60]

Pathophysiology

GBS affects the motor and sensory pathways of the peripheral nervous system, as well as the autonomic nervous system functions of the cranial nerves. The major finding in GBS (AIDP type) is a segmental demyelination process of the peripheral nerves. GBS is believed to be an autoimmune response to antibodies formed in response to a recent physiologic event. T cells migrate to the peripheral nerves, resulting in edema and inflammation. Macrophages then invade the area and break down the myelin.[54] Inflammation around this demyelinated area causes further dysfunction. Some axonal damage also occurs.

The myelin sheath of the peripheral nerves is generated by Schwann cells and acts as an insulator for the peripheral nerve. Myelin promotes rapid conduction of nerve impulses by allowing the impulses to jump along the nerve through the nodes of Ranvier. Disruption of the myelin fiber slows and may eventually stop the conduction of impulses along the peripheral nerves. In GBS the more thickly myelinated fibers of motor pathways and the cranial nerves are more severely affected than are the thinly myelinated sensory fibers of cutaneous pain, touch, and temperature.[31]

Once the temporary inflammatory reaction stops, myelin-producing cells begin the process of reinsulating the demyelinated portions of the peripheral nervous system. When remyelination occurs, normal neurologic function should return. In some patients the axon may be damaged during the inflammatory process. The degree of axonal damage is responsible for the degree of neurologic dysfunction that persists after recovery.[56]

Assessment and Diagnosis

Symptoms of GBS include motor weakness, paresthesias and other sensory changes, cranial nerve dysfunction (especially oculomotor, facial, glossopharyngeal, vagal, spinal accessory, and hypoglossal), and some autonomic dysfunction. The usual course of GBS begins with an abrupt onset of lower extremity weakness that progresses to flaccidity and ascends over hours to days. Motor loss usually is symmetric, bilateral, and ascending. The most severely affected patients have complete flaccidity of all peripheral nerves, including spinal and cranial nerves.[31]

The patient is admitted to the hospital when lower extremity weakness prevents mobility. Admission to the critical care unit is necessary when progression of the weakness threatens respiratory muscles. As the patient's weakness progresses, close observation is essential. Frequent assessment of the respiratory system, including ventilatory parameters such as inspiratory force and tidal volume, is necessary. The most common cause of death in patients with GBS is from respiratory arrest. As the disease progresses and respiratory effort weakens, intubation and mechanical ventilation are necessary. Continued, frequent assessment of neurologic deterioration is required until the patient reaches the peak of the disease and plateau occurs.[58]

The diagnosis of GBS is based on clinical findings plus CSF analysis and nerve conduction studies. The diagnostic finding is elevated CSF protein with normal cell count. The increased protein count is usually present after the first week but does not occur in approximately 10% of all cases.[54]

Nerve conduction studies that test the velocity at which nerve impulses are conducted show significant reduction, as the demyelinating process of the disease suggests.

Medical Management

With no curative treatment available, the medical management of GBS is limited. The disease simply must run its course, which is characterized by ascending paralysis that advances over 1 to 3 weeks and then remains at a plateau for 2 to 4 weeks.[54] The plateau stage is followed by descending paralysis and return to normal or near-normal function. The main focus of medical management is the support of bodily functions and the prevention of complications.

Plasmapheresis is often used in an attempt to limit the severity and duration of the syndrome. Plasmapheresis involves plasma exchanges or washes that remove the antibodies that cause GBS. Exchanges are given over 10 to 15 days. Controversy exists over the benefit of plasmapheresis. It is contraindicated in patients with hemodynamic instability. One study on the long-term benefit of plasmapheresis demonstrated that 71% of the treatment group versus 52% of the control group had full muscular strength recovery at 1 year.[61] Research also suggests that intravenous immunoglobulin (IVIG) has beneficial effects in treating GBS. IVIG is a blood product; close monitoring during its administration and during plasmapheresis is necessary.[58] No evidence supports one of these therapies over the other, but plasmapheresis costs $4000 less per patient.[62] Steroids have been used in GBS for their antiinflammatory effect, but no evidence supports this practice.[58,63]

Nursing Management

The nursing management of the patient with GBS incorporates a variety of nursing diagnoses and interventions (Box 17-11). The goal of nursing management is to support all normal body functions until patients can do so on their own. Although the condition is reversible, the patient with GBS requires extensive long-term care because

recovery can be a long process. **Nursing priorities for the patient with Guillain-Barré syndrome are directed toward** (1) **maintaining surveillance for complications,** (2) **initiating rehabilitation,** (3) **facilitating nutritional support,** (4) **providing comfort and emotional support,** and (5) **providing patient education**.

Maintaining Surveillance for Complications

Continuous assessment of the progressive paralysis associated with GBS is essential to timely intervention and the prevention of respiratory arrest and further neurologic insult. Once the patient is intubated and placed on mechanical ventilation, close observation for pulmonary complications (e.g., atelectasis, pneumonia, pneumothorax) is necessary. Autonomic dysfunction, or *dysautonomia*, can produce variations in heart rate and BP that can reach extreme values.[64,65] Hypertension and tachycardia may require β-blocker therapy. All GBS patients must be observed for this phenomenon.

Initiating Rehabilitation

Immobility may last for months in patients with GBS. The usual course of GBS involves an average of 10 days of symptom progression and 10 days of maximal level of dysfunction, followed by 2 to 48 weeks of recovery. Although GBS is usually completely reversible, the patient will require physical and occupational rehabilitation because of the problems of long-term immobility. Rehabilitation starts in the critical care area, with a multidisciplinary team designing and implementing an individualized plan for maximizing the patient's potential for rehabilitation.

Facilitating Nutritional Support

Nutritional support is implemented early in the course of GBS. Because recovery is a long process, adequate nutritional support will be a problem for an extended period. Nutritional support usually is accomplished through enteral feeding.

Providing Comfort and Emotional Support

Pain control is another important component in the care of the patient with GBS. Although patients may have minimal to no motor function, most sensory functions remain, causing patients considerable muscle ache and pain. Because of the length of this illness, a safe, effective, long-term solution to pain management must be identified. These patients also require extensive psychologic support. Although the illness is almost 100% reversible, lack of control over the situation, constant pain or discomfort, and the long-term nature of the disorder create coping difficulties for the patient. GBS does not affect the LOC or cerebral function. Patient interaction and communication are essential elements of the nursing management plan.

Providing Patient Education

Early in the patient's hospital stay, the patient and family must be taught about GBS and its different treatments. As the patient moves toward discharge, teaching focuses on the interventions to maximize the patient's rehabilitation potential. The patient's family must be encouraged to participate in the patient's care and to learn some basic rehabilitation techniques. In addition, the importance of participating in a neurologic rehabilitation program (if necessary) must be stressed.

Collaborative management of the patient with Guillain-Barré syndrome is outlined in Box 17-12.

CRANIOTOMY

A craniotomy is performed to gain access to portions of the central nervous system (CNS) inside the cranium, usually to allow removal of a space-occupying lesion such as a brain tumor (Table 17-2). Common procedures include tumor resection or removal, cerebral decompression, evacuation of hematoma or abscess, and clipping or removal of an aneurysm or AVM. Most patients who undergo craniotomy for tumor resection or removal do not require care in a critical care unit. Patients who do usually need intensive monitoring are at greater risk of complications because of underlying cardiopulmonary dysfunction or the surgical approach used (Box 17-13).

Preoperative Care

Protection of the integrity of the CNS is a major priority of care for the patient awaiting a craniotomy. Optimal arterial oxygenation, hemodynamic stability, and cerebral perfusion are essential to maintaining adequate cerebral oxygenation. Management of seizure activity is essential to controlling metabolic needs.

Detailed assessment and documentation of the patient's preoperative neurologic status are imperative for accurate postoperative evaluation. Specific attention is placed on identifying and describing the nature and extent of any pre-

operative neurologic deficits. When pituitary surgery is planned, thorough evaluation of endocrine function is necessary to prevent major intraoperative and postoperative complications.[66]

Current trends in health care demand judicious use of routine preoperative studies. Depending on the type of surgery and the general health of the patient, preoperative screening may include a complete blood count (CBC), blood urea nitrogen (BUN), creatinine, fasting blood sugar (FBS), chest radiograph, and ECG. A type and crossmatch for blood may also be ordered.

Preoperative teaching is necessary to prepare both the patient and family for what to expect in the postoperative period. A description of the intravascular lines and intracranial catheters used during the postoperative period allows the family to focus on the patient rather than be overwhelmed by masses of tubing. Some or all of the patient's hair is shaved off in the operating room, and a large, bulky, turbanlike craniotomy dressing is applied. Most patients experience some degree of postoperative eye or facial swelling and periorbital ecchymosis. An explanation of these temporary changes in appearance helps alleviate the shock and fear many patients and families experience in the immediate postoperative period.

All craniotomy patients require instruction to avoid activities known to produce sudden changes in ICP, including bending, lifting, straining, and Valsalva maneuver. Patients often elicit the Valsalva maneuver during repositioning in bed by holding their breath and straining with a closed epiglottis. Teaching the patient to continue to breathe deeply through the mouth during all position changes is an effective deterrent.

The patient undergoing transsphenoidal surgery requires preparation for the sensations associated with nasal packing. The patient often awakens with alarm because of the inability to breathe through the nose. Preoperative instruction in mouth breathing and avoidance of coughing, sneezing, or blowing of the nose facilitates postoperative cooperation.

The psychosocial issues associated with the prospect of neurosurgery cannot be overemphasized. Few procedures are as threatening as those involving the brain or spinal cord. For some patients the fear of permanent neurologic impairment may be as or more ominous than the fear of death. Steps to meet the needs of the patient, as well as the family, include collaboration with clergy and social services personnel, patient-controlled visitation, and provision of as much privacy as the patient's condition permits. Both the patient and the family must be provided with the opportunity to express their fears and concerns apart from each other as well as jointly.

Surgical Considerations

Whereas the emphasis in surgical approach for most other types of surgery is to gain adequate exposure of the surgical site, the neurosurgeon must select a route that also produces

---

Box 17-12 COLLABORATIVE Management

Guillain-Barré Syndrome

1. Support bodily functions.
   - Protect airway.
   - Provide ventilatory assistance as required.
2. Initiate treatments to limit duration of the syndrome.
   - Plasmapheresis
   - Intravenous immunoglobulin
3. Initiate nutritional support.
4. Maintain surveillance for complications.
   - Infections
   - Cardiac dysrhythmias
   - Blood pressure alterations
   - Temperature alterations
5. Provide comfort and emotional support.
6. Design and implement appropriate rehabilitation program.
7. Educate patient and family.

Table **17-2**   Tumor Types and Characteristics

Tumor	Clinical Features	Treatment/Prognosis
Glioblastoma multiforme (GM)	Often presents with nonspecific complaints and increased ICP. As tumor grows, focal deficits develop.	Rapidly progressive course, with poor prognosis. Total surgical removal usually not possible; response to radiation poor.
Astrocytoma	Presentation similar to GM, but course more protracted, often over several years; cerebellar astrocytoma, especially in children, may have more benign course.	Variable prognosis. By diagnosis, total excision usually impossible; tumor often not radiosensitive. In cerebellar astrocytoma, total excision often possible.
Medulloblastoma	Glioma most often seen in children. Generally arises from roof of fourth ventricle and leads to increased ICP, with brain stem and cerebellar signs; may seed subarachnoid space.	Treatment consists of surgery with radiation therapy and chemotherapy.
Ependymoma	Glioma arising from ependyma of ventricle, especially fourth; leads early to signs of increased ICP; arises also from central canal of spinal cord.	Tumor not radiosensitive and best treated surgically, if possible.
Oligodendroglioma	Slow-growing glioma, usually arises in cerebral hemisphere in adults. Calcification may be visible on radiograph.	Treatment is surgical and usually successful.
Brain stem glioma	Presents in childhood with cranial nerve palsies, then long-tract signs in limbs; signs of increased ICP occur late in course.	Tumor is inoperable. Treatment with irradiation and shunt for increased ICP.
Cerebellar hemangioblastoma	Presents with disequilibrium, ataxia of trunk or limbs, and signs of increased ICP; at times familial; may be associated with retinal and spinal lesions, polycythemia, and hypernephroma.	Treatment is surgical.
Pineal tumor	Presents with increased ICP, at times associated with impaired upward gaze (Parinaud syndrome) and other deficits indicating midbrain lesion.	Ventricular decompression by shunting, followed by surgical approach to tumor. Irradiation if tumor malignant. Prognosis depends on histopathologic findings and tumor extent
Craniopharyngioma	Originates from remnants of Rathke's pouch above sella turcica, depressing optic chiasm. May present at any age but usually in childhood, with endocrine dysfunction and bitemporal field deficits.	Treatment is surgical, but total removal may not be possible.
Acoustic neuroma	Most common initial symptom is ipsilateral hearing loss; subsequent symptoms may include tinnitus, headache, vertigo, facial weakness or numbness, and long-tract signs. May be familial and bilateral when related to neurofibromatosis. Most sensitive screening tests are MRI and brain stem AEP.	Treatment is by excision by translabyrinthine approach, craniectomy, or combination. Prognosis usually good.
Meningioma	Originates from dura mater or arachnoid; compresses rather than invades adjacent neural structures. Increasingly common with advancing age. Tumor size varies greatly; symptoms vary with tumor site.* Tumor usually benign; readily detected by CT; may lead to calcification and bone erosion visible on plain skull radiographs.	Treatment is surgical. Tumor may recur if removal is incomplete; patient may receive radiation with incomplete excision to decrease risk of recurrence.
Primary central lymphoma	Associated with AIDS and other immunodeficiency states. Presentation may be with focal deficits or disturbances of cognition and consciousness; may be indistinguishable from cerebral toxoplasmosis.	Treatment is by whole-brain irradiation. Chemotherapy may have adjunctive role. Prognosis depends on CD4 cell count at diagnosis.

From Gawlinski A, Hamwi D, editors: *Acute care nurse practitioner: clinical curriculum and certification review,* Philadelphia, 1999, Saunders.
*For example, unilateral exophthalmos (sphenoidal ridge), anosmia and optic nerve compression (olfactory groove).
ICP, Intracranial pressure; *MRI,* magnetic resonance imaging; *AEP,* auditory-evoked potential; *CT,* computed tomography; *AIDS,* acquired immunodeficiency syndrome.

Box **17-13** Common Neurosurgical Terms

Burr hole	Hole made into the cranium using a special drill.
Craniotomy	Surgical opening into skull.
Craniectomy	Removal of portion of skull without replacing it.
Cranioplasty	Plastic repair of skull.
Supratentorial	Above the tentorium, separating cerebrum from cerebellum.
Infratentorial	Below the tentorium; includes brain stem and cerebellum. An infratentorial surgical approach may be used for temporal or occipital lesions.

the least amount of disruption to the intracranial contents. Neural tissue is unforgiving. A significant portion of neurologic trauma and postoperative deficits is related to the surgical pathway through the brain tissue rather than to the procedure performed at the site of pathology. Depending on the location of the lesion and the surgical route chosen, either a transcranial or a transsphenoidal approach is used to open the skull.

Transcranial Approach

In the transcranial approach a scalp incision is made and a series of burr holes drilled into the skull to form an outline of the area to be opened. A special saw is then used to cut between the holes. In most cases the bone flap is left attached to the muscle to create a hinge effect. In some cases the bone flap is removed completely and either placed in the abdomen for later retrieval and implantation or discarded and replaced with synthetic material. Next the dura is opened and retracted. After the intracranial procedure, dura and bone flap are closed, muscles and scalp are sutured, and a turbanlike dressing is applied.[31]

Transsphenoidal Approach

The transsphenoidal approach is the technique of choice for removal of a pituitary tumor without extension into the intracranial vault.[67] This approach involves making a microsurgical entrance into the cranial vault through the nasal cavity. The sphenoid sinus is entered to reach the anterior wall of the sella turcica. The sphenoid bone and the dura are then opened to gain intracranial access. After tumor removal the surgical bed is packed with a small section of adipose tissue grafted from the patient's abdomen or thigh. After closure of the intranasal structures, nasal splints and soft packing or nasal tampons impregnated with antibiotic ointment are placed in the nasal cavities. Occasionally, epistaxis balloons are used instead. A nasal drip pad or mustache-type dressing is placed at the base of the nose to catch surgical drainage.[31]

The patient may be placed in a supine, prone, or even sitting position for a craniotomy procedure. A skull clamp con-

nected to skull pins is used to position and secure the patient's head throughout the surgery. During a transsphenoidal or transcranial approach into the infratentorial area, the patient's head is elevated during the surgery. This position places the patient at risk for an air embolism. Air can enter the vascular system either through the edges of the dura or a venous opening. Continuous Doppler monitoring of the patient's heart sounds allows immediate recognition of this complication. If air embolism occurs, an attempt may be made to withdraw the embolus from the right atrium through a central line. Flooding the surgical field with irrigation fluid and placing a moistened sterile surgical sponge over the surgical site creates an immediate barrier to any further air entrance.

Several other procedures are used intraoperatively during a craniotomy either to facilitate the surgery or to prevent surgical complications. Hypothermia is used to decrease the metabolic needs of the brain. Controlled hypotension lessens blood loss during resection of an AVM or cerebral aneurysm. Hyperventilation is used to reduce the size or bulk of the brain through reduced CBF.[31]

Postoperative Medical Management

Definitive management of the postoperative neurosurgical patient varies depending on the underlying reason for the craniotomy. During the initial postoperative period, management is usually directed toward the prevention of complications. Complications associated with a craniotomy include ICH, surgical hemorrhage, fluid imbalance, CSF leak, deep vein thrombosis, gastric stress ulceration, and pulmonary infection.

Intracranial Hypertension

Postoperative cerebral edema is expected to peak 48 to 72 hours after surgery. If the bone flap is not replaced at surgery, ICH will produce bulging at the surgical site. Close monitoring of the surgical site is important so that integrity of the incision can be maintained. Postcraniotomy management of ICH is usually accomplished through CSF drainage, hyperventilation, patient positioning, and steroid administration.

Surgical Hemorrhage

Surgical hemorrhage after a transcranial procedure can occur in the intracranial vault and is manifested by signs and symptoms of increasing ICP. Hemorrhage after a transsphenoidal craniotomy may be evident from external drainage, patient complaint of persistent postnasal drip, or excessive swallowing. Loss of vision after pituitary surgery is also indicative of evolving hemorrhage.[66] Postoperative hemorrhage requires surgical reexploration.

Fluid Imbalance

Fluid imbalance in the postcraniotomy patient usually results from a disturbance in production or secretion of antidiuretic hormone (ADH). ADH is secreted by the posterior pituitary (neurohypophysis) gland and stimulates the renal tubules and collecting ducts to retain water in response to low circulating blood volume or increased serum osmolality. Intraoperative trauma or postoperative edema of the pituitary gland or hypothalamus can result in insufficient ADH secretion. The outcome is unabated renal water loss even when blood volume is low and serum osmolality is high. This condition is known as *diabetes insipidus* (DI). The polyuria associated with DI is often greater than 200 ml/hour. Urine specific gravity of 1.005 or less and elevated serum osmolality provide evidence of insufficient ADH. The loss of volume may produce hypotension and inadequate cerebral perfusion. DI is usually self-limiting, with fluid replacement the only necessary therapy. In some patients, however, it may be necessary to administer IV vasopressin to control fluid loss.[31,68]

The *syndrome of inappropriate antidiuretic hormone* (SIADH) often occurs with neurologic insult and results from excessive ADH secretion. SIADH is manifested by inappropriate water retention with hyponatremia in the presence of normal renal function. Urine specific gravity is elevated, and urine osmolality is greater than serum osmolality. The dangers associated with SIADH include circulating volume overload and electrolyte imbalance, both of which may impair neurologic functioning. SIADH is usually self-limiting; the mainstay of treatment is fluid restriction.

Cerebrospinal Fluid Leak

Leakage of CSF results from an opening in the subarachnoid space, as evidenced by clear fluid draining from the surgical site. When occurring after transsphenoidal surgery, CSF leak is evidenced by excessive, clear drainage from the nose or persistent postnasal drip. To differentiate CSF drainage from postoperative serous drainage, a specimen is tested for glucose content. A CSF leak is confirmed by glucose values of 30 mg/dl or greater. Management of the patient with a CSF leak includes bed rest and head elevation. LP or placement of a lumbar subarachnoid catheter may be used to reduce CSF pressure until the dura heals. The risk of meningitis associated with CSF leak necessitates surgical repair to reseal the opening if necessary.[66]

Deep Vein Thrombosis

Deep vein thrombosis (DVT) has been reported to occur in 29% to 46% of all neurosurgical patients, compared with a 25% incidence in general surgical patients. Early research demonstrated a greater risk after removal of a supratentorial tumor and a twofold risk in patients whose surgery lasted for more than 4 hours.[67,69] Additional risk factors significantly associated with DVT development include preoperative leg weakness, longer preoperative intensive care unit (ICU) stay, longer recovery room time, longer postoperative ICU stay, more days on bed rest, and delay of postoperative mobility and activity.[70] Clinical manifestations of DVT include leg or calf pain, edema, localized tenderness, and pain with dorsiflexion or plantar flexion (Homans sign). Unfortunately the patient with a DVT is often asymptomatic, and the diagnosis is not made until the patient experiences a pulmonary embolism.

The primary treatment for DVT is prophylaxis. Graduated elastic stockings and sequential pneumatic compression boots or stockings are effective in reducing the incidence of DVT. These devices, alone or in combination, are often used in the care of the neurosurgical patient. Effectiveness is enhanced when these devices are initiated in the preoperative period. Low-dose heparin may also be used prophylactically in high-risk patients. A combination of all three therapies with the addition of postoperative use of an oscillating bed offers maximal DVT prophylaxis that is safe and effective for the neurosurgical patient.

If a DVT develops in the postcraniotomy patient, the physician must weigh the risk of therapeutic heparinization versus the risk of pulmonary embolism (PE). A DVT in the distal circulation below the knee is thought to carry a lower risk of PE than a DVT in the proximal circulation. Even when a PE occurs, the use of therapeutic heparin doses in the neurosurgical patient is controversial, and placement of a vena caval filter may be preferred.[66]

Stress Ulcers

Historically, stress ulcers have been a common complication in neurosurgical patients, especially in those requiring long-term mechanical ventilation. The most effective prophylactic measure for this complication is early enteral feeding. Histamine (H_2) antagonists and proton pump inhibitors are also used.

Pneumonia

The risk of pneumonia in the postoperative craniotomy patient is significantly increased if prolonged mechanical ventilation in the critical care unit is required. Adequate pulmonary hygiene and strict infection control measures are helpful to prevent this complication. Treatment consists of antibiotics and appropriate pulmonary management. Acute respiratory distress syndrome (ARDS) and neurogenic pulmonary edema may also occur in the postcraniotomy patient, possibly related to ICH.

Other complications after craniotomy include focal or generalized seizure activity, which is common and managed prophylactically with anticonvulsant therapy. Postoperative meningitis may result from surgical infection or CSF leak and is treated with antibiotics.[66] Cranial nerve dysfunction may occur either transiently or permanently as a result of surgical manipulation, edema, or anatomic disruption. Compression of the optic chiasm with complete or partial visual loss may result from migration of the adipose tissue packing placed in a pituitary tumor bed and requires surgical reexploration.[71]

Postoperative Nursing Management

The nursing management of the neurosurgical patient incorporates a variety of nursing diagnoses (Box 17-14). As in preoperative care, the primary goal of postcraniotomy nursing management is protection of the integrity of the CNS. **Nursing priorities for the postcraniotomy patient are directed toward (1) preserving adequate cerebral perfusion pressure, (2) promoting arterial oxygenation, (3) providing comfort and emotional support, (4) maintaining surveillance for complications, (5) initiating early rehabilitation, and (6) providing patient education.** Frequent neurologic assessment is necessary to evaluate accomplishment of these objectives and to identify and quickly intervene if complications do arise. Often a ventriculostomy is placed to facilitate ICP monitoring and CSF drainage.

Preserving Adequate Cerebral Perfusion

Nursing interventions to preserve cerebral perfusion include patient positioning, fluid management, and avoidance of postoperative vomiting and fever.

Positioning. Patient positioning is an important component of care for the postcraniotomy patient. The head of the bed should be elevated 30 to 45 degrees at all times to reduce the incidence of hemorrhage, facilitate venous drainage, and control ICP. Other positioning measures to control ICP include maintaining the patient's head in a neutral position at all times and avoiding neck or hip flexion. It is vital to adhere to these rules of positioning throughout all nursing activities, including linen changes and transporting the patient for diagnostic evaluation. Most craniotomy patients can still be turned from side to side within these restrictions, using pillows for support, except in some cases of extensive tumor removal, cranioplasty, and when the bone flap is not replaced. Specific orders from the surgeon must be obtained in these instances. The patient with an infratentorial incision may be restricted to only a very small pillow under the head to prevent strain on the incision. Avoidance of anterior or lateral neck flexion also protects the integrity of this type of incision.

Fluid Management. Fluid management is another important component of postcraniotomy care. Hourly monitoring of fluid intake and output facilitates early identification of fluid imbalance. Urine specific gravity must be measured if DI is suspected. Fluid restriction may be ordered

as a routine measure to lessen the severity of cerebral edema or as treatment for the fluid and electrolyte imbalances associated with SIADH.

Vomiting and Fever. Postoperative vomiting must be avoided to prevent sharp spikes in ICP and possibly surgical hemorrhage. Antiemetics are administered as soon as nausea is apparent. Early nutrition in the neurosurgical patient is beneficial. If the patient is unable to eat, enteral hyperalimentation via feeding tube is the preferred method of nutritional support and can be initiated as early as 24 hours after surgery.[72] Postoperative fever may also adversely affect ICP and increase the metabolic needs of the brain. Acetaminophen is administered orally, rectally, or via feeding tube. External cooling measures, such as a hypothermia blanket, may also be necessary.

Promoting Arterial Oxygenation

Routine pulmonary care is used to maintain airway clearance and prevent pulmonary complications. To prevent dangerous elevations in ICP, this care must be performed using proper technique and at intervals that are adequately spaced from other patient care activities. If pulmonary complications do arise, consideration must be given to maintaining adequate oxygenation during repositioning. It may be necessary to restrict turning to only the side that places the good lung down.

Providing Comfort and Emotional Support

Pain management in the postcraniotomy patient primarily involves control of headache. Small doses of IV morphine are used in the intensive care setting. As soon as oral analgesics can be tolerated, acetaminophen with codeine is used; both these analgesics cause constipation. Administration of stool softeners and initiation of a bowel program are important components of postcraniotomy care. Constipation is hazardous because straining to have a bowel movement can create significant elevations in BP and ICP.

Maintaining Surveillance for Complications

The postoperative neurosurgical patient is at risk for infection, corneal abrasions, and injury from falls or seizures.

Infection. Care of the incision and surgical dressings is specific to the institution and physician. The rule of thumb for a craniotomy dressing is to reinforce it as needed and change it only with a physician's order. Often a drain is left in place to facilitate decompression of the surgical site. If present, a ventriculostomy is treated as a component of the surgical site. All drainage devices must be secured to the dressing to prevent unintentional displacement with patient movement. Sterile technique is required to prevent infection and resultant meningitis.

Corneal Abrasions. Routine eye care may be necessary to prevent corneal drying and ulceration. Periorbital edema interferes with normal blinking and eyelid closure, which are essential to adequate corneal lubrication. Saline drops are instilled every 2 hours. If the patient remains in a coma state, covering the eyes with a polyethylene film extending over the orbits and eyebrows may be beneficial.[10]

Injury. The postcraniotomy patient may also experience periods of altered mentation. Protection from injury may require use of restraint devices. The side rails of the bed must also be padded to protect the patient from injury. Having a family member stay at the bedside or using music therapy is often helpful to keep the patient calm during periods of restlessness. In rare circumstances, neuromuscular blockade and sedation may be necessary to control patient activity and metabolic needs on a short-term basis.

Initiating Early Rehabilitation

Increased patient activity, including ambulation, is begun as soon as tolerated in the postoperative period. Rehabilitation measures and discharge planning may begin in the critical care unit but are beyond the scope of this chapter. Transfer to a general care or rehabilitation unit is usually accomplished as soon as the patient is considered to be stable and without complication.

Providing Patient Education

Preoperatively the patient and family should be taught about the precipitating event necessitating the need for the craniotomy and its expected outcome. The severity of the disease and the need for intensive care management postoperatively must be stressed. As the patient moves toward discharge, teaching focuses on medication instructions, incisional care including the signs of infection, and the signs and symptoms of increased ICP. If the patient has neurologic deficits, teaching focuses on the interventions to maximize the patient's rehabilitation potential, and the patient's family must be encouraged to participate in the patient's care and learn basic rehabilitation techniques. In addition, the importance of participating in a neurologic rehabilitation program must be stressed.

REFERENCES

1. Simon RS, Aminoff MJ, Greenberg DA: *Clinical neurology*, ed 4, Stamford, Conn, 1999, Appleton & Lange.
2. Sosnowski C, Ustik M: Early intervention: coma stimulation in the intensive care unit, *J Neurosci Nurs* 26:336, 1994.
3. Helwick LD: Stimulation programs for coma patients, *Crit Care Nurse* 14(4):47, 1994.
4. King DS: Central nervous system infections: basic concepts, *Nurs Clin North Am* 34:461, 1999.
5. Berger JR: Clinical approach to stupor and coma. In Bradley WG et al, editors: *Neurology in clinical practice*, ed 3, Newton, Mass, 2000, Butterworth-Heinemann.
6. Kofke WA: Neuropathophysiology. In Grenvik A et al, editors: *Textbook of critical care*, ed 4, Philadelpha, 2000, Saunders.
7. Stubgen JP, Plum F: Evaluation of coma. In Grenvik A et al, editors: *Textbook of critical care*, ed 4, Philadelpha, 2000, Saunders.
8. Jorgensen EO, Holm S: Prediction of neurological outcome after cardiopulmonary resuscitation, *Resuscitation* 41:145, 1999.
9. Snyder BD, Daroff RB: Anoxic and ischemic encephalopathies. In Bradley WG et al, editors: *Neurology in clinical practice*, ed 3, Newton, Mass, 2000, Butterworth-Heinemann.
10. Cortese D, Capp L, McKinley S: Moisture chamber versus lubrication for the prevention of corneal epithelial breakdown, *Am J Crit Care* 4:425, 1995.
11. Davis AE, White JJ: Innovative sensory input for the comatose brain-injured patient, *Crit Care Nurs Clin North Am* 7:351, 1995.
12. Jones R et al: Auditory stimulation effect on a comatose survivor of traumatic brain injury, *Arch Phys Med Rehabil* 75:164, 1994.
13. Zieger A: New research and considerations in managing minimally conscious coma patients, *Rehabilitation* 37:167, 1998.
14. Cooper JB et al: Right median nerve electrical stimulation to hasten awakening from coma, *Brain Inj* 13:261, 1999.
15. Duff DL, Wells DL: Postcomatose awareness/vegetative state following severe brain injury: a content methodology, *J Neurosci Nurs* 29:305,1997.
16. Guina FD et al: Sensorimotor stimulation of comatose patients, *Acta Med Croatica* 51:101, 1997.
17. Walker JS, Eakes GG, Siebelink E: The effects of familial voice interventions on comatose head-injured patients, *J Trauma Nurs* 5(2):41, 1998.
18. Schinner KM et al: Effects of auditory stimuli on intracranial pressure and cerebral perfusion pressure in traumatic brain injury, *J Neurosci Nurs* 27:348, 1995.
19. Kelley-Hayes M et al: The American Heart Association stroke outcome classification: executive summary, *Circulation* 97:2472, 1998.
20. Brown RD et al: A population-based study of first-ever and total stroke incidence rates in Rochester, Minnesota: 1990-1994, *Stroke* 31:279A, 2000.
21. American Heart Association: *Statistical supplement*, Dallas, 1996, The Association.
22. Chung C-S, Caplan LR: Neurovascular disorders. In Goetz CG, Pappert EJ, editors: *Textbook of clinical neurology*, Philadelphia, 1999, Saunders.
23. Sacco RL: Newer risk factors for stroke, *Neurology* 57:S31, 2001.
24. Hufnagel A et al: Stroke following chiropractic manipulation of the cervical spine, *J Neurol* 246:683, 1999.
25. Petty GW et al: Rates and predictors of cerebrovascular events among patients with valvular heart disease: a population-based study, *Stroke* 31:279A, 2000.
26. D'avila-Rom'an VG et al: Atherosclerosis of the ascending aorta is an independent predictor of long-term neurologic events and mortality, *J Am Coll Cardiol* 33:1308, 1999.
27. Rost NS et al: Plasma concentration of C-reactive protein and risk of ischemic stroke: the Framingham Study, *Stroke* 31:279A, 2000.
28. Grau AJ et al: Periodontitis as a risk factor for cerebral ischemia, *Stroke* 31:317A, 2000.
29. Hock NH: Brain attack: the stroke continuum, *Nurs Clin North Am* 34:689,1999.
30. Samples SD, Krieger DW: Acute ischemic stroke, *Curr Opin Crit Care* 6:77, 2000.
31. Barker E: *Neuroscience nursing*, ed 2, St Louis, 2002, Mosby.
32. Silverman IE, Restrepo L, Mathews G: Poststroke seizures, *Arch Neurol* 59:195, 2002.
33. Wityk RJ, Beauchamp NJ: Diagnostic evaluation of stroke *Neurol Clin* 18:357, 2000.
34. Becker K: Intensive care unit management of the stroke patient, *Neurol Clin* 18:439, 2000.
35. Adams JP et al: Guidelines for thrombolytic therapy for acute stroke: a supplement to the guidelines for the management of patients with acute ischemic stroke, *Circulation* 94:1167, 1996.
36. Lewandowski C, Barsan W: Treatment of acute ischemic stroke, *Ann Emerg Med* 37:202, 2001.
37. Schellinger PD et al: Thrombolytic therapy for ischemic stroke: a review. Part 1. Intravenous thrombolysis, *Crit Care Med* 29:1812, 2001.
38. Adams HP: Emergent use of anticoagulation for treatment of patients with ischemic stroke, *Stroke* 33:856, 2002.

39. Hanson SK et al: Should use of tPA for ischemic stroke be restricted to specialized stroke centers? *Stroke* 31:313A, 2000.

40. Mohr JP: Thrombolytic therapy for ischemic stroke: from clinical trials to clinical practice, *JAMA* 283:1189, 2000.

41. Adams HP et al: Guidelines for the management of patients with acute ischemic stroke: a statement for healthcare professionals from a special writing group of the Stroke Council, American Heart Association, *Circulation* 90:1588, 1994.

42. Hickenbottom SL, Barson WG: Acute ischemic stroke therapy, *Neurol Clin* 18:379, 2000.

43. Mayberg MR et al: Guidelines for the management of aneurysmal subarachnoid hemorrhage: a statement for healthcare professionals from a special writing group of the Stroke Council, American Heart Association, *Circulation* 25:2315, 1994.

44. Shpritz DW: Neurodiagnostic studies, *Nurs Clin North Am* 34:593, 1999.

45. Hunt WE, Hess RM: Surgical risks as related to time of intervention in the repair of intracranial aneurysms, *J Neurosurg* 28:14, 1968.

46. Solenski NJ et al: Medical complications of aneurysmal subarachnoid hemorrhage: a report of the multicenter, cooperative aneurysm study, *Crit Care Med* 23:1007, 1995.

47. Gruber A, Reinprecht IUM: Extracerebral organ dysfunction and neurologic outcome after aneurysmal subarachnoid hemorrhage, *Crit Care Med* 27:505, 1999.

48. Rusy KL: Rebleeding and vasospasm after subarachnoid hemorrhage: a critical care challenge, *Crit Care Nurse* 16(1):41, 1996.

49. Treggiari-Venzi MM, Suter PM, Romand JA: Review of medical prevention of vasospasm after aneurysmal subarachnoid hemorrhage: a problem of neurointensive care, *Neurosurgery* 48:249, 2001.

50. Finfer SR, Ferch R, Morgan MK: Barbiturate coma for severe, refractory vasospasm following subarachnoid hemorrhage, *Intensive Care Med* 25:406, 1999.

51. Thomas JE, Rosenwasser RH: Reversal of severe cerebral vasospasm in three patients after aneurysmal subarachnoid hemorrhage: initial observations regarding the use of intraventricular sodium nitroprusside in humans, *Neurosurgery* 44:48, 1999.

52. Gebel JM, Broderick JP: Intracerebral hemorrhage, *Neurol Clin* 18:419, 2000.

53. Broderick JP et al: Guidelines for the management of spontaneous intracerebral hemorrhage, *Stroke* 30:905, 1999.

54. Shields RW, Wilbourn AJ: Demyelinating disorders of the peripheral nervous system. In Goetz CG, Pappert EJ, editors: *Textbook of clinical neurology*, Philadelphia, 1999, Saunders.

55. Ang CW et al: Rapidly progressive, predominantly motor Guillain-Barré syndrome with antiGa1Nac-GD1a antibodies, *Neurology* 53:2122, 1999.

56. Ho T, Griffin J: Guillain-Barré syndrome, *Curr Opin Neurol* 12:389, 1999.

57. Toyka KV: Eighty three years of the Guillain-Barré syndrome: clinical and immunopathologic aspects, current and future treatments, *Rev Neurol (Paris)* 155:849, 1999.

58. Lindenbaum Y, Kissel JT, Mendell JR: Treatment approaches for Guillain-Barré syndrome and chronic inflammatory demyelinating polyradiculoneuropathy, *Neurol Clin* 19:187, 2001.

59. Keenlyside R, Brezman D: Fatal Guillain-Barré syndrome after the national influenza immunization program, *Neurology* 30:929, 1980.

60. D'Alessandro R, Casmiro M, Guarino M: Risk factors for Guillain-Barré syndrome: a population-based case-control study, *J Neurol* 246:1004, 1999.

61. French Cooperative Group on Plasma Exchange: Plasma exchange in Guillain-Barré syndrome: one year follow-up, *Ann Neurol* 32:94, 1992.

62. Nagpal S, Benstead T, Shumak K: Treatment of Guillain-Barré syndrome: a cost-effectiveness analysis, *J Clin Apheresis* 14(3):107, 1999.

63. Hughes RAC, van der Meche FGA: Corticosteroid treatment for Guillain-Barré syndrome, *Cochrane Syst Database Rev* 3, 1999 (online: update software).

64. Kihara M et al: A dysautonomia case of Guillain-Barré syndrome with recovery: monitored by composite autonomic scoring scale, *J Auton Nerv Syst* 73:186, 1998.

65. Pfeiffer G et al: Indicators of dysautonomia in severe Guillain-Barré syndrome, *J Neurol* 246:1015, 1999.

66. Couldwell WT, Simard MR, Weiss MH: Pituitary tumors. In Grossman RG, Loftus CM: *Principles of neurosurgery*, ed 3, Philadelphia, 1999, Lippincott-Raven.

67. Constantini S et al: Thromboembolic phenomena in neurosurgical patients operated upon for primary and metastatic brain tumors, *Acta Neurochir* 109:93, 1991.

68. Nickolaus MJ: Diabetes insipidus: a current perspective, *Crit Care Nurse* 19(6):18, 1999.

69. Valladeres JB, Hankinson J: Incidence of lower extremity deep vein thrombosis in neurosurgical patients, *Neurosurgery* 6:138, 1980.

70. Warbel A, Lewicki L, Lupica K: Venous thromboembolism: risk factors in the craniotomy patient population, *J Neurosci Nurs* 31:180, 1999.

71. McEwen DR: Transsphenoidal adenomectomy, *AORN J* 61:321, 1995.

72. Andrews BT: General management and intensive care of the neurosurgical patient. In Grossman RG, Loftus CM: *Principles of neurosurgery*, ed 3, Philadelphia, 1999, Lippincott-Raven.

KATHLEEN A. MENDEZ

18

Neurologic Therapeutic Management

Objectives

- Discuss the concept of cerebral autoregulation.
- Calculate cerebral perfusion pressure.
- Describe therapies typically used to treat intracranial hypertension.
- Identify the different types of intracranial pressure monitoring devices.
- List the four supratentorial herniation syndromes.

Despite the diversity of neurologic abnormalities, one aspect of the critical care management of patients with neurologic disorders is common to a wide variety of these pathologic conditions. This chapter focuses on the priority interventions used to manage the critically ill patient with intracranial hypertension.

ASSESSMENT OF INTRACRANIAL PRESSURE

Monro-Kellie Hypothesis

The intracranial space comprises three components: brain substance (80%), cerebrospinal fluid (CSF, 10%), and blood (10%). Under normal physiologic conditions, intracranial pressure (ICP) is maintained below 15 mm Hg mean pressure.[1] Essential to understanding the pathophysiology of ICP, the Monro-Kellie hypothesis proposes that an increase in volume of one intracranial component must be compensated by a decrease in one or more of the other components so that total volume remains fixed. This compensation, although limited, includes displacing CSF from the intracranial vault to the lumbar cistern, increasing CSF absorption, and compressing the low-pressure venous system[2] (Table 18-1).

Volume-Pressure Curve

When capable of compliance, the brain can tolerate significant increases in intracranial volume without much increase in ICP. The amount of intracranial compliance, however, does have a limit. Once this limit has been reached, a state of decompensation with increased ICP results. As the ICP rises, the relationship between volume and pressure changes, and small increases in volume may cause major elevations in ICP (Figure 18-1). The exact configuration of the volume-pressure curve and the point at which the steep rise in pressure occurs vary among patients. The configuration of this curve also is influenced by the cause and the rate of volume increases within the intracranial vault; for example, neurologic deterioration occurs more rapidly in a patient with an acute epidural hematoma than in a patient with a meningioma of the same size.[3]

Monitoring these changes in intracranial dynamics and continuous clinical assessment of the patient's neurologic status have proved beneficial in diagnosing and treating sustained rises in ICP. Such elevations of ICP often precede evidence of neurologic deterioration obtained through the clinical assessment.

Cerebral Blood Flow and Autoregulation

Cerebral blood flow (CBF) corresponds to the metabolic demands of the brain and is normally 50 ml/100 g of brain tissue/min. Although the brain makes up only 2% of body weight, it requires 15% to 20% of the resting cardiac output (CO) and 15% of the body's oxygen demands. The normal

Table 18-1	Mechanisms of Intracranial Pressure (ICP) Elevation

Pathophysiology	Example	Treatment
DISORDERS OF CEREBROSPINAL FLUID (CSF) SPACE		
Overproduction of CSF	Choroid plexus papilloma	Diuretics, surgical removal
Communicating hydrocephalus from obstructed arachnoid	Previous subarachnoid hemorrhage	Surgical drainage from lumbar intrathecal site
Noncommunicative hydrocephalus	Posterior fossa tumor obstructing aqueduct	Surgical drainage by ventricular drainage
Interstitial edema	Any of above	Surgical drainage of CSF
DISORDERS OF INTRACRANIAL BLOOD		
ICH causing increased ICP	Epidural hematoma	Surgical drainage
Vasospasm	Subarachnoid hemorrhage	Hypervolemia and hypertensive therapy Calcium channel antagonists
Vasodilation	Elevated $Paco_2$	Hyperventilation
Increasing cerebral blood volume and ICP	Hypoxia	Adequate oxygenation
DISORDERS OF BRAIN SUBSTANCE		
Expanding mass lesion with local vasogenic edema causing increased ICP	Brain tumor	Steroids Surgical removal
Ischemic brain injury with cytotoxic edema increasing ICP	Anoxic brain injury from cardiac or respiratory arrest	Resistant to therapy
Increased cerebral metabolic rate increasing cerebral blood flow and ICP	Seizures, hyperthermia	Anticonvulsant medications, especially barbiturates; control fever

Modified from Helfaer MA, Kirsch JR: *Crit Care Rep* 1:12, 1989.
ICH, Intracranial hypertension; *Paco2,* arterial carbon dioxide tension (partial pressure).

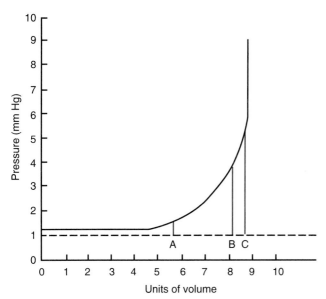

Figure 18-1   Intracranial volume-pressure curve. *A,* Pressure is normal, and increases in intracranial volume are tolerated without increases in intracranial pressure. *B,* Increases in volume may cause increases in pressure. *C,* Small increases in volume may cause larger increases in pressure.

brain has a complex capacity to maintain constant CBF, despite wide ranges in systemic arterial pressure, an effect known as *autoregulation.* Mean arterial pressure (MAP) of 50 to 150 mm Hg does not alter CBF when autoregulation is present. Outside the limits of this autoregulation, CBF becomes passively dependent on the perfusion pressure.[4]

Factors other than arterial blood pressure that affect CBF are conditions that result in acidosis, alkalosis, and changes in metabolic rate. Conditions that cause acidosis (e.g., hypoxia, hypercapnia, ischemia) result in cerebrovascular dilation. Conditions causing alkalosis (e.g., hypocapnia) result in cerebrovascular constriction. Normally, a reduction in metabolic rate (e.g., from hypothermia or barbiturates) decreases CBF, and increases in metabolic rate (e.g., from hyperthermia) increase CBF.[5]

Arterial blood gases (ABGs) exert a profound effect on CBF. Carbon dioxide (CO_2), which affects the pH of the blood, is a potent vasoactive substance. CO_2 retention (*hypercapnia*) leads to cerebral vasodilation, with increased cerebral blood volume, whereas *hypocapnia* leads to cerebral vasoconstriction and a reduction in cerebral blood volume. Prolonged hypocapnia, however, especially at an arterial partial pressure of carbon dioxide ($PaCO_2$) level less than 20 mm Hg, can produce cerebral ischemia. Low arterial partial pressure of oxygen (PaO_2) levels, especially below 40 mm Hg, lead to cerebral vasodilation, which increases the intracranial blood volume and can contribute to increased ICP. High PaO_2 levels have not been shown to affect CBF in either direction.[4]

Metabolic activity in the brain significantly influences CBF. Normally, when cerebral metabolic activity increases, CBF also increases to meet the demand. Any pathologic process that decreases CBF could lead to a mismatch between metabolic demand and blood supply, resulting in cerebral ischemia.[5]

Cerebral Perfusion Pressure

Measuring CBF in the clinical setting is difficult. Cerebral perfusion pressure (CPP), an estimated pressure, is the blood pressure gradient across the brain and is calculated as the difference between the incoming MAP and the opposing ICP on the arteries:

$$CPP = MAP - ICP$$

The CPP in the average adult is approximately 80 to 100 mm Hg, with a range of 60 to 150 mm Hg. The CPP must be maintained near 80 mm Hg to provide adequate blood supply to the brain. If the CPP drops below this point, ischemia may develop. A sustained CPP of 30 mm Hg or less usually results in neuronal hypoxia and cell death. When systemic MAP equals ICP, CBF may cease.[3]

Assessment Techniques
Signs and Symptoms

The numerous signs and symptoms of increased ICP include decreased level of consciousness (LOC), Cushing's triad (bradycardia, systolic hypertension, bradypnea), diminished brain stem reflexes, papilledema, decerebrate posturing (abnormal extension) and decorticate posturing (abnormal flexion), unequal pupil size, projectile vomiting, decreased pupillary reaction to light, altered breathing patterns, and headache.[6] Patients may exhibit one or all of these symptoms, depending on the underlying cause of the elevation in ICP. **One of the earliest and most important signs of increased ICP is a decrease in level of consciousness. This change must be reported immediately to the physician.**

Monitoring Sites

The four sites for monitoring ICP are the intraventricular space, subarachnoid space, epidural space, and parenchyma (Figure 18-2). Each site has advantages and disadvantages for monitoring ICP (Table 18-2). The type of monitor chosen depends on both the suspected pathologic condition and physician's preferences.[7,8]

Intraventricular Space. ICP monitoring is accomplished by placing a small catheter into the ventricular system; this procedure is known as a *ventriculostomy.* The catheter is inserted through a burr hole with the patient under local anesthesia and usually is placed in the anterior horn of the lateral ventricle. If possible, the side chosen for placement of the ventriculostomy is the nondominant hemisphere.

Subarachnoid Space. ICP monitoring is accomplished by placing a small, hollow bolt or screw into the subarach-

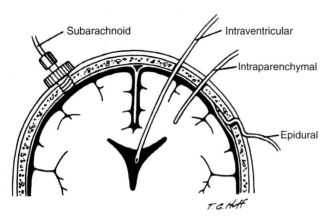

Figure 18-2 Intracranial pressure monitoring sites. (From Lee KR, Hoff JT: *Youman's neurological surgery*, ed 4, Philadelphia, 1996, Saunders.)

noid space. It is inserted though a burr hole, usually located in the front of the skull behind the hairline, with the patient under local anesthesia. Inserting this device is easier than inserting the ventriculostomy catheter.

Epidural Space. ICP monitoring is accomplished by placing a small fiberoptic sensor into the epidural space. It is also inserted through a burr hole while the patient is under local anesthesia. The physician strips the dura away from the inner table of the skull before inserting the epidural monitor.

Parenchyma. ICP monitoring is accomplished by placing a small fiberoptic catheter into the parenchymal tissue. After placing a subarachnoid bolt (as just described), a hole is punched in the dura and the catheter is inserted approximately 1 cm into the brain's white matter.

Intracranial Pressure Waves

The ICP pulse waveform is observed on a continuous, real-time pressure display and corresponds to each heartbeat. The waveform arises primarily from pulsations of the major intracranial arteries, receiving retrograde venous pulsations as well.[3]

Normal ICP Waveform. The normal ICP wave has three or more defined peaks (Figure 18-3). The first peak, or P_1, is called the *percussion wave*. Originating from the pulsations of the choroid plexus, P_1 has a sharp peak and is fairly consistent in its amplitude. The second peak, or P_2, is called the *tidal wave*. The tidal wave is more variable in shape and amplitude, ending on the dicrotic notch. The P_2 portion of the pulse waveform has been most directly linked to the state of decreased compliance. When the P_2 component is equal to or higher than P_1, decreased compliance occurs. Immediately after the dicrotic notch is the third wave, or P_3, called the *dicrotic wave*. After the dicrotic wave, the pressure usually tapers down to the diastolic position, unless retrograde venous pulsations add a few more peaks.[9,10]

A, B, and C pressure waves are not true waveforms (Figure 18-4). Rather, they are the graphically displayed trend data of ICP over time. These waves reflect spontaneous alterations in ICP associated with respiration, systemic blood pressure, and deteriorating neurologic status.[11]

A Waves. Also called *plateau waves* because of their distinctive shape, A waves are the most clinically significant of the three types. A waves usually occur in an already-elevated baseline ICP (greater than 20 mm Hg) and are characterized by sharp increases in ICP of 30 to 69 mm Hg, which plateau for 2 to 20 minutes and then return to baseline. The actual cause of A waves is unknown, but they may result from vasodilation and increased CBF, decreased venous outflow (and therefore increased cerebral blood volume), fluctuations in $PaCO_2$ (and therefore changes in cerebral blood volume), or decreased CSF absorption. B waves often precede A waves. Plateau waves are considered significant because of the reduced CPP associated with ICP in the 50 to 100 mm Hg range. Transient signs of intracranial hypertension, such as a decreased LOC, bradycardia, pupillary changes, or respiratory changes, may accompany these waves. Some research suggests that prolonged increases in ICP associated with plateau waves could result in transient as well as permanent cell damage from ischemia.

B Waves. B waves are sharp, rhythmic oscillations with a sawtooth appearance that occur every 30 seconds to 2 minutes and can raise the ICP from 5 to 70 mm Hg. B waves are a normal physiologic phenomenon that can occur in any patient, but they are amplified in states of low intracranial compliance. B waves appear to reflect fluctuations in cerebral blood volume. Decompensation of normal intracranial volume compensatory capacity is indicated by B waves with high amplitude (greater than 15 mm Hg pressure change from peak to trough of wave).

C Waves. C waves are smaller, rhythmic waves that occur every 4 to 8 minutes and at normal levels of ICP. C waves are related to normal fluctuations in respiration and systemic MAP. C waves are considered clinically insignificant.

MANAGEMENT OF INTRACRANIAL HYPERTENSION

Once intracranial hypertension (ICH) is documented, therapy must be prompt to prevent secondary insults. Although the exact pressure level denoting ICH remains uncertain, most current evidence suggests that ICP generally must be treated when it exceeds 20 mm Hg. All therapies are directed toward reducing the volume of one or more of the components (blood, brain, CSF) that lie within the intracranial vault. A major goal of therapy is to determine the cause of the elevated pressure and, if possible, to remove the cause.[2] In the absence of a surgically treatable mass lesion, ICH is treated medically. Nurses play an important role in rapid assessment and implementation of appropriate therapies for reducing ICP (Box 18-1).

Positioning and Other Nursing Activities

Positioning of the patient is a significant factor in the prevention and treatment of ICH. Head elevation has long

Table 18-2 Intracranial Pressure (ICP) Measuring Devices

Device	Location	Accuracy	Comments
Intraventricular catheter Fiberoptic transducer	Lateral ventricle of nondominant hemisphere	Excellent	May be difficult to insert, especially if ventricles are small or displaced. Therapeutic/diagnostic removal of cerebrospinal fluid (CSF) possible. Provides access for determination of volume-pressure relationship. May permit CSF leakage, but rapid CSF drainage may result in collapsed ventricle or subdural hematoma. May cause intracerebral bleeding or edema at cannula track. Infection rate 2%-5%. Fluid-filled system used if intraventricular catheter is placed.
Subarachnoid bolt	Subarachnoid space	Fair; unreliable at high ICP	Inexpensive, easy to insert; especially useful if ventricles are small. Does not penetrate brain; requires intact skull. Bolt can become occluded with clots or tissue; may require irrigation. Needs to be recalibrated frequently. CSF drainage not possible. Infection rate 1%-2%. Fluid-filled system used.
Epidural sensor or transducer	Between skull and dura	Variable	Easy to insert; least invasive (does not penetrate dura or brain). CSF drainage not possible. Infection rate less than 1%. Head position has no effect on pressure reading. Cannot be rezeroed once in place. Epidural pressure is slightly higher than intraventricular pressure.
Intraparenchymal transducer	1 cm into brain tissue	Excellent	Easy to insert. Unable to drain CSF or to test volume-pressure response (VPR). Catheter relatively fragile; avoid sharp kinks or pulls. Head position has no effect on pressure reading. Cannot be rezeroed once in place. Risk of intracerebral bleeding and infection.

From Dennison R: *Pass CCRN!*, ed 2, St Louis, 2000, Mosby.

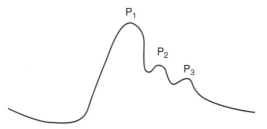

Figure 18-3 Components of normal intracranial pressure waveform. (From Barker E, editor: *Neuroscience nursing*, St Louis, 1994, Mosby.)

been advocated as a conventional nursing intervention to control ICP, presumably by increasing venous return. One recent study found that elevation of the bed at least 30 degrees did result in improvement in both ICP and CPP.[12] Although elevating the head of the bed does decrease ICP, this could, however, also decrease MAP and thus have an overall negative effect on CPP. Therefore the recent trend is to individualize the head position to maximize CPP and minimize ICP measurements.[13]

Positions that impede venous return from the brain cause elevations in ICP. Obstruction of jugular veins or an increase in intrathoracic or intraabdominal pressure is communicated as increased pressure throughout the open venous system, thereby impeding drainage from the brain and increasing ICP. Positions that decrease venous return from the head (e.g., Trendelenburg, prone, extreme flexion of hips, angulation of neck) must be avoided if possible. If changes to positions such as Trendelenburg are necessary to provide adequate pulmonary care, critical care nurses must closely monitor ICP and vital signs.[3]

Some routine nursing activities do affect ICP and can be harmful. Use of positive end-expiratory pressure (PEEP) greater than 20 cm H_2O pressure, coughing, suctioning, tight tracheostomy tube ties, and Valsalva maneuver have been associated with ICP increases. Cumulative increases in ICP have been reported when care activities are performed one after another. Conversely, family contact and gentle touch have been associated with decreases in ICP.[3,13,14]

Hyperventilation

Controlled hyperventilation has been an important adjunct of therapy for the patient with increased ICP. The rationale employed in hyperventilation is that if the $PaCO_2$ can be reduced from its normal level of 35 to 40 mm Hg to a range of 25 to 30 mm Hg in the patient with ICH, vasoconstriction of cerebral arteries, reduced CBF, and increased venous return will result. This practice is currently being reexamined. Increasing research indicates that severe or prolonged hyperventilation can actually reduce cerebral perfusion and lead to cerebral ischemia and infarction. Rather, the trend now is to maintain $PaCO_2$ levels on the lower side of normal (35 ±2 mm Hg) by carefully monitoring ABG measurements and by adjusting ventilator settings.[2,15,16]

Although hypoxemia must be avoided, excessively high levels of oxygen offer no benefit. In fact, increasing inspired oxygen concentrations above 60% may lead to toxic changes in lung tissue. The use of pulse oximetry has led to greater awareness of the circumstances, such as pain and anxiety, that can cause oxygen desaturation and therefore elevate ICP.[17]

Temperature Control

Directly proportional to body temperature, cerebral metabolic rate (CMR) increases 7% per degree centigrade of increase in body temperature.[16] This fact is significant because as the CMR increases, blood flow to the brain must increase to meet the tissue demands. To avoid the increase in blood volume associated with increased CMR, nurses must prevent hyperthermia in the patient with a brain injury. Antipyretics and cooling devices must be used when appropriate while the source of the fever is being determined.[15,16]

Conversely, hypothermia reduces CMR. Research done in patients with severe head injury who were unresponsive to barbiturate therapy for control of intractable ICH demonstrated a significant decrease in ICP when subjected to mild hypothermia between 32° and 35° C.[16]

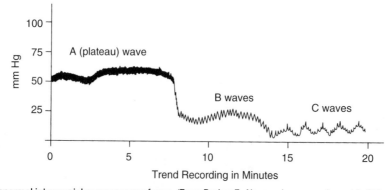

Figure 18-4 Abnormal intracranial pressure waveforms. (From Barker E: *Neuroscience nursing*, ed 2, St Louis, 2002, Mosby.)

Intracranial Hypertension

1. Position patient to achieve maximal intracranial pressure (ICP) reduction.
2. Reduce environmental stimulation.
3. Maintain normothermia.
4. Control ventilation to ensure a normal $Paco_2$ level (35 ±2 mm Hg).
5. Administer diuretic agents, anticonvulsants, sedation, analgesia, paralytic agents, and vasoactive medications to ensure central perfusion pressure (CPP) greater than 70 mm Hg.
6. Drain cerebrospinal fluid for ICP greater than 20 mm Hg.

$Paco_2$, Arterial carbon dioxide tension (partial pressure).

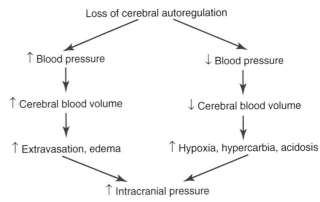

Figure 18-5   Loss of pressure autoregulation.

Blood Pressure Control

Maintenance of arterial blood pressure (BP) in the high-normal range is essential in the brain-injured patient. Inadequate perfusion pressure decreases the supply of nutrients and oxygen requirements for cerebral metabolic needs. On the other hand, too high BP increases cerebral blood volume and may increase ICP[16] (Figure 18-5).

Control of systemic hypertension may require nothing more than the administration of a sedative agent. Small, frequent doses may be sufficient to blunt noxious stimuli and prevent them from triggering rises in BP. When sedation proves inadequate in controlling systemic arterial hypertension, antihypertensive agents are used. Care must be taken in choosing these agents because many of the peripheral vasodilators (e.g., nitroprusside, nitroglycerin) also are cerebral vasodilators. However, all antihypertensives are believed to cause some degree of cerebral vasodilation. To reduce this vasodilating effect, co-treatment with β-blockers (e.g., metoprolol, labetalol) may be beneficial.[3]

Systemic hypotension should be treated aggressively with fluids to maintain a systolic BP greater than 90 mm Hg.[3] Crystalloids, colloids, and blood products can be used depending on the patient's condition.[14] Recent studies have demonstrated a positive effect on ICP and CPP with hypertonic saline.[18] If fluids fail to elevate the patient's BP adequately, inotropic agents may be necessary.[16]

Seizure Control

The incidence of posttraumatic seizures in the head-injured population has been estimated at 5%. Because of the risk of a secondary ischemic insult associated with seizures, many physicians prescribe anticonvulsant medications prophylactically. Seizures cause metabolic requirements to increase, which results in elevated CBF, cerebral blood volume, and ICP, even in paralyzed patients. If blood flow cannot match demand, ischemia develops, cerebral energy stores are depleted, and irreversible neuronal destruction occurs. The usual anticonvulsant regimen for seizure control includes phenytoin or phenobarbital, or both, in therapeutic doses.[17] Fast-acting short-duration agents such as lorazepam may be indicated for breakthrough seizures until therapeutic drug levels can be achieved.

Lidocaine

Various forms of sensory stimulation (e.g., tracheal intubation, endotracheal suctioning) may provoke marked increases in ICP and MAP. One therapy used to prevent cerebral ischemia and acute ICH has been administration of lidocaine through the endotracheal tube or through intravenous infusion before nasotracheal suctioning. Lidocaine is believed to be effective in blunting ICP spikes secondary to tracheal stimulation. Peak lidocaine concentrations are linearly related to the administered dose, and the rate of absorption depends on the vascularity of the site of administration.[19] Lidocaine is initially distributed to the lungs, then to the heart and kidneys, and then to muscle and adipose tissue.

Prophylactic administration of lidocaine before endotracheal suctioning is widely practiced. Lidocaine protects the patient from the associated increases in ICP that occur with suctioning. To prevent hypoxemia, suctioning should be limited to only if necessary. Suctioning should be preceded with hyperventilation using 100% oxygen, followed by a 10-second pass and limited to no more than two passes.[20]

Cerebrospinal Fluid Drainage

CSF drainage for ICH may be used with other treatment modalities. CSF drainage is accomplished by the insertion of a pliable catheter into the anterior horn of the lateral ventricle (ventriculostomy), preferably on the nondominant side. Such drainage can help support the patient through periods of cerebral edema by controlling spikes in ICP. One of the major advantages of the ventriculostomy is its dual role as both a monitoring device and a treatment modality. Because CSF provides a favorable medium for the development of infection, flawless aseptic technique must be followed during insertion and maintenance of the system. The ventricular system is connected to a drainage bag and is then maintained as a closed system for the period the ventriculostomy remains in place, usually 3 to 5 days[21] (Figures 18-6 and 18-7).

Diuretics
Osmotic Agents

Clinicians have known for decades that osmotic agents effectively reduce ICP. The mechanism by which these diuretics reduce ICP continues to be a subject of investigational interest. One theory is that these agents act by remaining relatively impermeable to the blood-brain barrier (BBB), thereby drawing water from normal brain tissue to plasma. The direction of flow is from the hypoconcentrated tissue to the hyperconcentrated cerebral vasculature. If the situation becomes reversed and the tissue becomes hyperconcentrated in relation to the cerebral vasculature, a rebound phenomenon could occur. Osmotic agents have little direct effect on edematous cerebral tissue situated in an area of a defective BBB; instead, these agents require an intact BBB for osmosis to occur.[2,22]

The most widely used osmotic diuretic is *mannitol*, a large molecule that is retained almost entirely in the extracellular compartment and has little to no rebound effect noted with other osmotic diuretics. Mannitol may improve perfusion to ischemic areas of the brain, producing cerebral vasoconstriction and resulting in a reduction of ICP.[2,22]

Perhaps the most common difficulty associated with the use of osmotic agents is the production of electrolyte disturbances. Careful attention must be paid to body weight and fluid and electrolyte stability. Serum osmolality must be kept between 300 and 320 mOsm/L. Hypernatremia and hypokalemia often are associated with repeated administration of osmotic agents. Central venous pressure readings must be monitored to prevent hypovolemia. Smaller doses of mannitol simplify fluid and electrolyte management, and their use is encouraged whenever possible.[17,22]

Nonosmotic Agents

Loop diuretics have also been used to decrease ICP. *Furosemide*, one such nonosmotic diuretic, may act differently from osmotic agents by pulling sodium and water from edematous areas and perhaps by decreasing CSF production. One advantage of furosemide administration over the use of osmotic diuretics is that its effect is not generally associated with increases in serum osmolality. Therefore electrolyte imbalances may not be as severe with the use of nonosmotic diuretics.[17]

Volume Maintenance

Administration of osmotic and loop diuretics can contribute to dehydration, thus precipitating a decrease in CPP. Optimally the patient should be maintained in a euvolemic state to optimize cerebral perfusion. Volume replacement strategies include fluid boluses, fluid replacements, and albumin administration. Intravenous (IV) fluids administered are typically isotonic and low in glucose to prevent

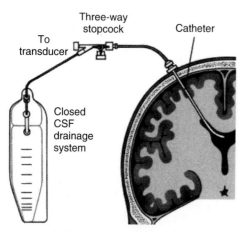

INTRAVENTRICULAR CATHETER

Figure 18-6 Intermittent drainage system. Intermittent drainage involves draining cerebrospinal fluid (*CSF*) via ventriculostomy when intracranial pressure (ICP) exceeds the upper pressure parameter set by physician. Intermittent drainage involves opening three-way stopcock to allow CSF to flow into drainage bag for brief periods (30 to 120 seconds) until ICP is below the upper pressure parameter. (From Barker E: *Neuroscience nursing*, ed 2, St Louis, 2002, Mosby.)

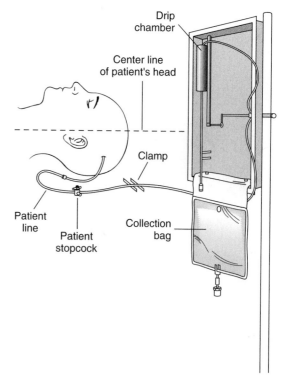

Figure 18-7 Continuous drainage system. Continuous drainage involves placing drip chamber of drainage system at a specified level above foramen of Monro (usually 15 cm). System is left open to allow continuous drainage of cerebrospinal fluid into the chamber (which drains into a collection bag) against a pressure gradient that prevents excessive drainage and ventricular collapse. (Courtesy Codman/Johnson & Johnson Professional, Raynham, Mass.)

gradient shifts across the BBB in the traumatically brain-injured patient.[14]

Control of Metabolic Demand

Any treatment modality that increases the incidence of noxious stimulation to the patient carries the potential for increasing ICP. Such noxious stimuli include pain, the presence of an endotracheal tube, coughing, suctioning, repositioning, bathing, and many other routine nursing interventions. Agents used to reduce metabolic demands include benzodiazepines (e.g., midazolam, lorazepam), IV sedative-hypnotics (e.g., propofol), opioid narcotics (e.g., fentanyl, morphine), and neuromuscular blocking agents (NMBAs; e.g., vecuronium, atracurium). These agents may be administered separately or in combination, via continuous drip or as an IV bolus, on an as-needed basis.

The preferred treatment regimen begins with the administration of benzodiazepines for sedation and narcotics for analgesia. If these agents fail to blunt the patient's response to noxious stimuli, propofol and/or an NMBA is added. The use of these medications is recommended only in patients who have an ICP monitor in place, because sedatives, narcotics, and NMBAs affect the reliability of neurologic assessment. NMBA use without sedation is not recommended; NMBAs cause skeletal muscle paralysis and have no analgesic effect, and they do not protect the patient from pain and the physiologic responses that can occur from pain-producing procedures.[14,17] If these agents fail to control the patient's ICP, barbiturate therapy is considered.

Barbiturate Therapy

Barbiturate therapy is a treatment protocol developed for the management of the patient with uncontrolled ICH who has not responded to the conventional treatments previously described.[2] The two most frequently used drugs in high-dose barbiturate therapy are *pentobarbital* and *thiopental*. The goal with either of these drugs is a reduction of ICP to 15 to 20 mm Hg while a MAP of 70 to 80 mm Hg is maintained. Patients are maintained on high-dose barbiturate therapy until ICP has been controlled within the normal range for 24 hours. Barbiturates must never be stopped abruptly but are tapered slowly over approximately 4 days.[3]

Complications of high-dose barbiturate therapy can be disastrous unless a specific and organized approach is used. The most common complications are hypotension, hypothermia, and myocardial depression. If allowed to persist unchecked, complications may cause secondary insults to an already damaged brain. *Hypotension*, the most common complication, results from peripheral vasodilation and can be compounded in an already dehydrated patient who has received large doses of an osmotic diuretic in an attempt to control ICP. Careful monitoring of fluid status by central venous pressure or a pulmonary artery catheter can help prevent this complication. *Myocardial depression* results from cardiac muscle suppression and can be avoided by frequent monitoring of fluid status,

CO, and serum drug levels. If an adequate CO cannot be maintained in the presence of normothermia, barbiturates must be reduced, regardless of serum levels.[2,3]

The major unresolved issue in the use of high-dose barbiturates is their effect on outcome after head injury. Several laboratory and clinical trials have been undertaken to address this issue. One trial demonstrated that most elevations of ICP could be controlled with aggressive use of standard therapies of ICP management. For the small subset of patients in whom standard therapy fails to achieve ICP control, judicious, carefully monitored and administered high-dose barbiturate therapy is beneficial.[23]

HERNIATION SYNDROMES

The goal of neurologic evaluation, ICP monitoring, and treatment of increased ICP is to prevent herniation. *Herniation* of intracerebral contents results in the shifting of tissue from one compartment of the brain to another and places pressure on cerebral vessels and vital function centers of the brain. If unchecked, herniation rapidly causes death as a result of the cessation of CBF and respirations.

Supratentorial Herniation

The four types of supratentorial herniation syndrome are uncal, central (transtentorial), cingulate, and transcalvarial[3,24] (Figure 18-8).

Uncal Herniation

Uncal herniation is the most common herniation syndrome. In uncal herniation a unilateral expanding mass lesion, usually of the temporal lobe, increases ICP, causing lateral displacement of the tip of the temporal lobe (uncus). Lateral displacement pushes the uncus over the edge of the tentorium, puts pressure on the oculomotor nerve (cranial nerve III) and posterior cerebral artery ipsilateral to the lesion, and flattens the midbrain against the opposite side. Clinical manifestations of uncal herniation include ipsilateral pupil

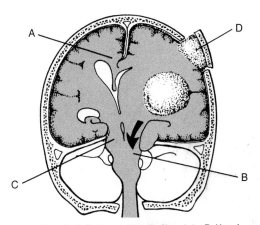

Figure 18-8   Supratentorial herniation. **A**, Cingulate. **B**, Uncal. **C**, Central. **D**, Transcalvarial.

dilation, decreased LOC, respiratory pattern changes leading to respiratory arrest, and contralateral hemiplegia leading to decorticate or decerebrate posturing. If no intervention occurs, uncal herniation results in fixed and dilated pupils, flaccidity, and respiratory arrest.

Central Herniation

In central, or *transtentorial*, herniation an expanding mass lesion of the midline, frontal, parietal, or occipital lobes results in downward displacement of the hemispheres, basal ganglia, and diencephalon through the tentorial notch. Central herniation often is preceded by uncal and cingulate herniation. Clinical manifestations of central herniation include loss of consciousness, small reactive pupils progressing to fixed dilated pupils, respiratory changes leading to respiratory arrest, and decorticate posturing progressing to flaccidity. In the late stages, uncal and central herniation syndromes affect the brain stem similarly.

Cingulate Herniation

Cingulate herniation occurs when an expanding lesion of one hemisphere shifts laterally and forces the cingulate gyrus under the falx cerebri. Cingulate herniation occurs often. When a lateral shift is noted on computed tomography (CT) scan, cingulate herniation has occurred. Little is known about the effects of cingulate herniation, and no clinical manifestations are present to assist in its diagnosis. Cingulate herniation is not in itself life threatening, but if the expanding mass lesion that caused cingulate herniation is not controlled, uncal or central herniation will follow.

Transcalvarial Herniation

Transcalvarial herniation is the extrusion of cerebral tissue through the cranium. In the presence of severe cerebral edema, transcalvarial herniation occurs through an opening from a skull fracture or craniotomy site.[3]

Infratentorial Herniation

The two infratentorial herniation syndromes are upward transtentorial herniation and downward cerebellar herniation.

Upward Transtentorial Herniation

Upward transtentorial herniation occurs when an expanding mass lesion of the cerebellum causes protrusion of the vermis (central area) of the cerebellum and the midbrain upward through the tentorial notch. Compression of the third cranial nerve (CN III) and diencephalon occurs. Blockage of the central aqueduct and distortion of the third ventricle obstruct CSF flow. Deterioration progresses rapidly.

Downward Cerebellar Herniation

Downward cerebellar herniation occurs when an expanding lesion of the cerebellum exerts pressure downward, sending the cerebellar tonsils through the foramen magnum. Compression and displacement of the medulla oblongata occur, rapidly resulting in respiratory and cardiac arrest.[3,24]

REFERENCES

1. McCance K, Huether S, editors: *Pathophysiology: the biologic basis for disease in adults and children*, ed 2, St Louis, 2002, Mosby.
2. Allen CH, Ward JD: An evidenced-based approach to management of increased intracranial pressure, *Crit Care Clin* 14:485, 1998.
3. Barker E: *Neuroscience nursing*, ed 2, St Louis, 2002, Mosby.
4. Goetz, CG, Pappert CJ: *Textbook of clinical neurology*, Philadelphia, 1999, Saunders.
5. Cunning S, Houdek L: Preventing secondary brain injuries, *Dimen Crit Care Nurs* 18(5):20, 1999.
6. Wall BM, Philips JP, Howard JC: Validation of increased intracranial pressure and high risk for increased intracranial pressure, *Nurs Diag* 5:74, 1994.
7. American Association of Neuroscience Nurses: *Intracranial pressure monitoring*, Clinical guideline series, Chicago, 1997, The Association.
8. Stewart-Amidei C: Neurologic monitoring in the ICU, *Crit Care Nurs Q* 21(3):47, 1998.
9. March K: Intracranial pressure monitoring and assessing intracranial compliance in brain injury, *Crit Care Nurs Clin North Am* 12:429, 2000.
10. Kirkness CJ et al: Intracranial pressure waveform analysis: clinical and research implications, *J Neurosci Nurs* 32:271, 2000.
11. McQuillan KA: Intracranial pressure monitoring: technical imperatives, *AACN Clin Issues Crit Care Nurs* 2:623, 1991.
12. Winkleman C: Effect of backrest position on intracranial and cerebral perfusion pressures in traumatically brain-injured adults, *Am J Crit Care* 9:373, 2000.
13. Simmons BJ: Management of intracranial hemodynamics in the adult: a research analysis of head positioning and recommendations for clinical practice and future research, *J Neurosci Nurs* 29:44, 1997.
14. Bader MK, Palmer S: Keeping the brain in the zone: applying the severe head injury guidelines to practice, *Crit Care Nurs Clin North Am* 12:413, 2000.
15. Ingis A, Tealdale G: Hyperventilation with increased intracranial pressure, *Crit Care Med* 23:983, 1995.
16. Wong FWH: Prevention of secondary brain injury, *Crit Care Nurse* 20(5):18, 2000.
17. Arbour R: Aggressive management of intracranial dynamics, *Crit Care Nurse* 18(3):30, 1998.
18. Qureshi AI, Suarez JI: Use of hypertonic saline solutions in treatment of cerebral edema and intracranial hypertension, *Crit Care Med* 28:3301, 2000.
19. Brucia JJ, Owen DC, Rudy EB: The effects of lidocaine on intracranial hypertension, *J Neurosci Nurs* 24:205, 1992.
20. Kerr M et al: Head-injured adults: recommendations for endotracheal suctioning, *J Neurosci Nurs* 25:86, 1993.
21. Cummings R: Understanding ventricular drainage, *J Neurosci Nurs* 24:84, 1992.
22. Paczynski RP: Osmotherapy: basic concepts and controversies, *Crit Care Clin* 13:105, 1997.
23. Lee M et al: The efficacy of barbiturate coma in the management of uncontrolled intracranial hypertension following neurosurgical trauma, *J Neurotrauma* 11:325, 1994.
24. Morrison CAM: Brain herniation syndromes, *Crit Care Nurs* 7(5):34, 1987.

UNIT SIX

RENAL ALTERATIONS

Renal Assessment and Diagnostic Procedures

Objectives

- Describe the priorities of the renal nursing assessment.
- Identify ways in which alterations of hemoglobin and hematocrit levels can signal fluid volume deficit or excess.
- Explain why elevation of blood urea nitrogen and serum creatinine signal renal dysfunction.

HISTORY

A renal history begins with a description of the "chief complaint," stated in the patient's own words. A description of the chief complaint includes the onset, location, duration, and factors that lessen or aggravate the problem.[1] The individual is encouraged to describe the effects of any treatment for the problem, medications taken to alleviate symptoms (both prescription and nonprescription), and any procedures performed to improve the problem. A careful history that explores symptoms fully is an essential component of the clinical assessment.

Predisposing factors for acute renal dysfunction are also elicited during the history, including use of over-the-counter medicines, recent infections requiring antibiotic therapy, newly prescribed medicines, and any diagnostic procedure that used radiopaque contrast media.[2] Nonsteroidal anti-inflammatory drugs (NSAIDs; e.g., ibuprofen), antibiotics (especially aminoglycosides), numerous prescription drugs (e.g., cyclosporine), and iodine-based dyes are potentially nephrotoxic; it is important to assess for these agents when an individual presents with renal-related symptoms. *Rhabdomyolysis* is another cause of acute renal dysfunction and occurs with severe muscle damage secondary to trauma or strenuous physical activity. Exercise-induced rhabdomyolysis is more likely in an individual who is unconditioned or poorly conditioned for extreme physical activity.[3]

Additional clues to renal dysfunction are a history of recent onset of nausea and vomiting and appetite loss caused by taste changes, because uremia often causes a metallic taste in the mouth.[2] Rapid weight gain of more than 2 to 3 pounds per day, sleeping on additional pillows, and sitting in a chair to sleep are signals of volume overload and potential kidney dysfunction. If the patient is not able to describe the symptoms, family members and significant nonrelatives can be approached for this information.

PHYSICAL EXAMINATION
Inspection

Nursing priorities for inspection of the patient with renal dysfunction focus on (1) bleeding, (2) volume depletion or overload, and (3) edema.

Bleeding

Visual inspection related to the kidneys generally focuses on the flank and abdomen. Renal injury in a trauma patient is suspected if a purplish discoloration is present on the flank (Grey-Turner sign) or near the posterior eleventh or twelfth rib.[1] Bruising, abdominal distention, and abdominal guarding may also signal renal trauma or a hematoma around a kidney.

Volume Depletion/Overload

Inspection is especially helpful in looking for signs of volume depletion or overload that might signal kidney problems. Fluid volume assessment is comprehensive and begins with an inspection of the patient's neck veins. The supine position facilitates normal venous distention. An absence of distention (or flat neck veins) indicates hypovolemia. If the neck veins remain distended more than 2 cm above the sternal notch when the bed is at 45 degrees, fluid overload is present.[1,4] Hand vein inspection is helpful in assessing volume status and is performed in two stages. First, the hand is held in a dependent position to observe for venous distention. Venous filling that takes longer than 5 seconds suggests hypovolemia. Second, the hand is elevated, and the distention should disappear within 5 seconds. If distention does not disappear within 5 seconds after the hand is elevated, fluid overload is suspected.

Assessment of skin turgor provides additional volume status data. To assess turgor, the skin over the forearm is picked up and released. Normal elasticity and fluid status allow an almost immediate return to shape after the skin is released. In fluid volume deficit, however, the skin remains raised and does not return to its normal position for several seconds (tenting). Because of the loss of skin elasticity in elderly persons, skin turgor assessment in the forearm is not an accurate fluid assessment technique. As an alternative, skin turgor is assessed in the shoulder area or anterior chest, which does retain elasticity in older persons.[4]

Inspection of the oral cavity, using a tongue blade, also provides clues to fluid volume status. When a true fluid volume deficit exists, the mucous membranes of the mouth become dry. However, mouth breathing can temporarily dry the mucous membranes as well. As a clue, dryness of the oral cavity is more indicative of fluid volume deficit than are complaints of a dry mouth.[4]

Edema

Edema is the presence of excess fluid in the interstitial space and can be a sign of volume overload. In the presence of volume excess, edema may be present in dependent areas of the body, such as the feet and legs of an ambulatory person or the sacrum of an individual confined to bed.

Although an important sign of volume overload, the presence of edema does not always indicate fluid overload because edema can result from disorders of other body systems. A loss of albumin from the vascular space can cause peripheral edema due to the loss of plasma oncotic pressure. A critically ill patient may have a low serum albumin level because of inadequate nutrition after surgery, a burn, or sepsis, and may exhibit edema due to hypoalbuminemia and not fluid overload. In addition, edema may signal circulatory difficulties. An individual who is fluid balanced but who has poor venous return may experience pedal edema after prolonged sitting in a chair with the feet dependent. Similarly, an individual with heart failure may experience edema because the left ventricle is unable to pump blood effectively through the vessels. The clinical priority is to assess all systems comprehensively.

Edema is assessed by applying fingertip pressure on the skin over a bony prominence, such as the ankle, tibial area (shin), or sacrum. If the indentation made by the fingertip does not disappear within 15 seconds, "pitting" edema is present. Pitting edema indicates increased interstitial volume and is generally not evident until a weight gain of approximately 10% has occurred. Dependent areas, such as the feet and sacrum, are the areas most likely to demonstrate edema in patients confined to a wheelchair or bed. The extent of edema may be measured by using a subjective scale of 1 to 4, with 1 indicating only minimal pitting and 4 indicating severe pitting.[1] Edema also may appear in the hands and feet, around the eyes, and in the face and cheeks.

Auscultation

Nursing priorities in auscultation of the patient with renal dysfunction focus on (1) the heart, (2) blood pressure, and (3) the lungs.

Heart

Auscultation of the heart requires not only assessing rate and rhythm but also listening for extra heart sounds (see Chapter 10). Fluid overload is often accompanied by a third or fourth heart sound, which is heard with the bell of the stethoscope.[1] The heart also is auscultated for the presence of a pericardial friction rub. A rub can best be heard at the third intercostal space to the left of the sternal border, with the individual leaning slightly forward.[1] A pericardial friction rub may result from uremia in a patient with renal failure. Increased heart rate (HR) alone offers little information about fluid volume status, but when combined with a low blood pressure (BP), may indicate hypovolemia.

Blood Pressure

Changes in BP and HR are very useful in assessing fluid volume deficit. Orthostatic vital sign measurements are assessed in the stable patient who can arise from bed. *Orthostatic hypotension* is defined as a drop in BP of more than 20 mm Hg or a rise in pulse rate of more than 20 beats/min from lying to sitting or from sitting to standing. Orthostatic measurements are used to evaluate the hemodynamic effects of blood loss, dehydration, unexplained syncope, and side effects of some antihypertensive medications in the stable patient.[5] The drop in BP occurs because a sufficient cardiac preload is not immediately available after the position change. HR increases in an attempt to maintain cardiac output (CO) and circulation. Orthostatic hypotension is uncomfortable for the patient and produces subjective feelings of weakness, dizziness, or faintness.

Lungs

Lung assessment is extremely important in gauging fluid status. Crackles indicate fluid overload. Dyspnea with mild exertion or dyspnea at night that prevents sleeping in a supine position or that awakens the individual from sleep suggests pooling of fluid in the lungs. Breathing patterns may also signal acid-base imbalances. Shallow, gasping breaths with periods of apnea reflect acidosis and severe acid-base imbalance.

Palpation

The nursing priority in palpation of the patient with renal dysfunction focuses on determining the size and shape of the kidney.

Determining Kidney Size/Shape

Although infrequently performed in critically ill patients, palpation of the kidneys in stable patients provides information about the kidneys' size and shape. Palpation of the kidneys is achieved through the *bimanual-capturing approach*, which is accomplished by the examiner placing one hand posteriorly under the flank of the supine patient with fingers pointing to the midline, while placing the opposite hand just below the rib cage anteriorly.[1] The patient is asked to inhale deeply while pressure is exerted to bring the hands together. As the patient exhales, the examiner may feel the kidney between the hands. After each kidney is palpated in this manner, the two should be compared for size and shape. Each kidney should be firm, smooth, and of equal size. A normal-sized left kidney is difficult to palpate. The right kidney is more easily palpated because it is displaced downward by the liver. Problems should be suspected if a mass (trauma or cancer) or an irregular surface (polycystic kidneys) is palpated, a size difference is detected, or the kidney extends significantly lower than the rib cage on either side.[1]

Percussion

Nursing priorities in percussion of the patient with renal dysfunction focus on (1) the kidneys and (2) the abdomen.

Kidneys

Percussion of a kidney is performed with the patient in a side-lying or sitting position, with the examiner's hand placed over the costovertebral angle (lower border of the rib cage on the flank).[1] The examiner strikes the back of the hand with the opposite fist. A dull, painless thud is normal. Pain may indicate infection (e.g., urinary tract infection extending into kidneys) or injury resulting from trauma. Traumatic injury to the kidneys should be assessed in the presence of a penetrating abdominal wound, with blunt abdominal trauma, or with fractured pelvis or ribs.

Abdomen

Percussing the abdomen with the patient in the supine position generally yields a dull sound (solid bowel contents or fluid) or a hollow sound (gaseous bowel).[1]

Ascites, in which fluid in the abdominal cavity causes distention of the abdomen, is an important observation in determining fluid overload. Differentiating ascites from distention caused by solid bowel contents is accomplished by producing a fluid wave. A *fluid wave* is elicited by exerting pressure to the abdominal midline while one hand is placed on the right or left flank.[1] Tapping the opposite flank produces a wave in the accumulated fluid that can be felt under the hands. Other signs of ascites include a protuberant, rounded abdomen and abdominal striae.

Individuals with renal failure may have ascites caused by volume overload. The volume-laden veins force fluid into the abdomen because of increased capillary hydrostatic pressures. However, ascites does not always represent fluid volume excess. Severe ascites in persons with compromised hepatic function has a different cause and occurs as a result of decreased plasma proteins and elevated portal vein pressure.

ADDITIONAL ASSESSMENT PARAMETERS
Fluid Balance

Nursing priorities for the patient undergoing fluid balance assessment focus on (1) weight, (2) intake and output, and (3) hemodynamic monitoring.

Weight

One of the most important assessments of renal and fluid status is the patient's weight. In the critical care unit, weight is monitored on every patient every day and is an important vital sign measurement. Significant fluctuations in body weight over 1 to 2 days indicate fluid gains and losses. Rapid weight gains or losses of more than 2 or 3 pounds per day generally indicate fluid rather than nutritional factors. One liter (1 L) of fluid equals 1 kg, or approximately 2.2 pounds.

Intake and Output

As with patient weight, intake and output (I&O) are monitored in all patients in the critical care unit. I&O can be compared with the patient's weight to evaluate the gain or loss of fluid. Urine output plus insensible fluid losses (perspiration, stool, water vapor from lungs) can vary from 750 to 2400 ml/day. When intake exceeds output (excessive intravenous fluid, decreased renal output), a positive fluid balance exists. In impaired renal function the positive fluid balance results in fluid volume overload. Conversely, if output exceeds intake (fever, increased respiration, profuse sweating, vomiting, diarrhea, gastric suction, diuretic therapy), a negative fluid balance exists and volume deficit results. During a 24-hour period, fever can increase skin and respiratory losses by as much as 75 ml/° F temperature rise.

Individuals with acute renal failure (ARF) often exhibit a decrease in urine output, or *oliguria* (less than 30 ml/hour or 400 ml/day). However, there may be a fairly normal or only slightly decreased urine output that reflects water removal without solute removal in the early phases of ARF. Therefore renal function cannot be accurately determined by urine output alone.

Hemodynamic Monitoring

Body fluid status is accurately reflected in measurements of cardiovascular hemodynamics. Measurements such as central venous pressure (CVP), pulmonary artery occlusion pressure (PAOP, "wedge" pressure), cardiac index (CI), and mean arterial pressure (MAP) provide a clear picture of the increases or decreases in vascular volume returning to and being ejected from the heart. Indeed, both volume depletion and overload are easily detected by use of the central venous or arterial catheters from which pressure measurements are obtained (Table 19-1).

Other Observations

Renal system dysfunction often leads to fluid and electrolyte imbalances. Some of the disturbances in fluid and electrolyte levels are accompanied by clinical manifestations (Box 19-1). Any sudden or slowly developing changes in mental status also must be investigated. Acidosis often results in disorientation. Lethargy, coma, and confusion may result from sodium, calcium, or magnesium excess or deficit. Apprehension or anxiety may be secondary to sodium deficit, a shift of fluid from the plasma to the interstitium, or respiratory changes caused by fluid volume overload.

Apathy and withdrawal from communicating with others often accompany hypovolemic states. Patients with renal failure manifest dramatic increases in electrolytes, intravascular fluids, and nitrogenous waste products.[2] The speed of onset will vary according to how rapidly (or slowly) the renal failure progresses and alters homeostasis.

LABORATORY ASSESSMENT
Serum Tests
Blood Urea Nitrogen

In addition to history and physical examination, laboratory data are extremely helpful in the diagnosis, management, and ongoing evaluation of renal system dysfunction. Blood urea nitrogen (BUN) is a by-product of protein and amino acid metabolism and increases as renal function deteriorates (normal is 9 to 20 mg/dl).[6] With renal dysfunction, BUN is elevated because of a decrease in the glomerular filtration rate (GFR) and therefore a fall in urea excretion. However, many other factors also affect the BUN value (e.g., malnutrition, dehydration, bleeding). Therefore BUN cannot be evaluated in isolation and is always considered with a known serum creatinine level.

Table **19-1**	Hemodynamic Assessment of Fluid Status	
Measurement	**Volume Depletion**	**Volume Overload**
CVP	<2 mm Hg	> 6 mm Hg
PAOP	<8 mm Hg	> 12 mm Hg
CI	<2.2 L/min/m²	> 4.4 L/min/m²
MAP	Decreased	Increased

CVP, Central venous pressure; *PAOP,* pulmonary artery occlusion pressure or "wedge pressure"; *CI,* cardiac index; *MAP,* mean arterial pressure; *mm HG,* millimeters of mercury; *L/min/m²,* liters per minute per meter squared body surface area.

Box **19-1**   Assessment of Fluid and Electrolyte Disturbances

FLUID STATUS
Skin turgor
Mucous membranes
Intake and output
Presence of edema/ascites
Diaphoresis
Low-grade fever
Neck and hand vein engorgement
Lung sounds—crackles
Dyspnea
Central venous pressure (CVP) <2 mm Hg, >6 mm Hg
Pulmonary artery occlusion pressure (PAOP) <8 mm Hg, >12 mm Hg
Tachycardia
Hypertension, hypotension
Cardiac index (CI) <2.2 L/min/m^2
S_3, S_4 heart sounds
Headache
Blurred vision
Vertigo on rising
Papilledema
Mental changes

ELECTROLYTE STATUS
Serum osmolality
Complete blood count (CBC)
Serum electrolyte level
Electrocardiogram (ECG) tracings (potassium, calcium, magnesium levels)
Behavioral and/or mental changes
Chvostek and Trousseau signs (calcium levels)
Changes in peripheral sensation (numbness, tremor)
Muscle strength
Gastrointestinal (GI) changes (nausea and vomiting)
Therapies that can alter electrolyte status (GI suction, diuretics, antihypertensives, calcium channel blockers)

Creatinine

Creatinine is a by-product of protein and normal cell metabolism and appears in serum in amounts proportional to the body muscle mass. Although slightly higher in men than women, the normal serum creatinine level is about 0.7 to 1.5 mg/dl.[6] Creatinine is easily excreted by the renal tubules and is not reabsorbed or secreted in the tubules. As with BUN, the creatinine level increases due to a drop in the GFR with renal failure. Serum creatinine levels are fairly constant and are affected by fewer factors than BUN. As a result, the serum creatinine level is a more accurate indicator of renal function than BUN. In general, the ratio of BUN to creatinine is 10:1. A change in the ratio can indicate renal dysfunction and help identify the etiology of the renal dysfunction.

Creatinine Clearance

Measuring the creatinine clearance—the amount of creatinine in the excreted urine and the amount of creatinine in the blood over 24 hours—provides accurate information about kidney function.[2] The normal value for urine creatinine clearance is 110 to 120 ml/min in men and 100 to 115 ml/min in women. Creatinine clearance is a direct indicator of the GFR; as renal function decreases, creatinine clearance decreases.[2]

The creatinine clearance can be measured by collecting the urine for a 24-hour period or, as is common in the critically ill patient, estimated using the Cockcroft-Gault formula (Box 19-2). The creatinine clearance is a useful parameter to monitor the severity and course of renal dysfunction (both decline and improvement in function) and is

Box **19-2**   Creatinine Clearance Calculations

Measured: 24-Hour Urine
(Urine creatinine × Volume of urine) ÷ Serum creatinine

Estimated: Cockcroft-Gault Formula
[(140 − Age) × Body weight (kg)] ÷ [72 × Plasma creatinine (mg/dl)]

For women, multiply above by 0.85.

widely used to determine changes in drug dosing because many drugs are excreted by the kidneys.[7]

Osmolality

The serum osmolality reflects the concentration or dilution of vascular fluid. The normal value is 280 to 300 mOsm/L (milliosmoles per liter).[6] When the serum osmolality level rises because of insufficient fluid intake or excessive losses, antidiuretic hormone (ADH) is released from the pituitary gland and stimulates increased water reabsorption by the kidneys. This expands the vascular space, produces more concentrated urine, and brings the serum osmolality back to a normal range. The opposite occurs as serum osmolality falls; ADH production is inhibited. The low serum ADH increases excretion of water by the kidneys, produces dilute urine, and brings serum osmolality back to normal. Measurement of serum osmolality is a useful parameter in determining fluid balance and fluid replacement therapy in critically ill patients.

Anion Gap

The anion gap is a calculation of the difference between the measurable *cations*, sodium (Na^+) and potassium (K^+), and the measurable *anions*, chloride (Cl^-) and bicarbonate (HCO_3^-).[4] The value represents the remaining infrequently measured anions present in the extracellular fluid (ECF), including phosphates, sulfates, ketones, and lactate. The clinical formula generally used in the calculation of the anion gap follows:

$$Na^+ - (Cl^- + HCO_3^-)$$

A normal anion gap is 1 to 12 mEq/L (milliequivalents per liter) and should not exceed 14 mEq/L. An increased anion gap level reflects acid overproduction or decreased excretion of acid products and correlates with serum pH measurement. An anion gap greater than 20 mEq/L indicates metabolic acidosis.

Hemoglobin and Hematocrit

The hemoglobin (Hgb) and hematocrit (Hct) levels can indicate increases or decreases in intravascular fluid volume. Hgb transports oxygen and carbon dioxide and is important in maintaining cellular metabolism and acid-base balance.[6] The Hct is the percentage of red blood cells (RBCs) in a volume of whole blood. An increase in the Hct in the presence of normal Hgb concentration suggests a fluid volume deficit with hemoconcentration. Conversely, a decreased Hct with a coexisting normal Hgb indicates fluid volume excess because of the dilutional effect of the extra fluid load. When both Hct and Hgb are low, potential causes are bleeding, anemias, liver damage, hemolytic reactions, and inadequate secretion of erythropoietin secondary to acute renal failure.[6,8] Hct and Hgb are always evaluated together in the critically ill patient.[8]

Albumin

Slightly more than 50% of the total plasma protein is serum albumin. Albumin is manufactured in the liver and is primarily responsible for the maintenance of *colloid osmotic pressure*, which functions to hold fluid in the vascular space. The blood vessel walls, because of their impermeability to plasma proteins, prevent albumin from leaving the vascular space. In some disease states, however, such as third-degree burns (cell membrane destruction), severe sepsis, or ARF resulting from the nephrotic syndrome (increased glomerular capillary permeability to protein), albumin escapes from the vascular space and enters the interstitial space. The result is peripheral and generalized edema and may progress to pulmonary edema.

Increased albumin levels are rare. The body uses a fixed amount of protein for energy and body cell replacement and converts excess protein into stored fat. If all plasma protein levels are elevated, fluid volume deficit (hemoconcentration) is suspected.

Urinalysis

Analysis of the urine provides excellent information about the patient's renal function and condition relative to fluids and electrolytes. Specific tests and abnormal indications are presented in Table 19-2.

Urine pH

Urine pH identifies the acidity or alkalinity of urine. The kidneys regulate acid-base balance; therefore more hydrogen ions are excreted than bicarbonate ions, creating the acidic urine. Changes in renal function and infection often produce changes in urine pH. An increase in urine acidity (decreased pH) indicates retention of sodium and acids by the body, which is present in acute intra-renal failure. Conversely, a decrease in urine acidity (increased pH or more alkaline) means the body is retaining bicarbonate.

Specific Gravity

Specific gravity measures the density or weight of urine compared with that of distilled water. Because urine is composed of solutes and substances suspended in water, the specific gravity is higher than water except in states where a very dilute urine is excreted, as in aggressive diuretic therapy.

Osmolality

The urine osmolality more accurately pinpoints fluid balance than the serum osmolality value. Serum osmolality reflects serum sodium concentration and therefore is subject to more influences than the urine osmolality. The simultaneous measurement of both serum and urine osmolality levels provides an accurate assessment of fluid status. Urine osmolality depends on reabsorption or excretion of water in the kidney tubules.[6] The urine osmolality level increases (and urine output decreases) during fluid volume deficit because of the retention of fluid by the body. Conversely, the urine osmolality level decreases (and urine output increases) during volume excess because fluid is excreted by the kidneys.

Glucose

Glucose normally is completely reabsorbed by the renal tubules; therefore the urine should be free of glucose. Transient appearance of glucose in the urine may be brought on by ingestion of a heavy carbohydrate load (patients receiving total parenteral nutrition), stress (trauma, surgery), or the renal changes that accompany pregnancy. Consistent *glycosuria* occurs during hyperglycemic episodes of diabetes when the renal threshold for glucose is exceeded (generally when the serum glucose reaches 180mg/dl) and the excess glucose spills into the urine. In renal failure (acute or chronic), glycosuria is not a reliable indicator of the level of hyperglycemia because of the erratic excretion of glucose by the damaged nephrons.

Protein

Protein, like glucose, normally is absent from urine because the large protein molecules are not filtered across an intact glomerular capillary membrane. Thus consistent appearance of protein in urine suggests compromise of the glomerular

Table 19-2   Urinalysis Results and Abnormal Indications

Test	Normal	Potential Causes	
		Increased Values	**Decreased Values**
pH	4.5-8.0	Alkalosis	Acidosis Intrarenal ARF
Specific gravity	1.003-1.030	Volume deficit Glycosuria Proteinuria Prerenal ARF (>1.020)	Volume overload
Osmolality	300-1200 mOsm/kg	Volume deficit Prerenal ARF (urine osmolality > serum osmolality)	Volume excess Intrarenal ARF (urine osmolality < serum osmolality)
Protein	30-150 mg/24 hr	Trauma Infection Intrarenal ARF Transient with exercise Glomerulonephritis	
Sodium	27-287 mEq/24 hr	High sodium diet Intrarenal ARF	Prerenal ARF
Creatinine	1-2 g/24 hr		Intrarenal ARF Chronic renal failure
Urea	6-17 g/24 hr		Intrarenal ARF Chronic renal failure
Myoglobin	Absent	Crush injury Rhabdomyolysis	
RBCs	0-5	Trauma Intrarenal ARF Infection Strenuous exercise Renal artery thrombus	
WBCs	0-5	Infection	
Bacteria	None-few	Infection	
Casts	None-few	RBC: Glomerular disease WBC: Glomerular disease, nephrotic syndrome, pyelonephritis Epithelial: glomerular disease	

ARF, Acute renal failure; *RBCs,* red blood cells; *WBCs,* white blood cells.

membrane and possible intrarenal damage. The amount of protein in the urine is often directly correlated with the severity of the damage and may exceed 4.0 g/day.

Electrolytes

Urine electrolytes are infrequently measured in the critical ill patient. To measure urine electrolyte levels, a 24-hour sample is often required, although a single specimen may also be used. Urine electrolyte levels are highly variable, and the electrolytes depend on the kidneys for adequate excretion. Consequently, changes in urine electrolyte levels strongly suggest renal failure and generally indicate intrarenal ARF.

Sediment

The presence of sediment such as epithelial cells and casts indicates problems related to the kidneys and can be helpful in identifying the etiology of ARF. In prerenal ARF the kid-

neys are not damaged and urine sediment is normal. In intrarenal ARF, however, the kidney tubules are damaged and urine sediment is abnormal, containing casts and epithelial cells. *Casts* are shells or clumps of cellular breakdown or protein materials that form in the renal tubular system and are washed out in the urine flow.

Hematuria

Both obvious and microscopic hematuria may signal renal damage. Visibly bloody urine indicates bleeding within the urinary tract or renal trauma. Microscopic hematuria may occur normally after strenuous exercise or insertion of a urinary drainage catheter but should disappear in 48 hours.

DIAGNOSTIC ASSESSMENT

Relevant diagnostic procedures used to evaluate the patient with renal dysfunction are presented in Table 19-3.

Table **19-3** Renal Diagnostic Studies

Study	Purposes	Comments
Computed tomography (CT) scan	Provides a view of kidneys, retroperitoneal space, bladder, prostate Evaluates kidney size Evaluates kidney for tumors, abscesses, and obstruction	No special preparation. Can be safely used in patients with renal failure. Contrast medium may be used.
Cystometrogram	Evaluates pressure exerted against wall of bladder to evaluate bladder tone	No special preparation required. Urinary catheter inserted and saline instilled into bladder. Postprocedure monitor for clinical indications of urinary tract infection.
Cystoscopy	Visualizes bladder and urethra for identification pathology	*Preprocedure:* NPO after midnight if general anesthesia to be used. Administer sedative if prescribed. No special preparation required. *Postprocedure:* Pink-tinged urine is normal but gross hematuria is abnormal; monitor urine output. Encourage fluids.
Intravenous pyelogram (IVP)	Evaluates position, size, shape, and location of kidneys Provides visualization of internal kidney (parenchyma, calices, pelvis) Evaluates filling of renal pelvis Outlines ureters and bladder Identifies presence of cysts and tumors Identifies obstruction and congenital abnormality	Also called *excretory urogram.* Contraindicated in renal insufficiency, multiple myeloma, pregnancy, congestive heart failure, sickle cell disease. Bowel preparation (e.g., cathartics as prescribed). NPO for 8 hours before test. *Contrast media used:* Check for allergy to iodine before study. Monitor for allergic reaction and ensure hydration postprocedure.
Kidneys, ureters, and bladder (KUB)	Outlines kidneys, ureters, bladder Evaluates size, shape, and position of kidneys Identifies location of calculi	Also called *flat plate of abdomen.* Bowel preparation (e.g., cathartics) may be prescribed if to be followed by IVP.
Magnetic resonance imaging (MRI)	Differentiates between cyst and solid mass Identifies infarction, trauma, and obstruction	More specific than renal ultrasonography or CT scan because MRI shows subtle density changes. Cannot be used in patients with any implanted metallic device, including pacemakers. No special preparation required.
Nephrotomogram	Evaluates segments of kidney at different levels Differentiates between cysts and solid mass	Bowel preparation (e.g., cathartics) as prescribed. NPO for 8 hours before study. *Contrast media used:* Check for allergy to iodine before study. Monitor for allergic reaction and ensure hydration postprocedure.
Renal angiography	Evaluates renal vasculature Identifies renal artery stenosis Identifies cysts, tumors, infarction, and trauma	Bowel preparation (e.g., cathartics) as prescribed. NPO for 8 hours before test. Sedative usually prescribed before procedure. *Contrast media used: As above.*

Procedure	Purpose	Nursing Considerations
		Postprocedure: Keep affected extremity (catheter placed) immobilized in straight position for 6-12 hours. Monitor arterial puncture point for hemorrhage or hematoma, neurovascular status of affected limb, and for indications of systemic emboli.
Renal biopsy	Obtains tissue specimen for microscopic evaluation	Performed open or closed. Clotting profile evaluated and type/crossmatch for 2 units of blood preprocedure. Usually not performed if patient has only one functioning kidney (unless to evaluate possible transplant rejection). Closed biopsy contraindicated in bleeding abnormalities, polycystic disease, neoplasm, hydronephrosis, urinary tract infection, uncooperative patient. *Postprocedure:* Maintain pressure dressing and bed rest for 24 hours. Observe for hematuria, flank pain, and hypotension.
Renal radionuclide scan (renogram)	Evaluates position, size, shape, and location of kidneys Identifies obstruction, abscesses, cysts, and tumors Evaluates renal perfusion Evaluates glomerular filtration, tubular function, and excretion Assesses status of renal transplant	Assure patient that amount of radioactive material is minimal. Do not schedule within 24 hours after IVP. Ask patient to void before scan. Encourage fluids postprocedure.
Retrograde pyelogram	Evaluates position, size, shape, and location of kidneys Outlines ureters and bladder Identifies presence of cysts and tumors Identifies obstruction	Does not require the kidney to excrete the dye, so may be used in patients with renal insufficiency. Bowel preparation (e.g., cathartics) as prescribed. NPO for 8 hours before test. *Contrast media used:* Check for allergy to iodine before study. Monitor for allergic reaction and ensure hydration postprocedure. Monitor patient for clinical indications of urinary tract infection or sepsis.
Ultrasonography	Evaluates fluid vs. solid mass Identifies obstruction Identifies cysts, abscesses, tumors, and polycystic kidney disease Identifies hemorrhage Identifies urinary tract obstruction and leaks	No special preparation required. Can be safely used in patients with renal failure. Contrast media may be used.
Voiding cystourethrography	Identifies abnormalities of lower urinary tract to determine presence of reflux and residual urine	No special preparation required. Encourage fluids postprocedure.

From Dennison R: *Pass CCRN!*, ed 2, St Louis, 2000, Mosby.

A *renal biopsy* provides tissue (nephron) specimen for microscopic evaluation. Renal biopsy is not performed frequently in the critical care unit but is useful in determining unclear causes of ARF.

Nursing Management

The nursing management of a patient undergoing a diagnostic procedure involves a variety of nursing interventions. **Nursing priorities are directed toward (1) preparing the patient physically and psychologically for the procedure, (2) monitoring the patient's responses during the procedure, and (3) assessing the patient after the procedure.**

Preparing the patient includes asking questions about allergies, specifically to radiopaque contrast dye, describing the procedure and what the experience "will feel like," answering any questions, and contacting the physician if the patient is not fully informed about the purpose, risks, and benefits of the procedure. The patient may need to go to a diagnostic area (e.g., radiography) or be repositioned in bed for a procedure in the intensive care unit. Assessment of the critically ill patient's physiologic responses to the procedure usually includes monitoring the electrocardiogram, BP, and CVP and using the 1 to 10 pain scale if the person can speak, as well as a sedation/anxiety scale. Postprocedural monitoring focuses on potential complications and medication for discomfort. **Any evidence of bleeding or decompensation in vital signs or renal function must be reported to the physician immediately.**

REFERENCES

1. Seidel HM et al: *Mosby's guide to physical examination*, ed 5, St Louis, 2003, Mosby.
2. Richard C: Assessment of renal structure and function. In Lancaster L, editor: *Core curriculum for nephrology nursing*, ed 4, Pitman, NJ, 2001, American Nephrology Nurses Association.
3. Fishbane S: Exercise-induced renal and electrolyte changes, *Physician Sportsmed* 23:39, 1996.
4. Metheny NM: *Fluid and electrolyte balance: nursing considerations*, ed 4, Philadelphia, 2000, Lippincott.
5. Roper M: Back to basics: assessing orthostatic vital signs, *Am J Nurs* 96(8):43, 1996.
6. Fischbach F: *A manual of laboratory diagnostic tests*, ed 6, Philadelphia, 2000, Lippincott.
7. Simonson M: Measurement of glomerular filtration rate. In Hricik D et al, editors: *Nephrology secrets*, Philadelphia, 1999, Hanley & Belfus.
8. Pearl RG, Pohlman A: Understanding and managing anemia in critically ill patients, *Crit Care Nurs*, Dec supplment: 1-16, 2002

JUDITH K. GLANN MITCHELL

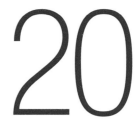

Renal Disorders and Therapeutic Management

Objectives

- List the etiologies of acute renal failure.
- Describe the stages of acute tubular necrosis.
- Identify the priorities of nursing management in acute renal failure.
- Discuss or explain the differences among hemodialysis, peritoneal dialysis, and continuous renal replacement therapy.

evolve Be sure to check out the free exercises on-line at *http://evolve.elsevier.com/Urden/priorities/*

ACUTE RENAL FAILURE

Acute renal failure (ARF) is characterized by an sudden decline in glomerular filtration rate (GFR), with subsequent retention of metabolic waste products from protein catabolism (i.e. azotemia) and an inability to maintain electrolyte and acid-base homeostasis.[1,2] This change in renal function also disturbs the regulation of fluid volume. *Oliguria*, or a urine output less than 400 ml/day, is a classic finding in ARF.[2] Oliguria occurs in up to one half of patients admitted to critical care units, depending on the specific patient population.[1,2]

Once ARF is diagnosed, mortality is high, ranging from 50% to 80%.[3] Many patients have multiple system problems, such as low cardiac output (CO), shock, or systemic sepsis, that impacts not only the kidneys but other vital organs as well. Sepsis causes 30% to 70% of deaths in patients with acute renal tubular necrosis.[3] In the critically ill patient, renal recovery is significantly associated with the recovery of all body systems.

At this time there is no standardized definition of ARF.[4] An international committee is developing a biochemical definition and classification system for acute renal dysfunction because of the more than 35 separate definitions in the renal literature. For the purposes of understanding the etiology of acute renal dysfunction in this chapter, ARF is classified into three categories according to location of the insult relative to the kidney: prerenal intrarenal, and postrenal (Box 20-1).[2] The term *azotemia* is used to describe an acute rise in blood urea nitrogen (BUN).

Prerenal azotemia is a physiologic response to an insult that occurs before blood reaches the kidney. This results in renal hypoperfusion, but initially the integrity of the kidney's nephron structure and function is preserved. The low-flow state, or hypoperfusion, decreases the GFR, leading to oliguria. The nephrons remain normal, and a return to normal renal function is possible with prompt treatment of the underlying cause of the prerenal condition.[1] Critical care patients are at risk from a cascade of events that may precipitate prerenal azotemia (Box 20-1).

Intrarenal azotemia is the physiologic response to an ischemic or toxic insult that occurs at the site of the nephrons.[3] It may involve both the glomeruli and the tubular epithelium. When the internal filtering structures are affected, this is known as *acute tubular necrosis*.

Postrenal azotemia is caused by the disruption of the urine flow from beyond the kidney in the remainder of the urinary tract. It affects fewer than 5% of critical care patients.[4]

ACUTE TUBULAR NECROSIS

Acute tubular necrosis (ATN) results from either nephrotoxic or ischemic injury that damages the renal tubular epithelium and, in severe cases, extends to the basement membrane.[1] Injury that is limited to the epithelial layer recovers sooner than injury that also involves the basement membrane.

Epidemiology and Etiology

ATN is the most common form of intrarenal failure, making up approximately 75% of cases, and accounts for the vast majority of cases of hospital-acquired ARF.[1,3,5] Damage to the cellular structures in this area prevents normal concentration of urine, filtration of wastes, and regulation of acid-base, electrolyte, and water balance. The renal tubular cells are constantly at risk for damage because of their normally high blood flows, high oxygen requirements, and the constant reabsorption and secretion of metabolites. A number of disorders can result in ATN, and several contributing factors often work together to bring about tubular damage.[1] Common causes of ATN are divided into two categories: ischemic injury and nephrotoxic injury[2] (Box 20-2).

Ischemic Acute Tubular Necrosis

Ischemic damage secondary to inadequate perfusion impairs the tubular membranes, causing non-uniform patchy areas of tubular cell damage and cast formation. Ischemic necrosis results when the low blood flow episode is prolonged and is worsened by renal hypoperfusion or dehydration.[2]

Toxic Acute Tubular Necrosis

Toxic damage results from nephrotoxins, usually drugs; chemical agents; or bacterial endotoxins, which cause uniform, widespread damage. Because the basement membrane is not injured as severely as with ischemic ATN, the healing is more rapid, the layer of the membrane can regenerate, and

---

Box **20-1**	Etiology of Acute Renal Failure

PRERENAL

Dehydration, severe
Hypotension
Cardiac failure, impaired
Anesthesia, surgery (increased renal vascular resistance)
Embolism, thrombosis (bilateral, renal vascular obstruction)
Sepsis

INTRARENAL

Acute tubular necrosis
Acute glomerulonephritis
Acute pyelonephritis
Acute cortical necrosis

POSTRENAL

Urethral obstructions (stenosis, calculi)
Renal calculi
Prostatic disease
Bladder obstruction, infection, neurogenic problem

From Stark JS: *Crit Care Clin North Am* 10:159, 1998.

Box 20-2   Acute Tubular Necrosis: Toxic versus Ischemic Origins

ISCHEMIC INJURY
Massive hemorrhage
Severe dehydration
Severe, prolonged hypotension
Shock: cardiogenic, hypovolemic, septic
Sepsis
Major trauma, crush injuries
Transfusion reaction
Postpartum/obstetric complications: severe toxemia, abruptio placentae, placenta previa, uterine rupture

NEPHROTOXIC INJURY
Rhabdomyolysis
Nephrotoxic medications: aminoglycosides (gentamicin, amikacin), cephalosporins, antimicrobials, antineoplastic agents, amphotericin B, analgesics containing phenacetin
Heavy metals: lead, arsenic, mercury, uranium
Radiocontrast media
Insecticides, pesticides, fungicides
Carbon tetrachloride
Methanol
Street drugs (e.g., phencyclidine, PCP)

From Stark JS: *Crit Care Clin North Am* 10:159, 1998.

full recovery from ATN and resumption of renal function in less than 8 days is more likely.[2,5]

Pathophysiology

The mechanisms responsible for tubular dysfunction in ischemic ATN are multifactorial. When "cellular debris" accumulates in the nephron tubular lumen, an obstruction will occur if there is not adequate flow of filtrate through the nephron. The obstruction is made up of casts and sloughing tissue and exacerbated by interstitial edema. Filtration ceases when tubular hydrostatic pressure rises to match GFR. This decreases the formation of urine because of the nonavailability of filtrate to process.[6] The result is more tubular cell swelling, obstruction, decreased capillary blood flow, and finally, further ischemia and cell injury. The clinical course of ATN progresses through four phases.

Phases of Acute Tubular Necrosis
Onset Phase

The onset (initiating) phase is the period from when an insult occurs until cell injury. Ischemic injury is evolving during this time. The GFR is decreased because of impaired renal blood flow and decreased glomerular ultrafiltration pressure. This disrupts the integrity of the tubular epithelium, which back-leaks the glomerular filtrate. This phase lasts from hours to days, depending on the cause, with toxic factors causing the phase to last longer. If treatment is initiated during this time, irreversible damage can be alleviated.

A longer course of recovery reflects the presence of more extensive tubular injury.[5]

Oliguric/Anuric Phase

The oliguric/anuric phase, the second phase of ATN, lasts 5 to 8 days in the nonoliguric patient and 10 to 16 days in the oliguric patient.[6] The accumulation of necrotic cellular debris in the tubular space blocks the flow of urine and causes damage to the tubular wall and basement membranes. Also, a back-leak phenomenon occurs because damage in the tubular wall causes the glomerular filtrate to flow passively into the renal tissue rather than be passed out as urine through the ureters and bladder.[2] Oliguria is encountered more often in ischemic damage and is a sign that the damage is more extensive and severe.[2] Mortality in patients with nonoliguric ATN is 25%, but mortality is 66% if oliguria is present.[1] During the oliguric/anuric phase, GFR is greatly reduced, which leads to increased levels of BUN (azotemia), elevated serum creatinine levels, electrolyte abnormalities (hyperkalemia, hyperphosphatemia, hypocalcemia), and metabolic acidosis.[1,5]

Diuretic Phase

The third phase, the diuretic phase, lasts 7 to 14 days and is characterized by an increase in GFR and sometimes polyuria with a urine output as high as 2 to 4 L/day.[1,5] If the patient is receiving hemodialysis during this phase, the polyuria will not be evident because excess volume will be removed by dialysis. During the diuretic phase the tubular obstruction has passed, but edema and scarring are present and have not completely covered the necrotic area.[2] Thus tubular function returns slowly, and tubular reabsorption may not increase as quickly as GFR. The kidneys can clear volume but not solutes, which, with a large diuresis, can lead to volume depletion.[1]

Recovery Phase

The last phase of ATN is the recovery or convalescent phase. Both oliguric and nonoliguric patients will increase their urine output if they enter the recovery stage. During this stage, renal function slowly returns to normal or near normal, with GFR 70% to 80% of normal within 1 to 2 years.[7] However, if significant renal parenchymal damage has occurred, BUN and creatinine levels may never return to normal.[1] For patients surviving ATN, approximately 62% will recover normal renal function, 33% will be left with residual renal insufficiency, and at least 5% will require long-term hemodialysis.[7]

ASSESSMENT AND DIAGNOSIS
Laboratory Assessment

Once acute renal disease is suspected, the presence or degree or renal dysfunction is assessed using both urine and blood analysis (Table 20-1). Most of the serum electrolytes will become increasingly elevated as ARF develops[2]

Table **20-1**	Laboratory Evaluation (Urinalysis) of Acute Renal Failure					
Condition	**Volume**	**Specific Gravity**	**Sodium**	**Sediment**		**BUN/Cr Ratio**
Prerenal	≤30 ml/hr	>1.020	<10 mEq/L	Normal		>25:1
Intrarenal	Oliguria or nonoliguria	1.010	>40 mEq/L	Erythrocyte or tubular casts		10:1
Postrenal	Oliguria to anuria	1.0-1.010	1-40 mEq/L	+Bacteriology possible		10:1

From Stark JS: Acute renal failure: focus on advances in acute tubular necrosis, *Crit Care Clin North Am* 10(2):159-170, 1998.
Cr, Creatinine; *anuria*, urine volume less than 100 ml/24 hr; *oliguria*, urine volume 100-400 ml/24 hr.

(Table 20-2). Clinical findings associated with specific electrolyte imbalances are listed in Table 20-3. Normal and abnormal urinalysis findings and significance are summarized in Chapter 19.

An estimation of the GFR is made using the plasma creatinine concentration and less often in critically ill patients by the urinary creatinine clearance. These tests are used clinically to assess the degree of renal impairment and to follow the course of the disease. Other signs of disease progression include decreased urine output, increased urine sediment, increased protein excretion, and elevated blood pressure.[2,3,6]

Blood Urea Nitrogen

BUN is not the most reliable indicator of renal damage. Although it reflects cellular damage, BUN is easily changed by protein intake, blood in the gastrointestinal (GI) tract, cell catabolism, and fluid volume changes. A *BUN/creatinine ratio* may be evaluated to determine the cause of the acute renal dysfunction (see Table 20-1). In prerenal failure the level of BUN is greatly elevated relative to the serum creatinine value.

Serum Creatinine

Creatinine is a by-product of muscle metabolism. It reflects renal damage because it is almost totally excreted by the renal tubules. Elevated levels of serum creatinine reflect damage to 50% or more of the nephrons.

Creatinine Clearance

If the patient is making sufficient urine, the urinary creatinine clearance can be measured. A normal urine creatinine

clearance is 120 ml/min, but this value decreases with renal failure. Critical care patients in ARF do not make sufficient urine; therefore the serum creatinine level is assessed daily.

Fractional Excretion of Sodium

The fractional excretion of sodium (FENa) in the urine is measured early in the course to differentiate between a prerenal condition and ATN.[3,9] A FENa value below 1% (in the absence of diuretics) suggests prerenal compromise, where reabsorption of almost all the filtered sodium is an appropriate response to decreased renal perfusion. In comparison, a value of 1% to 2% may be seen with either disorder, whereas a value above 2% urinary sodium usually indicates ATN.[9]

Urinary sodium is also measured in mEq/L (milliequivalents per liter). The interpretation of results is similar to the FENa. Urinary sodium less than 10 Eq/L (low) indicates a prerenal condition. Urinary sodium greater than 40 mEq/L suggests an intrarenal cause[2] (see Table 20-1).

Radiologic Findings

Sonography, tomography, and angiography can help pinpoint causal mechanisms and even help differentiate between acute diseases and chronic renal failure. It is important to be aware that radiologic contrast media have been implicated in the development and worsening of renal disorders.[10] Patients with a history of coronary artery disease, diabetes, or renal disease can develop acute renal problems when contrast medium is not adequately cleared because of an already-compromised circulatory or renal system.[11]

Hemodynamic Monitoring and Fluid Balance

Hemodynamic monitoring is important for the analysis of fluid volume status in the critically ill patient with ARF. Hemodynamic monitoring includes surveillance of central venous pressure (CVP), pulmonary artery occlusion pressure (PAOP), CO, and cardiac index (CI).[12] Less "high-tech" but also important is a daily weight and clinical assessment.[13] The patient's weight is indicative of fluid gains or losses over 1 to 2 days. Additional signs and symptoms, such

Table **20-2**	Normal Serum Electrolyte Values
Electrolyte	**Normal Value**
Sodium	135-145 mEq/L
Potassium	3.5-5.0 mEq/L
Chloride	98-108 mEq/L
Calcium	8.5-10.5 mg/dl *or* 4.5-5.8 mEq/L
Phosphorus	2.7-4.5 mg/dl
Magnesium	1.5-2.5 mEq/L
Bicarbonate	24-28 mEq/L

Table **20-3** Serum Electrolytes in Acute Renal Failure

Electrolyte Disturbance	Serum Value	Clinical Findings
POTASSIUM		
Hypokalemia	<3.5 mEq/L	Muscular weakness Cardiac irregularities on ECG Abdominal distention and flatulence Paresthesia Decreased reflexes Anorexia Dizziness, confusion Increased sensitivity to digitalis
Hyperkalemia	>5.0 mEq/L	Irritability and restlessness Anxiety Nausea and vomiting Abdominal cramps Weakness Numbness and tingling (fingertips and circumoral) Cardiac irregularities on ECG
SODIUM		
Hyponatremia	<135 mEq/L	Disorientation Muscle twitching Nausea/vomiting, abdominal cramps Headaches, dizziness Seizures, postural hypotension Cold clammy skin Decreased skin turgor Tachycardia Oliguria
Hypernatremia	>145 mEq/L	Extreme thirst Dry sticky mucous membranes Altered mentation Seizures (later stages)
CALCIUM		
Hypocalcemia	<8.5 mg/dl or <4.5 mEq/L	Irritability Muscular tetany, muscle cramps Decreased cardiac output (decreased contraction) Bleeding (decreased ability to coagulate) ECG changes Positive Chvostek/Trousseau signs
Hypercalcemia	>10.5 mg/dl or >5.8 mEq/L	Deep bone pain Excessive thirst Anorexia Lethargy, weakened muscles
MAGNESIUM		
Hypomagnesemia	<1.4 mEq/L	Choroid/athetoid muscle activity Facial tics, spasticity Cardiac dysrhythmias
Hypermagnesemia	>2.5 mEq/L	CNS depression Respiratory depression Lethargy Coma Bradycardia ECG changes

Continued

Table **20-3** Serum Electrolytes in Acute Renal Failure—cont'd

Electrolyte Disturbance	Serum Value	Clinical Findings
PHOSPHATE		
Hypophosphatemia	<3.0 mg/dl	Hemolytic anemias Depressed white cell function Bleeding (decreased platelet aggregation) Nausea/vomiting Anorexia
Hyperphosphatemia	>4.5 mg/dl	Tachycardia Nausea, diarrhea, abdominal cramps Muscle weakness, flaccid paralysis Increased reflexes
CHLORIDE		
Hypochloremia	<98 mEq/L	Hyperirritability Tetany or muscular excitability Slow respirations
Hyperchloremia	>108 mEq/L	Weakness, lethargy Deep rapid breathing Possible unconsciousness (later stages)
ALBUMIN		
Hypoalbuminemia	<3.8 g/dl	Muscle wasting Peripheral edema (fluid shift) Decreased resistance to infection Poorly healing wounds

ECG, Electrocardiogram; CNS, central nervous system.

as thirst, decreased skin turgor, and lethargy, suggest extracellular fluid (ECF) depletion. Abdominal girth is measured for ascites, and the patient is assessed frequently for pitting edema over bony prominences and in dependent body areas.

Medical Management

Treatment goals for patients experiencing ARF focus on compensating for the deterioration of renal function. Over the past four decades, mortality from ATN has remained at more than 80%.[3] Medical interventions for ARF are directed toward three goals: (1) prevention, (2) correcting the causative mechanism, and (3) promoting regeneration of the remaining renal functional capacity. Clinical interventions are based on the three causes of ARF.

Prevention

The only truly effective remedy for ARF is prevention. For effective prevention the patient's risk for ARF must be assessed as described below.

Underlying Chronic Kidney Disease. The incidence of chronic kidney disease (CKD) in the United States is estimated to be 11% (19.2 million adults).[14] Recent clinical practice guidelines for management of end-stage renal

disease (ESRD) have classified renal dysfunction into five stages.[15] Because of the large numbers of adults with renal dysfunction (diagnosed or not), renal function must be assessed on all critically ill patients at risk for fluid and electrolyte imbalance. The numeric population estimates in each stage of renal dysfunction are shown in Table 20-4. Hypertension and diabetes predispose an individual to CKD. Older age is another key predictor because 11% of individuals older than 65 years without hypertension or diabetes have stage 3 or worse CKD.[14]

Risk of Acute Renal Failure. A classification to determine risk of ARF has been proposed using the acronym RIFLE: risk, injury, failure, loss, and ESRD.[16] The RIFLE system classifies patients into categories of risk based on GFR criteria, urine output, or previous loss of renal function (Table 20-5).

Prevention Strategies. Principles of prevention include avoiding the use of nephrotoxic drugs in elderly patients and in patients with renal insufficiency or CKD[14,15] and avoiding nonsteroidal antiinflammatory drugs (NSAIDs) for pain relief in patients taking antibiotics or recovering from major surgery.[17] Delaying the use of intravascular x-ray contrast medium until the patient is rehydrated will help preserve kidney function in the high-risk patient.[10,11]

Table **20-4**   Chronic Kidney Disease/Decreased Kidney Function by Stage in Adult U.S. Population

Stage	Population Affected	GFR (ml/min/1.73 m^2)/Diagnosis
1	9 million (3.3%)	Normal; persistent albuminuria
2	5.3 million (3.0%)	60 to 89; persistent albuminuria
3	7.6 million (4.3%)	30 to 59
4	400,000 (0.2%)	15 to 29
5	300,000 (0.2%)	Kidney failure

Data from Coresh J et al: *Am J Kidney Dis* 41:1. 2003.

Table **20-5**   RIFLE Criteria for Acute Renal Dysfunction

RIFLE	Serum CR/GFR Criteria	Urine Output Criteria
Risk	Cr increased 1.5 times above normal *or* GFR decreased more than 25%	<0.5 ml/kg/hr for 6 hours
Injury	Cr increased 2.0 times above normal *or* GFR decreased more than 50%.	<0.5 ml/kg/hr for 12 hours
Failure	Cr increased 3.0 times above normal *or* GFR decreased more than 75%.	<0.5 ml/kg/hr for 24 hours *or* anuria for 12 hours
Loss	Persistent acute renal failure (ARF); complete loss of renal function for more than 4 weeks	
ESRD	End-stage renal disease	

Data from *Acute Dialysis Quality Initiative Newsletter*, Summer-Fall 2002.
GFR, Glomerular filtration rate; CR, creatinine; *anuria*, urine volume less than 100 ml/24 hr.

Fluid Balance

Prerenal failure is caused by decreased perfusion and is often associated with trauma, hemorrhage, hypotension, and major fluid losses. Fluid resuscitation is the only treatment shown to prevent renal failure in these conditions.[18]

The objectives of fluid replacement are to replace fluid and electrolyte losses and to prevent ongoing loss. Maintenance intravenous (IV) fluid therapy is initiated when oral (PO) fluid intake is inadvisable.[1] Maintenance fluids are calculated with consideration for individual body surface area. Adults require approximately 1500 ml/m^2/24 hr; fever, burns, and trauma significantly increase fluid requirements. Other important criteria when calculating fluid volume replacement include baseline metabolism, environmental temperature, and humidity. The rate of replacement depends on cardiopulmonary reserve, adequacy of renal function, fluid balance, ongoing loss, and type of fluid replaced.[16]

Crystalloids and Colloids. Crystalloids and colloids refer to two different types of IV fluids used for volume management in critically ill patients. Crystalloid solutions, which are balanced salt solutions, are in widespread use for both maintenance infusion and replacement therapy. Crystalloid fluids include normal saline solution (0.9 NaCl); half-strength saline solution (0.45 NaCl), and lactated Ringer's (LR) solution (Table 20-6). LR solution should be avoided in patients with renal failure as it may increase hyperkalemia due to the electrolyte additives. A noncrystalloid

solution that may be infused is dextrose (5% or 10%) in water (D$_5$W, D$_{10}$W).

Colloids are solutions containing oncotically active particles that are employed to expand intravascular volume to achieve and maintain hemodynamic stability. Albumin (5% and 25%) and hetastarch are colloid solutions (Table 20-6). Colloids expand intravascular volume and the effect can last as long as 24 hours. The goal is to optimize PAOP or "wedge" pressure, raise mean arterial pressure (MAP), and increase cardiac output (CO) and cardiac index (CI) to a therapeutic level.

Adequacy of IV fluid replacement depends on strict ongoing evaluation and frequent adjustment. Frequent monitoring of serum electrolyte levels is required, and strictly regulated intake and output are correlated with daily weight records. Finally, hemodynamic readings are frequently undertaken. If, following a fluid challenge, the increase in CVP is only minimal, this implies additional fluid replacement is required. Continued decreases in CVP, PAOP, and CI indicate ongoing volume losses. Significant rises in CVP and PAOP, with a fall in CI, may indicate hypervolemia with underlying cardiac failure.

Fluid Restriction. Fluid restriction constitutes a large part of the medical treatment for renal failure. Fluid restriction is used to prevent circulatory overload and development of interstitial edema when excess volume cannot be removed by the kidneys. The fluid requirements are calculated on the basis of daily urine volumes and insensible

Table **20-6** Frequently Used Intravenous Solutions

Solution	Electrolytes	Indications
CRYSTALLOIDS*		
Dextrose in water (D$_5$W)—isotonic	None	Maintain volume. Replace mild loss. Provide minimal calories.
Normal saline solution (0.9% NaCl)	Sodium 154 mEq/L Chloride 154 mEq/L Osmolality 308 mEq/L	Maintain volume. Replace mild loss. Correct mild hyponatremia.
Half-strength saline solution (0.45% NaCl)	Sodium 77 mEq/L Chloride 77 mEq/L	Free water replacement. Correct mild hyponatremia. Free water/electrolyte replacement (fluid/electrolyte-restricted conditions).
Lactated Ringer's solution	Sodium 130 mEq/L Potassium 4 mEq/L Calcium 2.7 mEq/L Chloride 107 mEq/L Lactate 27 mEq/L pH 6.5	Fluid and electrolyte replacement (contraindicated for patients with renal or liver disease or in lactic acidosis).
COLLOIDS		
5% Albumin (Albumisol)	Albumin 50 g/L Sodium 130-160 mEq/L Potassium 1 mEq/L Osmolality 300 mOsm/L Osmotic pressure 20 mm Hg pH 6.4 to 7.4	Volume expansion. Moderate protein replacement. Achievement of hemodynamic stability in shock states.
25% Albumin (salt-poor)	Albumin 240 g/L Globulins 10 g/L Sodium 130-160 mEq/L Osmolality 1500 mOsm/L pH 6.4 to 7.4	Concentrated form of albumin sometimes used with diuretics to move fluid from tissues into the vascular space for diuresis.
Hetastarch	Sodium 154 mEq/L Chloride 154 mEq/L Osmolality 310 mOsm/L Colloid osmotic pressure 30-35 mm Hg	Synthetic polymer (6% solution) used for volume expansion. Hemodynamic volume replacement after cardiac surgery, burns, sepsis.
Low-molecular-weight dextran (LMWD)	Glucose polysaccharide molecules with average molecular weight of 40,000; no electrolytes	Volume expansion and support (contraindicated for patients with bleeding disorders).
High-molecular-weight dextran (HMWD)	Glucose polysaccharide molecules with average molecular weight of 70,000; no electrolytes	Used prophylactically in some cases to prevent platelet aggregation; available in either saline or glucose solutions.

*For the crystalloid solutions that contain electrolytes, specific concentrations of electrolytes and pH will vary according to the manufacturer.

losses. Obtaining daily weights and keeping accurate intake and output records are essential. Renal failure patients are usually restricted to 1 liter of fluid per 24 hours if urine output is 500 ml or less. Insensible losses range from 500 to 750 ml/day.

Fluid Removal. Intrarenal failure promotes the introduction of increased amounts of water, solutes, and potential toxins into the circulation; thus prompt measures are needed to decrease their levels. Diuretics are used to stimulate the urine output. However, hemodialysis or hemofiltration is the treatment of choice, particularly if volume overload creates pulmonary and cardiac compromise. Severe hyperkalemia almost always necessitates hemodialysis because of the life-threatening cardiac dysrhythmias resulting from hyperkalemia. Hemodialysis also may be initiated for severe azotemia when other treatments are contraindicated.

Electrolyte Balance

Potassium. Electrolyte levels require frequent observation, especially in the critical phases of renal failure (see Table 20-3). Potassium may quickly reach levels of 6.0 milliequivalents per liter (mEq/L) and above. Specific ECG changes are associated with hyperkalemia, specifically peaked T waves, a widening of the QRS interval, and ultimately, ventricular tachycardia or fibrillation. If hyperkalemia is present, all potassium supplements are stopped.[19] If the patient is producing urine, IV diuretics can be administered. Acute hyperkalemia can be treated temporarily by IV insulin and glucose. An infusion of 100 ml of 50% dextrose accompanied by 20 units of regular insulin forces potassium out of the serum and into the cells. Sodium bicarbonate (40 to 160 mEq) may be infused to promote greater excretion of potassium in the urine, particularly if the serum pH is below 7.10. Finally, sodium polystyrene sulfonate (Kayexalate), a cation-exchange resin, is mixed in water and sorbitol and given orally, rectally, or through a nasogastric (NG) tube. The resin binds potassium in the bowel, which eliminates it in the feces. Kayexalate and dialysis are the only permanent methods of potassium removal.[19]

Sodium. Dilutional hyponatremia, associated with renal failure is not uncommon (see Table 20-3). It can be corrected over a few days with fluid restriction. Sodium levels may be raised more rapidly during dialysis by changing the amount of sodium in the dialysate bath.

Calcium and Phosphorus. Calcium levels are reduced (hypocalcemia) in renal failure (see Table 20-3). This reduction results from multiple factors, including hyperphosphatemia. At the renal level, calcium and phosphorus are regulated in part by parathyroid hormone (PTH). Normally, PTH helps calcium be reabsorbed into the proximal tubule and distal nephron and promotes excretion of phosphate by the kidney to maintain homeostasis. Medications that bind phosphorus in the GI tract (e.g., aluminum hydroxide) are administered orally or via NG tube. Phosphorus occurs in many foods and unless eliminated will pass from the GI tract into the bloodstream. The binding agent is taken with a meal, and once the dietary phosphorus is bound to a secondary substance in the bowel, it is eliminated from the body with stool. This lowers the serum phosphorus level and increases the calcium blood level. Most calcium is bound to protein in the bloodstream. The metabolically active, nonbound portion is known as the *ionized calcium*. Maintaining adequate calcium stores is important and is achieved by administration of calcium supplements, vitamin D preparations, and synthetic calcitriol.

Nutrition

The renal diet restricts the electrolytes potassium, sodium, and phosphorus. It also limits protein intake to control azotemia (increased BUN). Fluids are limited. By contrast, carbohydrates are encouraged, to provide energy for metabolism and healing.[20]

Medications

The first step is to eliminate any nephrotoxic medications. Second, if drugs are eliminated through the kidneys, it is important to decrease the frequency of administration (e.g., from every 6 hours to every 12 hours) or to decrease the dose and to monitor the serum concentration by measuring serum drug levels.[17]

Diuretics. Diuretics are used to stimulate urinary output in the fluid overloaded patient with functioning kidneys. Care must be taken in their use to avoid the creation of secondary electrolyte abnormalities. Diuretic therapy is thought to increase renal blood flow, GFR, and intratubular pressure. The loop diuretic *furosemide* (Lasix) is the most frequently employed diuretic. It may be prescribed as a bolus dose or as a continuous infusion; concurrent use of furosemide preceded by synergistic thiazide diuretics, such as metolazone, is also seen. Newer agents that may increase diuresis include the natriuretic peptides (ANP and BNP), which work by stimulating natriuretic receptors in the myocardium, and fenoldopam (Corlopam), a selective dopamine receptor agonist that vasodilates the systemic and renal vasculature. Osmotic diuretics (Mannitol) are also prescribed to decrease fluid overload and improve urine output. Once renal failure with oliguria is present, diuretics do not appear to promote renal recovery.[21]

Dopamine. Low dose dopamine (2 to 3 mcg/kg/min) also known as "renal dose dopamine" is frequently infused to stimulate renal blood flow. Dopamine is effective in increasing urine output in the short term, but dopamine renal-receptor tolerance to the drug is theorized to develop in the critically ill patients who are most at risk for development of ARF.[22] A recent meta-analysis found that renal dose dopamine did not prevent onset of ARF and did not decrease the need for dialysis or reduce mortality.[23] At this point the proof for routine use of low-dose dopamine for the prevention of renal failure remains anecdotal only.[24]

Nursing Management

Nursing management of ARF patients involves a variety of nursing diagnoses (Box 20-3). **Nursing priorities for the patient with acute renal disease are directed toward (1) recognizing risk factors for development of acute renal failure, (2) preventing infectious complications, (3) optimizing fluid balance, (4) avoiding electrolyte imbalance, (5) preventing anemia, and (6) providing patient education.**

Recognizing Risk Factors

Some individuals have an increased risk of developing ARF as a complication during their hospitalization, and the alert critical care nurse recognizes potential risk factors and acts as a patient advocate.[14,15] Patients at risk include elderly persons because GFR may be decreased, dehydrated patients because hypoperfusion of the kidneys may lead to ischemic ATN, patients with increased creatinine levels before their hospitalization, and patients undergoing a radiologic procedure involving contrast dye.[10,11]

Preventing Infectious Complications

The critical care patient with ARF is at risk for infectious complications.[3] Signs of infection, such as increased white blood cell (WBC) count, redness at a wound or IV site, or increased temperature, are always a cause for concern. A urinary catheter is inserted to facilitate accurate urine measurement and patient comfort. However, any indwelling catheter is a potential source for infection.[3] Therefore, if the patient stops making large quantities of urine, the catheter is removed and a scheduled "straight catheterization" is performed to minimize the risk of infection from an indwelling catheter and drainage system. This method allows the patient's bladder to be emptied but the catheter does not remain in place. Pulmonary hygiene is maintained by asking the patient to cough and deep-breathe frequently if they are awake and alert. If intubated and ventilated, frequent turning, endotracheal suctioning, and frequent mouth care become mandatory. If the patient is immobile, changes of position and observation of potential sites for skin breakdown help avoid creating sites for infection.

Optimizing Fluid Balance

Assessment of fluid balance is often done on an hourly basis in the critically ill patient who has hemodynamic lines inserted. Hemodynamic values (HR, BP, CVP, PAOP, CO, CI) and daily weights are correlated with the intake and output. Urine output is measured hourly, via a catheter and drainage bag, throughout all phases of ARF, particularly in response to diuretics. Any fluid removed with dialysis is recorded in the fluid balance. Recognition of the clinical signs and symptoms of fluid overload is important. Excess fluid will move from the vascular system into the peripheral tissues (dependent edema), abdomen (ascites), the lungs (crackles, pulmonary edema and pleura effusions), around the heart (pericardial effusion), and into the brain (intracranial swelling).

Avoiding Electrolyte Imbalance

Hyperkalemia, hypocalcemia, hyponatremia, hyperphosphatemia, and acid-base imbalances all occur during ARF (see Table 20-3).[2] Clinical manifestations of these electrolyte imbalances must be prevented and their associated side effects controlled. The imbalances that are the most potential hazards are hyperkalemia and hypocalcemia, which can result in life-threatening cardiac dysrhythmias. Dilutional hyponatremia may develop as fluid overload worsens in the patient with oliguria. Monitoring the serum sodium level is important to prevent this complication. Hyperphosphatemia results in severe pruritus. Nursing care is directed at soothing the itching by performing frequent skin care with emollients, discouraging scratching, and administering phosphate-binding medications. The acid-base imbalances that occur with renal failure are monitored by arterial blood gas (ABG) analysis. The goal of treatment is to maintain the pH within the normal range.

Preventing Anemia

Anemia is an expected side effect of renal failure that occurs because the kidney no longer produces the hormone *erythropoietin*. Thus the bone marrow is not stimulated to produce red blood cells (RBCs). Care is taken to prevent blood loss in the patient with ARF, and blood withdrawal is minimized as much as possible. Irritation of the GI tract from metabolic waste accumulation is expected, and GI bleeding is a possibility. Stool, NG drainage, and emesis are routinely tested for occult blood. Anemia is treated pharmacologically by the administration of epoetin alfa (Procrit, Epogen) to stimulate erythrocyte production by the bone marrow and, if required, by RBC transfusion.[25]

Providing Patient Education

It is vital to provide accurate and uncomplicated information to the patient and family about ARF, including its prognosis, treatment, and possible complications. Education of the patient can be challenging because elevations of BUN and creatinine can negatively impact level of consciousness. Also, sleep-rest disorders and emotional upset often occur as complications of ARF and can disrupt short-term memory. Encouraging the patient and family to voice concerns, frustrations, or fears and allowing the patient to control some aspects of the acute care environment and treatment also are essential.

Collaborative Management

Management of the patient with acute renal dysfunction is complex and requires the expertise of many different health care clinicians (Box 20-4). Recently developed clinical guidelines[15] and those in process[16] can be used to guide the health care team in determining priority interventions for this high-risk group of patients.

DIALYSIS

A wide range of options are available for the treatment of ARF, including hemodialysis, peritoneal dialysis, and continuous renal replacement therapy (CRRT).[1,3]

Hemodialysis

Hemodialysis roughly translates as "separating from the blood." Indications and contraindications for hemodialysis are listed in Box 20-5. As a treatment, hemodialysis literally separates and removes from the blood the excess electrolytes, fluids, and toxins by use of a dialyzer (Figure 20-1). Although efficient in removing chemicals, it does not remove all metabolites. Furthermore, electrolytes, toxins, and fluids increase between treatments, requiring hemodialysis on a regular basis. Each dialysis treatment takes 3 to 4 hours. In the acute phases of renal failure, dialysis is performed daily. The dialysis frequency gradually decreases to three times per week as the patient moves into a more chronic phase of renal failure.

Hemodialyzer

Hemodialysis works by circulating blood outside the body through synthetic tubing to a dialyzer, which consists of hol-

---

Box 20-5 Indications and Contraindications for Hemodialysis

INDICATIONS

Blood urea nitrogen (BUN) > 90 mg/dl
Serum creatinine > 9 mg/dl
Hyperkalemia
Drug toxicity
Intravascular and extravascular fluid overload
Metabolic acidosis
Symptoms of uremia
- Pericarditis
- Gastrointestinal bleeding
Mental changes
Contraindications to other forms of dialysis

CONTRAINDICATIONS

Hemodynamic instability
Inability to anticoagulate
Lack of access to circulation

---

low-fiber tubes. The dialyzer is sometimes described as an "artificial kidney" (Figure 20-2). While the blood flows through the membranes, which are semipermeable, a fluid "dialysate bath" bathes the membranes and, through osmosis and diffusion, performs exchanges of fluid, electrolytes, and toxins from the blood to the bath, where toxins and dialysate then pass out of the artificial kidney. The blood and the dialysate bath are shunted in opposite directions (countercurrent flow) through the dialyzer to match the osmotic and chemical gradients at the most efficient level for effective dialysis.

Ultrafiltration

To remove fluid, a positive hydrostatic pressure is applied to the blood and a negative hydrostatic pressure is applied to the dialysate bath. The two forces together, called *transmembrane pressure*, pull and squeeze the excess fluid from the blood. The difference between the two values (expressed in millimeters of mercury [mm Hg]) represents the transmembrane pressure and results in fluid extraction, known as *ultrafiltration*, from the vascular space.

Anticoagulation

Either heparin or sodium citrate is added to the system just before the blood enters the dialyzer to anticoagulate the blood within the dialysis tubing. Without an anticoagulant the blood will clot because its passage through the foreign tubular substances of the dialysis machine activates the clotting mechanism. Heparin can be administered either by bolus injection or intermittent infusion. It has a short half-life and its effects subside within 2 to 4 hours. If necessary, the effects of heparin are easily reversed with the antidote protamine. Citrate can also be infused as an anticoagulant via intermittent bolus or continuous infusion.

Box 20-4 COLLABORATIVE Management

Acute Renal Failure (ARF)

1. **Assess risk of renal failure.**
   - Assess baseline renal function on all patients at risk for development of ARF.
2. **Protect the kidneys.**
   - If patient has preexisting renal dysfunction, avoid nephrotoxic drugs, limit exposure to radiologic contrast dye, and avoid both hypotension and hypovolemia.
3. **Monitor urine output.**
   - Intervene for low urine output before patient is oliguric or anuric for several hours (see Table 20-5).
4. **Supply nutrition.**
   - Oral, enteral, or parenteral nutrition is needed to combat catabolism in critically ill patient with renal dysfunction.
5. **Provide renal replacement.**
   - If patient has lost renal function during acute illness, replace kidney function with hemodialysis or CRRT as indicated.

CRRT, Continuous renal replacement therapy.

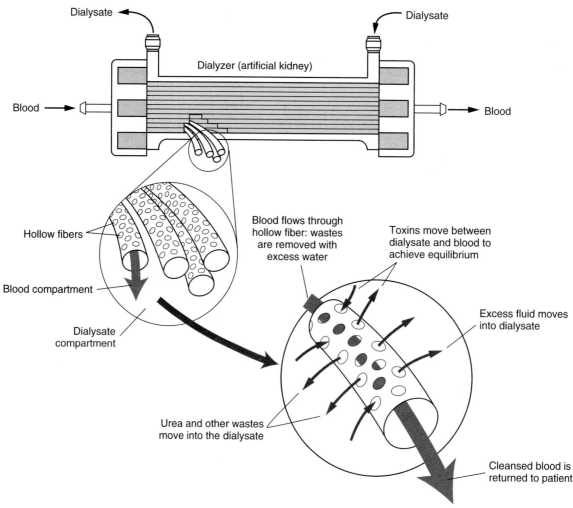

Dialysate

Dialysate

Dialyzer (artificial kidney)

Blood

Blood

Hollow fibers

Blood flows through
hollow fiber: wastes
are removed with
excess water

Toxins move between
dialysate and blood to
achieve equilibrium

Blood compartment

Excess fluid moves
into dialysate

Dialysate
compartment

Urea and other wastes
move into the dialysate

Cleansed blood is
returned to patient

Figure 20-1   Hemodialyzer.

Vascular Access

Hemodialysis requires access to the bloodstream. Various types of temporary and permanent devices are in clinical use. It is important for patient safety to be able to recognize these different vascular access devices and to properly care for them. The following section discusses temporary vascular access catheters used in the acute hospital environment and permanent methods used for long-term hemodialysis.

Temporary Acute Access. *Subclavian* and *femoral* veins are catheterized when short-term access is required or when existing vascular access is nonfunctional in a patient requiring immediate hemodialysis. Both subclavian and femoral catheters are routinely inserted at the bedside. Most temporary catheters are venous only. Blood flows out towards the dialyzer and flows back to the patient via the same vein. A dual-lumen venous catheter is the most commonly seen. It has a central partition running the length of the catheter. The outflow catheter section pulls the blood flow through openings that are proximal to the inflow openings on the

opposite side. This design avoids dialyzing the same blood just returned to the area (recirculation), which would severely reduce the procedure's efficiency. A silicone rubber, dual-lumen catheter with a polyester cuff designed to decrease catheter-related infections is also available.

Permanent Vascular Access. The common denominator in pernament vascular access devices is a connection to the arterial circulation and a return conduit to the venous circulation.

Arteriovenous Fistula. The arteriovenous (AV) fistula is created by surgically visualizing a peripheral artery and vein; creating a side-by-side opening in the artery and the vein; and joining the two vessels together. The high arterial flow creates a swelling of the vein, or a pseudoaneurysm, at which point (when healed) a large-bore needle can be inserted to obtain arterial outflow to the dialyzer. Inflow is accomplished through a second large-bore needle inserted into a peripheral vein distal to the fistula (Figure 20-3, A). If the patient's vessels are adequate, fistulas are the preferred

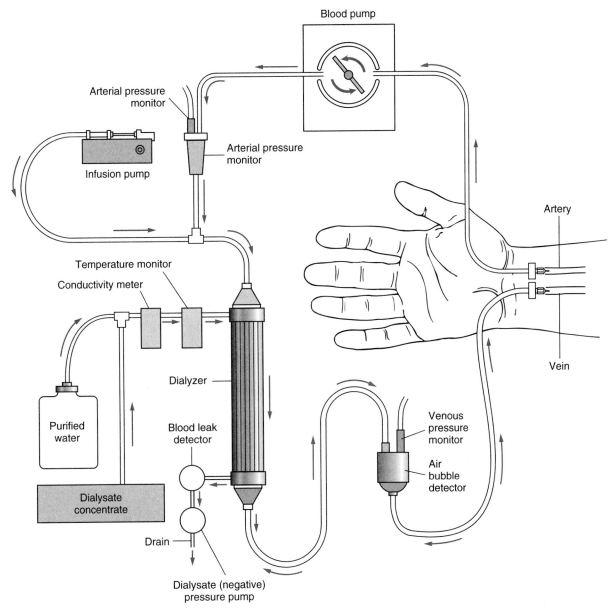

Figure 20-2 Components of a hemodialysis system.

mode of access because of the durability of blood vessels, relatively few complications, and less need for revision compared with other access methods. However, an initial disadvantage of a fistula concerns the time required for development of sufficient arterial flow to enlarge the new access. The time lag until the fistula can be used for dialysis can be long, often requiring weeks to months.

Caring for a patient with a fistula has some important nursing priorities to ensure the ongoing viability of the vascular access and safety of the limb (Table 20-7). The critical care nurse frequently assesses the quality of blood flow through the fistula. A patent fistula has a thrill when palpated gently with the fingers and a bruit if auscultated with a stethoscope. The extremity should be pink and warm to the

touch. No blood pressure measurements, IV infusions, or laboratory phlebotomy are performed on the arm with the fistula.

Arteriovenous Grafts. AV grafts are the most often used access for treating chronic renal failure. The graft is a tube formed of Gortex, which is surgically implanted in the limb. The area is surgically opened, and an artery and a vein are located. A tunnel is created in the tissue where the graft is placed. Anastomoses are made with the graft ends connected to the artery and vein. The blood is allowed to flow through the graft, and the surgical area is closed. The graft creates a raised area that looks like a large peripheral vein just under the skin and peripheral tissue layers (Figure 20-3, B). Two large-bore needles are used for outflow and inflow to

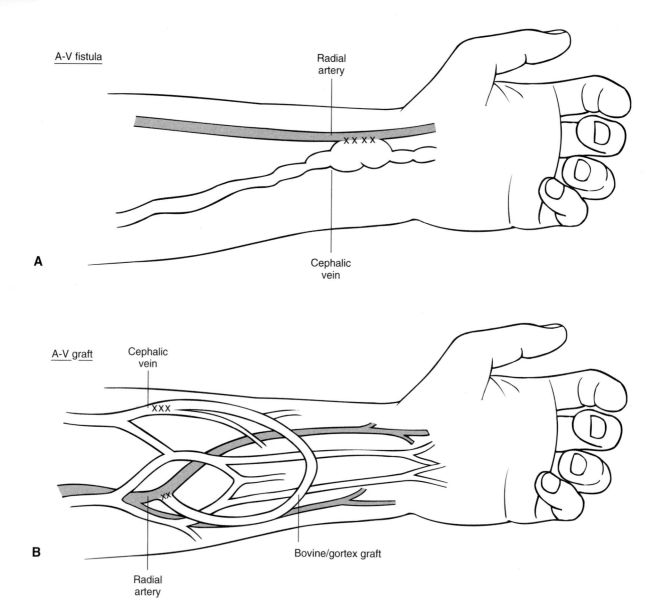

A-V fistula

Radial
artery

x x x x

A

Cephalic
vein

A-V graft

Cephalic
vein

xxx

xx

B

Radial
artery

Bovine/gortex graft

Figure 20-3   Methods of vascular access for hemodialysis. **A,** Arteriovenous fistula between vein and artery. **B,** Internal synthetic graft connects artery and vein.

the graft. For both grafts and fistulas, after needle removal at the end of the hemodialysis treatment, firm pressure must be applied to stem bleeding (Table 20-7).

Medical Management

Medical management involves the decision to place a vascular access device and then to choose the most appropriate type and location for each patient. Patients in the critical care setting require vascular access if they suffer from ARF and require hemodialysis. The exact quantity of fluid and/or solute removal to be achieved via hemodialysis is determined individually for each patient by clinical examination and review of all relevant laboratory results.

Nursing Management

Nursing priorities for the patient with acute renal failure receiving hemodialysis are directed toward (1) maintaining hemodialysis vascular access, (2) monitoring patient hemodynamic stability during dialysis, and (3) providing education about the disease process and treatment plan to patient and family.

Continuous Renal Replacement Therapy

Continuous renal replacement therapy (CRRT) is a newer mode of dialysis that has many similarities to traditional hemodialysis. CRRT has the advantage of being a continuous therapy lasting 12 hours or longer, where the venous

Table 20-7 Complications and Nursing Management of Arteriovenous Fistula/Graft

Type	Complications	Nursing Management
Fistula	Thrombosis Infection Pseudoaneurysm Vascular steal syndrome Venous hypertension Carpal tunnel syndrome Inadequate blood flow	Teach patients to avoid wearing constrictive clothing on limbs containing access. Teach patients to avoid sleeping on or prolonged bending of accessed limb. Use aseptic technique when cannulating access. Avoid repetitious cannulation of one segment of access. Offer comfort measures, such as warm compresses and ordered analgesics, to lessen pain of vascular steal. Teach patients to develop blood flow in the fistulas through exercises (squeezing a rubber ball) while applying mild impedance to flow just distal to the access (at least once per day for 10-15 minutes). Avoid too-early cannulation of new access.
Graft	Bleeding Thrombosis False aneurysm formation Infection Arterial or venous stenosis Vascular steal syndrome	Teach patients to avoid wearing constrictive clothing on accessed limbs. Avoid repeated cannulation of one segment of access. Use aseptic technique when cannulating access. Monitor for changes in arterial or venous pressure while patients are on dialysis. Provide comfort measures to reduce pain of vascular steal (e.g., warm compresses, analgesics as ordered).

blood is circulated through a highly porous hemofilter.[26] Unlike traditional hemodialysis, it is rare to use an artery to vein catheter system today; blood access and return is through a venous catheter in the majority of cases. The CRRT system allows for continuous fluid removal from the plasma, the amount ranging from 5 to 45 ml/minute, depending on the particular CRRT system used, plus removal of urea, creatinine, and electrolytes (Table 20-8 and Figure 20-4). The removed fluid is described as *ultrafiltrate*. In an ideal situation the hydrostatic pressure exerted by a mean arterial blood pressure (MAP) greater than 70 mm Hg would propel a continuous flow of blood through the hemofilter to remove fluid and solute. However, because many critically ill patients are hypotensive and cannot provide adequate flow through the hemofilter, an electric roller pump "milks" the tubing to augment flow. If large amounts of fluid are to be removed, IV replacement solutions are infused. Indications and contraindications for CRRT are described in Box 20-6.

Because controlled removal and replacement of fluid are possible over many hours or days with CRRT, hemodynamic stability is maintained. This makes CRRT highly advantageous for use in the patient with multisystem problems. The possible forms of CRRT are (1) slow continuous ultrafiltration (SCUF), (2) continuous venovenous hemofiltration (CVVH), and (3) continuous venovenous hemodialysis (CVVHD). The decision as to which type of therapy to initiate is based on myriad factors, including clinical assessment, metabolic status, severity of uremia, and whether a particular treatment modality is available at that institution.

Slow Continuous Ultrafiltration

SCUF, as the name implies, slowly removes fluid, 100 to 300 ml/hr, through a process of ultrafiltration. This consists of an exchange of fluid, solutes, and solvents across a semipermeable membrane.[27] Because small amounts of fluid are removed via this process, it is a suitable choice for patients with acute heart failure and diminished renal perfusion who are unresponsive to diuretics. SCUF is an infrequent clinical choice, primarily because it requires both arterial and venous access for effective functioning.

Continuous Venovenous Hemofiltration

Continuous hemofiltration is indicated when the patient's clinical condition warrants removal of significant volumes of fluid and solutes. Fluid is removed by ultrafiltration in volumes of 5 to 20 ml/min or 7 to 30 L/24 hr.[16] Increased removal

Table 20-8 Comparison of Continuous Renal Replacement Therapy Methods

Type	Ultrafiltration Rate	Fluid Replacement	Indication
SCUF	100-300 ml/hr	None	Fluid removal
CVVH	500-800 ml/hr	Predilution or postdilution, calculating hourly net loss	Fluid removal, moderate solute removal
CVVHD	500-800 ml/hr	Predilution or postdilution, subtracting dialysate, then calculating hourly net loss	Fluid removal, maximum solute removal

SCUF, Slow continuous ultrafiltration; *CVVH,* continuous venovenous hemofiltration; *CVVHD,* continuous venovenous hemodialysis.

of solutes such as urea, creatinine, and other nonprotein-bound toxins is accomplished by increasing flow through the hemofilter via the addition of a prehemofilter replacement fluid (Figure 20-4, *B*). Although arterial vascular access was often required when CRRT was first developed, systems that circulate only venous blood are currently used.

As with other CRRT systems, the blood outside the body is anticoagulated and the ultrafiltrate is drained off either by gravity or by the addition of negative-pressure suction into a large drainage bag. Because large volumes of fluid may be removed in CVVH, some of the removed ultrafiltrate volume must be replaced hourly with a continuous infusion to avoid intravascular dehydration. Replacement fluids may consist of standard solutions of bicarbonate, potassium-free LR solution, acetate, or dextrose. Electrolytes such as potassium, sodium, calcium chloride, magnesium sulfate, and sodium bicarbonate also may be added.[14] The following formula (with example) can be used to calculate the volume removed from the patient:

$$\text{Ultrafiltrate in bag} - (\text{CVVH replacement fluid} + \text{IV/oral/NG intake}) = \text{Output}$$
$$1000\ ml - 800\ ml = 200\ ml/hr\ output$$

Continuous Venovenous Hemodialysis

CVVHD is technically different from the two previously described methods because of a slow (15 to 30 ml/min) countercurrent drainage flow on the membrane side of the hemofilter (Figure 20-4, *C*). Countercurrent flow is through the hemodialyzer. *Countercurrent* means the blood flows in one direction and the dialysate flows in the opposite direction. This increases the clearance of uremic toxins and makes it more like traditional hemodialysis.[27] This is the most efficient form of CRRT. As with other types of CRRT and dialysis, while arterial access is always possible, venous-only vascular access is the most common choice today.

CVVHD is indicated for patients who require large-volume removal for severe uremia or critical acid-base imbalances or who are diuretic-resistant. A MAP of at least 70 mm Hg is desirable for effective volume removal and dialysis, and it is most effective when used over days, not hours. The use of replacement fluid is optional and depends on the patient's clinical condition and plan of care. The critical care nurse is responsible for calculating the hourly intake and output, noting fluid trends, and replacing excessive losses. This therapy is ideal for hemodynamically unstable patients in the critical care setting because they do not experience the abrupt fluid and solute changes that can accompany standard hemodialysis treatments.[26]

Complications

Complications associated with CRRT are listed in Table 20-9.[27,28]

Medical Management

The choice of which blood purification to use in ARF is a medical decision. Age, gender, and preexisting chronic conditions are of little help in determining the need for hemofiltration or hemodialysis.[29] Often the acute clinical diagnosis, physician preference, availability of the CRRT machine, and knowledgeable physicians and nurses at the hospital are the deciding factors. Infectious complications are associated with a grave prognosis. Dialysis is prescribed for almost anyone who develops severe ARF unless the patient is clearly dying.

Intermittent hemodialysis or CCRT is usually begun before the BUN level exceeds 90 mg/dl or the creatinine exceeds 9 mg/dl. Whether daily treatment is more effective than treatment every other day is controversial.

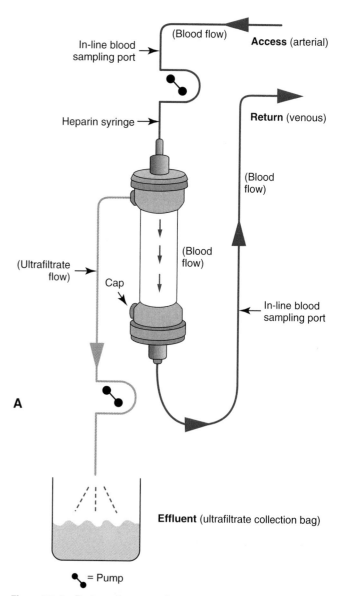

Figure 20-4   For legend see opposite page.

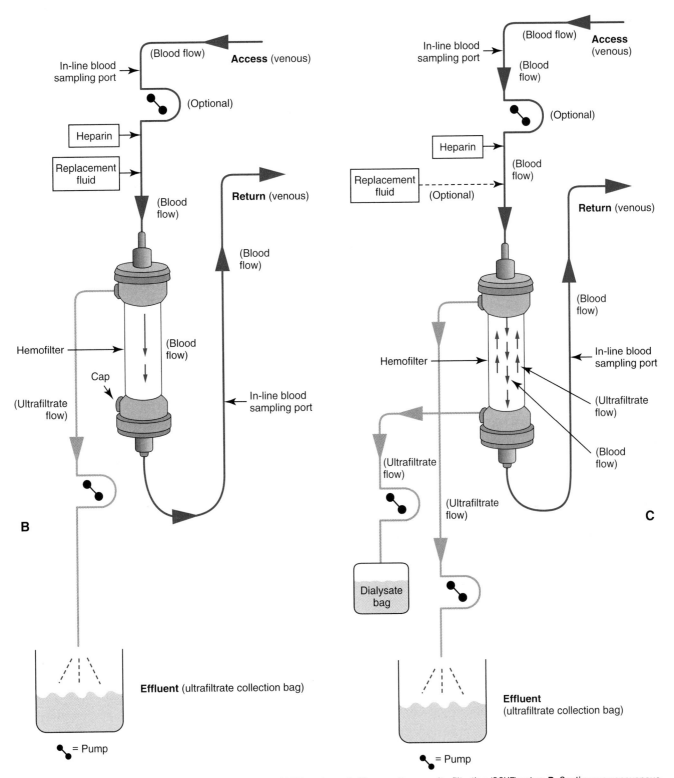

Figure 20-4, cont'd   Continuous renal replacement therapy (CRRT) systems. **A**, Slow, continuous ultrafiltration (SCUF) setup. **B**, Continuous venovenous hemofiltration (CVVH). **C**, Continuous venovenous hemofiltration dialysis (CVVHD).

Box **20-6**	Indications and Contraindications for CRRT

INDICATIONS

Need for large fluid volume removal in hemodynamically unstable patient

Hypervolemic or edematous patients unresponsive to diuretic therapy

Patients with multiple organ dysfunction syndrome

Ease of fluid management in patients requiring large daily fluid volume

- Replacement for oliguria
- TPN administration

Contraindications to hemodialysis and peritoneal dialysis

Inability to be anticoagulated

CONTRAINDICATIONS

Hematocrit >45%

Terminal illness

CRRT, Continuous renal replacement therapy; *TPN,* total parenteral nutrition, > greater than.

The patient's serum creatinine, BUN, and fluid volume status are the deciding factors. CRRT is often prescribed when the BUN level is approximately 60 mg/dl. CRRT is more effective in the early stages of ARF. If severe electrolyte imbalance or fluid overload is present, even earlier intervention may be required.

Nursing Management

Critical care nurses play a vital role in monitoring the patient receiving hemodialysis and hemofiltration. **Nursing priorities are directed toward (1) monitoring fluid intake and output, (2) preventing and detecting potential complications** (e.g., bleeding, hypotension), **(3) trending electrolyte laboratory values, (4) supervising safe operation of CRRT equipment,** and **(5) providing patient and family education.**

Peritoneal Dialysis

Peritoneal dialysis (PD) is a modality used in patients with chronic kidney disease. When a PD-dependent patient is admitted to the critical care unit with an unrelated acute illness, PD is continued. PD is not an intervention used for acute renal failure.[30] PD involves the introduction of sterile dialyzing fluid through an implanted catheter into the abdominal cavity. The dialysate bathes the peritoneal membrane, which covers the abdominal organs and overlies the capillary beds that support the organs. By the processes of osmosis, diffusion, and active transport, excess fluid and solutes travel from the peritoneal capillary fluid through the capillary walls, through the peritoneal membrane, and into the dialyzing fluid. After a selected period the fluid is drained out of the abdomen by gravity (Figure 20-5). The process is then repeated at regular prescribed intervals.[31]

Indications for PD include uremia, volume overload, electrolyte imbalances, hemodynamic instability, lack of access to circulation, and removal of high-molecular-weight toxins. In the critical care unit, patients who have PD at home may be admitted with a nonrenal critical illness but will continue to receive PD for chronic renal failure in the critical care unit (Box 20-7).

The peritoneal membrane's structure and capillary blood flow to the peritoneum account for the relatively slow nature of PD. The small capillary pores, the capillary membrane, the interstitium, the mesothelium of the peritoneum, and the fluid film layers in the capillary and the peritoneal cavity provide formidable barriers to fluid and solute passage.

The volume of dialysate instilled into the abdomen affects the clearance. Normally, the patients are well versed in the amount, type, and frequency of dialysate to be infused into their abdomen with subsequent drainage by gravity into a "waste" bag. The primary nursing duty is to avoid contamination of the access point and monitor patient's vital signs during this process. The dialysate should be instilled at body temperature to be comfortable, provide some vasodilation, and provide increased solute transport in the peritoneum. The length of time the solution remains in the peritoneal cavity (*dwell time*) and the solution composition affect the outcome. The dwell time affects the amount of fluid removed from the peritoneal capillaries, although a longer dwell time will not remove proportionately more fluid because of osmotic equilibration across the membranes. The various glucose concentrations of the dialysate provide for different rates of fluid removal.

Catheter Placement

Most catheters have four segments: an external segment outside the abdomen, a tunnel segment that passes through subcutaneous tissue and muscle, a cuff for stabilization at the peritoneal membrane, and an internal segment with numerous holes for fast delivery and drainage of dialysate (Figure 20-6). The infusion and removal of the dialysate fluid are sterile procedures.

The most significant risk to the patient with PD is development of peritonitis secondary to intraabdominal contamination and infection. The critical care nurse must be acutely aware of the signs and symptoms of systemic infection, such as a sudden rise in WBCs, increased temperature and malaise. At the same time the nurse remains vigilant for signs of localized catheter or abdominal infection manifested by catheter site redness, site swelling, abdominal tenderness, or cloudy ultrafiltrate following the dwell time.

Medical Management

PD is used for long-term chronic renal failure. It is almost never used as a first-line acute care intervention. If a chronic renal failure patient uses PD at home then medical management will continue during the acute care hospitalization.

Table **20-9** Complications Associated With CRRT

Complication	Etiology	Clinical Manifestations	Nursing Management
Decreased ultrafiltration rate	Hypotension Dehydration Kinked lines Bending of catheters Clotting of filter	Ultrafiltration rate decreased Minimal flow through blood lines	Observe filter and arteriovenous system. Control blood flow. Control coagulation time. Position patient on back. Lower height of collection container.
Filter clotting	Obstruction Insufficient heparinization	Ultrafiltration rate decreased, despite height of collection container being lower	Control heparinization. Maintain continuous heparinization. Call physician. Remove system. Prime catheters with heparin. Prime new system; connect it. Start predilution with 1000 ml saline 0.9% solution per hour. Do not use three-way stopcocks.
Hypotension	Increased ultrafiltration rate Blood leak Disconnection of one of lines	Bleeding	Control amount of ultrafiltration. Control access sites. Clamp lines. Call physician.
Fluid and electrolyte changes	To much/too little removal of fluid Inappropriate replacement of electrolytes Inappropriate dialysate	Changes in mentation ↑ or ↓ CVP, ↑ or ↓ PAOP, ECG change ↑ or ↓ BP and heart rate Abnormal electrolyte levels	Observe for: • Changes in CVP/PAOP. • Changes in vital signs. • ECG changes resulting from electrolyte abnormalities. Monitor output values every hour. Control ultrafiltration.
Bleeding	System disconnection ↑ Heparin dose	Oozing from catheter insertion site or connection	Monitor ACT no less than once every hour. Adjust heparin dose within specifications to maintain ACT. Observe dressing on vascular access for blood loss. Observe for blood in filtrate (filter leak).
Access dislodgment or infection	Catheter or connections not secured Break in sterile technique Excessive patient movement	Bleeding from catheter site or connections Inappropriate flow/infusion Fever Drainage at catheter site	Observe access site at least once every 2 hours. Ensure that clamps are available within easy reach at all times. Observe strict sterile technique when dressing vascular access.

CRRT, Continuous renal replacement therapy; *CVP,* central venous pressure; *PAOP,* pulmonary artery occlusion pressure or "wedge" pressure; *BP,* blood pressure; *ECG,* electrocardiogram; *ACT,* activated coagulation time.

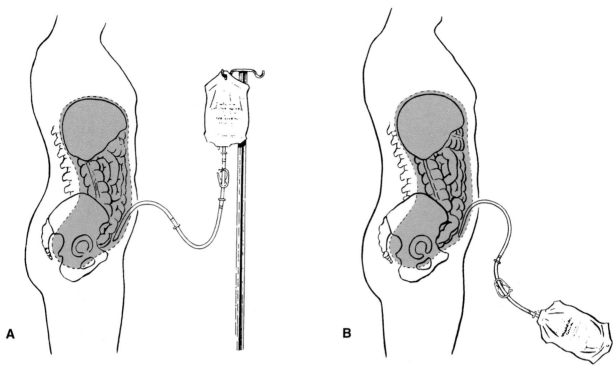

Figure 20-5   Peritoneal dialysis. **A**, Inflow. **B**, Outflow (drains by gravity). (From Thompson JM et al: *Mosby's clinical nursing*, ed 4, St Louis, 1997, Mosby.)

Box **20-7**   **Indications and Contraindications for Peritoneal Dialysis**

INDICATIONS

Uremia
Volume overload
Electrolyte imbalances
Hemodynamic instability
Lack of access to circulation
Removal of high-molecular-weight toxins
Patients with nonrenal critical illness receiving peritoneal dialysis for chronic renal failure
Severe cardiovascular disease
Inability to anticoagulate
Contraindication to hemodialysis

CONTRAINDICATIONS

Recent abdominal surgery
History of abdominal surgeries with adhesions and scarring
Significant pulmonary disease
Need for rapid fluid removal
Peritonitis

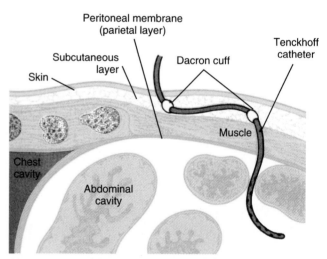

Figure 20-6   Tenckhoff catheter used in peritoneal dialysis. (From Lewis SM, Heitkemper MM, Dirksen SR: *Medical-surgical nursing assessment and management of clinical problems*, ed 5, St Louis, 2000, Mosby.)

This reason for the hospitalization is often for a condition unrelated to the kidneys.

Nursing Management

Nursing management of the patient receiving peritoneal dialysis is directed toward prevention and detection of complications related to PD (Table 20-10). **Nursing priorities focus on observing for signs and symptoms of infection, (2) monitoring fluid volume status, (3) infusing the dialysate fluid, (4) observing drainage of the ultrafiltrate fluid, and (5) preventing complications with the PD catheter.**

Table **20-10**   Complications Associated with Peritoneal Dialysis

Complication	Nursing Management
Peritonitis	Assess for signs and symptoms: cloudy effluent, abdominal pain, rebound tenderness, nausea and vomiting, fever. Obtain effluent sample for culture. Administer antibiotics as ordered. Teach patient/family signs and symptoms and prevention.
Exit site infection	Monitor site daily for signs and symptoms of infection: induration, erythema, purulence, hyperthermia. Increase daily cleaning of site. Apply topical antibiotics as ordered (controversial). Teach patient/family to avoid agents such as creams and lotions around exit site.
Catheter-tunnel infection	Assess for signs and symptoms of infection: pain along tunnel, induration for several centimeters away from catheter, erythema leading away from exit site, drainage at exit site or as tunnel is "milked" toward exit site. Teach patient/family signs and symptoms of infection. Teach patient/family to avoid pulls or tugs on catheter or trauma to exit site. Emphasize need to maintain cleansing regimen at exit site.
Fluid obstruction	Change position of patient (standing, lying, side-lying, knee-chest). Relieve patient's constipation. Irrigate the catheter. Ensure that sufficient fluid is in abdomen (sometimes requires a residual reservoir of approximately 50 ml).
Rectal pain	Ensure a sufficient reservoir of fluid. Use slow infusion rate.
Shoulder pain	Ensure that all air is primed from infusion tubing. Attempt draining the effluent with patient in knee-chest position. Administer mild analgesics as ordered.
Hernia	Monitor for increase in size of or pain in area of hernia. Decrease volume of exchanges as ordered. Dialyze with patients in the supine position. Use abdominal binder or support for patients (as long as not binding on catheter exit site). Avoid initiation of peritoneal dialysis until exit site healing has taken place (approximately 1 to 2 weeks) if possible.
Fluid overload	Increase use of hypertonic solutions. Decrease oral (PO) fluid intake. Shorten dwell times. Weigh patients frequently. Monitor lung sounds and peripheral edema.
Dehydration	Assess patients for decreased skin turgor, muscle cramps, hypotension, tachycardia, and dizziness. Discontinue hypertonic solutions. Increase PO fluid intake. Lengthen dwell times.
Blood-tinged effluent	Monitor for change in effluent color (clear yellow to pink or rusty). Administer heparin, as ordered, to avoid fibrin formation. Obtain patient history about catheter trauma and patient activity before appearance of complication.

PHARMACOLOGY

Diuretics are prescribed frequently in the critical care setting because they are used to increase water excretion via the kidneys. These medications are usually administered by IV bolus, although they are also effective by continuous direct infusion. As urine output declines, diuretics are prescribed to increase urine flow through the renal tubules.

Many medications are eliminated from the body by renal excretion. In determining whether renal failure will affect drug clearance from the body, the amount of unchanged drug that is excreted by the kidney is considered. The health care team must look at the dose, interval between doses, metabolites and combination of medications to avoid accumulation of drug in the serum.

The critical care nurse is cognizant of those drugs that are eliminated by the kidney and that are dialyzed during hemodialysis. The molecular weight of medications, the higher water solubility of some medications that makes them easily removed by dialysis, or the ability of the medications to bind with proteins and therefore not be removed by dialysis are factors that affect the serum blood level of the medication.

REFERENCES

1. Racusen LC: Pathology of acute renal failure: structure/function correlations, *Adv Ren Replace Ther* 4(2):3, 1997.
2. Stark, JS: Acute renal failure: focus on advances in acute tubular necrosis, *Crit Care Nurs Clin North Am* 10:159, 1998.
3. Esson ML, Schrier RW: Diagnosis and treatment of acute tubular necrosis, *Ann Intern Med* 137:744, 2002.
4. Kellum JA et al: Developing a consensus classification system for acute renal failure, *Curr Opin Crit Care* 8:509, 2002.
5. Marini J, Wheeler A: *Critical care medicine: the essentials*, ed 2, Baltimore, 1997, Williams & Wilkins.
6. Sheridan AM, Bonventre JV: Cellular biology and molecular mechanisms of injury in ischemic acute renal failure: current opinions in nephrology, *Hypertension* 9:427, 2000.
7. Liano F et al: The spectrum of acute renal failure in the intensive care unit compared with that seen in other settings, *Kidney Inst Suppl* 66:516, 1998.
8. Rhan, KH, Heidenreich, S, Bruckner: How to assess glomerular function and damage in humans, *J Hypertens* 17:309, 1999.
9. Liano F, Pascual J: Epidemiology of acute renal failure: a prospective, multicenter, community-based study. Madrid Acute Renal Failure Study, *Kidney Int* 50:811, 1996.
10. Guitterez NV et al: Determinants of serum creatinine trajectory in acute contrast nephropathy, *J Interv Cardiol* 15:349, 2002.
11. Freeman RV et al: Nephropathy requiring dialysis after percutaneous coronary intervention and the critical role of an adjusted contrast dose, *Am J Cardiol* 90:1068, 2002.
12. El-Shahawy MA et al: Severity of illness scores and the outcome of acute tubular necrosis, *Int Urol Nephrol* 32:185, 2000.
13. Mitchell S: Estimated dry weight (EDW): aiming for accuracy, *Nephrol Nurs J* 29:421, 2002.
14. Coresh J et al: Prevalence of chronic kidney disease and decreased kidney function in the adult U.S. population. Third National Health and Nutrition Examination Survey, *Am J Kidney Dis* 41:1, 2003.
15. Clinical practice guidelines for chronic kidney disease: evaluation, classification, and stratification: K/DOQI executive summary, *Am J Kidney Dis* 39(2 suppl):17, 2002.
16. *Acute Dialysis Quality Initiative Newsletter*, Summer-Fall 2002.
17. Haney SL: Drug use in renal failure, *Crit Care Nurs Clin North Am* 14:77, 2002.
18. Mehta RL, Clark WC, Schetz M.: Techniques for assessing and achieving fluid balance in acute renal failure, *Curr Opin Crit Care* 8:535, 2002.
19. Ahee P, Crowe AV: The management of hyperkalemia in the emergency department, *J Accid Emerg Med* 17:181, 2000.
20. Druml W: Nutritional management of acute renal failure, *Am J Kidney Dis* 37(suppl 2):89, 2001.
21. Mehta RL et al: Diuretics, mortality, and nonrecovery of renal function in acute renal failure, *JAMA* 288:2547, 2002.
22. Ichai C et al: Comparison of the renal effects of low to high doses of dopamine and dobutamine in critically ill patients: a single-blind randomized study, *Crit Care Med* 28:921, 2000.
23. Kellum JA, Decker JM: Use of dopamine in acute renal failure: a meta-analysis, *Crit Care Med* 29:1526, 2001.
24. Bellomo R et al: Low-dose dopamine in patients with early renal dysfunction: a placebo-controlled randomised trial. Australian and New Zealand Intensive Care Society (ANZICS) Clinical Trials Group, *Lancet* 356:2139, 2000.
25. Pearl RG, Pohlman A: Understanding and managing anemia in critically ill patients, *Crit Care Nurse* (suppl):1, 2002.
26. Mehta RL: Continuous renal replacement therapies in acute renal failure setting: current concepts, *Adv Ren Replace Ther* 4(2 suppl):81, 1997.
27. Craig M: Continuous venous to venous hemofiltration: implementing and maintaining a program: examples and alternatives, *Crit Care Nurs Clin North Am* 10:219, 1998.
28. Headrick CL: Adult/pediatric CVVH: the pump, the patient, the circuit, *Crit Care Nurs Clin North Am* 10:197, 1998.
29. Forni LG, Hilton PJ: Continuous hemofiltration in the treatment of acute renal failure, *N Engl J Med* 336:1303, 1997.
30. Daugirdas JT: Peritoneal dialysis in acute renal failure: why the bad outcome? *N Engl J Med* 347:933, 2002.
31. Bernardini J: Everything I wanted to know about peritoneal dialysis: nursing application at a United States center, *Perit Dial Int* 19:595, 1999.

UNIT SEVEN

GASTROINTESTINAL ALTERATIONS

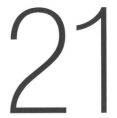

KATHLEEN M. STACY

Gastrointestinal Assessment and Diagnostic Procedures

Objectives

- Identify the components of a gastrointestinal (GI) history.
- Describe inspection, palpation, percussion, and auscultation of the patient with GI dysfunction.
- Discuss the clinical significance of laboratory tests used in assessment of GI disorders.
- Identify key diagnostic procedures used in assessment of the patient with GI dysfunction.
- Discuss the nursing management of a patient undergoing a GI diagnostic procedure.

Assessment of the critically ill patient with gastrointestinal dysfunction includes a review of the patient's health history, a thorough physical examination, and an analysis of the patient's laboratory data. Numerous invasive and noninvasive diagnostic procedures may also be performed to assist in the identification of the patient's disorder. This chapter focuses on priority clinical assessments, laboratory studies, and diagnostic tests for the critically ill patient with GI dysfunction.

CLINICAL ASSESSMENT

A thorough clinical assessment of the patient with GI dysfunction is imperative for the early identification and treatment of GI disorders. Once completed, the assessment serves as the foundation for developing the management plan for the patient. The assessment process can be brief or can involve a detailed history and examination, depending on the nature and immediacy of the patient's situation.[1]

HISTORY

Taking a thorough and accurate history is extremely important to the assessment process. The patient's history provides the foundation and direction for the rest of the assessment. The overall goal of the patient interview is to expose key clinical manifestations that will facilitate the identification of the underlying cause of the illness. This information will then assist in the development of an appropriate management plan.[2]

The initial presentation of the patient determines the rapidity and direction of the interview. For a patient in acute distress, the history should be curtailed to just a few questions about the patient's chief complaint and precipitating events. For a patient in no obvious distress, the history focuses on four areas: (1) review of the patient's *present illness*; (2) overview of the patient's *general GI status*, including previous GI diagnostic studies and interventional procedures; (3) examination of the patient's *personal and social history*, including dietary habits, nutritional status, bowel characteristics (stool descriptions), alcohol intake, and dependence on laxatives or enemas; and (4) survey of the patient's *family history*, including metabolic disorders, malabsorption syndromes, and cancer of the GI tract.[3,4]

PHYSICAL EXAMINATION

The physical assessment helps establish baseline data about the physical dimensions of the patient's situation.[3] The *abdomen* is divided into four quadrants—left upper, right upper, left lower, and right lower—with the umbilicus as the middle point, to facilitate the identification of the location of examination findings (Figure 21-1 and Box 21-1). The assessment proceeds when the patient is as comfortable as possible and in the supine position; however, the position may need readjustment if it elicits pain. To prevent stimulation of GI activity, the order for the assessment should be changed to inspection, auscultation, percussion, and palpation.[4]

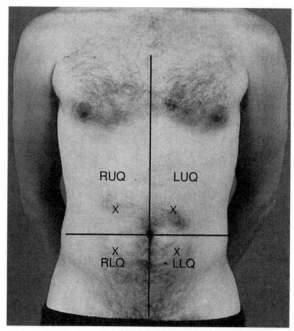

Figure 21-1 Anatomic mapping of four quadrants of the abdomen. *X* indicates correct placement of stethoscope in each quadrant. *RUQ*, Right upper quadrant; *LUQ*, left upper quadrant; *RLQ*, right lower quadrant; *LLQ*, left lower quadrant. (From Barkauskas V et al: *Health and physical assessment*, ed 3, St Louis, 2002, Mosby.)

Inspection

Inspection should be performed in a warm, well-lighted environment with the patient in a comfortable position with the abdomen exposed. Although assessment of the GI system classically begins with inspection of the abdomen, the patient's oral cavity also must be inspected to determine any unusual findings. Abnormal findings of the mouth include joint tenderness, inflammation of the gums, missing teeth, dental caries, poorly fitting dentures, and mouth odor.[5]

The skin is observed for pigmentation, lesions, striae, scars, petechiae, signs of dehydration, and venous pattern. Pigmentation may vary considerably within normal range because of race and ethnic background, although the abdomen is generally lighter in color than other, exposed areas of the skin. Abnormal findings include jaundice, skin lesions, and a tense and glistening appearance of the skin. Previous striae (stretch marks) are generally silver in color, whereas pink-purple striae may indicate Cushing's syndrome.[4] A bluish discoloration of the umbilicus (Cullen's sign) or of the flank (Turner's sign) suggests intraperitoneal bleeding.[1]

The abdomen is observed for contour (noting if it is flat, slightly concave, or slightly round), for symmetry, and for movement. Marked distention is an abnormal finding. In particular, ascites may cause generalized distention and bulging flanks. Asymmetric distention may be indicative of organ enlargement or a mass. Peristaltic waves should not be visible except in very thin patients. In the case of intestinal obstruction, hyperactive peristaltic waves may be noted. Pulsation in the epigastric area is frequently a normal

Box 21-1   Anatomic Correlates of Four Abdominal Quadrants

RIGHT UPPER QUADRANT	LEFT UPPER QUADRANT
Liver and gallbladder	Left lobe of liver
Pylorus	Spleen
Duodenum	Stomach
Head of pancreas	Body of pancreas
Right adrenal gland	Left adrenal gland
Portion of right kidney	Portion of left kidney
Hepatic flexure of colon	Splenic flexure of colon
Portions of ascending and transverse colon	Portions of transverse and descending colon
RIGHT LOWER QUADRANT	**LEFT LOWER QUADRANT**
Lower pole of right kidney	Lower pole of left kidney
Cecum and appendix	Sigmoid colon
Portion of ascending colon	Portion of descending colon
Bladder (if distended)	Bladder (if distended)
Ovary and salpinx	Ovary and salpinx
Uterus (if enlarged)	Uterus (if distended)
Right spermatic cord	Left spermatic cord
Right ureter	Left ureter

From Barkauskas V et al: *Health and physical assessment*, ed 3, St Louis, 2002, Mosby.

finding, but increased pulsation may be indicative of an aortic aneurysm. Symmetric movement of the abdomen with respirations is usually seen in men.[4,5]

Auscultation

Nursing priorities in auscultation of the patient with gastrointestinal dysfunction focus on (1) identifying bowel sounds and (2) determining the presence of bruits.

Auscultation of the abdomen provides clinical data regarding the status of the motility of the bowel. Initially the examiner must listen with the diaphragm of the stethoscope below and to the right of the umbilicus. Proceeding methodically through all four quadrants, the examiner lifts and places the diaphragm of the stethoscope lightly against the abdomen. Normal bowel sounds include high-pitched, gurgling sounds that occur approximately every 5 to 15 seconds or at a rate of 5 to 34 times each minute. Colonic sounds are low pitched and have a rumbling quality. A venous hum may also be audible at times[6] (Table 21-1).

Table 21-1   Abnormal Abdominal Sounds

Sound	Description	Causes
Borborygmi	Hyperactive bowel sounds; loud and prolonged	Hunger Gastroenteritis Early intestinal obstruction
Bowel sounds	High-pitched, tinkling sounds	Intestinal air/fluid under pressure; characteristic of early intestinal obstruction
Decreased bowel sounds	Hypoactive bowel sounds; infrequent, abnormally faint	Possible peritonitis or ileus
Absence of bowel sounds	Confirmed only after auscultation of all four quadrants and continuous auscultation for 5 minutes	Temporary loss of intestinal motility, as with complete ileus
Friction rubs	High-pitched sounds over liver/spleen (RUQ/LUQ), synchronous with respiration	Pathologic conditions (e.g., tumors, infection) that cause inflammation of organ's peritoneal covering
Bruits	Audible swishing sounds over aorta, iliac, renal, and femoral arteries	Abnormality of blood flow (requires additional evaluation to determine specific disorder)
Venous hum	Low-pitched, continuous sound	Increased collateral circulation between portal and systemic venous systems

From Doughty DB, Jackson DB: *Gastrointestinal disorders*, St Louis, 1993, Mosby.
RUQ, Right upper quadrant; *LUQ*, left upper quadrant.

Abnormal findings include the absence of bowel sounds throughout a 5-minute period, extremely soft and widely separated sounds, and increased sounds with a high-pitched, loud rushing sound (peristaltic rush). Absent bowel sounds may occur as a result of inflammation, ileus, electrolyte disturbances, and ischemia. Bowel sounds may be increased with diarrhea and early intestinal obstruction.[6] The abdomen should also be auscultated for the presence of bruits using the bell of the stethoscope. Bruits are created by turbulent flow over a partially obstructed artery and are always considered an abnormal finding. The aorta, right and left renal arteries, and iliac arteries should be auscultated.[5,6]

Percussion

The nursing priority in percussion of the patient with gastrointestinal dysfunction focuses on the abdomen.

Percussion is used to elicit information about deep organs, such as the liver, spleen, and pancreas. Because the abdomen is a sensitive area, muscle tension may interfere with this part of the assessment. Because percussion often helps relax tense muscles, it is performed before palpation. Percussion, in the absence of disease, is most helpful in delineating the position and size of the liver and spleen. Percussion also assists in the detection of fluid, gaseous distention, and masses in the abdomen.[5]

Percussion should proceed systematically and lightly in all four quadrants. Normal findings include tympany over the stomach when empty, tympany or hyperresonance over the intestine, and dullness over the liver and spleen. Abnormal areas of dullness may indicate an underlying mass. Solid masses, enlarged organs, and a distended bladder also produce areas of dullness. Dullness over both flanks may be indicative of ascites and requires further assessment.[6]

Palpation

Nursing priorities in palpation of the patient with gastrointestinal dysfunction focus on light and deep palpation of the abdominal area.

Palpation is the assessment technique most useful in detecting abdominal pathologic conditions. Both light and deep palpation of each organ and quadrant should be completed. *Light* palpation assesses the depth of skin and fascia, which has a depth of palpation of approximately 1 cm. *Deep* palpation assesses the rectus abdominis muscle and is performed bimanually to a depth of 4 to 5 cm. Deep palpation is most helpful in detecting abdominal masses. Areas in which the patient complains of tenderness should be palpated last.[6]

Normal findings include no areas of tenderness or pain, no masses, and no hardened areas. Persistent involuntary guarding may indicate peritoneal inflammation, particularly if it continues even after relaxation techniques are used. Rebound tenderness, in which pain increases with quick release of the palpated area, is indicative of an inflamed peritoneum.[4]

LABORATORY STUDIES

The value of various laboratory studies used to diagnose and treat diseases of the GI system has been emphasized often. No single study, however, provides an overall picture of the various organs' functional state. Also, no single value is predictive by itself. Laboratory studies used in the assessment of GI function, liver function, and pancreatic function are found in Tables 21-2, 21-3, and 21-4, respectively.

Table 21-2 Selected Laboratory Studies of Gastrointestinal Function

Test	Normal Findings	Clinical Significance of Abnormal Findings
Stool studies	Resident microorganisms: clostridia, enterococci, *Pseudomonas*, a few yeasts	Detection of *Salmonella typhi* (typhoid fever), *Shigella* (dysentery), *Vibrio cholerae* (cholera), *Yersinia* (enterocolitis), *Escherichia coli* (gastroenteritis), *Staphylococcus aureus* (food poisoning), *Clostridium botulinum* (food poisoning), *Clostridium perfringens* (food poisoning), *Aeromonas* (gastroenteritis)
	Fat: 2-6 g/24 hr	Steatorrhea (increased values) from intestinal malabsorption or pancreatic insufficiency
	Pus: none	Large amounts of pus associated with chronic ulcerative colitis, abscesses, anal-rectal fistula
	Occult blood: none (orthotoludine, guaiac test)	Positive tests associated with bleeding
	Ova and parasites: none	Detection of *Entamoeba histolytica* (amebiasis), *Giardia lamblia* (giardiasis), worms
D-Xylose absorption	5-hr urinary excretion: 4.5 g/L Peak blood level: >30 mg/dl	Differentiation of pancreatic steatorrhea (normal D-xylose absorption) from intestinal steatorrhea (impaired D-xylose absorption)
Gastric acid stimulation	11-20 mEq/hr after stimulation	Detection of duodenal ulcers, Zollinger-Ellison syndrome (increased values); gastric atrophy, gastric carcinoma (decreased values)
Culture and sensitivity of duodenal contents	No pathogens	Detection of *Salmonella typhi* (typhoid fever)

Modified from McCance KL, Huether SE: *Pathophysiology: the biologic basis for disease in adults and children*, ed 4, St Louis, 2002, Mosby.

Table **21-3**   Common Laboratory Studies of Liver Function

Test	Normal Value	Interpretation
SERUM ENZYMES		
Alkaline phosphatase	13-39 U/ml	Increases with biliary obstruction and cholestatic hepatitis
Aspartate transferase (AST)*	5-40 U/ml	Increases with hepatocellular injury
Alanine transferase (ALT)†	5-35 U/ml	Increases with hepatocellular injury
Lactate dehydrogenase (LDH)	200-500 U/ml	Isoenzyme LD_5 elevated with hypoxic and primary liver injury
5'-Nucleotidase	2-11 U/ml	Increases with increased alkaline phosphatase, cholestatic disorders
BILIRUBIN METABOLISM		
Serum bilirubin		
• Indirect (unconjugated)	<0.8 mg/dl	Increases with hemolysis (lysis of red blood cells)
• Direct (conjugated)	0.2-0.4 mg/dl	Increases with hepatocellular injury or obstruction
Total	<1.0 mg/dl	Increases with biliary obstruction
Urine bilirubin	0	Decreases with biliary obstruction
Urine urobilinogen	0-4 mg/24 hr	Increases with hemolysis or shunting of portal blood flow
SERUM PROTEINS		
Albumin	3.3-5.5 g/dl	Reduced with hepatocellular injury
Globulin	2.5-3.5 g/dl	Increases with hepatitis
Total	6-7 g/dl	
Albumin/globulin (A/G) ratio	1.5:1-2.5:1	Ratio reverses with chronic hepatitis or other chronic liver disease
Transferrin	250-300 mcg/dl	Liver damage with decreased values; iron deficiency with increased values
Alpha-fetoprotein (AFP)	6-20 ng/ml	Elevated values in primary hepatocellular carcinoma
BLOOD-CLOTTING FUNCTIONS		
Prothrombin time (PT)	11.5-14 seconds or 90%-100% of control	Increases with chronic liver disease (cirrhosis) or vitamin K deficiency
Partial thromboplastin time (PTT)	25-40 seconds	Increases with severe liver disease or heparin therapy
Bromsulphalein (BSP) excretion	<6% retention in 45 minutes	Increased retention with hepatocellular injury

From McCance KL, Huether SE: *Pathophysiology: the biologic basis for disease in adults and children*, ed 4, St Louis, 2002, Mosby.
*Also aspartate aminotransferase; previously serum glutamic-oxaloacetic transaminase (SGOT).
†Also alanine aminotransferase; previously serum glutamic-pyruvic transaminase (SGPT).

Table **21-4**   Common Laboratory Studies of Pancreatic Function

Test	Normal Value	Clinical Significance
Serum amylase	60-180 Somogyi units/ml	Elevated levels with pancreatic inflammation
Serum lipase	1.5 Somogyi units/ml	Elevated levels with pancreatic inflammation
		May be elevated with other conditions; differentiates with amylase, isoenzyme study
Urine amylase	35-260 Somogyi units/hr	Elevated levels with pancreatic inflammation
Secretin test	Volume 1.8 ml/kg/hr HCO_3^- concentration: >80 mEq/L HCO_3^- output: >10 mEq/L/30 sec	Decreased volume with pancreatic disease (secretin stimulates pancreatic secretion)
Stool fat	2-5 g/25 hr	Measures fatty acids; decreased pancreatic lipase increases stool fat

From McCance KL, Huether SE: *Pathophysiology: the biologic basis for disease in adults and children*, ed 4, St Louis, 2002, Mosby.
HCO_3^-, Bicarbonate.

DIAGNOSTIC PROCEDURES

The various diagnostic procedures used to evaluate the patient with GI dysfunction are presented in Table 21-5.[4]

Nursing Management

The nursing management of a patient undergoing a diagnostic procedure involves a variety of interventions. **Nursing**

Table **21-5** Abdominal Diagnostic Procedures

Procedure	Evaluates	Comments
Barium enema (also called lower GI series)*	Visualizes movement, position, and filling of various segments of colon after installation of barium by enema Diagnoses colorectal lesions, diverticulitis, inflammatory bowel disease, strictures, fistulas Evaluates colon size, length, patency	Low-fiber diet for 1-3 days before study. Bowel preparation with bowel irrigation (e.g., GoLytely) and cathartics. NPO for 8-12 hours before study. Cathartics must be given after study. Contraindicated if bowel perforation or obstruction exists.
Barium swallow, upper GI series, and small bowel follow-through*†	Visualizes position, shape, and activity of esophagus, stomach, duodenum, and jejunum Diagnoses esophageal lesions/varices or motility disorders, hiatal hernia, gastric ulcers/tumors, small bowel obstruction, small bowel lesions, Crohn's disease Evaluates gastric and small bowel motility	Bowel preparation with bowel irrigation (e.g., GoLytely) and cathartics. NPO for 8-12 hours before study. Cathartics must be given after study. Contraindicated if bowel perforation or obstruction exists.
Angiography (celiac or mesenteric)	Evaluates portal vasculature Diagnoses source of GI bleeding Evaluates cirrhosis, portal hypertension, vascular damage resulting from trauma, intestinal ischemia, tumors May be used to treat GI bleeding using vasopressin	Bowel preparation (e.g., cathartics) as prescribed. NPO for 8 hours before study. Sedative usually prescribed before procedure. If contrast media used: • Check for allergy to iodine before study. • Monitor for allergic reaction after procedure. • Ensure hydration after procedure. After procedure, keep affected extremity (catheter placed) immobilized in straight position for 6-12 hours. Monitor arterial puncture point for hemorrhage or hematoma. Monitor neurovascular status of affected limb. Monitor for indications of systemic emboli.
Cholecystography (oral, intravenous, common bile duct)	Assesses gallbladder function, patency of biliary system, and presence of gallstones	PTC contraindicated in patients with bleeding disorders. Fatty meal day before study, but fat-free evening meal. Enema may be given evening before study. NPO 8-12 hours before study. Check for allergy to iodine before study.
Percutaneous transhepatic cholangiography (PTC)	Diagnoses extrahepatic/intrahepatic jaundice, biliary calculi, biliary obstruction, common bile duct injury	Contrast medium administered orally evening before study; intravenously immediately before study; injected percutaneously into bile duct or directly into common bile duct during surgery. Monitor for allergic reaction after procedure. Ensure hydration after procedure. After PTC, monitor for clinical indications of bile leakage, hemorrhage, or peritonitis.
Computed tomography (CT) of abdomen	Diagnoses tumors, pancreatic cancer or cysts, pancreatitis, biliary tract disorders, obstructive versus nonobstructive jaundice, cirrhosis, liver metastases, ascites, lymph node metastases, aneurysm Evaluates vasculature and focal points found on nuclear scans Used to direct biopsy of tumors or aspiration of abscess	No special preparation required. Contrast medium may be used; if used: • Check for allergy to iodine before study. • Monitor for allergic reaction after procedure. • Ensure hydration after procedure.

Procedure	Diagnostic Use	Nursing Implications
Endoscopic retrograde cholangio-pancreatography (ERCP)	Diagnoses biliary stones, ductal stricture, ductal compression, neoplasms of pancreas and biliary system Evaluates patency of biliary and pancreatic ducts, jaundice, pancreatitis, cholecystitis, hepatitis	Same as for esophagogastroduodenoscopy. Contraindicated if patient uncooperative or if bilirubin >3.5 mg/dl. Monitor for clinical indications of pancreatitis (most common complication) after study. Monitor for clinical indications of sepsis.
Endoscopy • Esophagogastro-duodenoscopy (EGD) • Colonoscopy • Proctosigmoidoscopy	Directly visualizes mucosa of areas in GI tract EGD can be extended to visualize pancreas and gallbladder EGD diagnoses esophagitis, esophageal ulcers/strictures/varices, hiatal hernia, gastritis, gastric ulcers, pyloric obstruction, pernicious anemia, foreign bodies, duodenal inflammation/ulcers; evaluates esophageal/gastric motility, bleeding, lesions, anastomoses. Esophagoscopy or gastroscopy used therapeutically: sclerosis of varices Proctosigmoidoscopy diagnoses rectosigmoid cancer, strictures, polyps, inflammatory processes, hemorrhoids; evaluates bleeding from rectosigmoid area and surgical anastomoses Colonoscopy diagnoses diverticular disease, obstruction, strictures, radiation injury, polyps, neoplasms, bleeding, ischemia Colonoscopy or sigmoidoscopy used therapeutically: polyp removal Biopsies may be taken during any endoscopic procedure	Sedation may be prescribed, especially for colonoscopy. Bowel preparation with gastric irrigation (e.g., GoLYTELY) and cathartics required before lower GI endoscopy. NPO 4-8 hours before study. Keep NPO until gag reflex returns if sedated. Monitor closely after procedure for clinical indications of perforation and hemorrhage.
Flat plate of abdomen	Diagnoses perforated viscus, paralytic ileus, mechanical obstruction, intraabdominal mass Evaluates distribution of visceral gas (and identifies free air in peritoneum indicative of bowel perforation) Evaluates organ size	No preparation required.
Liver biopsy	Obtains tissue specimen for microscopic evaluation Diagnoses liver disease or malignancy	May be performed open or closed. • Open biopsy done in surgery. • Closed biopsy may be done at bedside; contraindicated if platelets <100,000/mm³. Clotting profile evaluated before procedure. Patient must be cooperative because must take deep breath and hold for closed biopsy. Type/crossmatch 2 U blood before procedure. NPO for 4-8 hours before study. After procedure, position patient on right side for 2 hours; apply pressure dressing, and patient on bed rest for 24 hours. Observe for: • Hemorrhage: hypotension, dyspnea (subphrenic hematoma) • Pneumothorax: dyspnea, chest pain, diminished breath sounds on right, hypoxemia • Sepsis: fever, leukocytosis, rebound tenderness

*Meglumine diatrizoate (Gastrografin) may be used, especially if bowel perforation is suspected.
†Ordered according to which area or areas need to be evaluated (e.g., "upper GI with small bowel follow-through" means stomach, pylorus, duodenum; "barium swallow with upper GI" means esophagus, stomach, pylorus.

Continued

Table **21-5** Abdominal Diagnostic Procedures—cont'd

Procedure	Evaluates	Comments
Liver scan	Diagnoses cirrhosis, hepatitis, tumors, abscesses, cysts, tuberculosis	No preparation required.
Magnetic resonance imaging (MRI)	Evaluates liver, biliary tree, pancreas, spleen Differentiates cyst from solid mass Diagnoses hepatic metastasis Evaluates abscesses, fistulas, source of GI bleeding Used for staging of colorectal cancer	Cannot be used in patients with implanted metallic device, including pacemakers. No special preparation required. Cannot be done if patient mechanically ventilated.
Paracentesis	Analysis of fluid removed during peritoneal tap Diagnoses intraperitoneal bleeding with diagnostic peritoneal lavage	After tap, monitor for: • Peritoneal leakage • Clinical indications of infection, peritonitis
Percutaneous transhepatic portography	Diagnoses esophageal varices and visualizes portal venous circulation	As for angiography.
Radionuclide imaging (hepatobiliary scintigraphy) • HIDA scan • PIPIDA scan	Diagnoses hepatocellular disease, hepatic metastasis, biliary disease, lower GI bleeding, gastric reflux	NPO 2 hours before study.
Schilling test	Evaluates ileal absorption of vitamin B_{12} Diagnoses pernicious anemia caused by intrinsic factor deficiency and inadequate ilial absorption of intrinsic factor–vitamin B_{12} complex	Intramuscular (IM) vitamin B_{12} and oral radioactive B_{12} are given, and 24-hour urine specimen is collected.
Ultrasound of abdomen	Evaluates pancreas, biliary ducts, gallbladder, liver Identifies tumor, abdominal abscesses, hepatocellular disease, splenomegaly, pancreatic or splenic cysts Differentiates obstructive from nonobstructive jaundice	All barium must have been cleared from GI tract before ultrasonography. NPO for 8 hours before study. If for evaluation of gallbladder: fat-free meal evening before study.

From Dennison RD: *Pass CCRN!*, ed 2, St Louis, 2000, Mosby.
GI, Gastrointestinal; *NPO*, nothing by mouth.

priorities are directed toward (1) **preparing the patient psychologically and physically for the procedure**, (2) **monitoring the patient's responses to the procedure**, and (3) **assessing the patient after the procedure**. Preparing the patient includes teaching the patient about the procedure, answering any questions, and transporting/positioning the patient for the procedure. Monitoring the patient's responses to the procedure includes observing the patient for signs of pain, anxiety, or hemorrhage and monitoring vital signs. Assessing the patient after the procedure includes observing for complications of the procedure and medicating the patient for any postprocedural discomfort. Evidence of GI bleeding must be reported immediately to the physician and emergency measures to maintain circulation initiated.

REFERENCES

1. O'Toole MT: Advanced assessment of the abdomen and gastrointestinal problems, *Nurs Clin North Am* 24:771, 1990.
2. Gehring PE: Physical assessment begins with a history, *RN* 54(11):26, 1991.
3. Seidel HM et al: *Mosby's guide to physical examination*, ed 5, St Louis, 2003, Mosby.
4. Barkauskas V et al: *Health and physical assessment*, ed 3, St Louis, 2002, Mosby.
5. Thompson JM et al: *Mosby's clinical nursing,* ed 5, St Louis, 2002, Mosby.
6. O'Hanlon-Nicholas T: Basic assessment series: gastrointestinal system, *Am J Nurs* 98(4):48, 1998.

KATHLEEN M. STACY

22

Gastrointestinal Disorders and Therapeutic Management

Objectives

- Describe the etiology and pathophysiology of the major gastrointestinal (GI) disorders seen in the intensive care unit.
- Identify the clinical manifestations of GI disorders.
- Explain the treatment of GI disorders.
- Discuss the nursing priorities for managing a patient with GI dysfunction.
- Outline the use and care of GI tubes.

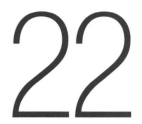 Be sure to check out the free exercises on-line at *http://evolve.elsevier.com/Urden/priorities/*

Understanding the pathology of a disease, the areas of assessment on which to focus, and the usual medical management allows the critical care nurse to anticipate and plan nursing interventions more accurately. This chapter focuses on gastrointestinal disorders most often seen in the critical care environment.

ACUTE GASTROINTESTINAL HEMORRHAGE

Gastrointestinal hemorrhage is a medical emergency that remains a common complication of critical illness[1] and results in almost 300,000 hospital admissions yearly.[2] Despite advances in medical knowledge and nursing care, mortality for acute GI bleeding has not changed in more than 50 years and remains at 7% to 10%.[2]

Etiology

Gastrointestinal hemorrhage occurs from bleeding in the upper or lower GI tract. The ligament of Treitz is the anatomic division used to differentiate between the two sites. Thus bleeding proximal to the ligament is considered to be *upper* GI in origin, and bleeding distal to the ligament is considered to be *lower* GI in origin[3,4] (Box 22-1). The three main causes of GI hemorrhage seen in the intensive care unit are peptic ulcer disease, stress-related erosive syndrome, and esophagogastric varices.

Peptic Ulcer Disease

Peptic ulcer disease (gastric and duodenal ulcers), resulting from the breakdown of the gastromuscosal lining, is the leading cause of upper GI hemorrhage, accounting for

---

Box **22-1**	Causes of Acute Gastrointestinal (GI) Hemorrhage

UPPER GI TRACT
Peptic ulcer disease
Stress-related erosive syndrome
Esophagogastric varices
Mallory-Weiss tear
Esophagitis
Neoplasm
Aortoenteric fistula
Angiodysplasia

LOWER GI TRACT
Diverticulosis
Angiodysplasia
Neoplasm
Inflammatory bowel disease
Trauma
Infectious colitis
Radiation colitis
Ischemia
Aortoenteric fistula
Hemorrhoids

---

approximately 50% of cases.[5] Normally, protection of the gastric mucosa from the digestive effects of gastric secretions is accomplished in three ways. First, the gastroduodenal mucosa is coated by a glycoprotein mucus, which forms a gel that prevents the back diffusion of acid and pepsin and helps to maintain a mucosal-luminal pH gradient. Second, gastroduodenal epithelial cells secrete bicarbonate, which augments the actions of the glycoprotein mucus in maintaining this pH gradient. Third, gastroduodenal epithelial cells are protected structurally against damage from acid and pepsin because they are connected by tight junctions that help prevent acid penetration. Through these mechanisms, gastroduodenal mucosal pH is maintained above 6.0, even when the luminal pH is as low as 1.5.[6]

Peptic ulceration occurs when these protective mechanisms cease to function, thus allowing gastroduodenal mucosal breakdown. Once the mucosal lining is penetrated, gastric secretions autodigest the layers of the stomach, resulting in damage to the mucosal and submucosal layers of the stomach or duodenum. This results in damage to blood vessels and subsequent hemorrhage. The two main causes of disruption of gastroduodenal mucosal resistance are nonsteroidal antiinflammatory drugs (NSAIDs) and the bacterial action of *Helicobacter pylori*.[7]

Stress-Related Erosive Syndrome

Stress-related erosive syndrome (SRES), also known as a *stress ulcer* or *hemorrhagic gastritis*, is a term used to describe the gastric mucosal abnormalities often found in the critically ill patient. These abnormalities develop rapidly within hours of admission and range from superficial mucosal erosions to deep ulcers and are usually limited to the stomach. SRES occurs through the same pathophysiologic mechanisms as peptic ulcer disease, but the main cause of disruption of gastric mucosal resistance is increased acid production and decreased mucosal blood flow resulting in ischemia and degeneration of the mucosal lining. Patients at risk include those in high–physiologic-stress situations, as with extensive burns, severe trauma, major surgery, shock, and acute neurologic disease. GI hemorrhage is estimated to occur in 1% to 30% of patients who develop SRES, with an associated mortality of 30% to 80%. SRES is the second leading cause of upper GI hemorrhage, accounting for approximately 20% of cases.[3,8]

Esophagogastric Varices

Esophagogastric varices are engorged and distended blood vessels of the esophagus and proximal stomach that develop from portal hypertension secondary to *hepatic cirrhosis*, a chronic disease of the liver that results in damage to the liver sinusoids. Without adequate sinusoid function, resistance to portal blood flow is increased, and pressures within the liver increase. This leads to a rise in portal venous pressure (portal hypertension), causing collateral circulation to divert portal blood from areas of high pressure within the liver to adjacent areas of low pressure outside the liver, such as into the veins of the esophagus, spleen, intestines, and stomach. The tiny, thin-walled vessels of the esophagus and proximal stomach that receive this diverted blood lack sturdy mucosal protection. The vessels become engorged and dilated, forming gastroesophageal varices that are vulnerable to damage from gastric secretions, resulting in subsequent rupture and hemorrhage.[9,10] Rupture and hemorrhage occur in 19% to 40% of the patients with varices and have an associated mortality of 40% to 70%.[2,9]

Pathophysiology

Gastrointestinal hemorrhage is a life-threatening disorder characterized by acute, massive GI bleeding. Regardless of the etiology, acute GI hemorrhage results in hypovolemic shock, initiation of the shock response, and development of multiple organ dysfunction syndrome if left untreated[6] (Figure 22-1). However, the most common cause of death in GI hemorrhage is exacerbation of the underlying disease, not intractable hypovolemic shock.

Assessment and Diagnosis

The initial clinical presentation of the patient with acute GI hemorrhage is that of a patient in hypovolemic shock; the clinical presentation varies depending on the amount of blood lost[6] (Table 22-1). Hematemesis, hematochezia, and melena are the hallmarks of GI hemorrhage.[3,11]

The patient vomiting blood is usually bleeding from a source above the duodenojejunal junction because reverse peristalsis is seldom sufficient to cause hematemesis if the bleeding point is below this area. *Hematemesis* may be bright red or have a coffee-grounds appearance, depending on the amount of gastric contents at the time of bleeding and the length of time the blood has been in contact with gastric secretions. Gastric acid converts bright-red hemoglobin to brown hematin, accounting for the coffee-grounds appearance of the emesis. Bright-red emesis results from profuse bleeding with little contact with gastric secretions.

The presence of blood in the GI tract results in increased peristalsis and diarrhea. *Hematochezia* (bright-red stools) results from massive lower GI hemorrhage and, if rapid enough, upper GI hemorrhage. *Melena* (black, tarry, or dark-red stools) results from digestion of blood from an upper GI hemorrhage and may take several days to clear after the bleeding has stopped.

Laboratory Studies

Laboratory tests can help determine the extent of bleeding, although the patient's hemoglobin (Hgb) and hematocrit (Hct) are poor indicators of the severity or rapidity of blood loss. As whole blood is lost, plasma and red blood cells (RBCs) are lost in the same proportion; thus if the patient's Hct is 45% before a bleeding episode, it will still be 45% several hours later. Redistribution of plasma from the extravas-

cular to the intravascular space may take as long as 72 hours and thus as long for the patient's Hgb and Hct to drop.[2]

Diagnostic Procedures

To isolate the source of bleeding, an urgent fiberoptic endoscopy is usually undertaken. If performed within 12 hours of the bleeding event, endoscopy has a 90% to 95% accuracy rate. Before endoscopy the patient must be hemodynamically stabilized and the area to be visualized cleared of blood.[2] A tagged RBC study or angiography may be done when endoscopy fails to identify the source of bleeding or if it is impossible to view the GI tract clearly because of continued active bleeding.[11,12]

Medical Management

To reduce mortality related to GI hemorrhage, patients at risk should be identified early and interventions implemented to reduce gastric acidity and support the gastric mucosal defense mechanisms. Management of the patient at risk for GI hemorrhage should include prophylactic administration of pharmacologic agents for gastric acid neutralization. These agents include antacids, histamine (H$_2$) antagonists, cytoprotective agents, and proton-pump inhibitors.[1-3]

Stabilization

The initial treatment priority is the restoration of adequate circulating blood volume to treat or prevent shock. This is accomplished with intravenous (IV) infusions of crystalloids, blood, and blood products.[2,5] A central venous catheter[5] or pulmonary artery catheter[2] may be necessary to provide a more decisive guide to fluid replacement therapy, particularly in patients at risk for developing cardiac failure. Supplemental oxygen therapy is initiated to increase oxygen delivery and improve tissue perfusion.[2,5] Intubation may be necessary in the patient at risk for aspiration or to facilitate gastric lavage. A large nasogastric (NG) tube should be inserted and lavaged with water or normal saline until clear. Lavaging is used to confirm the diagnosis of active bleeding; to slow the bleeding; and to prepare the esophagus, stomach, and proximal duodenum for endoscopic evaluation.[4] A urinary drainage catheter should be inserted to monitor urine output.[2]

Control Bleeding

Interventions to control bleeding are the second priority for the patient with GI hemorrhage.

Peptic Ulcer Disease. In the patient with GI hemorrhage related to peptic ulcer disease, bleeding hemostasis may be accomplished through endoscopic thermal therapy or endoscopic injection therapy. *Endoscopic thermal therapy* uses heat to cauterize the bleeding vessel, whereas *endoscopic injection therapy* uses a variety of agents (e.g., hypertonic saline, epinephrine, dehydrated alcohol) to induce localized vasoconstriction of the bleeding vessel. Intraarterial infusion of

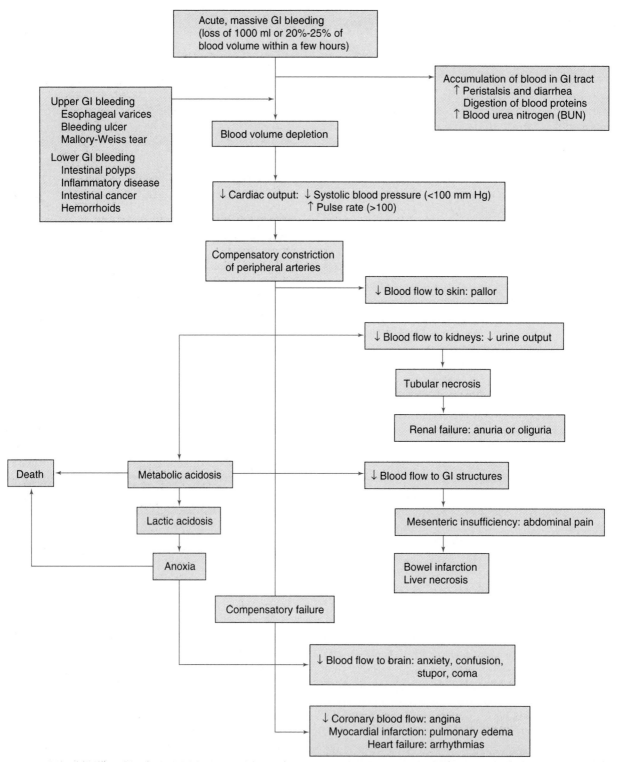

Figure 22-1 Pathophysiology of acute gastrointestinal hemorrhage. (From McCance KL, Huether SE: *Pathophysiology: the biologic basis for disease in adults and children*, ed 4, St Louis, 2002, Mosby.)

vasopressin into the gastric artery or intraarterial injection of an embolizing agent (e.g., Gelfoam pledgets, stainless steel coils, platinum microcoils, polyvinyl alcohol particles) can also be performed during arteriography to control bleeding once the site has been identified.[13] Intraarterial administra-

tion of vasopressin is less effective for duodenal lesions because of the dual blood supply of the duodenum.[2]

Stress-Related Erosive Syndrome. In the patient with GI hemorrhage caused by SRES, bleeding hemostasis may be accomplished through intraarterial infusion of vasopressin

Table 22-1 Clinical Classification of Hemorrhage

Class	Blood Loss	Clinical Signs/Symptoms
1	≤15%	Pulse rate normal or <100 beats/min (supine) Capillary refill <3 seconds Urine output adequate (30-35 ml/hr) Orthostatic hypotension Apprehension
2	15%-30%	Pulse rate increased (>100 beats/min) Capillary refill sluggish Pulse pressure decreased Blood pressure normal (supine) Tachypnea Urine output low (25-30 ml/hr)
3	30%-40%	Pulse rate 120+ beats/min (supine) Hypotension Cool and pale skin Confusion Hyperventilation Urine output low (5-15 ml/hr)
4	≥40%	Profound hypotension Pulse rate 140+ beats/min Confusion, lethargy Urine output minimal

From Klein DG: *AACN Clin Issues Crit Care Nurs* 1:508, 1990.

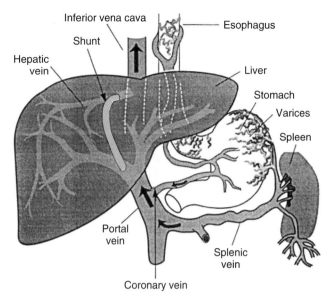

Figure 22-2   Anatomic location of transjugular intrahepatic portosystemic shunt (TIPS). (From Vargas HE, Gerber D, Abu-Elmagd K: *Surg Clin North Am* 79:1, 1999.)

and intraarterial embolization. Endoscopic therapies have been of minimal benefit because of the diffuse nature of the disease.[3]

Esophagogastric Varices. In acute variceal hemorrhage, control of bleeding may be initially accomplished through pharmacologic and endoscopic therapies. IV vasopressin, somatostatin, and octreotide have been shown to reduce portal venous pressure and slow variceal hemorrhaging by constricting the splanchnic arteriolar bed.[9,10] Two common endoscopic therapies are injection therapy and variceal ligation. Endoscopic injection therapy (also referred to as *sclerotherapy*) controls bleeding through injection of a sclerosing agent in or around the varices. This creates an inflammatory reaction that induces vasoconstriction and results in the formation of a venous thrombosis. During *endoscopic variceal band ligation*, latex bands are placed around the varices to create an obstruction to stop the bleeding.[9,10]

If these initial therapies fail, esophagogastric balloon tamponade and *transjugular intrahepatic portosystemic shunting* (TIPS) may become necessary. Balloon tamponade tubes (e.g., Sengstaken-Blakemore, Linton, Minnesota) halt hemorrhaging by applying direct pressure against bleeding vessels while decompressing the stomach[9,10] (see Figure 22-4). In a TIPS procedure, a channel between the systemic and portal venous systems is created to redirect portal blood, thereby reducing portal hypertension and decompressing the varices to control bleeding[10,14] (Figure 22-2).

Surgical Intervention

The patient who remains hemodynamically unstable despite volume replacement may need urgent surgery.

Peptic Ulcer Disease. The surgical procedure of choice to control bleeding from peptic ulcer disease is vagotomy and pyloroplasty. The vagus nerve to the stomach is severed, thus eliminating the autonomic stimulus to the gastric cells and reducing hydrochloric acid production. Because the vagus nerve also stimulates motility, a pyloroplasty is performed to provide for gastric emptying.[13]

Stress-Related Erosive Syndrome. Operative procedures to control bleeding from SRES include total gastrectomy, which is performed when bleeding is generalized, and oversew of the ulcers, which is performed when bleeding is localized. A *total gastrectomy* involves the complete removal of the stomach with anastomosis of the esophagus to the jejunum. During an *oversew of the ulcers* the bleeding vessel is ligated and the ulcer crater is closed.[13]

Esophagogastric Varices. Surgical procedures to control bleeding gastroesophageal varices include portacaval shunt, mesocaval shunt, and splenorenal shunt (Figure 22-3).[14] These shunt procedures are also referred to as *decompression procedures* because they result in the diversion of portal blood flow away from the liver and decompression of the portal system. The *portacaval* shunt procedure has two variations. An *end-to-side* portacaval shunt procedure involves the ligation of the hepatic end of the portal vein with subsequent anastomosis to the vena cava. During a *side-to-side* portacaval shunt procedure the side of the portal vein is anastomosed to the side of the vena cava. A *mesocaval* shunt procedure involves the insertion of a graft between the superior mesenteric artery and the vena cava.

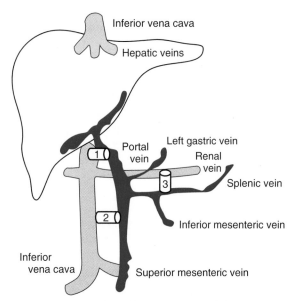

Figure 22-3 Anatomy of portal venous system and sites in which surgical anastomoses are made to shunt blood from the portal (*dark*) to the systemic (*light*) venous circulation. Sites used for surgical portal decompression: *1*, portacaval shunt; *2*, mesocaval shunt; *3*, splenorenal shunt. (From Luketic VA, Sanyal AJ: *Gastroenterol Clin North Am* 29:387, 2000.)

During a distal *splenorenal* shunt procedure the splenic vein is detached from the portal vein and anastomosed to the left renal vein.[13,14]

Nursing Management

All critically ill patients should be considered at risk for stress ulcers and thus GI hemorrhage. Routine assessments should include gastric fluid pH monitoring every 2 hours, with a goal of keeping the pH greater than 4.0.[3] Gastric pH measurements, either via litmus paper or direct NG tube probes, may be used to assess gastric fluid pH and the need for or effectiveness of prophylactic agents. In addition, patients at risk should be assessed for the presence of bright-red or coffee-grounds emesis, bloody NG aspirate, and bright-red, black, or dark-red stools. Any signs of bleeding should be promptly reported to the physician.[1]

Nursing management of a patient experiencing acute GI hemorrhage incorporates a variety of nursing diagnoses (Box 22-2). **Nursing priorities are directed toward (1) administering volume replacement, (2) controlling the bleeding, (3) providing comfort and emotional support, (4) maintaining surveillance for complications, and (5) educating the patient and family.**

Administering Volume Replacement

Measures to facilitate volume replacement include obtaining IV access and administering prescribed fluids and blood products. Two large-diameter peripheral IV catheters should be inserted to facilitate the rapid administration of prescribed fluids.[2,11]

Controlling Bleeding

One measure to control active bleeding is *gastric lavage*, used to decrease gastric mucosal blood flow and evacuate blood from the stomach. A large-bore NG tube is inserted in the stomach, which is irrigated with normal saline or water until the returned solution is clear. It is important to keep accurate records of the amount of fluid instilled and aspirated to ascertain the true amount of bleeding. Historically, iced saline was favored as a lavage irrigant. Research has shown, however, that low-temperature fluids shift the oxyhemoglobin dissociation curve to the left, decrease oxygen delivery to vital organs, and prolong bleeding time and prothrombin time. Iced saline also may further aggravate bleeding; therefore room-temperature water or saline is the currently preferred irrigant for use in gastric lavage.[4]

Maintaining Surveillance for Complications

The patient also should be continuously observed for signs of gastric perforation. Although a rare complication, gastric perforation constitutes a surgical emergency. Signs and symptoms include sudden, severe, generalized abdominal pain, with significant rebound tenderness and rigidity. Perforation should be suspected when fever, leukocytosis, and tachycardia persist despite adequate volume replacement.[4]

Educating Patient and Family

Early in the hospital stay the patient and family should be taught about acute GI hemorrhage and its causes and treatments. As the patient moves toward discharge, teaching should focus on the interventions necessary for preventing the recurrence of the precipitating disorder. If an alcohol abuser, the patient should be encouraged to stop drinking and should be referred to an alcohol cessation program.

Collaborative management of the patient with acute GI hemorrhage is outlined in Box 22-3.

ACUTE PANCREATITIS

Acute pancreatitis is an acute inflammation of the pancreas that produces exocrine and endocrine dysfunction that may also involve surrounding tissues and remote organ systems. In approximately 80% of patients it takes the form of *edematous*

Box **22-3** COLLABORATIVE Management

Acute Gastrointestinal Hemorrhage

1. Initiate fluid resuscitation to achieve hemodynamic stability.
   - Crystalloids
   - Colloids
   - Blood and blood products
2. Determine the etiology of the bleeding.
   - Gastric lavage
3. Control bleeding
   - Endoscoptic interventions
   - Vasopression, somatostatin, octreotide
   - Esophagogastric balloon tube
   - Transjugular intrahepatic portosystemic shunting
   - Surgery
4. Provide comfort and emotional support.
5. Maintain surveillance for complications.
   - Hypovolemic shock
   - Gastric perforation

interstitial pancreatitis, whereas the other 20% develop *severe acute necrotizing pancreatitis*.[15] The severity of acute pancreatitis can be estimated with Ranson's criteria (Box 22-4). If the patient has up to two factors present, predicted mortality is 2%; with three or four factors, 15% mortality; with five or six factors, 40% mortality; and with seven or eight factors, 100% predicted mortality.[15,16]

Etiology

The two most common causes of acute pancreatitis are *biliary disease* (gallstones) and *alcoholism*. Other less common causes include surgical trauma, hyperparathyroidism, vascular disease, and the use of certain drugs (Box 22-5). In 10% to 20% of patients with acute pancreatitis, no etiologic factor can be determined.[17-19]

Pathophysiology

In acute pancreatitis the normally inactive digestive enzymes become prematurely activated within the pancreas itself, creating the central pathophysiologic mechanism of acute pancreatitis, namely *autodigestion*.[17] The enzymes become activated through a variety of mechanisms, including obstruction or damage to the pancreatic duct system, alterations in the secretory processes of acinar cells, infection, ischemia, and other unknown factors.[20]

Trypsin is the enzyme that becomes activated first and initiates the autodigestion process by triggering the secretion of the proteolytic enzymes kallikrein, chymotrypsin and elastase and phospholipase A and lipase. Release of *kallikrein* and *chymotrypsin* results in increased capillary membrane permeability, leading to fluid leaking into the interstitium and the development of edema and relative hypovolemia. *Elastase* activation causes dissolution of the elastic fibers of blood vessels and ducts, leading to hemorrhage. *Phospholipase A*, in the presence of bile, digests the phospholipids of cell membranes, causing severe pancreatic and adipose tissue necrosis. *Lipase* flows into the damaged tissue and is absorbed into the systemic circulation, resulting in fat necrosis of the pancreas and surrounding tissues.[21]

The extent of injury to the pancreatic cells determines which form of acute pancreatitis will develop. If injury to the pancreatic cells is mild without necrosis, edematous pancreatitis develops; this form of acute pancreatitis is self-limiting. If injury to the pancreatic cells is severe with necrosis, severe acute necrotizing pancreatitis develops.[17] Pancreatic injury also results in the release of systemic inflammatory mediators, which can lead to the development of *systemic inflammatory response syndrome* (SIRS).[21] Local tissue injury results in infection, abscess and pseudocyst formation, disruption of the pancreatic duct, and severe hemorrhage with shock.[17]

Box **22-4**   Ranson's Criteria for Estimating Severity of Acute Pancreatitis

AT ADMISSION	DURING INITIAL 48 HOURS OF HOSPITALIZATION
Age >55 years	Fall in hematocrit >10% with hydration or hematocrit <30%
Hypotension	Necessity for massive fluid and colloid replacement
Abnormal pulmonary findings	Hypocalcemia (<8 mg/dl)
Abdominal mass	Pao_2 <60 mm Hg with or without acute respiratory distress syndrome
Hemorrhagic or discolored peritoneal fluid	Hypoalbuminemia (<3.2 mg/dl)
Increased serum LDH levels (>350 U/L)	Base deficit >4 mEq/L
AST >250 U/L	Azotemia
Leukocytosis (>16,000/mm^3)	
Hyperglycemia (>200 mg/dl; no diabetic history)	
Neurologic deficit (confusion, localizing signs)	

From Latifi R, McIntosh JK, Dudrick SJ: *Surg Clin North Am* 71:583, 1991.
LDH, Lactate dehydrogenase; *AST*, aspartate transferase; *Pao$_2$*, arterial oxygen partial pressure (tension).

Box **22-5** Causes of Acute Pancreatitis

Toxins: Ethyl alcohol, methyl alcohol, scorpion venom, parathion
Biliary disease: Stones, sludge, common bile duct obstruction
Drugs: Sulfonamides, thiazide diuretics, furosemide, estrogens, tetracycline, pentamidine, procainamide, salicylates, steroids, cyclosporine, amphetamines, nonsteroidal antiinflammatory drugs, valproic acid, azathioprine, allopurinol
Infection: Bacterial, viral, parasitic
Trauma: Abdominal, surgical, endoscopic
Hypercalcemia, hyperparathyroidism
Hyperlipidemia
Tumors
Ischemia
Transplant
Vasculitis
Pregnancy
Hypothermia
Sphincter of Oddi dysfunction
Systemic lupus erythematosus
Ampullary stenosis
Idiopathic

From Steer ML: In Taylor MB, editor: *Gastrointestinal emergencies,* Baltimore, 1992, Williams & Wilkins.

Assessment and Diagnosis

The clinical manifestations of acute pancreatitis range from mild to severe and often mimic other disorders. Epigastric to midabdominal pain may vary from mild and tolerable to severe and incapacitating. Many patients report a twisting or knifelike sensation that radiates to the low dorsal region of the back. Nausea, vomiting, or both may accompany the pain. The patient may obtain some comfort by leaning forward or by lying down with knees drawn up. Other clinical findings include fever, diaphoresis, weakness, tachypnea, hypotension, and tachycardia. Depending on the extent of fluid loss and hemorrhage, the patient may exhibit signs of hypovolemic shock.[17,21]

Physical Examination

The results of physical assessment usually reveal hypoactive bowel sounds and abdominal tenderness, guarding, distention, and tympany. Uncommon inspection findings that could indicate pancreatic hemorrhage include Grey Turner's sign (gray-blue discoloration of flank) and Cullen's sign (discoloration of umbilical region). A palpable abdominal mass is indicative of the presence of a pseudocyst or abscess.[17,21]

Laboratory Studies

Assessment of laboratory data usually demonstrates elevated levels of serum amylase and lipase. Serum lipase is more pancreas specific than amylase and a more accurate marker for acute pancreatitis. Amylase is present in other body tissues, and other disorders (e.g., cerebral trauma, mumps, renal insufficiency, burns, shock) may contribute to an elevated level. Unlike other serum enzymes, however, amylase is excreted in urine, and this clearance increases with acute pancreatitis. Measurement of urinary versus serum amylase should be considered in light of the patient's creatinine clearance. In addition, serum amylase may be elevated for only 2 days in mild cases. If the patient delays seeking treatment and the amylase level is not measured within 2 to 7 days after onset of symptoms, a normal level (false-negative result) may be noted. Leukocytosis, hypocalcemia, hyperglycemia, hyperbilirubinemia, and hypoalbuminemia may also be present[17] (Table 22-2).

Diagnostic Procedures

An abdominal ultrasound is obtained as part of the diagnostic evaluation to determine the presence of biliary stones. In addition, a contrast-enhanced computed tomography (CT) scan is obtained to evaluate the overall status of the pancreas and to differentiate between edematous and necrotizing pancreatitis.[15,17,21]

Medical Management

Fluid Management

Intravenous crystalloids and colloids are administered immediately to prevent hypovolemic shock and maintain hemodynamic stability. In severe forms of acute pancreatitis, a pulmonary artery catheter is used to guide ongoing fluid management. Total parenteral nutrition (TPN) should be started as soon as possible in all patients who will have oral feeding withheld for more than 7 days.[15] Electrolytes are monitored closely, and abnormalities such as hypocalcemia, hypokalemia, and hypomagnesemia are treated. If hyperglycemia develops, exogenous insulin is given. Supplemental oxygen to support oxygen delivery to the tissues is also initiated.[17,21]

Systemic Complications

Acute pancreatitis can affect every organ system, and recognition and treatment of systemic complications are crucial to management of the patient (Box 22-6). The most serious complications are hypovolemic shock, acute respiratory distress syndrome (ARDS), acute renal failure (ARF), and GI hemorrhage. Hypovolemic shock is the result of relative hypovolemia resulting from third spacing of intravascular volume and vasodilation caused by the release of inflammatory immune mediators. These mediators also contribute to the development of ARDS and ARF. Other possible pulmonary complications include pleural effusions, atelectasis, and pneumonia. Stress ulcers and bleeding gastroesophageal varices (in the alcoholic patient) can precipitate the development of GI hemorrhage.[17]

Local Complications

Local complications include infected pancreatic necrosis and pancreatic pseudocyst.[17] The necrotic areas of the

Table 22-2 Laboratory Tests and Diagnostic Procedures in Acute Pancreatitis

Laboratory Study	Finding in Pancreatitis
Serum amylase	Elevated
Serum isoamylase	Elevated
Urinary amylase	Elevated
Serum lipase (if available)	Elevated
Serum triglycerides	Elevated
Glucose	Elevated
Calcium	Decreased
Magnesium	Decreased
Potassium	Decreased or increased
Albumin	Decreased
White blood cell (WBC) count	Elevated
Bilirubin	May be elevated
Liver enzymes	May be elevated
Prothrombin time (PT)	Prolonged
Arterial blood gases (ABGs)	Hypoxemia, metabolic acidosis

RADIOGRAPHIC

Abdominal computed tomography (CT)
Ultrasonography (US)
Magnetic resonance imaging (MRI)
Endoscopic retrograde cholangiopancreatography (ERCP)
Abdominal radiographs (flat plate, upright or decubitus)
Chest radiographs (posteroanterior, lateral)

From Krumberger JM: *Crit Care Nurs Clin North Am* 5:185, 1993.

Box 22-6 Complications of Acute Pancreatitis

RESPIRATORY

Early hypoxemia
Pleural effusion
Atelectasis
Pulmonary infiltration
Acute respiratory distress syndrome
Mediastinal abscess

CARDIOVASCULAR

Hypotension
Pericardial effusion
ST segment–T wave changes

RENAL

Acute tubular necrosis
Oliguria
Renal artery or vein thrombosis

HEMATOLOGIC

Disseminated intravascular coagulation
Thrombocytosis
Hyperfibrinogenemia

ENDOCRINE

Hypocalcemia
Hypertriglyceridemia
Hyperglycemia

NEUROLOGIC

Fat emboli

Psychosis
Encephalopathy

OPHTHALMOLOGIC

Purtscher's retinopathy—sudden blindness

DERMATOLOGIC

Subcutaneous fat necrosis

GASTROINTESTINAL/HEPATIC

Hepatic dysfunction
Obstructive jaundice
Erosive gastritis
Paralytic ileus
Duodenal obstruction
Pancreatic
• Pseudocyst
• Phlegmon
• Abscess
• Ascites
Bowel infarction
Massive intraperitoneal bleed
Perforation
• Stomach
• Duodenum
• Small bowel
• Colon

From Ranson JHC: In Taylor MB, editor: *Gastrointestinal emergencies*, Baltimore, 1992, Williams & Wilkins.

pancreas can lead to the development of a widespread pancreatic infection (*infected pancreatic necrosis*). Prophylactic antibiotics are initiated to prevent infection in the patient with suspected necrotizing pancreatitis.[22] Once the patient develops infected necrosis, however, surgical debridement is necessary.[17] The procedure of choice is a *necrosectomy*, which entails careful debridement of the necrotic tissue in and around the pancreas. It often requires several reoperations to remove all the necrotic tissue.[23]

A *pancreatic pseudocyst* is a collection of pancreatic fluid enclosed by a nonepithelialized wall[15] resulting from an obstruction in the main pancreatic duct.[17] A pancreatic pseudocyst (1) may resolve spontaneously; (2) may rupture, resulting in peritonitis; (3) may erode a major blood vessel, resulting in hemorrhage; (4) may become infected, resulting in abscess; or (5) may invade surrounding structures, resulting in obstruction.[17] Treatment involves drainage of the pseudocyst surgically,[23] endoscopically,[24] or percutaneously.[25]

Nursing Management

Nursing management of the patient with pancreatitis incorporates a variety of nursing diagnoses (Box 22-7). **Nursing priorities are directed toward (1) minimizing pancreatic stimulation, (2) providing comfort and emotional support, (3) maintaining surveillance for complications, and (4) educating the patient and family.**

Minimizing Pancreatic Stimulation

Theoretically, minimizing pancreatic stimulation is thought to inhibit or slow down the autodigestion process and thus improve outcome.[18] Interventions to suppress pancreatic stimulation include bed rest and restricting all oral food and fluids. Oral feedings should not be resumed until the patient is pain-free and amylase levels return to normal. In the past, nasogastric suction was also recommended, but this intervention has not been shown to improve patient outcome and should be avoided unless the patient has gastric distention or is at risk for aspiration.[17]

Providing Comfort and Emotional Support

Pain management is a major priority in acute pancreatitis because the patient may be in severe pain. Administration of analgesics to achieve pain relief is essential. For years, meperidine (Demerol) was considered the preferred agent in the patient with acute pancreatitis because morphine could produce spasms at the sphincter of Oddi. This belief is now being seriously questioned because morphine is a more effective analgesic than meperidine and has been found to have minimal effects on the sphincter of Oddi. As long as pancreatic stimulation is controlled, spasms are no longer an issue.[17] Positioning the patient in the knee-chest position and implementing measures to rest the pancreas also assist in pain control. Relaxation techniques may augment analgesia.

Maintaining Surveillance for Complications

The patient must be routinely monitored for signs of local or systemic complications (see Box 22-6). Intensive monitoring of each of the organ systems is imperative because organ failure is a major indicator of the severity of pancreatitis. In addition, the patient must be closely monitored for signs and symptoms of a pancreatic infection, which include abdominal pain and tenderness, fever, and increased white blood cell count.[15,17]

Educating Patient and Family

Early in the patient's hospital stay the patient and family should be taught about acute pancreatitis and its causes and treatment. As the patient moves toward discharge, teaching should focus on the interventions necessary for preventing the recurrence of the precipitating disorder. If the patient has sustained permanent damage to the pancreas, the patient will require teaching specific to diet modification and supplemental pancreatic enzymes. Diabetes education also may be necessary. If an alcohol abuser, the patient should be encouraged to stop drinking and should be referred to an alcohol cessation program.

Collaborative management of the patient with pancreatitis is outlined in Box 22-8.

FULMINANT HEPATIC FAILURE

Fulminant hepatic failure (FHF) is a medical emergency best described as severe acute liver failure (*hepatocellular necrosis*)

---

nursing diagnosis
priorities   Box **22-7**

Acute Pancreatitis

- Acute Pain related to transmission and perception of cutaneous, visceral, muscular, ischemia impulses
- Deficient Fluid Volume related to relative fluid loss
- Decreased Cardiac Output related to alterations in preload
- Anxiety related to threat to biologic, psychologic, and/or social integrity
- Deficient Knowledge: Discharge Regimen related to lack of previous exposure to information

---

Box **22-8** COLLABORATIVE Management

Acute Pancreatitis

1. Ensure adequate circulating volume.
2. Provide nutritional support.
3. Correct metabolic alterations.
4. Minimize pancreatic stimulation.
5. Provide comfort and emotional support.
6. Maintain surveillance for complications.
   - Multiple organ dysfunction syndrome

accompanied by *hepatic encephalopathy*. FHF is associated with mortality as high as 80% and generally occurs in patients without preexisting liver disease, although it is occasionally seen in those with compensated chronic liver disease. Because liver transplantation is one of the few definitive treatments for FHF, the patient should be transferred to a critical care unit and strongly considered for referral to a major medical center where transplant services are available.[26-28]

Etiology

The causes of FHF include infections, drugs, toxins, hypoperfusion, metabolic disorders, and surgery (Box 22-9). Patients are usually healthy before onset of symptoms because FHF tends to occur in those with no known liver history. Therefore a thorough medication and health history is imperative to determine a possible etiology. The patient should be questioned about exposure to environmental toxins, hepatitis, IV drug use, and sexual history. Viral hepatitis, drug toxicity, poisoning, and metabolic disorders such as Reye's syndrome and Wilson's disease, should be considered.[28]

Pathophysiology

FHF is a syndrome characterized by development of acute liver failure over 1 to 3 weeks, followed by development of hepatic encephalopathy within 8 weeks, in a patient with a previously healthy liver. Generally the interval between the actual failure of the liver and the onset of hepatic encephalopathy is less than 2 weeks. The underlying cause is massive necrosis of the hepatocytes.[26-28]

Acute liver failure results in a number of derangements, including impaired bilirubin conjugation, decreased production of clotting factors, depressed glucose synthesis, and decreased lactate clearance. This results in jaundice, coagulopathies, hypoglycemia, and metabolic acidosis. Other effects of acute liver failure include increased risk of infection and altered carbohydrate, protein, and glucose metabolism. Hypoalbuminemia, fluid and electrolyte imbalances, and acute portal hypertension contribute to the development of ascites.[26-28] Hepatic encephalopathy is thought to result from failure of the liver to detoxify various substances in the bloodstream and may be worsened by metabolic and electrolyte imbalances.[29]

The patient also may experience a variety of other complications, including cerebral edema, cardiac dysrhythmias, acute respiratory failure, and ARF. Cerebral edema develops as a result of breakdown of the blood-brain barrier and astrocyte swelling. Hypoxemia, acidosis, electrolyte imbalances, and cerebral edema can precipitate the development of cardiac dysrhythmias. Acute respiratory failure, progressing to ARDS, can result from pulmonary edema, aspiration pneumonia, and atelectasis. ARF may be caused by acute tubular necrosis, hypotension, and hemorrhage.[26-28]

Assessment and Diagnosis

Early recognition of FHF is extremely important. The diagnosis should include potentially reversible conditions (e.g., autoimmune hepatitis) and should differentiate FHF from decompensating chronic liver disease. Prognostic indicators such as coma grade, serum bilirubin, prothrombin time

---

Box **22-9** **Causes of Fulminant Hepatic Failure**

INFECTIONS
Hepatitis A, B, C, D, E, non-A, non-B, non-C
Herpes simplex virus (types 1 and 2)
Epstein-Barr virus
Varicella-zoster virus
Dengue fever virus
Rift Valley fever virus

DRUGS/TOXINS
Industrial substances (chlorinated hydrocarbons, phosphorus)
Amanita phalloides (mushrooms)
Aflatoxin (herb)
Medications (isoniazid, rifampin, halothane, methyldopa, tetracycline, valproic acid, monoamine oxidase inhibitors, phenytoin, nicotinic acid, tricyclic antidepressants, isoflurane, ketoconazole, trimethoprim-sulfamethoxazole, sulfasalazine, pyrimethamine, octreotide)
Acetaminophen toxicity
Cocaine

HYPOPERFUSION
Venous obstructions

Budd-Chiari syndrome
Veno-occlusive disease
Ischemia

METABOLIC DISORDERS
Wilson's disease
Tyrosinemia
Heat stroke
Galactosemia

SURGERY
Jejunoileal bypass
Partial hepatectomy
Liver transplant failure

OTHER
Reye's syndrome
Acute fatty liver of pregnancy
Massive malignant infiltration
Autoimmune hepatitis

(PT), coagulation factors, and pH should be noted and potential etiologies investigated.[26]

Signs and symptoms of FHF include headache, hyperventilation, jaundice, personality changes, palmar erythema, spider nevi, bruises, and edema. The patient should be evaluated for the presence of asterixis and "liver flaps," best described as the inability to sustain voluntarily a fixed position of the extremities. Asterixis is best demonstrated by having the patient extend the arms and dorsiflex the wrists, resulting in downward flapping of the hands. Hepatic encephalopathy is assessed using a grading system that stages the encephalopathy according to the patient's clinical manifestations (Box 22-10).[29] Diagnostic findings include elevated serum bilirubin, aspartate transferase (AST), alkaline phosphatase, serum ammonia, and decreased serum albumin. Arterial blood gases (ABGs) reveal respiratory alkalosis and/or metabolic acidosis. Hypoglycemia, hypokalemia, and hyponatremia also may be present.[26]

Factors I (fibrinogen), II (prothrombin), V, VII, IX, and X are produced exclusively by the liver. Of these, prothrombin may be the most useful test in the evaluation of acute FHF because levels may be 40 to 80 seconds above control values. Decreased levels of plasmin and plasminogen and increased levels of fibrin and fibrin split products also are noted. Platelet counts may be decreased to $80,000/mm^3$ or less.[26]

Medical Management

Medical interventions are directed toward management of the multisystem impact of FHF.

Ammonia Levels

Neomycin or lactulose is administered to remove or decrease production of nitrogenous wastes in the large intestine. *Neomycin*, given orally or rectally, reduces bacterial flora of the colon, which aids in decreasing ammonia formation by decreasing bacterial action on protein in the feces. Side effects include renal toxicity and hearing impairment. *Lactulose*, a synthetic ketoanalogue of lactose split into lactic acid and acetic acid in the intestine, is given orally, via NG tube, or as a retention enema. The result is the creation of an acidic environment that decreases bacterial growth.

Lactulose also traps ammonia and has a laxative effect that promotes expulsion.[29]

Complications

Bleeding is best controlled through prevention. Because patients with FHF are at risk for acute GI hemorrhage, stress ulcer prophylaxis is essential. If the patient develops active bleeding, vitamin K, fresh-frozen plasma (to maintain reasonable PT), and platelet transfusions are necessary. Metabolic disturbances (e.g., hypoglycemia, metabolic acidosis, hypokalemia, hyponatremia) should be monitored and treated appropriately. Prophylactic antibiotic administration may be initiated because the patient is at high risk for an infection.[26-28]

The development of cerebral edema necessitates the need for intracranial pressure (ICP) monitoring. Mannitol (although not suggested for patients experiencing associated renal failure), albumin, and hyperventilation may be used to decrease ICP. If renal failure develops, continuous renal replacement therapy should be initiated. Intubation and mechanical ventilation are necessary as hypoxemia develops. Hemodynamic instability is a common complication requiring fluid administration and vasoactive medications to avoid prolonged episodes of hypotension.[26-28]

If FHF continues and the patient shows no immediate signs of improvement or reversal, the patient should be considered for a liver transplant. Prompt referral to a transplant center should be a high priority for patients experiencing FHF.[27]

Nursing Management

Nursing management of the patient with fulminant hepatic failure incorporates a variety of nursing diagnoses (Box 22-11). **Nursing priorities are directed toward (1) protecting the patient from injury, (2) providing comfort and emotional support, (3) maintaining surveillance for complications, and (4) educating the patient and family.**

Box **22-10**	Staging of Hepatic Encephalopathy

I	Euphoria or depression, mild confusion, slurred speech, disordered sleep rhythm; slight asterixis and normal EEG
II	Lethargy, moderate confusion; marked asterixis and abnormal EEG
III	Marked confusion, incoherent speech, sleeping but arousable; asterixis present and abnormal EEG
IV	Coma; initially responsive to noxious stimuli, later unresponsive; asterixis absent and abnormal EEG

EEG, Electroencephalogram.

---

nursing diagnosis priorities   Box **22-11**

Fulminant Hepatic Failure

- Impaired Gas Exchange related to ventilation/perfusion mismatching or intrapulmonary shunting
- Decreased Cardiac Output related to alterations in preload
- Decreased Intracranial Adaptive Capacity related to failure of normal compensatory mechanisms
- Ineffective Renal Tissue Perfusion related to decreased renal blood flow
- Compromised Family Coping related to critically ill family member
- Deficient Knowledge: Discharge Regimen related to lack of previous exposure to information

Protecting Patient from Injury

Use of benzodiazepines and other sedatives is discouraged in the FHF patient because of the "masking" of pertinent neurologic changes and further potentiation of hepatic encephalopathy. These patients are often very difficult to manage because they may be extremely agitated and combative. Physical restraint is generally required to prevent patient injury.

Maintaining Surveillance for Complications

As the neurologic condition worsens, respiratory depression and arrest can occur quickly. Continuous arterial saturation monitoring and ABG analysis are helpful in assessing adequacy of respiratory efforts. A thorough neurologic assessment should be performed at least every hour.

Educating Patient and Family

Early in the patient's hospital stay the patient and family should be taught about fulminant hepatic failure and its causes and treatment. As the patient moves toward discharge, teaching should focus on the interventions necessary for preventing the recurrence of the precipitating etiology. If the patient is considered a liver transplant candidate, the patient and family will need specific information regarding the procedure and care. Liver transplant evaluation may include screening for medical contraindications, human immunodeficiency virus (HIV) serology, anticipated compliance, and assessment of the social support system. Psychiatric and other specialty team consults are necessary for a thorough evaluation of the patient's suitability for a transplant.

Collaborative management of the patient with fulminant hepatic failure is outlined in Box 22-12.

THERAPEUTIC MANAGEMENT
Gastrointestinal Intubation

Because GI intubation is used so often in critical care units, it is important for nurses to know the clinical indications and responsibilities inherent in tube use. The four categories of GI tubes are based on function: nasogastric suction tubes, long intestinal tubes, esophagogastric balloon tamponade tubes, and feeding tubes. Feeding tubes are discussed in Chapter 6.

Nasogastric Suction Tubes

NG suction tubes (e.g., Levin, Salem sump) remove fluid regurgitated into the stomach, prevent accumulation of swallowed air, may partially decompress the bowel, and reduce the patient's risk for aspiration. NG tubes also can be used for collecting specimens and administering tube feedings. The tube is passed through the nose into the nasopharynx and then down through the pharynx into the esophagus and stomach. The length of time the NG tube remains in place depends on its use. The tube is then placed to gravity, low intermittent suction, or low continuous suction, or in rare instances is clamped.

Nursing management is focused on preventing complications common to this therapy, such as ulceration and necrosis of the nares, esophageal reflux, esophagitis, esophageal erosion and stricture, gastric erosion, and dry mouth and parotitis from mouth breathing. In addition, interference with ventilation and coughing, aspiration, and loss of fluid and electrolytes can be critical problems. Interventions include irrigating the tube every 4 hours with normal saline, ensuring the blue air vent of the Salem sump is patent and maintained above the level of the patient's stomach, and providing frequent mouth and nares care.

Long Intestinal Tubes

Miller-Abbott, Cantor, Johnston, and Baker are examples of long intestinal tubes that are placed either preoperatively or intraoperatively. The long length allows removal of contents from the intestine that cannot be accomplished by an NG tube. These tubes can decompress the small bowel and can splint the small bowel intraoperatively or postoperatively. Because progression of the tubes depends on bowel peristalsis, their use is contraindicated in patients with paralytic ileus and severe mechanical bowel obstruction.

Interventions used in the care of the patient with a long intestinal tube are similar to those with an NG tube. The patient should be observed for (1) gaseous distention of the balloon section, which makes removal difficult; (2) rupture of the balloon or spillage of mercury into the intestine; (3) overinflation of the balloon, which can lead to intestinal rupture; and (4) reverse intussusception if the tube is removed rapidly. Intestinal tubes should be removed slowly; usually 6 inches of the tube is withdrawn every hour.

Esophagogastric Balloon Tamponade Tubes

Currently three different types of balloon tamponade tubes are available. The *Sengstaken-Blakemore* tube has three lumens: one for the gastric balloon, one for the esophageal balloon, and one for gastric suction (Figure 22-4, *A*). The *Linton* tube also has three lumens, for the gastric balloon, gastric suction, and esophageal suction (Figure 22-4, *B*).

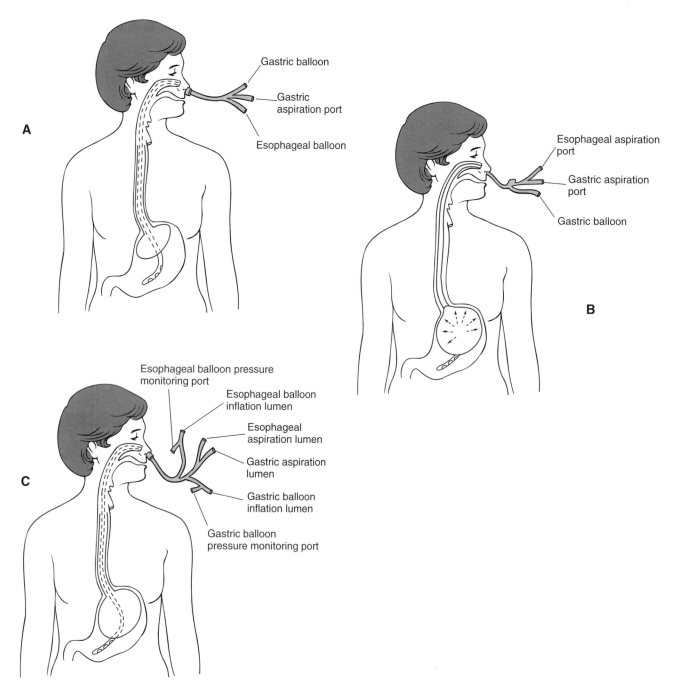

Figure 22-4 Esophageal tamponade balloons. **A**, Sengstaken-Blakemore tube. **B**, Linton tube. **C**, Minnesota tube.

The *Minnesota* tube has four lumens, for the gastric balloon, esophageal balloon, gastric suction, and esophageal suction (Figure 22-4, C). The Minnesota tube is preferable to the other tubes because it offers both a gastric and an esophageal balloon and allows suction to be applied both above and below the balloons (in the stomach and in the esophagus).[30]

Balloon tamponade tubes are inserted by the physician. Once the tube is passed into the stomach and placement is assessed, the gastric balloon is inflated with 250 to 300 ml of air (or as specified by the tube manufacturer). The tube is then placed under tension so that the gastric balloon places pressure on the gastroesophageal junction. Two to three pounds of tension is usually applied using a helmet with a constant-traction spring device. Once secured in place, the esophageal balloon is inflated to a pressure of 25 to 45 mm Hg. Low intermittent suction is applied to both the gastric and esophageal ports. Once the patient's bleeding has stopped for 24 hours, the esophageal balloon is deflated, and

patient safety ——————————— Box 22-13

Esophagogastric Balloon Tamponade Tubes

- Balloon migration is a potentially life-threatening complication of balloon tamponade therapy.
- If gastric balloon is allowed to deflate slowly or it ruptures, esophageal balloon migrates upward, where it can occlude patient's airway. If patient develops respiratory distress, gastric and esophageal balloon ports must be cut immediately.

if rebleeding does not occur over the next 24 hours, the gastric balloon is deflated. If no further bleeding occurs, the tube is removed 24 hours later.[30]

Nursing management of the patient with a balloon tamponade tube includes monitoring for rebleeding and observing for complications of the tube. The most common complication is pulmonary aspiration, which can be limited by emptying the stomach and placing an endotracheal tube before passing the balloon tamponade tube. Additional complications include esophageal erosion and rupture, balloon migration, and nasal necrosis (Box 22-13).[30]

Transjugular Intrahepatic Portosystemic Shunt

A transjugular intrahepatic portosystemic shunt (TIPS) is an angiographic interventional procedure for decreasing portal hypertension. Recent data suggest that TIPS is advocated in (1) patients with portal hypertension who are also experiencing active bleeding or poor liver reserve, (2) transplant patients, and (3) patients with other surgical risks.[14] The TIPS procedure is usually performed by a gastroenterologist, vascular surgeon, or interventional radiologist.

Portal hypertension is first confirmed by direct measurement of the pressure in the portal vein (gradient greater than 10 mm Hg). Cannulation is achieved through the internal jugular vein, and an angiographic catheter is advanced into the middle or right hepatic vein. The midhepatic vein is then catheterized, and a new route is created connecting the portal and hepatic veins, using a needle and guidewire with a dilating balloon. An expandable stainless steel stent is then placed in the liver parenchyma to maintain that connection (see Figure 22-2). The increased resistance in the liver is therefore bypassed.[32]

TIPS may be performed on patients with bleeding varices or refractory bleeding varices or as a "bridge" to liver transplant if the candidate becomes hemodynamically unstable. Postprocedural care should include observation for overt (cannulation site) or covert (intrahepatic site) bleeding, hepatic or portal vein laceration (resulting in rapid loss of blood volume), and inadvertent puncture of surrounding organs. Other complications include bile duct trauma, stent migration, and stent thrombosis.[31] Portal hypertension recurs in 90% of patients, whereas stent stenosis occurs in 20% to 50% of patients.[32]

REFERENCES

1. Liolios A, Oropello JM, Benjamin E: Gastrointestinal complications in the intensive care unit, Clin Chest Med 20:329, 1999.
2. Kupfer Y, Cappell MS, Tessler S: Acute gastrointestinal bleeding in the intensive care unit: the intensivist's perspective, Gastroenterol Clin North Am 29:275, 2000.
3. Beejay U, Wolfe MM: Acute gastrointestinal bleeding in the intensive care unit: the gastroenterologist's perspective, Gastroenterol Clin North Am 29:309, 2000.
4. Zuckerman GR, Prakash C: Acute lower intestinal bleeding. Part II. Etiology, therapy, and outcomes, Gastrointest Endosc 49:228, 1999.
5. Fallah MA, Prakash C, Edmundowicz S: Acute gastrointestinal bleeding, Med Clin North Am 84:1183, 2000.
6. McCance KL, Huether SE: Pathophysiology: the biologic basis for disease in adults and children, ed 4, St Louis, 2002, Mosby.
7. Smoot DT, Go MF, Cryer B: Peptic ulcer disease, Prim Care 28:487, 2001.
8. Fennerty MB: Pathophysiology of the upper gastrointestinal tract in the critically ill patient: rationale for the therapeutic benefits of acid suppression, Crit Care Med 30:S351, 2002.
9. Luketic VA, Sanyal AJ: Esophageal varices. I. Clinical presentation, medical therapy, and endoscopic therapy, Gastroenterol Clin North Am 29:337, 2000.
10. Sharara AI, Rockey DC: Medical progress: gastroesophageal variceal hemorrhage, N Engl J Med 345:669, 2001.
11. Zimmerman HM, Curfman KL: Acute gastrointestinal bleeding, AACN Clin Issues 8:449, 1997.
12. Zuckerman GR, Prakash C: Acute lower intestinal bleeding. Part I. Clinical presentation and diagnosis, Gastrointest Endosc 48:606, 1999.
13. Stabile BE, Stamos MJ: Surgical management of gastrointestinal bleeding, Gastroenterol Clin North Am 29:189, 2000.
14. Luketic VA, Sanyal AJ: Esophageal varices. II. TIPS (transjugular intrahepatic portosystemic shunt) and surgical therapy, Gastroenterol Clin North Am 29:387, 2000.
15. Banks PA: Practice guidelines for acute pancreatitis, Am J Gastroenterol 92:377, 1997.
16. Triester SL, Kowdley KV: Prognostic factors in acute pancreatitis, J Clin Gastroenterol 34:167, 2002.
17. Krumberger JM: Acute pancreatitis, Aliso Viejo, Calif, 1998, American Association of Critical-Care Nurses.
18. Hale AS, Moseley MJ, Warner SC: Treating pancreatitis in the acute care setting, Dimens Crit Care Nurs 19(4):15, 2000.
19. Bank S, Indaram A: Causes of acute and recurrent pancreatitis: clinical considerations and clues to diagnosis, Gastroenterol Clin North Am 28:571, 1999.
20. Karne S, Gorelick FS: Etiopathogenesis of acute pancreatitis, Surg Clin North Am 79:699, 1999.
21. Wrobleski DM, Barth MM, Oyen LJ: Necrotizing pancreatitis: pathophysiology, diagnosis, and acute care management, AACN Clin Issues 10:464, 1999.
22. Ratschko M, Fenner T, Lankisch PG: The role of antibiotic prophylaxis in the treatment of acute pancreatitis, Gastroenterol Clin North Am 28:641, 1999.
23. Cooperman AM: Surgical treatment of pancreatic pseudocysts, Surg Clin North Am 81:411, 2001.
24. Venu RP et al: Endoscopic transpapillary drainage of pancreatic abscess: technique and results, Gastrointest Endosc 51:391, 2000.
25. Neff R: Pancreatic pseudocysts and fluid collections: percutaneous approach, Surg Clin North Am 81:399, 2001.
26. Gill RQ, Sterling RK: Acute liver failure, J Clin Gastroenterol 33:191, 2001.
27. Riordan SM, Williams R: Fulminant hepatic failure, Clin Liver Dis 4:25, 2000.

28. Shakil AO, Mazariegos GV, Kramer DJ: Fulminant hepatic failure, *Surg Clin North Am* 79:77, 1999.

29. Jones EA: Pathogenesis of hepatic encephalopathy, *Clin Liver Dis* 4:467, 2000.

30. Society of Gastroenterology Nurses and Associates Core Curriculum Committee: *Gastroenterology nursing: a core curriculum*, ed 2, St Louis, 1998, Mosby.

31. Bouley G et al: Transjugular intrahepatic portosystemic shunt: an alternative, *Crit Care Nurse* 16(1):26, 1996.

32. Carr-Locke DL et al: Technology assessment status evaluation: transvenous intrahepatic portosystemic shunt (TIPS), *Gastrointest Endosc* 47:584, 1998.

EIGHT

ENDOCRINE ALTERATIONS

JOANN M. CLARK

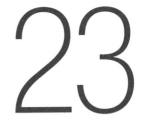

Endocrine Assessment and Diagnostic Procedures

Objectives

- Identify the components of an endocrine history.
- Describe clinical findings in patients with pancreatic and posterior pituitary dysfunction.
- Delineate the clinical significance of laboratory tests in assessment of endocrine disorders.
- Outline important diagnostic procedures for detection of endocrine dysfunction.

Assessment of the patient with endocrine dysfunction is a systematic process that incorporates both the history and the physical examination. Most of the endocrine glands are deeply encased in the human body. Although the placement of the glands provides security for the glandular functions, their resulting inaccessibility limits clinical examination. Nevertheless, the endocrine glands can be assessed indirectly. The critical care nurse who understands the metabolic actions of the hormones produced by endocrine glands assesses the physiology of the gland by monitoring that gland's target tissue (Figure 23-1). This chapter describes clinical and diagnostic evaluation of the pancreas and the posterior pituitary gland.

HISTORY

The initial presentation of the patient determines the rapidity and direction of the interview. For a patient in acute distress the history is curtailed to only a few questions about the patient's chief complaint and precipitating events. For the patient without obvious distress the endocrine history focuses on four priority areas: (1) review of present illness, (2) overview of general endocrine status, (3) examination of general health status, and (4) survey of lifestyle. Data collection in the endocrine history for diabetes complications is outlined in Box 23-1.

PANCREAS
Physical Assessment

Insulin, which is produced by the pancreas, is responsible for glucose metabolism. The clinical assessment provides information about pancreatic functioning. Clinical manifestations of abnormal glucose metabolism often manifest as hyperglycemia, which is the initial assessment priority for the patient with pancreatic dysfunction.

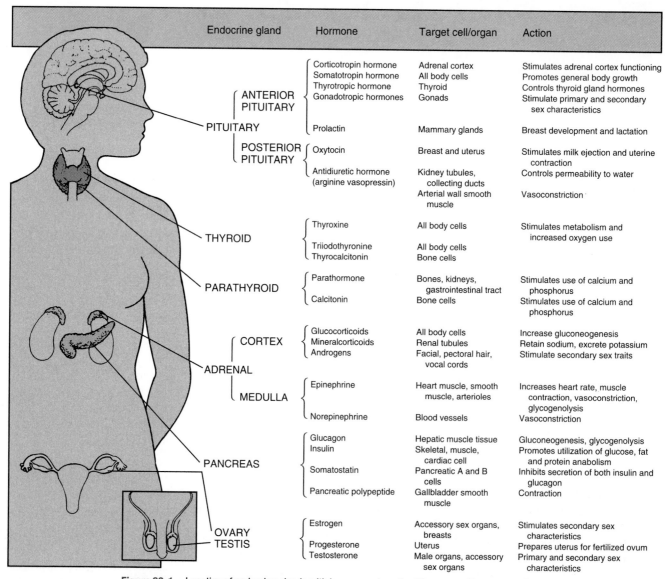

Endocrine gland	Hormone	Target cell/organ	Action
ANTERIOR PITUITARY	Corticotropin hormone	Adrenal cortex	Stimulates adrenal cortex functioning
	Somatotropin hormone	All body cells	Promotes general body growth
	Thyrotropic hormone	Thyroid	Controls thyroid gland hormones
	Gonadotropic hormones	Gonads	Stimulate primary and secondary sex characteristics
PITUITARY	Prolactin	Mammary glands	Breast development and lactation
POSTERIOR PITUITARY	Oxytocin	Breast and uterus	Stimulates milk ejection and uterine contraction
	Antidiuretic hormone (arginine vasopressin)	Kidney tubules, collecting ducts	Controls permeability to water
		Arterial wall smooth muscle	Vasoconstriction
THYROID	Thyroxine	All body cells	Stimulates metabolism and increased oxygen use
	Triiodothyronine	All body cells	
	Thyrocalcitonin	Bone cells	
PARATHYROID	Parathormone	Bones, kidneys, gastrointestinal tract	Stimulates use of calcium and phosphorus
	Calcitonin	Bone cells	Stimulates use of calcium and phosphorus
ADRENAL CORTEX	Glucocorticoids	All body cells	Increase gluconeogenesis
	Mineralcorticoids	Renal tubules	Retain sodium, excrete potassium
	Androgens	Facial, pectoral hair, vocal cords	Stimulate secondary sex traits
ADRENAL MEDULLA	Epinephrine	Heart muscle, smooth muscle, arterioles	Increases heart rate, muscle contraction, vasoconstriction, glycogenolysis
	Norepinephrine	Blood vessels	Vasoconstriction
PANCREAS	Glucagon	Hepatic muscle tissue	Gluconeogenesis, glycogenolysis
	Insulin	Skeletal, muscle, cardiac cell	Promotes utilization of glucose, fat and protein anabolism
	Somatostatin	Pancreatic A and B cells	Inhibits secretion of both insulin and glucagon
	Pancreatic polypeptide	Gallbladder smooth muscle	Contraction
OVARY	Estrogen	Accessory sex organs, breasts	Stimulates secondary sex characteristics
	Progesterone	Uterus	Prepares uterus for fertilized ovum
TESTIS	Testosterone	Male organs, accessory sex organs	Primary and secondary sex characteristics

Figure 23-1   Location of endocrine glands with hormones, target cell/organ, and hormone action.

Box 23-1 Endocrine History for Diabetic Complications

CURRENT HEALTH STATUS

Recent history of severe infection, surgical wound, or traumatic injury (Body may not be able to adjust to increased insulin needs resulting from sudden physiologic changes.)

Recent/current signs and symptoms
- Unexplained changes in weight, thirst, or hunger
- Headache, blurred vision
- Long-standing, unhealed infection
- Vaginitis, pruritus
- Leg pain, numbness

Unexplained change in urinary patterns (daytime/nighttime, frequency, volume)
- Energy/stamina changes
- Endurance level
- Weakness
- Unexplained, excessive fatigue

Behavior/mental changes (Also ask family member or significant other for input.)
- Memory loss
- Disorientation

HISTORY OF PRESENT ILLNESS

Onset, characteristics, and course

Chronic illness (Physiologic or psychologic stress could increase endogenous glucose.)

Recent treatment as possible source of exogenous glucose
- Hyperalimentation
- Peritoneal dialysis
- Hemodialysis

Medications, prescription and over-the-counter preparations (Pharmacologic agents can alter pancreatic function by either increasing or decreasing release of endocrine hormones. Drugs also may interfere with hormonal action at receptor sites on target cell.)

PAST HISTORY

Previous pancreatic surgery

Patient ever been told that:
- Had too much sugar in the urine?
- Had too much sugar in the blood?
- Would probably develop too much sugar later in life?

If "yes" to any question above:
- What treatment (if any) was prescribed?
- Is patient currently following such a treatment?

FAMILY HISTORY

Has a family member ever been diagnosed with diabetes or sugar in the blood?

If so, how did family member treat the condition?

Hyperglycemia

Because severe hyperglycemia affects a variety of body systems, all systems are assessed. The patient may complain of blurred vision, headache, weakness, fatigue, drowsiness, anorexia, nausea, and abdominal pain. On *inspection* the patient has flushed skin, polyuria, polydipsia, vomiting, and evidence of dehydration. Progressive deterioration in the level of consciousness, from alert to lethargic or comatose, is observed as the hyperglycemia exacerbates. If ketoacidosis occurs the patient's breathing becomes deep and rapid (Kussmaul respirations) and the breath may have a fruity odor. *Auscultation* of the abdomen reveals hypoactive bowel sounds. *Palpation* elicits abdominal tenderness. *Percussion* reveals diminished deep tendon reflexes. Because hyperglycemia results in osmotic diuresis, the patient's fluid volume status is assessed. Signs of dehydration include tachycardia, orthostatic hypotension, and poor skin turgor.

Laboratory Studies

Pertinent laboratory tests for pancreatic function measure the short- and long-term serum glucose levels, which can identify precursor states to type 2 diabetes and diagnose presence of the disease. Laboratory studies also measure the amount of insulin produced by the pancreatic B cells and the effectiveness of insulin in transporting glucose from the bloodstream into the cell. Additional tests that determine the residual effects of incomplete glucose uptake and use by the cells include serum osmolality and ketone levels.[1,2]

Glucose

The National Diabetes Data Group and the World Health Organization revised the criteria used to diagnose diabetes mellitus.[3,4] A normal fasting glucose range is from 70-110 milligrams per deciliter (mg/dl). A fasting glucose between 110 and 126 mg/dl identifies *impaired fasting glucose tolerance*, a condition implying increased risk to develop type 2 diabetes and coronary heart disease.[3] Fasting blood (plasma) glucose level greater than 126 mg/dl in an asymptomatic individual is diagnostic for diabetes.[3,4] Recent clinical practice guidelines list three ways to diagnose diabetes. For example, one instance of symptoms with casual (nonfasting) plasma glucose greater than 200 mg/dl (11.1 millimoles per liter [mmol/L]), confirmed *on a subsequent day* by (1) fasting plasma glucose (FPG) greater than 126 mg/dl (7.0 mmol/L), *or* (2) oral glucose tolerance test (OGTT) with plasma glucose greater than 200 mg/dl at 2 hours after glucose load, *or* (3) symptoms with casual (nonfasting) plasma glucose greater than 200 mg/dl, warrants the diagnosis of diabetes.[4]

The circulating blood (plasma) glucose level is derived from three sources: exogenous intake of glucose, release of glycogen stores (*glycogenolysis*), and conversion of noncarbohydrate sources to glucose (*gluconeogenesis*). The circulating glucose level also depends on the peripheral uptake of glucose and the functioning of the liver and its role in gluconeogenesis. Consistently elevated glucose levels signal both an increase in glucagon production and an insufficient amount of effective insulin.[5]

Glycosylated Hemoglobin

A normal glycosylated hemoglobin level is 4% to 6%, with an acceptable level of 7% or less.[6] This laboratory test provides information about the average amount of glucose that has been present in the patient's bloodstream over the previous 3 to 4 months.[6] During the 120-day life span of red blood cells (erythrocytes), the hemoglobin within each cell binds to the available blood glucose through a process known as *glycosylation*. Typically, 4% to 6% of hemoglobin contains the glucose group HbA$_{1c}$. The HbA$_{1c}$ test result provides useful information about the degree of hyperglycemia over time.[3,6] This value correlates with specific blood glucose levels (Table 23-1).

Glycated Serum Proteins

Serum fructosamine level, a newer and less frequently used test, measures the glycosylation of the serum protein albumin. Albumin has a much shorter half-life than glucose, and the test reflects glycemic levels of the preceding 2 to 4 weeks. This test is a useful measure for patients who have a hemoglobin abnormality, such as hemolytic anemia. Normal serum fructosamine levels are 1.5 to 2.4 mmol/L when serum albumin level is 5 grams per deciliter (g/dl).[3,6]

Serum Ketones

In a serum blood test, normal ketone level is 2 to 4 mg/dl of blood and normal acetone 0.3 to 2.0 mg/dl of blood. Ketones are by-products of fat metabolism. In most cases, when the body uses carbohydrate as its main source of energy, the liver completes fat metabolism and minimal or no ketones are found in the blood. Elevated blood ketones (ketonemia) are also detected by a fruity, sweet-smelling odor on the exhaled

breath. This odor is the result of the body's attempt to keep the pH within the normal range. A sweet-smelling breath occurs when the lungs release carbon dioxide in an attempt to decrease the accumulated acids.[1]

Urine Ketones

Normally ketones are not present in the urine. In the absence of glucose, fats are burned for energy. In diabetic ketoacidosis, fat breakdown (lipolysis) occurs so rapidly that fat metabolism is incomplete and ketone bodies (acetone, β-hydroxybutyric acid, and acetoacetic acid) collect in the blood (*ketonemia*) and are excreted in the urine (*ketonuria*).[7]

PITUITARY GLAND

The pituitary gland, recessed in the base of the cranium, is not accessible to physical assessment. The critical care nurse must therefore be aware of the systemic effects of a normally functioning pituitary to be able to identify dysfunction. One essential hormone formed in the hypothalamus but secreted through the posterior pituitary gland is *antidiuretic hormone* (ADH), also known as *vasopressin*.

Physical Assessment

ADH controls the amount of fluid lost and retained within the body. Acute dysfunction of the posterior pituitary or the hypothalamus can result in insufficient or excessive ADH production. Thus the clinical signs of posterior pituitary dysfunction often manifest as fluid volume deficit (insufficient ADH production) or fluid volume excess (excessive ADH production).

Nursing priorities in assessment of the patient with fluid volume imbalance and endocrine dysfunction focus on (1) **assessing hydration status,** (2) **evaluating vital signs,** and (3) **measuring the patient's weight and intake/output level.**

Assessing Hydration Status

The nurse determines the effectiveness of ADH production by conducting a hydration assessment. A hydration assessment includes observations of skin integrity, skin turgor, and buccal membrane moisture. Moist, shiny buccal membranes indicate satisfactory fluid balance. Skin turgor that is resilient and returns to its original position in less than 3 seconds after being pinched or lifted indicates adequate skin elasticity. Skin over the forehead, clavicle, and sternum is the most reliable for testing tissue turgor because it is less affected by aging and thus more easily assessed for changes related to fluid balance. A well-hydrated patient has skin in the groin and axilla that is slightly moist to touch.

Other indicators that the patient's hydration status is adequate for metabolic demands include a balanced intake and output and absence of thirst. Absence of thirst, however, is not a reliable indicator of dehydration in those with decreased thirst mechanisms, such as the elderly or critically ill patients. Absence of abrupt changes in mental status may

Table **23-1**	Correlation between Hemoglobin (Hb) A$_{1c}$ and Blood (Plasma) Glucose	
	Mean Plasma Glucose	
HbA$_{1c}$ (%)	**(mg/dl)**	**(mmol/L)**
6	135	7.5
7	170	9.5
8	205	11.5
9	240	13.5
10	275	15.5
11	310	17.5
12	345	19.5

Data from American Diabetes Association: Tests of glycemia in diabetes, *Diabetes Care* 26(suppl):106, 2003.

also indicate normal hydration. Other indicators of normal hydration include absence of edema, stable weight, and urine specific gravity that falls within the normal range (1.005 to 1.030).

Evaluating Vital Signs

Changes in heart rate, blood pressure (BP), and central venous pressure (when available) are useful to determine fluid volume status. BP and pulse are monitored frequently. Decreased BP with increased pulse is characteristic of hypovolemia, whereas elevated blood pressure and a rapid, bounding pulse may indicate hypervolemia. *Orthostatic hypotension*, which occurs when intravascular fluid volume decreases, is identified by a drop in systolic BP of 20 millimeters of mercury (mm Hg) or a drop in diastolic BP of 10 mm Hg when the patient changes position from lying to standing.

Measuring Weight and Intake/Output

Daily weight changes coincide with fluid retention and fluid loss. Sudden changes in weight could result from a change in fluid balance; 1 liter (L) of fluid retained or lost is equal to approximately 2.2 pounds or 1 kilogram (Kg) of weight gained or lost. To use weight as a true determinant of the fluid balance, all extraneous variables are eliminated, and the same scale is used at the same time each day. Precise measurement and notation of intake and output are used as criteria for fluid replacement therapy.

Laboratory Assessment

No single diagnostic test identifies dysfunction of the posterior pituitary gland. Diagnosis usually is made through an array of laboratory tests combined with the clinical profile of the patient.

Serum Antidiuretic Hormone

The result of a blood test for normal levels of serum ADH is 1 to 5 pg/ml (picogram; 5 pg = five trillionths of a gram).[6] To prepare the patient for the test, all drugs that may alter the release of ADH are withheld for a minimum of 8 hours. Common medications that affect ADH levels include morphine sulfate, lithium carbonate, chlorothiazide, carbamazepine, oxytocin, and certain neoplastic and anesthetic agents. Nicotine, alcohol, both positive-pressure and negative-pressure ventilation, and emotional stress also influence the ADH levels and must be considered in the interpretation of values.[8]

The test, read by comparing serum ADH levels with the blood and urine osmolality, is helpful in differentiating the *syndrome of inappropriate antidiuretic hormone* (SIADH) from central *diabetes insipidus* (DI). The presence of increased ADH in the bloodstream compared with a low serum osmolality and elevated urine osmolality confirms the diagnosis of SIADH. Reduced levels of serum ADH in a patient with high serum osmolality, hypernatremia, and reduced urine concentration signal central DI.[9]

Urine and Serum Osmolality

Values for serum osmolality in the bloodstream range from 280 to 300 mOsm/kg H_2O (milliosmoles per kilogram of water).[7] *Osmolality* measurements determine the concentration of dissolved particles in a solution. In a healthy person a change in the concentration of solutes triggers a chain of events to maintain adequate serum dilution. Urine osmolality in the person with normal kidneys is highly dependent on fluid intake. With high fluid intake, particle dilution is low but will increase if fluids are restricted, and therefore the expected range for urine osmolality is wide, ranging from 50 to 1400 mOsm/kg.[8]

Increased serum osmolality stimulates the release of ADH, which in turn reduces the amount of water lost through the kidney. Body fluid thereby is retained to dilute the particle concentration in the bloodstream. Decreased serum osmolality inhibits the release of ADH, the kidney tubules increase their permeability, and fluid is eliminated from the body in an attempt to regain normal concentration of particles in the bloodstream. The most accurate measures of the body's fluid balance are obtained when urine and blood samples are collected simultaneously.

Vasopressin Stimulation Test

The ADH test is used to differentiate between *neurogenic* DI (central) and *nephrogenic* (kidney) DI.[7] Five units of aqueous vasopressin (Pitressin) is administered subcutaneously to the patient, followed by measurement of urine volume and osmolality every 30 minutes for 2 hours. The patient with normal posterior pituitary functioning responds to the exogenous ADH by reabsorbing water at the renal tubule and raising the urine osmolality slightly. In severe central DI, where the pituitary is affected, the urine osmolality shows a significant rise (more concentrated), which indicates that the cell receptor sites on the renal tubules are responsive to vasopressin. Test results in which urine osmolality remains unchanged indicate nephrogenic DI, suggesting renal dysfunction because the kidneys are no longer responsive to ADH.[9]

Diagnostic Procedures

In addition to laboratory tests, radiographic examination, computed tomography (CT), and magnetic resonance imaging (MRI) are used to diagnose structural lesions such as cranial bone fractures, tumors, or blood clots in the region of the pituitary. Although these procedures do not diagnose DI or SIADH, they are useful in uncovering the likely underlying cause.

Radiographic Examination

A basic x-ray examination of the inferior skull views the sella turcica and surrounding bone formation. Bone fractures or tissue swelling at the base of the brain, which are apparent on a radiograph, suggest interference with the vascular supply and nerve impulses to the hypothalamic-pituitary system. Dysfunction can occur if the hypothalamus, infundibular stalk, or pituitary is impaired.

Computed Tomography

CT scan of the base of the skull identifies pituitary tumors, blood clots, cysts, nodules, or other soft tissue masses. This rapid procedure causes no discomfort except that it requires the patient to lie perfectly still. CT studies can be performed with radiopaque contrast or "without contrast" (sodium iodine solution). The contrast dye is given intravenously to highlight the hypothalamus, infundibular stalk, and pituitary gland. This dye may cause allergic reactions in iodine-sensitive persons, and the patient must be carefully questioned about iodine allergy before the test. Size and shape of sella turcica and position of hypothalamus, infundibular stalk, and pituitary are identified.

Magnetic Resonance Imaging

MRI enables the radiologist to visualize internal organs and cellular characteristics of specific tissue. MRI uses a magnetic field rather than radiation to produce high-resolution cross-sectional images. The soft brain tissue and surrounding cerebrospinal fluid (CSF) makes the brain especially suited to MRI scanning. Although not a definitive diagnostic test

for posterior pituitary hormonal imbalance, MRI may identify anatomic disruption of the gland and the surrounding area to uncover a primary cause of DI or SIADH.

REFERENCES

1. Buse JB, Polonsky KS, Burant CF: Disorders of carbohydrate and lipid metabolism. In Larsen PR et al: *Williams textbook of endocrinology*, ed 10, Philadelphia, 2003, Saunders.
2. Pourmotabbed G, Kitabchi AE: Hypoglycemia, obstetrics and gynecology, *Obstet Gynecol Clin North Am* 28(2):383-400, 2001.
3. Peterson KA: Diabetes mamagement in the primary care setting, *Am J Med,* Oct 28, 2003:113(suppl 6A):365-405.
4. American Diabetes Association: Report of the expert committee on the diagnosis and classification of diabetes mellitus, *Diabetes Care* 26(suppl):S5-S20, 2003.
5. McCowen KC: Stress-induced hyperglycemia, *Crit Care Clin* 17(1):107-124, 2001.
6. American Diabetes Association: Tests of glycemia in diabetes, *Diabetes Care* 26(suppl):S106-S108, 2003.
7. American Diabetes Association: Standards of medical care for patients with diabetes mellitus, *Diabetes Care* 26(suppl):S33-S50, 2003.
8. Pagana KD, Pagana TJ: *Mosby's diagnostic and laboratory test reference*, ed 6, St Louis, 2003, Mosby.
9. Holcomb SS: Diabetes insipidus, *Dimens Crit Care Nurs* 21(3):94-97, 2002.

J O A N N   M .   C L A R K

24

Endocrine Disorders and Therapeutic Management

Objectives

- Summarize the endocrine responses to the stress of critical illness.
- Describe the etiology and pathophysiology of diabetes and other endocrine disorders.
- Identify the clinical manifestations of select endocrine disorders.
- Explain the treatment of diabetes and other endocrine disorders.
- Discuss the nursing priorities for managing a patient with endocrine dysfunction.

evolve Be sure to check out the free exercises on-line at *http://evolve.elsevier.com/Urden/priorities/*

The endocrine system is almost invisible when it functions well and causes widespread upset whenever an organ is suppressed or hyperstimulated. This results in a wide spectrum of possible disorders; some are rare, whereas others are frequently encountered in the critical care unit. This chapter focuses on the stress of critical illness, diabetes and associated complications, and symptoms manifested with malfunction of the posterior pituitary gland.

STRESS AND CRITICAL ILLNESS

Physiologic changes occur when the individual is confronted with the reality or the threat of illness, trauma, or psychologic stress. These changes are initiated when the body mobilizes energy to the cardiopulmonary system, endocrine system, nervous system, liver, and muscles in an attempt to protect itself from harm. Other systems, such as the reproductive, integumentary, and genitourinary systems, are slowed to conserve energy. The body's response to stress, which is often seen in critically ill patients, has a particularly profound effect on both the endocrine and the nervous systems[1-4] (Table 24-1).

DIABETES MELLITUS

Diabetic complications and ensuing mortality have risen dramatically in the United States over the past 20 years. The U.S. Centers for Disease Control and Prevention (CDC) identified a 58.1% increase in diabetes-related mortality from 1979 to 1997. However, age-adjusted mortality from diabetes decreased 1.2% from 1999 to 2000.[5] This trend reversal may be related to applied information from two long-term studies, the Diabetes Control and Complications Trial of 1995 on type 1 diabetes mellitus (DM) and the United Kingdom Prospective Diabetes Study of 1998 on type 2 DM. These studies demonstrate that lifestyle changes and use of medications that lead to consistently normal glucose levels reduce the risk of life-threatening complications and mortality (Table 24-2).[6]

There are two distinct types of DM: *type 1* describes insulin-dependent diabetes mellitus (IDDM), and *type 2* identifies individuals who manufacture an insufficient amount of insulin or who are unable to use the insulin produced, formerly referred to as non–insulin-dependent diabetes mellitus (NIDDM). The two diseases are different in nature, etiology, treatment, and prognosis.[7]

Type 1 Diabetes

Type 1 DM is an autoimmune disease resulting in progressive destruction of the beta cells of the islets of Langerhans in the pancreas (pancreatic islets). Multiple antibodies target and destroy the beta cells, rendering them incapable of secreting insulin and regulating intracellular glucose. Lack of insulin impairs carbohydrate, protein, and fat metabolism. Treatment with exogenous insulin replacement restores normal entry of glucose into the cells. The range of insulin replacements available is expanding, and it is essential that critical care nurses are knowledgeable about this class of medications (Table 24-3). Without insulin, the rapid breakdown of noncarbohydrate substrate, particularly fat, leads to ketonemia, ketonuria, and diabetic ketoacidosis, a life-threatening complication associated with type 1 DM.

Type 2 Diabetes

The widespread difference in the number of people with type 2 DM among various cultures suggests a critically important environmental component to its epidemiology. Type 2 is prevalent in industrialized wealthy countries and is rare in poor nations. Type 2 is characterized by an imbalance between insulin production and use. Pancreatic beta cells are present and functioning but produce either ineffective or insufficient insulin. A compounding factor is an "insulin resistance" in abdominal organ and peripheral muscle cells to the entry of insulin and glucose. This creates a clinical paradox in which elevated serum insulin levels and hyperglycemia are present at the same time.

The majority of people with type 2 diabetes are overweight or obese adults, as demonstrated by a body mass index (BMI) that exceeds 30.[7] The first step in treatment is a change in diet and an exercise regimen. The diet should contain less than 30% calories from fat, lower sugar intake, and an increased quantity of whole grains, vegetables, and fruits. The exercise program is tailored to the individual but might start with 30 minutes of brisk walking each day if the person was previously sedentary.

If the serum glucose level is not normalized by these interventions, oral antidiabetic drugs are prescribed. These drugs are not oral forms of insulin because insulin would be destroyed by gastric juices. The oral agents are classified as *insulin secretogogues*, which stimulate secretion of insulin; *insulin sensitizers*, which improve the effect of insulin at the liver and reduce resistance to insulin; and α-*glucosidase inhibitors*, which slow digestion of ingested carbohydrates and delay glucose absorption. The number of oral antidiabetic agents is increasing rapidly, and the critical care nurse must be familiar with this category of drugs[8-10] (Table 24-4). After a time the oral agents may fail to increase sensitivity at the cell receptor site, and the patient then requires insulin to control blood sugar levels.

A serious complication of type 2 DM that often requires admission to a critical care unit is hyperglycemic hyperosmolar nonketotic syndrome. This severe, sustained elevation of glucose levels leads to a serum hyperosmolality and, if left untreated, progresses to cellular dehydration, coma and death.[11]

Table 24-1 Endocrine Responses to Stress

Gland/Organ	Hormone	Response/Physical Examination
Adrenal cortex	Cortisol	↑ Insulin resistance → ↑ glycogenolysis → ↑ glucose circulation ↑ Hepatic gluconeogenesis → ↑ glucose available ↑ Lipolysis ↑ Protein catabolism ↑ Sodium → ↑ water retention to maintain plasma osmolality by movement of extravascular fluid to intravascular space ↓ Connective tissue fibroblasts → poor wound healing
	Glucocorticoid	↓ Histamine release → suppresses immune system ↓ Lymphocytes, monocytes, eosinophils, basophils ↑ Polymorphonuclear leukocytes → ↑ infection risk ↑ Glucose ↓ Gastric acid secretion
	Mineralocorticoids	↑ Aldosterone → ↓ sodium excretion → ↓ water excretion → ↑ intravacular volume ↑ Potassium excretion → hypokalemia → ↑ Hydrogen ion excretion → metabolic alkalosis
Adrenal medulla	Epinephrine	↑ Endorphins → ↓ pain
	Norepinephrine, epinephrine	↑ Metabolic rate to accommodate stress response ↑ Liver glycogenolysis → ↑ glucose ↑ Insulin (cells are insulin resistant) ↑ Cardiac contractility ↑ Cardiac output ↑ Dilation of coronary arteries ↑ Blood pressure ↑ Heart rate ↑ Bronchodilation → ↑ respirations ↑ Perfusion to heart, brain, lungs, liver, and muscle ↓ Perfusion to periphery of body ↓ Peristalsis
	Norepinephrine	↑ Peripheral vasoconstriction ↑ Blood pressure ↑ Sodium retention ↑ Potassium excretion
Pituitary	All hormones	↑ Endogenous opioids → ↓ pain
Anterior pituitary	Adrenocorticotropic hormone	↑ Aldosterone → ↓ sodium excretion → ↓ water excretion → ↑ intravascular volume ↑ Cortisol to ↑ blood volume
	Growth hormones	↑ Protein anabolism of amino acids to protein ↑ Lipolysis → ↑ gluconeogenesis
Posterior pituitary	Antidiuretic hormone	↑ Vasoconstriction ↑ Water retention → restoration of circulating blood volume ↓ Urine output ↑ Hypoosmolality
Pancreas	Insulin	Insulin resistance → hyperglycemia
	Glucagon	Directly opposes action of insulin → ↑ glycolysis ↑ Glucose for fuel ↑ Glycogenolysis ↑ Gluconeogenesis ↑ Lipolysis
Thyroid	Thyroxine	↓ Routine metabolic demands during stress
Gonads	Sex hormones	Energy and oxygen supply diverted to brain, heart, muscles, and liver

↑, Increased; →, causes; ↓, decreased.

Table 24-2	Blood Glucose Levels	
Patient Status	**(mg/dl)**	**mmol/L**
Hypoglycemia	<60	
Normal FPG	>70-110	>1-6.1
Impaired FPG	>110-<126	6.1-7.0
Fasting FPG diagnostic of diabets	>126	>7.0
Non-FPG diagnostic of diabetes	>200	>11.1

Data from *Diabetes Care* 26(suppl):5, 2003.
FPG, Fasting plasma glucose

DIABETIC KETOACIDOSIS
Epidemiology and Etiology

Diabetic ketoacidosis (DKA) is a significant community health problem with a major financial impact. Of DKA episodes, 20% occur in persons with newly diagnosed diabetes, whereas the other 80% occur after the diagnosis has been made. DKA may develop over several hours in a person who has established diabetes. In an undiagnosed diabetic patient, it may take days to develop and signal an abrupt onset of the disease. Of all deaths attributed to diabetes, 9% to 14% result from DKA.[7] Many deaths occur not from the ketoacidotic state, but from late complications, such as pneumonia, myocardial infarction, and infection.[7,12] Mortality from DKA is three times higher in the nonwhite than the white population.[5]

Ketoacidosis is a result of untreated hyperglycemia, ketosis, and acidemia. Counterregulatory hormones, such as glucagon, growth hormone, cortisol, and catecholamines, respond in an attempt to reverse the imbalance but only add to the continuing cycle by adding more glucose into the serum (Box 24-1).

Changes in self-management of diabetes can create an imbalance between metabolic demand and the exogenous insulin supply. For example: a decrease in insulin intake, an increase in dietary intake, or a decrease in routine exercise without adequate adjustment in insulin or diet will alter the serum blood sugar. Life cycle changes, such as growth spurts in the adolescent, require an increase in insulin intake, as do surgery, infection, and trauma. Emotional stress can increase glucose levels by releasing epinephrine, norepinephrine, or both, which triggers increased production of glucose. The patient may be continuing a routine insulin dose that is now inadequate for the required rate of glucose entry at the cellular level.

DKA can also develop in patients who use the subcutaneous (SQ) insulin pump. This device provides tighter glucose control than SQ injections. Improper functioning resulting in insulin leakage or pump failure[12] initially causes subtle changes in glucose levels. The person, believing that the pump adequately controls the serum glucose, attributes the physical symptoms to extraneous health problems.

Tending to trust the functioning of the pump, the individual delays testing serum glucose and urine ketone levels while DKA is progressively developing.

Pathophysiology
Insulin Deficiency

Insulin is the metabolic key to the transfer of glucose from the bloodstream into the cell, where it can be used immediately for energy or stored for use at a later time. Without insulin, glucose remains in the bloodstream, and cells are deprived of their energy source. A complex pathophysiologic chain of events follows (Figure 24-1). The release of glucagon is stimulated when insulin is ineffective in providing the cells with glucose for energy. Glucagon increases the amount of glucose in the bloodstream by breaking down stored glucose (glycogenolysis) and converting noncarbohydrate molecules into glucose (gluconeogenesis). Blood glucose levels for the patient in DKA typically range from 300 to 800 milligrams per deciliter (mg/dl) of blood. Elevated blood glucose levels alone do not define DKA; the major determining factor is the presence of ketoacidosis.

Hyperglycemia

Hyperglycemia increases the plasma osmolality, and blood becomes hyperosmolar. Cellular dehydration occurs as the hyperosmolar extracellular fluid draws the more dilute intracellular and interstitial fluid into the vascular space in an attempt to return the plasma osmolality to normal. Dehydration stimulates catecholamine production in an effort to provide emergency support. Catecholamine output stimulates further glycogenolysis, lipolysis, and gluconeogenesis, pouring glucose into the bloodstream.

Fluid Volume Deficit

Excessive urination (*polyuria*) and *glycosuria* (sugar in the urine) occur as a result of the osmotic diuresis. The excess glucose, filtered at the glomeruli, cannot be reabsorbed at the renal tubule and "spills" into the urine. The unreabsorbed solute exerts its own osmotic pull in the renal tubules, and less water is returned to circulation through the collecting ducts. As a result, large volumes of water, along with sodium, potassium, and phosphorus, are excreted in the urine, causing a fluid volume deficit.[13]

Ketoacidosis

As DKA progresses, noncarbohydrate molecules are converted into glucose (gluconeogenesis). Ketoacidosis occurs as ketoacid end products accumulate in the blood. Rapid, incomplete fatty acid metabolism releases highly acidic substances (acetoacetic acid, β-hydroxybutyric acid) into the bloodstream (*ketonemia*) and the urine (*ketonuria*).

Acid-Base Balance

The patient with moderate to severe DKA typically has a pH between 7.20 and 7.36.[14] Acid ketones dissociate and

Text continued on p. 399

Table **24-3**   Parenteral Insulin for Diabetes Mellitus*

Insulin	Route	Action	Onset/Peak/Duration	Special Considerations
Regular (crystalline zinc)	IV or SQ	Insulin replacement therapy Regulates storage and metabolism of protein, carbohydrate, and fats Potent hypoglycemic	In 1 hr/2-4 hr/5-8 hr	Only type of insulin suitable for IV use. Also available as regular insulin, human. Do not use if cloudy, colored, or unusually viscous. Prepared from bovine, pork, and human sources; source determined by patient sensitivity; human source has least intolerance. Potential drug interactions. Side effect: hypoglycemia.
Lispro	SQ	Insulin replacement	10-15 min/45-60 min/1.5-3.5 hr	First available synthetic insulin almost *immediately* absorbed. Shorter duration of action than regular insulin; should be used with longer-acting insulin. Reliable treatment of postprandial hyperglycemia with decreased risk of hypoglycemia.
Zinc suspension (Lente, Semilente)	SQ†	Insulin replacement hormone	1-3 hr/8-12 hr/18-28 hr	Also available as insulin zinc, human suspension.
Isophane suspension (NPH)	SQ†	Insulin replacement hormone	3-4 hr/6-12 hr/18-28 hr	Also available as isophane insulin, human.
Zinc suspension (Ultralente)	SQ†	Insulin replacement hormone Extended action	4-6 hr/18-24 hr/36 hr	Also available as extended insulin zinc, human.
Isophane Human suspension Human injection	SQ†	Rapid and intermediate acting	Varies according to combination	50% isophane human with 50% human (Humulin 50/50). 70% isophane human with 30% human injection (Humulin 70/30) and Novolin. 75% isophane human with 25% human injection (Humalog Mix 75/25).
Lantus	SQ†	Long-acting basal insulin Longer acting than NPH or Ultralente	Does not produce peak concentrations; relatively constant concentrations over 24 hours	Synthetic, also called *insulin glargine*; differs from human insulin by three amino acids, slowing release over 24 hours. Less incidence of hypoglycemia and weight loss.

*Parenteral refers to a route other than by mouth (PO). Dosages are individualized according to patient's age and size.
†Not for IV use.
IV, Intravenous; *SQ,* subcutaneous.

Table **24-4** Oral Medications for Type 2 Diabetes Mellitus

Drug	Dosage	Action	Onset/Duration	Special Consideration
FIRST-GENERATION HYPOGLYCEMICS				
Tolbutamide (Orinase)	0.5-2.0 g bid-tid	Stimulates release of insulin	Rapid absorption 30 min-1 hr/ 3-5 hr/6-12 hr	Contraindicated in pregnancy; parenteral insulin maintains glucose within normal limits. Metabolized in liver; excreted in kidneys. Renal insufficiency: start with lower dose; observe for signs of hypoglycemia. Numerous drug interactions; only a few are related.
Tolazamide (Tolinase)	0.1-1.0 g single dose or bid	Hypoglycemic	4 hr/4 hr/10 hr	
Chlorpropamide (Diabinese)	0.1-0.5 g single dose	Hypoglycemic Antidiuretic	1 hr/2-4 hr/48 hr	Disulfiram-like reaction with alcohol. Frequent monitoring for patients with fluid retention or cardiac dysfunction.
SECOND-GENERATION HYPOGLYCEMICS				
Glipizide (Glucotrol, Glucotrol XL)	5-10 mg bid 5-20 mg bid	Hypoglycemic	1 hr/1-3 hr/12-24 hr	
Glyburide (Micronase, Diabeta, Glynase PresTab)	5 mg single dose or bid 3-6 mg qd	Hypoglycemic	1 hr/4 hr/18-24 hr	
Glimepiride (Amaryl)	1-4 mg qd	Hypoglycemic	Duration 24 hr	
SECRETAGOGUES				
Nateglinide (Starlix)	120 mg tid (1-30 minutes before meals)	Hypoglycemic	Peak <1 hr	*Contraindications:* • Pregnancy, breast-feeding • Children • Hepatic disorders Dose may need to be adjusted with increased glucose during times of stress (infection, surgery, trauma).
Repaglinide (Prandin)	0.5-4.0 mg before meals; maximum dose: 16 mg/24 hr	Binds to potassium on pancreatic beta cells; increase insulin secretion		Nonsulfonylurea; useful in patients with sulfa allergies.
BIGUANIDE				
Metformin (Glucophage)	Max: 500-2550 mg divided dose	Sensitizer Antihyperglycemic Suppresses hepatic glucose production	1-3 hr/24 hr/24-48 hr	Temporarily withhold if patient having contrast radiography. Adverse effects: lactic acidosis, GI upset. Nonsulfonylurea; directly lowers serum glucose by reducing hepatic output. Promotes weight loss. *Contraindications:* • Pregnancy • Renal failure

THIAZOLIDINEDIONES

Drug	Dosage	Action	Onset	Notes / Considerations
Pioglitazone (Actos)	15-45 mg	Enhances insulin action by increasing sensitivity of cell receptors to exogenous and endogenous insulin	Peak 2-3 hr	• Renal insufficiency • Acute/chronic acidosis • Diabetic ketoacidosis • Hepatic dysfunction • Excessive alcohol intake Patients with type 2 currently receiving therapy whose hyperglycemia is inadequately controlled (HbA$_{1c}$ >8.5%) despite >30 U insulin qd.
Rosiglitazone (Avandia)	4-8 mg			Take with meals to increase absorption. Reduces BP and triglycerides. Increases LDL and fluid retention. Administration with oral contraceptives reduces efficacy of both drugs by 30%.

α-GLUCOSIDASE INHIBITORS (CARBOHYDRATE INHIBITORS)

Drug	Dosage	Action	Onset	Notes / Considerations
Acarbose (Precose)	Initial 25 mg tid with meals Maximum 100 mg tid with meals	Inhibits activity of intestinal enzymes that metabolize CHO. Reduces postprandial glucose mobilization	Peak 2-3 hr	With "first bite" each meal. First drug to reduce effectively postprandial glucose. Delays CHO digestion by blocking absorption of complete CHOs in small intestine. Does not promote weight loss; CHO absorbed in distal small intestine and perhaps colon. No apparent effect on lactose absorption, so lactose (not sucrose) substances should be used to treat hypoglycemia. Side effects: flatulence, abdominal pain, diarrhea; minimized with slow titration. Not recommended in severe renal impairment; safety in pregnancy not established.
Miglitol (Glyset)	50-100 mg tid Initial 25 mg qd, adjust bi-weekly per GI tolerance		Peak 2-3 hr	Same as for acarbose. Administration with digoxin reduces average plasma concentration of digoxin. Administration with propranolol or ranitidine greatly reduces bioavailability of these two drugs. Do not take concomitantly with digestive enzymes (e.g., amylase, pancreatin).

COMBINATION

Drug	Dosage	Action	Onset	Notes / Considerations
Glyburide and metformin (Glucovance)	1.25 mg/250 mg 2.5 mg/500 mg 5.0 mg/500 mg	Initial or second-line therapy. Glyburide stimulates insulin secretion. Metformin decreases glucose production and absorption.		See glyburide and metformin. Common side effects: diarrhea, nausea, upset stomach.

Second-generation hypoglycemics in this table are considered second-generation *oral* hypoglycemics and are more potent. Dosage is lower than for the first-generation drugs, but fewer side effects are associated with the second-generation agents.

bid, Twice daily; *qd*, daily; *tid*, three times daily; *BP*, blood pressure; *LDL*, low-density lipoprotein; *CHO*, carbohydrate.

Box 24-1 Etiology of Diabetic Ketoacidosis

DECREASED EXOGENOUS INSULIN INTAKE

Undiagnosed
Lack of knowledge, poor compliance
- New diabetic patient
- Omission of dose
- Insufficient dose to meet glucose requirement (e.g., hyperalimentation)

Malfunctioning insulin pump
Drugs
- Phenytoin
- Thiazide/sulfonamide diuretics

INCREASED ENDOGENOUS GLUCOSE

Diabetes management changes

- Decreased exercise without decreasing food or increasing insulin
- Increased dietary intake

Sympathetic nervous system responses
- Stressful events
  - Injury
  - Surgery
  - Infections: respiratory tract, urinary tract, pancreatitis
  - Emotional trauma

Increased glucagon
Increased growth hormone
Drugs
- Steroid therapy
- Epinephrine/norepinephrine

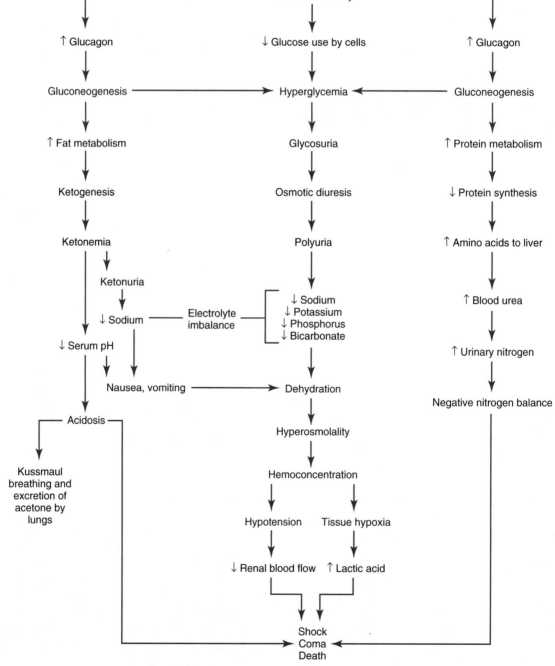

Figure 24-1 Pathophysiology of diabetic ketoacidosis (DKA).

yield hydrogen ions (H^+) that accumulate and cause a drop in serum pH. Breathing becomes deep and rapid (Kussmaul respirations) to release carbonic acid in the form of carbon dioxide. Acetone is exhaled, giving the breath its characteristic "fruity" odor.

Gluconeogenesis

Gluconeogenesis stimulates mobilization of protein as catabolism increases. Protein is broken down and converted to glucose in the liver. Continuous, uninterrupted gluconeogenesis leaves no reserve protein available for synthesis and repair of vital body tissues. Nitrogen accumulates as protein is metabolized to urea. Urea, added to the bloodstream, increases the osmotic diuresis and accentuates the dehydration.

Assessment and Diagnosis
Clinical Presentation

DKA has a predictable clinical presentation. It is usually preceded by patient complaints of malaise, headache, polyuria (excessive urination), polydipsia (excessive thirst), and polyphagia (excessive hunger). Nausea, vomiting, extreme fatigue, dehydration, and weight loss follow. Central nervous system depression, with changes in the level of consciousness, can lead quickly to coma.[15]

The patient with DKA may be stuporous or unresponsive, depending on the degree of fluid-balance disturbance. The physical examination reveals evidence of dehydration, including flushed dry skin, dry buccal membranes, and skin turgor that takes longer than 3 seconds to return to its original position after the skin has been lifted. Often, "sunken eyeballs," resulting from the lack of fluid in the interstitium of the eyeball, are observed. Tachycardia and hypotension may signal profound fluid losses. Kussmaul air hunger reveals the "fruity" odor of acetone. Normal or subnormal body temperature exists despite volume depletion. An increased temperature at this point may indicate the presence of infection.

Laboratory Findings

Considering the complexity and potential seriousness of DKA, the diagnosis is straightforward. With a known diabetic patient, urine ketones and bedside finger-stick blood sugar determinations provide rapid confirmation of ketoacidosis.

In a critically ill young adult without a previous history of diabetes, these same laboratory findings support a diagnosis of diabetes. Most likely, a second clinical condition (e.g., infection) has unmasked the latent diabetes and must also be diagnosed and treated.

Medical Management

Diagnosis of DKA is based on the combination of presenting symptoms, patient history, medical history (type 1 diabetes), precipitating factors if known, and results of serum glucose and urine ketone testing. Once diagnosed, DKA requires aggressive medical and nursing management to prevent progressive decompensation. The goals of treatment are to (1) reverse dehydration, (2) replace insulin and promote the cellular use of glucose, (3) break the ketoacidotic cycle, (4) prevent circulatory collapse, and (5) replenish electrolytes. In addition to vigorous medical treatment, the practitioner investigates the precipitating causes of ketoacidosis. Unless the precipitating factors are known and resolved, DKA probably will recur. After 10 to 12 hours of effective treatment, the patient's hydration and neurologic and metabolic status should improve drastically.

Reverse Hydration

The patient with DKA is significantly dehydrated and may have lost 5% to 10% of body weight in fluids. A fluid deficit up to 12 liters (L) may be present, creating symptoms of severe dehydration. Aggressive fluid replacement is provided to rehydrate both the intracellular and the extracellular compartments and prevent circulatory collapse.[15] Either isotonic or hypotonic intravenous (IV) solution can be used for volume replacement; no consensus exists among practitioners as to which one is preferable. Initially, normal physiologic saline solution may be given to reverse the vascular deficit, hypotension, and extracellular fluid losses. Half-strength normal saline may then be used if the individual is not in shock and has an elevated serum osmolality greater than 350 mOsm/L (milliosmoles per liter).[16] During the first hour of treatment, 1 L is infused, although the rate varies depending on urine output, secondary illnesses, and precipitating factors. To dilute the serum osmolality, infusions of half-strength sodium chloride may follow the initial saline replacement. Because the water deficit exceeds the sodium loss, half-strength sodium chloride can be given at a rate of 300 to 500 milliliters per hour (ml/hr) until serum osmolality returns to normal and blood glucose levels decrease.

Once the serum glucose level decreases to about 200 mg/dl, the infusing solution is often changed again to a 50/50 mix of isotonic or hypotonic saline and 5% dextrose. IV glucose becomes necessary to replenish depleted cellular glucose as the circulating serum glucose level falls. This will prevent unexpected hypoglycemia in the period before the patient is eating, while insulin administration continues.

Administer Insulin and Promote Cellular Glucose Use

Insulin is given simultaneously with IV fluids. The body requires insulin to move glucose inside the cells (Table 24-3). In DKA this is usually a continuous infusion of regular insulin. Frequent determinations of the patient's blood sugar and adjustments using a "regular insulin sliding scale" are requested (Table 24-5). Typically, as the acuity of the patient's condition improves, the scale is designed so that the insulin requirement is decreased from a "stress" or

Table **24-5** Regular Insulin Sliding Scale			
Glucose[*/†] (Patient status)	Mild (Thin, NPO, or elderly)	Moderate (Average weight, eating)	Aggressive (Steroid therapy of infection)
60-150	No insulin	No insulin	No insulin
150-200	1 unit	3 units	4 units
201-250	2 units	5 units	6 units
251-300	4 units	7 units	10 units
301-350	6 units	9 units	12 units
351-400	8 units	11 units	15 units
>400	Call physician		

[*]Goal is to maintain blood glucose level between 70 and 150 milligrams per deciliter (mg/dl).
[†]When blood glucose level is below 200 mg/dl, ensure patient is eating or receiving adequate IV glucose to avoid hypoglycemia.
Sliding scale insulin requirements must be individualized to each patient clinical condition.

aggressive level to lower values. Initially testing of the blood sugar can be as frequent as hourly, decreasing to every 4 hours between tests as the patient's blood sugar levels stabilize and approach normal[9,10]

Recognize Insulin Resistance

Patients who do not respond to insulin may have a problem with insulin resistance at the cell receptor site. If the serum glucose level does not fall as expected, a more aggressive approach is required. An example of one therapeutic approach is to administer a one-time IV bolus of 0.3 unit per kilogram of body weight (U/kg) to saturate the insulin cell receptor sites. This is followed by an IV infusion of low-dose insulin, 0.1 U/kg/hr (approximately 5 U/hr), until acidosis is reversed. Blood glucose testing on a scheduled frequent basis is mandatory during any IV insulin infusion.

Break Ketoacidotic Cycle

Replacement of fluid volume and insulin will break the ketotic cycle. In the presence of insulin, glucose will enter the cells, and the body will cease to convert fats into glucose. The stress cycle is broken as fluid volume is replenished. DKA can create a metabolic acidosis that can be severe.

Adequate hydration and insulin replacement will usually correct the acidosis, and replacement of lost bicarbonate is no longer routine for the patient with DKA. In severe acidotic states (pH less than 7.0), however, bicarbonate is prescribed and stopped when the pH level reaches 7.20.[16-18] An indwelling arterial line provides access for hourly sampling of arterial blood gases (ABGs) to evaluate pH and bicarbonate.

Prevent Circulatory Collapse

The symptoms of hypovolemia associated with DKA result from the glycemic diuresis and lack of oral fluid intake once the individual's neurologic status is compromised. Aggressive IV volume replacement will raise blood pressure (BP) and central venous pressure (CVP) and slow heart rate (HR). Low cardiac output (CO) and BP cause systemic vasocon-

striction, leading to tissue ischemia, infarction, and lactic acidosis from inadequate blood supply. Aggressive IV fluid replacement is required to rehydrate intracellular and extracellular compartments and prevent circulatory collapse.

Replenish Electrolytes

Hypokalemia may occur as insulin promotes the return of potassium into the cell and acidosis is reduced. Replacement of potassium begins as soon as the serum potassium falls below normal. Frequent verification of the serum potassium level is required for the DKA patient receiving fluid resuscitation and insulin therapy. Insulin treatment also precipitates hypophosphatemia as serum phosphate returns into the interior of the cell. Although the need to administer phosphate currently is debated, its use may improve tissue oxygenation and promote the renal excretion of hydrogen ions.[13]

Nursing Management

Nursing management of the patient with diabetic ketoacidosis incorporates a variety of nursing diagnoses (Box 24-2).

nursing diagnosis
priorities   Box **24-2**

Diabetic Ketoacidosis (DKA)

- Decreased Cardiac Output related to alterations in preload
- Readiness for Enhanced Fluid Balance related to absolute loss
- Anxiety related to threat to biologic, psychologic, and/or social integrity
- Disturbed Body Image related to functional dependence on life-sustaining technology
- Ineffective Coping related to situational crisis and personal vulnerability
- Powerlessness related to lack of control over current situation and/or disease progression
- Deficient Knowledge: Discharge Regimen related to lack of previous exposure to information

Nursing priorities are directed toward (1) **administering prescribed fluids, insulin, and electrolytes**; (2) **monitoring the patient's response to therapy**; (3) **providing comfort and emotional support**; (4) **maintaining surveillance for complications**; and (5) **providing patient education**.

Administering Fluids, Insulin, and Electrolytes

Rapid IV fluid replacement requires the use of a volumetric pump. Insulin is given intravenously to the severely dehydrated patient with DKA to ensure absorption when inadequate tissue perfusion is present. Throughout the insulin therapy, both patient response and laboratory data are assessed for changes relating to glucose levels. In most patients, serum glucose levels decline approximately 100 mg/dl/hr. When the blood glucose level falls to about 200 mg/dl, a 5% dextrose solution is infused to prevent hypoglycemia. At this time, insulin dose per hour may also be decreased. Administration of regular insulin drip is not discontinued until ketoacidosis subsides, as identified by the ABGs.[10] Insulin is given subcutaneously when glucose levels, dehydration, and hypotension are reversed and the patient is in stable condition with an oral diet.

Monitoring Response to Therapy

Accurate intake and output (I&O) measurements must be maintained to record the body's use of fluid. Measuring hourly urine output is an indicator of renal functioning and also provides information to prevent overhydration or underhydration. Vital signs, especially HR, hemodynamic values, and BP, are continuously monitored to assess cardiac response to the fluid replacement. Evidence that fluid replacement is effective includes normal CVP, decreased HR, and normal pulmonary artery pressure (PAP). Further evidence of hydration includes a change from the previously weak, thready pulse to a pulse that is strong and full. A change from a previously low BP to a gradual elevation of systolic BP is also an indicator of hydration. Respirations are assessed frequently for changes in rate, depth, and fruity "acetone" odor.

Once ketonuria is established and treatment initiated, ABG testing is performed to evaluate the DKA. Serum osmolality is monitored, and blood urea nitrogen (BUN) and creatinine levels are assessed for possible renal impairment related to decreased kidney perfusion.

Maintaining Surveillance for Complications

The patient in DKA may experience a variety of complications, including fluid volume overload, hypoglycemia or hyperglycemia, hyperkalemia or hypokalemia, hyponatremia, and cerebral edema. In addition, the patient is at risk for infection and for complications related to endotracheal intubation, ventilation, or nasogastric tube placement.

Fluid Volume Overload. Fluid overload from rapid volume infusion is a serious complication that can occur in the patient with a compromised cardiovascular system, renal system, or both. Neck vein engorgement, dyspnea without exertion, and elevated CVP and PAP, as well as moist lung sounds, signal circulatory overload. Reduction in the rate and volume of infusion, elevation of the head, and administration of oxygen may be required to manage the increased intravascular volume. Hourly urine measurement is mandatory to assess renal output and adequacy of fluid replacement.

Hyperglycemia. Signs of hypoglycemia, such as unexpected behavioral changes, diaphoresis, and tremors, occur after relative drop in glucose level. If hypoglycemia occurs, insulin is stopped and the physician notified immediately. The physical and emotional stressors that the patient experiences during the stay in the critical care unit may induce rebound hyperglycemia. The patient should be closely monitored for signs of hyperglycemia, such as Kussmaul respirations, dry skin, and acetone breath odor (Box 24-3).

Hypoglycemia. Hypoglycemia is defined as serum glucose level below 60 mg/dl. Most acute care hospitals have specific procedures for the hypoglycemic patient. For example, if hypoglycemia is detected by finger-stick point-of-care testing at the bedside, a blood sample is sent to the laboratory as a verification, the physician is notified immediately, and replacement glucose is administered either intravenously or by mouth, depending on the patient's clinical diagnosis (Box 24-3).

Hypokalemia/Hyperkalemia. Hypokalemia can occur within the first 4 hours of rehydration and insulin treatment. Continuous cardiac monitoring is required because

Box 24-3	Clinical Manifestations of Hypoglycemia and Hyperglycemia

HYPOGLYCEMIA	HYPERGLYCEMIA
Restlessness	Excessive thirst
Apprehension	Excessive urination
Weakness	Weakness
Irritability	Listlessness
Trembling	Mental fatigue
Diaphoresis	Flushed, dry skin
Pallor	Itching
Headache	Headache
Hunger	Hunger
Paresthesia	Nausea
Difficulty thinking	Vomiting
Loss of coordination	Abdominal cramps
Difficulty walking/talking	Dehydration
Visual disturbances	Weak, rapid pulse
Hypertension	Postural hypotension
Blurred vision	Hypotension
Double vision	Acetone breath odor
Tachycardia	Kussmaul respirations
Shallow respirations	Rapid breathing
Changes in level of consciousness	Changes in level of consciousness
• Seizures	• Stupor
• Coma	• Coma

potassium affects the heart's electrical condition. Hypokalemia is depicted on the cardiac monitor by ventricular dysrhythmias, prolonged QT interval, flattened or depressed T wave, and depressed ST segments. Hyperkalemia occurs with acidosis or with overaggressive administration of potassium replacement in patients with renal insufficiency. Severe hyperkalemia is noted on the cardiac monitor by a large, peaked T wave, flattened P wave, and broad "slurred" QRS complex. Ventricular fibrillation can follow (Box 24-4).

Hyponatremia. Sodium is eliminated from the body as a result of the osmotic diuresis and compounded by the vomiting and diarrhea that occur during DKA. Clinical manifestations of hyponatremia include abdominal cramping, apprehension, postural hypotension, and unexpected behavioral changes. Sodium chloride is infused as the initial IV solution. Maintenance of the saline infusion depends on clinical manifestations of sodium imbalance plus serum laboratory values.

Cerebral Edema. Changes in the patient's neurologic status may be insidious. Alterations in level of consciousness, pupil reaction, and motor function may be the result of fluctuating glucose levels and cerebral fluid shifts. Confusion and sudden complaints of headache are ominous signs that may signal cerebral edema. These observations require immediate action to prevent neurologic damage. Neurologic assessments are performed every hour or as needed during the acute phase. Assessment of level of consciousness serves as the cerebral index of the patient's response to the rehydration therapy.

Risk for Infection. Skin care takes on new dimensions for the patient with DKA. Dehydration, hypovolemia, and hypophosphatemia interfere with oxygen delivery at the cell site and contribute to inadequate perfusion and tissue breakdown. Patients must be repositioned every hour to relieve capillary pressure and promote adequate perfusion to body tissues. The typical patient with type 1 DM is either of normal weight or underweight. Bony prominences must be assessed for tissue breakdown and the patients body weight repositioned every 1 to 2 hours. Irritation of skin from adhesive tape, shearing force, and detergents should be avoided. Maintenance of skin integrity prevents unwanted portals of entry for microorganisms.

Oral care, including lip balm, helps keep lips supple and prevents cracking. Prepared sponge sticks or moist gauze pads can be used to moisten oral membranes of the unconscious patient. Swabbing the mouth moistens the tissue and displaces the bacteria that collect when saliva, which has a bacteriostatic action, is curtailed by dehydration. The conscious patient removes bacteria and provides oral comfort with frequent tooth brushing and oral rinsing.

Strict sterile technique is used to maintain all IV systems. All venipuncture sites are checked every 4 hours for signs of inflammation, phlebitis, or infiltration. Strict surgical asepsis is used for all invasive procedures. Careful sterile technique is used if urinary catheterization is necessary to obtain urine samples for testing. Urinary catheter care is provided every 8 hours.

Providing Patient Education

It is important to be aware of the knowledge level and compliance history of patients with previously diagnosed diabetes to formulate an appropriate teaching plan. Learning objectives include a definition of hyperglycemia and its causes, harmful effects, and symptoms. Additional objectives include a definition of DKA and its causes, symptoms, and harmful consequences. The patient and family are expected to learn the principles of diabetes management. They must also learn the warning signs to report to the attention of a health care practitioner. Education of the patient, family, or other support persons to achieve knowledge-based, independent self-management of blood sugar level and avoidance of diabetes-related complications are the ultimate goals of the teaching process.

In all aspects of patient care management, health care professionals work as a team, with the major collaborative goal of providing the best possible outcome for each patient (Box 24-5).

| Box **24-4** | Clinical Manifestations of Hypokalemia and Hyperkalemia |

HYPOKALEMIA	**HYPERKALEMIA**
Generalized muscle weakness	Impaired muscle activity
Fatigue	• Weakness
Diminished to absent reflexes	• Muscle pain/cramps
Decreased GI motility	Increased GI motility
• Anorexia	• Nausea
• Abdominal distention	• Diarrhea
• Paralytic ileus	• Intestinal colic
Vomiting	Oliguria
Hypotension	Dizziness
Decreased stroke volume	Bradycardia
Dysrhythmias	Ventricular fibrillation
Weak pulse	Irritability
Respiratory muscle weakness	ECG changes
• Shallow respirations	• Flattened P wave
• Shortness of breath	• Large, peaked T wave
Apathy	• Broad, slurred QRS complex
Drowsiness	
Depression	
Irritability	
Tetany	
Coma	
ECG changes	
• Prolonged QT interval	
• Flattened, depressed T wave	
• Depressed ST segment	

Box 24-5 COLLABORATIVE Management

Diabetic Ketoacidosis (DKA)

1. Frequently monitor and treat elevated blood glucose levels.
2. Prevent complications related to potential acidosis and electrolyte imbalance.
3. Refer patient for diabetes education once recovery from the acute hyperglycemic episode is ensured.

HYPERGLYCEMIC HYPEROSMOLAR NONKETOTIC SYNDROME

Epidemiology and Etiology

Hyperglycemic hyperosmolar nonketotic syndrome (HHNS) is often a lethal complication of type 2 DM. The hallmarks of HHNS are extremely high levels of plasma glucose with resulting elevations in hyperosmolality and osmotic diuresis. Ketosis is absent or mild. Inability to replace fluids lost through diuresis or severe diarrhea leads to profound dehydration and changes in level of consciousness. Exact mortality figures are unknown. Deaths previously caused by HHNS were probably attributed to comorbid conditions. Mortality estimates from HHNS are as high as 60%. The extremely elevated serum glucose, plus minimal or absent ketosis, distinguishes HHNS from DKA (Table 24-6).

HHNS occurs when the pancreas produces a relatively insufficient amount of insulin for the high levels of glucose that flood the bloodstream. HHNS primarily affects older obese persons with underlying cardiovascular conditions (Box 24-6). The patient may have type 2 NIDDM treated with diet and oral hypoglycemic agents. HHNS also can occur in persons with previously undiagnosed and therefore untreated DM. In either situation, some of the manufactured insulin may be effective in admitting glucose into the cells for energy. There is a major difference between DKA and HHNS. In HHNS, protein and fats are not used to create new supplies of glucose to the same degree as in DKA, and the ketotic cycle is either never started or does not occur until the glucose is extremely elevated.

The extreme hyperglycemia of HHNS can be precipitated by the stress of any major illness, such as myocardial infarction, pneumonia, other major infection, trauma, burns, or fractures. The syndrome also may be precipitated by medical interventions that may increase the serum glucose levels iatrogenically. Such treatments include total parental nutrition (TPN), high-calorie enteral feedings,

Table 24-6   Comparison of Diabetic Ketoacidosis (DKA) and Hyperglycemic Hyperosmolar Nonketotic Syndrome (HHNS)

	DKA	HHNS
Cause	Insufficient exogenous glucose for glucose needs	Insufficient exo/endogenous insulin for glucose needs
Onset	Sudden (hours)	Slow, insidious (days, weeks)
Precipitating factors	Noncompliance with type 1 DM, illness, surgery, decreased activity	Elderly patients with recent acute illness; therapeutic procedures
Mortality	9%-14%	10%-50%
Population affected	Type 1 DM patients	Type 2 DM patients, age >65 years
Clinical manifestations	Dry mouth, polydipsia, polyuria, polyphagia, dehydration, dry skin, hypotension, weakness, mental confusion, tachycardia, changes in level of consciousness	
	Ketoacidosis; air hunger, acetone breath odor, respirations deep and rapid, nausea, vomiting	No ketosis, no breath odor, respirations rapid and shallow, usually mild nausea/vomiting
LABORATORY TESTS		
Serum glucose	300-800 mg/dl	600-2000 mg/dl
Serum ketones	Strongly positive	Normal or mildly elevated
Serum pH	<7.3	Normal*
Serum osmolality	<350 mOsm/L	>350 mOsm/L
Serum sodium	Normal or low	Normal or elevated
Serum potassium	Normal, low, or elevated (total body K$^+$ depleted)	Low, normal, or elevated
Serum bicarbonate	<15 mEq/L	Normal
Serum phosphorus	Low, normal, or elevated (may decrease after insulin therapy)	Low, normal, or elevated (may decrease after insulin therapy)
Urine acetone	Strong	Absent or mild

*Except if lactic acidosis develops. With severe HHNS, lactic acidosis may result from dehydration and severe tissue hypoperfusion and ischemia.
DM, Diabetes mellitus.

Box **24-6** **Etiology of Hyperglycemic Hyperosmolar Nonketotic Syndrome (HHNS)**

INSUFFICIENT INSULIN

Diabetes mellitus
Pancreatic disease
Pancreatectomy
Pharmacologic
- Phenytoin
- Thiazide/sulfonamide diuretics

INCREASED ENDOGENOUS GLUCOSE

Acute stress
- Extensive burns
- Myocardial infarction
- Infection
Pharmacologic
- Glucocorticoids
- Steroids
- Sympathomimetics
- Thyroid preparations

INCREASED EXOGENOUS GLUCOSE

Hyperalimentation (total parenteral nutrition)
High-calorie enteral feedings
Hemodialysis
Peritoneal dialysis

hemodialysis, and peritoneal dialysis when glucose is in the dialysate. Prescription medications that interfere with pancreatic insulin production may also precipitate HHNS, including phenytoin, thiazide diuretics, and diazoxide.

Pathophysiology

HHNS represents a deficit of insulin and an excess of glucagon (Figure 24-2). Reduced insulin levels prevent the movement of glucose into the cells, thus allowing glucose to accumulate in the plasma. The decreased insulin triggers glucagon release from the liver, and hepatic glucose is poured into the circulation. As the number of glucose particles increases in the blood, serum hyperosmolality increases. In an effort to decrease the serum osmolality, fluid is drawn from the intracellular compartment (inside the cells) into the vascular bed. Profound intracellular volume depletion occurs if the patient's thirst sensation is absent or decreased.

Hemoconcentration persists despite removal of large amounts of glucose in the urine (glycosuria). The glomerular filtration and elimination of glucose by the kidney tubules is ineffective in reducing the serum glucose level sufficiently to maintain normal glucose levels. The hyperosmolality and reduced blood volume stimulate release of antidiuretic hormone (ADH) to increase the tubular reabsorption of water. ADH, however, is powerless in overcoming the osmotic pull exerted by the glucose load. Excessive fluid volume is lost at the kidney tubule with simultaneous loss of potassium, sodium, and phosphate in the urine. This chain of events results in progressively worsening hypovolemia.

Hypovolemia reduces renal circulation, and oliguria develops. Although this process conserves water and preserves the blood volume, it prevents further glucose loss, and hyperosmolality increases. Ketosis is absent or mild in HHNS. However, the patient with HHNS with an extremely elevated serum glucose (greater than 1000 mg/dl) can develop a metabolic acidosis secondary to dehydration, poor tissue perfusion, and lactic acid accumulation (see Table 24-6).

The sympathetic nervous system reacts to the body's stress response to try to restore homeostasis. Epinephrine, a potent stimulus for gluconeogenesis, is released, and additional glucose is added to the bloodstream. Unless the glycemic diuresis cycle is broken with aggressive fluid replacement, the intracellular dehydration affects fluid and oxygen transport to the brain cells. Central nervous system dysfunction may result and lead to coma. Hemoconcentration increases the blood viscosity, which may result in clot formation, thromboemboli, and cerebral, cardiac, and pleural infarcts.[12]

Assessment and Diagnosis

HHNS has a slow, subtle onset. Initially the symptoms may be nonspecific and may be ignored or attributed to the patient's concurrent disease processes. History reveals polyuria, polydipsia (depending on patient's thirst sensation), and advancing weakness. Medical attention may not be obtained for these nonspecific, nonacute symptoms until the patient is unable to take sufficient fluids to offset the fluid losses. Progressive dehydration follows and leads to mental confusion, convulsions, and coma.

Clinical Manifestations

The physical examination may reveal a profound fluid deficit. Signs of severe dehydration include longitudinal wrinkles in the tongue, decreased salivation, and decreased CVP, with increases in HR and respirations (Kussmaul air hunger is not present). Neurologic status is variable, but as the serum glucose climbs (e.g., above 1500 mg/dl), level of consciousness is affected. Without intervention, obtundation and coma will occur.

Laboratory Studies

Serum glucose levels are strikingly elevated, often double the values seen in DKA, and can reach 2000 mg/dl in some patients. Serum osmolality may be greater than 340 mOsm/kg,[19] averaging 320 mOsm/kg. Elevated hematocrit and depleted potassium and phosphorus levels result from the osmotic diuresis.

Point-of-care finger-stick testing of glucose at the bedside is the usual method for frequent monitoring of the serum blood sugar. Insulin replacement is then prescribed according to the blood sugar result[7] (see Tables 24-2 and 24-5). Some electrolytes also can be tested at the bedside (potassium, sodium, ionized calcium) but generally require an arte-

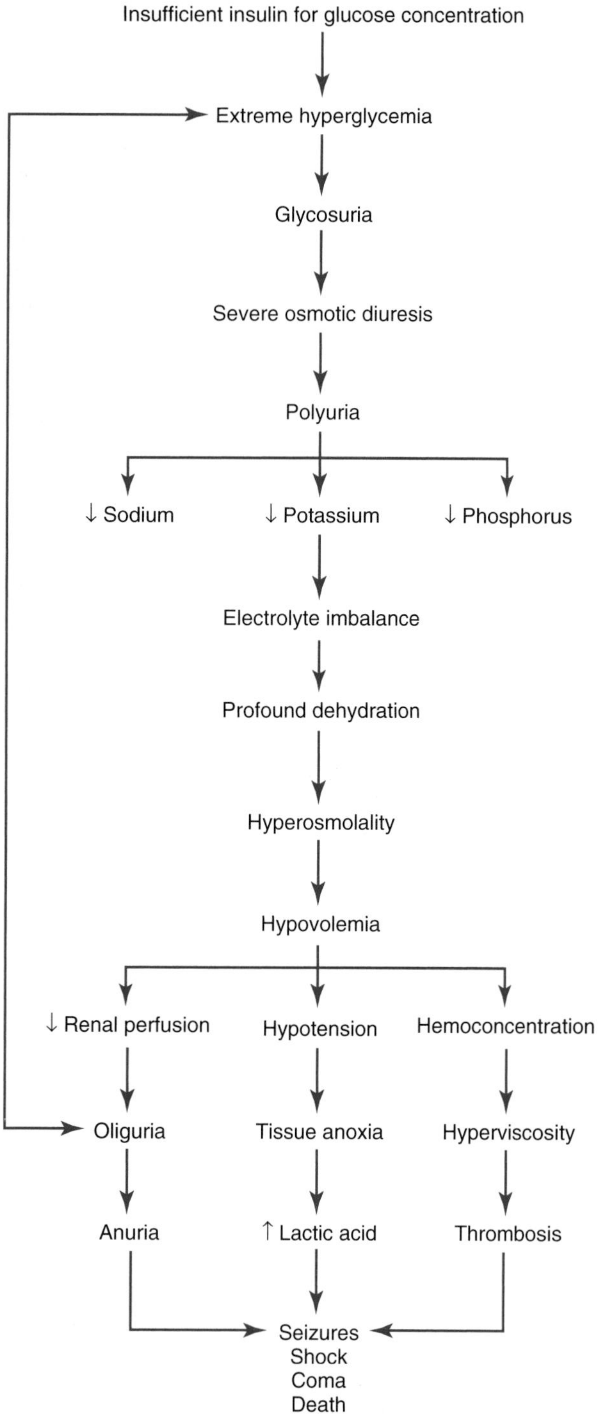

Figure 24-2 Pathophysiology of hyperglycemic hyperosmolar nonketotic syndrome (HHNS).

rial line for frequent blood access. If point-of-care testing is not available, traditional serial laboratory tests keep the clinician apprised of the fluctuating serum electrolyte levels and provide the basis for electrolyte replacement. Intracellular potassium usually is depleted as dehydration progresses. With potassium replacement, the increased

potassium in the extracellular fluid quickly reenters the cells when insulin is administered. Phosphate levels also are carefully monitored and replaced according to insulin activity and laboratory studies.

Elevated BUN and creatinine levels suggest kidney impairment as a result of the severe reduction in renal circulation.

Metabolic acidosis usually is absent at lower glucose levels. Acidosis may result from starvation ketosis, relative increase in lactic acid, or azotemia caused by impaired renal function.[12]

Medical Management

Medical management is necessary to interrupt the glycemic diuresis and to prevent vascular collapse. The underlying stimulus of HHNS must be discovered and treated. The same basic principles used to treat DKA are used for the patient with hyperglycemic hyperosmolar coma: rehydration, electrolyte replacement, restoration of insulin/glucagon ratio, and prevention or treatment of circulatory collapse.

Rehydration

The primary intervention is rapid rehydration. The fluid deficit may be as much as 150 ml/kg of body weight. The average 150-pound adult can lose more than 7 to 10 L of fluid[10] and perhaps 5 to 10 milliequivalants per kilogram (mEq/kg) of sodium a day.[20] Debate continues as to whether isotonic or hypotonic solutions are more appropriate for treating the severe fluid deficit. The consensus is to use physiologic normal saline solution (0.9%) initially, for the first 2 L,[15,20] especially for the patient undergoing circulatory collapse.[12] Once BP is within normal range for the patient, a hypotonic solution may follow. Half-strength hypotonic saline solution (0.45%) can be used subsequently to reduce the serum osmolality. The patient may need replacement of 6 to 10 L of fluid in the first 10 hours.

Another parameter for changing from 0.9% to 0.45% is the serum sodium level. Patients with sodium levels equal to or less than 140 mEq/L receive 0.9% normal saline solution. Patients with levels greater than 140 mEq/L receive 0.45% normal saline solution. Sodium input should not exceed the amount required to replace the losses. Careful monitoring of serum sodium is recommended to avoid a sodium-water imbalance and hemolysis as the hemoconcentration is reduced.[20] To prevent hypoglycemia, the hydrating solution is changed to 5% dextrose in water, in 0.9% saline solution, or in 0.45% saline solution when the serum glucose level falls to approximately 200 mg/dl.

Insulin Administration

IV insulin is given to facilitate the cellular use of glucose.[12] Muscle, liver, and adipose cells tend to be very receptive to exogenous insulin. Also in the patient with HHNS, insulin needs are low relative to the severity of the hyperglycemia.

Methods to lower the glucose level vary. One method is initially to administer 10 to 15 units of regular insulin as an IV bolus, followed by an insulin drip. Regular insulin infusing at the rate of 0.1 units/kg/hr mimics the normal physiologic secretion of 30 units/day, which includes upsurges at mealtime.[21] Once glucose levels are at or below 200 mg/dl, insulin treatment is discontinued.

Electrolyte Replacement

Increasing the circulating levels of insulin with therapeutic doses of IV insulin will promote the rapid return of potassium and phosphorus into the cell. Potassium imbalances disturb the electrocardiographic (ECG) tracings (see Chapter 11). Serial laboratory tests keep the clinician apprised of the fluctuating serum electrolyte levels and provide the basis for electrolyte replacement. Intracellular potassium usually is depleted as dehydration progresses. Potassium replacement (usually potassium chloride) in the extracellular fluid quickly enters the cells when insulin is administered. Phosphate levels also are carefully monitored and replaced according to serum levels and insulin activity.

Nursing Management

Nursing management of the patient with hyperglycemic hyperosmolar nonketotic syndrome incorporates a variety of nursing diagnoses (Box 24-7). **Nursing priorities are directed toward (1) administering prescribed fluids, insulin, and electrolytes; (2) monitoring the patient's response to therapy; (3) providing comfort and emotional support; (4) maintaining surveillance for complications; and (5) providing patient education.**

Administering Fluids, Insulin, and Electrolytes

Rigorous fluid replacement and low-dose insulin administration are best controlled with electronic volumetric pump devices. Electrolyte replacement orders are based on the patient's response to the treatment plan.

Monitoring Response to Therapy

Accurate I&O measurements must be maintained to record the body's use of fluid. Hourly urine output measures renal functioning and provides information to prevent overhydration or insufficient volume replacement. Hemodynamic monitoring includes central venous pressure (CVP), and pulmonary artery pressures (PAP) and wedge pressure if a PA catheter has been inserted. These pressures are used to evaluate the degree of dehydration, the effective-

---

nursing diagnosis priorities   Box **24-7**

Hyperglycemic Hyperosmolar Nonketotic Syndrome (HHNS)

- Decreased Cardiac Output related to alterations in preload
- Deficient Fluid Volume related to absolute loss
- Anxiety related to threat to biologic, psychologic, and/or social integrity
- Deficient Knowledge: Discharge Regimen related to previous lack of exposure to information

ness of the hydration therapy, and the patient's fluid tolerance. Symptoms of circulatory overload include elevated CVP and PAP levels, tachycardia, bounding pulse, dyspnea, tachypnea, lung crackles, and engorged neck veins. Decreasing CO is signaled by hypotension and urine output less than 0.5 ml/kg/hr. Because a preexisting cardiopulmonary or renal problem may exist in the elderly patient, the hemodynamic criteria must be based on the values normal for that patient's age and current medical condition. The critical care nurse is alerted for the clinical manifestations of fluid overload while rehydrating the patient with preexisting cardiac or pulmonary disease.

Tests for blood glucose are initially performed every 60 minutes at the bedside to determine the effectiveness of treatment. Arterial blood gases (ABG) are measured to assess oxygenation and acid-base status.

Maintaining Surveillance for Complications

The patient in HHNS may experience a variety of complications, including dehydration, fluid volume overload, hypoglycemia or hyperglycemia, hyperkalemia or hyperkalemia, and seizures. In addition, the patient is at risk for infection. Often an underlying history of cardiovascular disease may be known or latent, creating a high risk of cardiovascular complications for HHNS patients.

Providing Patient Education

As the patient's condition improves and the patient and family receive assistance regarding coping strategies, readiness to learn becomes a priority. Most teaching will occur after the patient has left the critical care unit. Teaching topics include a description of type 2 diabetes and how it relates to HHNS, dietary restrictions, exercise requirements, medication protocols, home testing of blood glucose, signs and symptoms of hyperglycemia and hypoglycemia, foot care, and lifestyle modifications if cardiovascular disease is present.

Because HHNS is an acute condition superimposed upon the chronic health problem of type 2 DM, many health professionals are involved in the care and work collaboratively to restore homeostasis for each patient (Box 24-8).

Box 24-8 COLLABORATIVE Management

Hyperglycemic Hyperosmolar Nonketotic Syndrome (HHNS)

1. Frequently monitor and treat elevated blood glucose levels.
2. Prevent complications related to potential electrolyte imbalance.
3. Treat any comorbidities that may cause problems (infection, cardiac, renal or pulmonary disease).
4. Refer patient for diabetes education once recovery from the acute hyperglycemic episode is ensured.

DIABETES INSIPIDUS (ANTIDIURETIC HORMONE HYPOSECRETION)

Diabetes insipidus (DI) occurs because of insensitivity to ADH or insufficient release of ADH from the posterior pituitary gland. ADH normally stimulates the kidney tubules to reabsorb filtered water when the body needs to increase fluid stores. ADH stimulates the tubules to increase permeability to water when particles in the bloodstream increase in number (rising osmolality) or when blood pressure falls.[22] Persons with inadequate ADH develop extremely high serum osmolality because of the massive water loss through the kidneys. If the patient is alert, an intense thirst and the passage of excessively large quantities of very dilute urine are warning signs of the disease.[23,24]

Etiology

DI is categorized into three types according to cause: central, nephrogenic, and psychogenic (Box 24-9). Only central DI is frequently seen in the critical care unit.

Central Diabetes Insipidus

Central DI occurs when the synthesis and release of ADH are interrupted. It is further divided into primary and secondary categories. *Primary* DI occurs when structural abnormalities

---

Box 24-9 Etiology of Diabetes Insipidus (DI)

CENTRAL DI
Primary
ADH deficiency from hypothalamic-hypophyseal malformation
- Congenital defect
- Idiopathic

Secondary
ADH deficiency from destruction to hypothalamic-hypophyseal system
- Trauma
- Infection
- Surgery
- Primary neoplasms
- Metastatic malignancies
- Autoimmune response

NEPHROGENIC DI
Inability of kidney tubules to respond to circulating ADH
- Decrease or absence of ADH receptors
- Cellular damage to nephron, especially loop of Henle
- Kidney damage (e.g., hydronephrosis, pyelonephritis, polycystic kidney)
- Untoward response to drug therapy (e.g., lithium carbonate, demeclocycline)

PSYCHOGENIC DI
Rare form of water intoxication
- Compulsive water drinking

ADH, Antidiuretic hormone.

in the hypothalamus, infundibular stalk, and posterior pituitary prevent the release of ADH. Primary DI may result from an inherited familial disorder, may have a congenital cause, or may occur without apparent cause. *Secondary* DI occurs as a result of a pathologic condition of the posterior pituitary. Surgery or irradiation to the pituitary gland, traumatic head injury, tumors (malignant and benign), and infections (e.g., encephalitis, tuberculosis, meningitis) can interfere with pituitary structure and physiology and compromise the release of ADH. Secondary DI also can occur in critically ill patients after a head injury or neurosurgery.

Nephrogenic Diabetes Insipidus

Nephrogenic DI results from the inability of the kidney nephrons to respond to circulating ADH. This may result from diseased kidneys with insensitive or inadequate numbers of receptors on the nephron. Some drugs cause nephrogenic DI by decreasing the responsiveness of the kidney tubules to ADH. Long-term lithium carbonate use is a common cause of nephrogenic DI.[22]

Psychogenic DI

Psychogenic DI is a rare form of the disease that occurs with compulsive drinking of more than 5 L of water a day. Long-standing psychogenic DI closely mimics nephrogenic DI because the kidney tubules develop decreased responsiveness to ADH as a result of prolonged conditioning to hypotonic urine.

Pathophysiology

The purpose of ADH in the body is to maintain normal blood osmolality and circulating blood volume. Injury to the hypothalamus, infundibular stalk, or posterior pituitary can disrupt the normal secretion of ADH. Without ADH the kidney tubules prevent the reabsorption of urinary substrate, and an excessive amount of water is lost from the body. This condition is known as *diabetes insipidus*. Although there are three types of DI, this discussion focuses on central DI, the condition encountered in the critical care unit with neurosurgery or head injury (Figure 24-3).

In DI, as free water is excreted in urine, the serum osmolality rises, and excessive sodium concentration (hyperna-

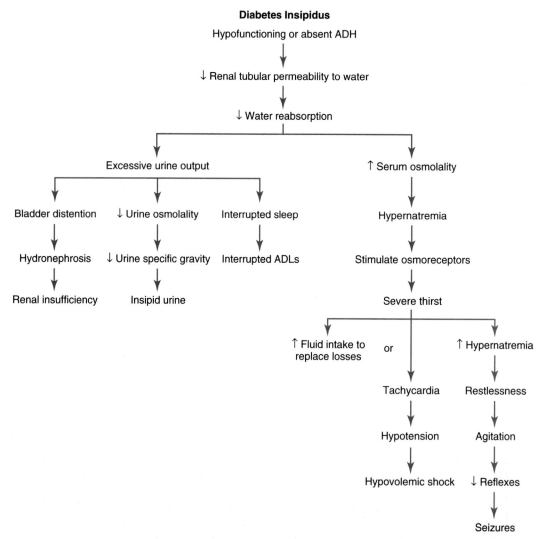

Figure 24-3 Pathophysiology of diabetes insipidus (DI). *ADH*, Antidiuretic hormone; *ADLs*, activities of daily living.

tremia) in the vascular space stimulates the thirst receptors. Polyuria develops as the kidneys fail to reabsorb tubular fluid and concentrate the urine. Extremely dilute urine is excreted, and the body is depleted of the fluid necessary for hydration. Urine osmolality and specific gravity decrease. Normally, rising serum osmolality triggers the synthesis and release of ADH. In DI, however, no ADH is released, or the ADH released is ineffective or insufficient. Without ADH, the kidney tubules are incapable of conserving enough water to reduce serum sodium.

As the extracellular dehydration ensues, hypotension and hypovolemic shock can occur. If the person is alert, extreme thirst and polydipsia permit the individual to replace lost fluids by drinking lots of water. This excessive intake of water reduces the serum osmolality to a more normal level and prevents dehydration. In the person with decreased level of consciousness, the polyuria leads to severe hypernatremia, dehydration, decreased cerebral perfusion, seizures, loss of consciousness, and death.

Assessment and Diagnosis

Diagnostic tests used to establish the presence of DI evaluate the body's innate ability to balance fluid and electrolytes and are not specific to the endocrine system. The most common tests include a comparison of serum osmolality, urine osmolality, and serum sodium values. Serum osmolality has a narrow normal range, 280 to 300 mOsm/kg; severe DI can raise serum osmolality to 330 mOsm/kg.[25] Urine osmolality can fluctuate between 300 and 800 mOsm/kg, with extremes ranging from 50 to 1400 mOsm/kg.[22-24] For greatest accuracy the urine sample should be collected and tested simultaneously with the blood sample. DI should be suspected in the unconscious patient with hypoosmotic polyuria when the serum sodium level reaches 143 mEq/L before more serious problems with hemoconcentration develop.[25]

Serum testing of the level of ADH is one diagnostic step. Normal serum ADH levels range from 1 to 20 pg/ml (picogram; 5 pg = five trillionths of a gram).[26] Alternatively, to test for the underlying cause of the DI, exogenous ADH (vasopressin) is administered intravenously, after which simultaneous urine and blood osmolality tests are recorded. The patient must be hemodynamically monitored because the ADH can precipitate hypertension and vasospasm. Patients with cardiac dysfunction are particularly at risk for complications.[27]

Medical Management

Immediate management of the patient with DI requires an aggressive approach. Treatment goals include restoration of circulating volume and replacement of ADH, plus treatment of the primary condition that is creating the interference in ADH circulation.

Volume Restoration

Fluid replacement is provided in the initial phase of the treatment to prevent circulatory collapse. Patients who are able to drink are given voluminous amounts of fluid orally to balance output. For those unable to take sufficient fluids orally, hypotonic IV solutions are rapidly infused and carefully monitored to restore the hemodynamic balance. The amount of fluid lost to the body can be estimated based on normal fluid stores and usual body weight, using the following formula:

$$\text{Body water deficit (L)} = 0.6 \text{ (kg wt)} - \frac{(\text{Serum sodium} - 140)}{140}$$

The formula assumes that 60% of an individual's weight is fluid, although this is not always exact.[28] The resulting liters of body water deficit can then be used for planning replacement fluids to restore the hemodynamic balance.

ADH Replacement

Medications have been used successfully to treat DI[9,18,22] (Table 24-7). Patients with primary and secondary DI who are unable to synthesize ADH require exogenous ADH (*vasopressin*) replacement therapy. One form of the hormone available for short-term substitution is aqueous Pitressin Synthetic, administered intramuscularly or subcutaneously or applied topically to the nasal mucosa. Onset of antidiuresis is rapid and lasts up to 8 hours. This drug constricts smooth muscle and can elevate systemic blood pressure. Water intoxication also can occur if the dose is higher than the therapeutic level.

Another drug for patients with mild forms of DI is a synthetic analog of ADH, *desmopressin* (DDAVP). It is administered parenterally or topically via the nasal mucosa (not inhaled). The drug has fewer side effects than other ADH/vasopressin preparations. Desmopressin has minimal effects on the smooth muscle tissue and rarely causes hypertension.

Nursing Management

Nursing management of the patient with diabetes insipidus incorporates a variety of nursing diagnoses (Box 24-10). **Nursing priorities are directed toward (1) administering prescribed fluids and medications, (2) monitoring the patient's response to therapy, (3) providing comfort and emotional support, (4) maintaining surveillance for complications, and (5) providing patient education.**

Administering Fluids and Medications

Rapid IV fluid replacement requires the use of a volumetric pump. Initially, a hypotonic IV solution is used to replace fluids lost and reduce the serum hyperosmolality. ADH replacement is accomplished with extreme caution in the patient with a history of cardiac disease because ADH may cause hypertension and overhydration. At the first signs of cardiovascular impairment, the drug is discontinued and fluid intake restricted until urine specific gravity is less than 1.015 and polyuria resumes.

Table **24-7** Pharmacologic Management of Diabetes Insipidus (DI)

Drug	Dosage	Actions	Special Considerations
Desmopressin acetate (DDAVP, nasal spray, Rhinal tube, Rhinyle drops, Stimate)	Nasal: 10-40 mcg at bedtime or in divided doses 10 mg/0.1 ml; 100 mg/ml Parenteral: 2-4 mg twice daily	Treatment of central DI Antidiuretic: Increases water reabsorption in nephron Prevents/controls polydipsia, polyuria Preferred treatment for chronic, Long-term DI	Few side effects. Observe for nasal congestion, upper respiratory infection, allergic rhinitis. Monitor intake/output, urine osmolality, serum sodium.
Vasopressin (Pitressin Synthetic, Pressyn)	Parenteral, intramuscular, intravenous, subcutaneous, intraarterial Topical: nasal mucosa	Treatment of central DI Antidiuretic Promotes reabsorption of water at kidney tubule Decreases urine output Increases urine osmolality Diagnostic aid Increases gastrointestinal peristalsis	Monitor fluid volume often, especially in elderly patients. Assess cardiac status. May precipitate angina, hypertension, or myocardial infarction if increased dose given to patient with cardiac history. Parenteral extravasation may cause skin necrosis.
Lypressin (Diapid)	Intranasal: 1-2 sprays (7-14 mcg) each nostril four times daily	Treatment of central DI Synthetic antidiuretic hormone Increases reabsorption of sodium and water in nephron	Proper instillation important for absorption and action. Patient sits upright while holding bottle upright for administration. Repeat sprays (>2-3) ineffective, wasteful; if dose increased to 2-3 sprays, shorten time between dosing. Cough, chest tightness, shortness of breath.
Thiazide diuretics	Varies according to diuretic chosen, patient's size and age	Treatment of nephrogenic DI Leads to mild fluid depletion; increased water/sodium reabsorbed in proximal nephron; less fluid travels to distal nephron, excreting less water	Varies according to diuretic chosen.
Anti-compulsive disorder medications, anxiolytics, psychopharmacologic medications	Varies	Treatment of psychogenic DI	Varies according to medication chosen.

Diabetes Insipidus (DI)

- Deficient Fluid Volume related to compromised regulatory mechanism
- Decreased Cardiac Output related to alterations in preload
- Anxiety related to threat to biologic, psychologic, and/or social integrity
- Deficient Knowledge: Discharge Regimen related to lack of previous exposure to information

Monitoring Response to Therapy

Critical assessment and management of the fluid status are the most important initial concerns for the patient with DI. Monitoring of HR, BP, CVP, and PA pressures (if PA catheter in place) provide early indications of response to fluid volume replacement. I&O measurement, condition of buccal membranes, skin turgor, daily weights, presence of thirst, and temperature provide a basic assessment list that is vital for the patient unable to regulate fluid needs and losses. Simultaneous urine and blood specimens for osmolality, sodium, and potassium levels are collected and results relayed to the physician as necessary.

Providing Comfort and Emotional Support

The patient who is unable to satisfy sensations of thirst or to complete any task or self-care activity without the need to urinate is confused and frightened. For patients who are able to verbalize their fears, having a nurse be interested and nonjudgmental may help reduce the emotional turmoil. The nurse must recognize the patient's reluctance to engage in any activity because of the polyuria. An indwelling urinary catheter can relieve anxiety in this regard.

Maintaining Surveillance for Complications

The most dangerous potential complication is hypertension and vasospasm of cardiac, cerebral, or mesenteric arterial vessels secondary to vasopressin or Pitressin therapy. A less serious complication is constipation from fluid loss, treated with dietary fiber, stool softeners, or both. Conversely, diarrhea may accompany abdominal cramping and intestinal hyperactivity associated with vasopressin therapy. Untoward effects are brought to the attention of the physician for dose modification.

Providing Patient Education

Educating the patient and the family about the disease process and how it affects thirst, urination, and fluid balance will encourage patients to participate in their care and reduce the feelings of hopelessness. Patients who are discharged with the disease are taught, along with their families, the signs and symptoms of dehydration, overhydration, procedures for accurate daily weight, and urine specific gravity measurement. Printed information pertaining to drug actions, side effects, dosages, and timetable is provided, as well as an outline of factors that need to be reported to the physician.

Diabetes insipidus is a life-threatening condition. The collaborative assessment and clinical skills of all health care professionals with a clear plan of care is essential to achieve optimal outcomes for each patient (Box 24-11).

SYNDROME OF INAPPROPRIATE SECRETION OF ANTIDIURETIC HORMONE (ADH HYPERSECRETION)

The opposite of DI is the syndrome of inappropriate secretion of antidiuretic hormone (SIADH). The patient with SIADH has ADH secreted into the bloodstream exceeding the amount needed to maintain blood volume and serum osmolality. Excessive water is reabsorbed at the kidney tubule, leading to dilutional hyponatremia.

Etiology

Many of the numerous causes of SIDAH are observed in patients who are critically ill. Central nervous system injury or disease interfering with the normal functioning of the hypothalamic-pituitary system may cause SIADH. A common cause is malignant bronchogenic oat cell carcinoma. This type of malignant cell is capable of synthesizing and releasing ADH regardless of the body's needs. Other carcinomas capable of this autonomous production of ADH involve the pancreas, prostate, duodenum, and thymus. ADH levels are also elevated with use of positive-pressure ventilators that decrease venous return to the thorax, simultaneously stimulating pulmonary baroreceptors to release and increase levels of ADH (Box 24-12).

Pathophysiology

ADH (vasopressin) is a powerful, complex polypeptide compound. When released into the circulation by the posterior pituitary gland, ADH regulates water and electrolyte balance in the body. In SIADH, profound fluid and electrolyte disturbances result from the unsolicited, continuous release of the hormone into the bloodstream (Figure 24-4). Rather than providing a water balance within the body, excessive ADH stimulates the kidney tubules to retain fluid regardless of need. This results in severe overhydration.

Box **24-11** COLLABORATIVE Management

Diabetes Insipidus (DI)

1. Recognize potential for DI in any neurologic or head injury patient.
2. Monitor urine output hourly, and treat DI promptly.
3. Administer antidiuretic hormone (ADH; e.g., Pitressin) to control DI.
4. Provide education after acute hospitalization regarding rationale for ADH replacement.

Box **24-12** Etiology of Syndrome of Inappropriate Secretion of Antidiuretic Hormone (SIADH)

Malignant disease associated with autonomous production of ADH
- Bronchogenic oat cell carcinoma
- Pancreatic adenocarcinoma
- Duodenal, bladder, ureter, and prostatic carcinomas
- Lymphosarcoma, Ewing sarcoma
- Acute leukemia, Hodgkin disease
- Cerebral neoplasm, thymoma

Central nervous system diseases that interfere with hypothalamic-hypophyseal system and increase production/release of ADH
- Head injury
- Brain abscess
- Hydrocephalus
- Pituitary adenoma
- Subdural hematoma
- Subarachnoid hemorrhage
- Cerebral atrophy
- Guillain-Barré syndrome
- Tuberculosis, meningitis
- Purulent meningitis
- Herpes simplex encephalitis
- Acute intermittent porphyria

Neurogenic stimuli capable of increasing ADH
- Decreased glomerular filtration rate
- Physical and/or emotional stressors
  - Pain
  - Fear
  - Trauma
  - Surgery
  - Myocardial infarction
  - Acute infection
  - Hypotension
  - Hemorrhage
  - Hypovolemia

Pulmonary diseases believed to stimulate the baroreceptors and increase ADH
- Pulmonary tuberculosis

- Viral and bacterial pneumonia
- Empyema
- Lung abscess
- Chronic obstructive lung disease
- Status asthmaticus
- Cystic fibrosis

Endocrine disturbances that hormonally influence ADH
- Myxedema
- Hypothyroidism
- Hypopituitarism
- Adrenal insufficiency (Addison disease)

Medications that mimic, increase the release of, or potentiate ADH
- Hypoglycemics
  - Insulin
  - Tolbutamide
  - Chlorpropamide
- Potassium-depleting thiazide diuretics
- Tricyclic antidepressants
  - Imipramine
  - Amitriptyline
- Phenothiazines
  - Fluphenazine
  - Thioridazine
- Thioxanthenes
  - Thiothixene
  - Chlorprothixene
- Chemotherapeutic agents
  - Vincristine
  - Cyclophosphamide
- Narcotics
- Carbamazepine
- Clofibrate
- Acetaminophen
- Nicotine
- Oxytocin
- Vasopressin
- Anesthetics

Excessive ADH dramatically alters the extracellular fluid's sodium balance. The overhydration causes a dilutional hyponatremia and reduces the sodium concentration to critically low levels. In the healthy adult, hyponatremia inhibits the release of ADH; however, in SIADH the increased levels of circulating ADH are unrelated to the serum sodium. Aldosterone production from the adrenal glands is also suppressed. Serum hypoosmolality leads to a shift of fluid from the extracellular fluid space into the intracellular fluid compartment (inside the cells) in an attempt to equalize osmotic pressure. Because minimal sodium is present in this fluid, edema usually does not result. Without ADH and aldosterone, water is retained, urine output is diminished, and further sodium is excreted in the urine. The urine has an increased osmolality from the decreased water excretion. Urinary concentration is also elevated by excess sodium in the urine. It is believed that despite the serum hyponatremia, the increased release of ADH promotes sodium loss through the kidneys into the urine.

Assessment and Diagnosis
Clinical Manifestations

The clinical manifestations of SIADH relate to the excess fluids in the extracellular compartment and the proportionate dilution of the circulating sodium. Although edema usually is not present, slight weight gain may occur from the expanded extracellular fluid volume. Early clinical manifestations of dilutional hyponatremia include lethargy, anorexia, nausea, and vomiting. The water and sodium imbalance progresses, with the sodium levels dropping below 120 mEq/L.[16] Progressively deteriorating neurologic signs of hyponatremia then predominate, and the patient is admitted to the critical care unit. Symptoms of severe hyponatremia include the inability to concentrate, mental

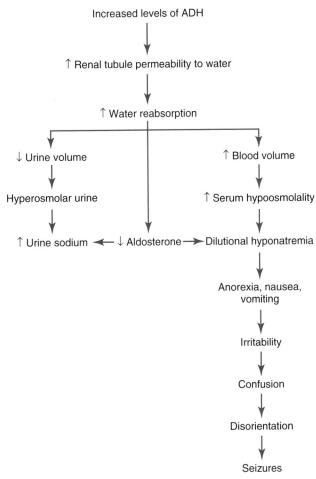

Increased levels of ADH

↑ Renal tubule permeability to water

↑ Water reabsorption

↓ Urine volume   ↑ Blood volume

Hyperosmolar urine   ↑ Serum hypoosmolality

↑ Urine sodium ◄— ↓ Aldosterone —► Dilutional hyponatremia

Anorexia, nausea, vomiting

Irritability

Confusion

Disorientation

Seizures

Figure 24-4   Pathophysiology of syndrome of inappropriate secretion of antidiuretic hormone (SIADH). *ADH,* Antidiuretic hormone.

confusion, apprehension, seizures, decreased level of consciousness, coma, and death.

Laboratory Values

SIADH presents with very dilute serum and very concentrated urine output. Laboratory values confirm this clinical picture. In SIADH the serum is hypoosmolar (less than 275 mOsm/kg) with low serum sodium (less than 135 mEq/L) and a urine osmolality greater than would be expected of such hypotonic blood. The urine sodium level is typically greater than 20 mEq/L, congruent with the concentrated urine output. A comparison of the typical laboratory values associated with SIADH versus those in DI is presented in Table 24-8.

Table 24-8   Laboratory Values and Intake/Output for Patients with DI and SIADH

Value	Normal	DI	SIADH
Serum ADH	1-5 pg/ml	Central: decreased Nephrogenic or psychogenic: may be normal	Elevated
Serum osmolality	280-300 mOsm/L	>300 mOsm/L	<250 mOsm/L
Serum sodium	135-145 mEq/L	>145 mEq/L	<120 mEq/L
Urine osmolality	300-1400 mOsm/L	<300 mOsm/L	Increased
Urine specific gravity	1.005-1.030	<1.005	>1.030
Urine output	1.0-1.5 L/24 hr	30-40 L/24 hr	Below normal
Fluid intake	1.0-1.5 L/24 hr	≥50 L/24 hr	Unchanged

DI, Diabetes insipidus; *SIADH,* syndrome of inappropriate antidiuretic hormone.

Medical Management

In the critical care unit, SIADH often occurs as a secondary disease. Ideally, recognition and treatment of the primary disease will reduce the production of ADH. If the patient is receiving any of the chemical agents suspected of causing the disease, discontinuing the drug may return ADH levels to normal (see Box 24-12).

Fluid Restriction

The medical therapy that is the most successful (along with treatment of the primary disease) is simple reduction of fluid intake. This is done most successfully for the patient with a moderate increase in the body fluid volume with hyponatremia. Although fluid restrictions are calculated on the basis of individual needs and losses, a general criterion is to restrict fluids to 500 ml less than average daily output.

Sodium Replacement

Patients with severe hyponatremia (less than 115 mEq/L) experience severe neurologic symptoms, even seizures. An infusion of 3% to 5% hypertonic saline solution is designed to replenish the serum sodium without adding extra volume. However, hypertonic saline solution is dangerous if administered too quickly, and extreme caution is required. An IV rate that provides 1 to 2 ml/kg/hr is considered safe to raise serum sodium levels by up to 12 mEq/day for the first 24 to 48 hours.[29,30] Furosemide (Lasix) may also be added to increase the diuresis of free water and to prevent development of pulmonary edema.

Medications

Certain classes of drugs decrease the output of ADH from the pituitary gland, and other drugs reduce the effectiveness of ADH on the kidney tubule. Narcotic antagonists, such as oxilorphan and butorphanol, are used to reduce the secretion of ADH. These drugs, however, do not seem to be effective for patients with SIADH caused by lung malignancies. Patients with lung malignancies are treated with demeclocycline, an antibacterial tetracycline, and lithium carbonate. These drugs inhibit the tubule response to ADH and decrease the water reabsorption at the tubules.

Nursing Management

Nursing management of the patient with SIADH incorporates a variety of nursing diagnoses (Box 24-13). **Nursing priorities are directed toward (1) administering and restricting prescribed fluids, (2) maintaining surveillance for complications, and (3) providing patient education.**

Administering/Restricting Fluids

Thorough, astute nursing assessments are required for care of the patient with SIADH, while an attempt is made to correct the fluid and sodium imbalance; the systemic effects of hyponatremia occur rapidly and can be lethal. Frequent

assessment of the patient's hydration status is accomplished with serial measurements of urine output, blood and urine sodium levels, urine specific gravity, and urine and blood osmolality. Accurate I&O measurement is required to calculate fluid replacement for the patient with excessive ADH. All fluids are restricted. Intake that equals urine output may be given until serum sodium level returns to normal. Frequent mouth care through moistening the buccal membrane may give comfort during the period of fluid restriction. The patient is weighed daily to gauge fluid retention or loss. Weight gain signifies continual fluid retention, whereas weight loss indicates loss of body fluid.

Constipation is a frequent complication of decreased fluid intake. Cathartics or low-volume hypertonic enemas may be given to stimulate peristalsis. Tap water or hypotonic enemas should never be given because the water in the enema solution may be absorbed through the bowel and potentiate water intoxication.

Maintaining Surveillance for Complications

The patient's neurologic status, especially level of consciousness, should be evaluated every 1 to 2 hours. Seizure precautions for the patient with SIADH are provided regardless of the degree of hyponatremia. Serum sodium levels may fluctuate rapidly, and neurologic impairment may occur with no apparent warning. The patient's altered neurologic response also may be influenced by the acuity of the primary disease (central nervous system disease) and not solely by the result of low sodium levels. Seizure precautions include nursing actions to protect the patient from injury (padded side rails, bed in low position when patient is unattended) and to provide an open airway (oral airway, head turned to side without forcibly restraining the patient, suction apparatus). Oxygen may be required if there is pulmonary congestion or edema than interferes with alveolar gas exchange. Oxygen is administered if needed to maintain a saturation level greater than 92%.

Providing Patient Education

Rapidly occurring changes in the patient's neurologic status may frighten visiting family members. Sensitivity to the family's unspoken fears can be shown by words that express empathy and by providing time for the patient and family to communicate their feelings. The nurse may discuss the

Box 24-14 COLLABORATIVE Management

Syndrome of Inappropriate Secretion of Antidiuretic Hormone (SIADH)

1. Recognize potential for SIADH in vast array of clinical situations.
2. Monitor urine output hourly, serum sodium, and fluid status (CVP), and treat SIADH promptly.

course of SIADH, its effect on water balance, the reasons for fluid restrictions, and the family's role in treating SIADH. Teaching the patient and the family to be alert to severe thirst and to measure I&O, along with parameters on when to notify the physician, will encourage independence and involve the family in the patient's care.

SIADH is a complex condition. Effective clinical management requires the skills of many health care professionals working as a team with clear goals (Box 24-14).

REFERENCES

1. Vasa FR, Molitch ME: Endocrine problems in the chronically critically ill patient, *Clin Chest Med* 22(1):193-208, 2001.
2. Van den Berghe G: Neuroendocrine pathobiology of chronic critical illness. *Crit Care Clin* 18(3):509-528, 2002.
3. Cone RD et al: Neuroendocrinology. In Larsen PR et al, editors: *Williams textbook of endocrinology*, ed 10, Philadelphia, 2003, Saunders.
4. Habib KE, Gold PW, Chrousos GP: Neuroendocrinology of stress, *Endocrinol Metab Clin* 30(3):695-728, 2001.
5. American Diabetes Association: *Diabetes 2001 Vital Statistics*, American Diabetes Association, 2001.
6. Cefalu WT: Evaluation of alternative strategies for optimizing glycemia: progress to date, *Am J Med* 113(suppl 6A):23S-35S, 2002.
7. American Diabetes Association: Standards of medical care for patients with diabetes mellitus, *Diabetes Care* 26(suppl):S33-S50, 2003.
8. Edleman SV, Henry RR: *Diagnosis and management of type 2 diabetes*, ed 4, Caddo, Okla, 2001, Professional Communications.
9. Kizior R, Hodgson BB: *Saunders drug handbook for health professions*, ed 2, Philadelphia, 2002, Saunders.
10. Pugh MJ: Differential adoption of pharmacotherapy recommendations for type 2 diabetes by generalists and specialists, *Med Care Res and Rev* 60(2):178-200, 2003.
11. Trence DL, Hirsch IB: Hyperglycemic crises in diabetes mellitus type 2, *Endocrinol Metab Clin North Am* 30(4):817-831, 2001.
12. Powers AC: Diabetes mellitus. In Braunwald E et al, editors: *Harrison's principles of internal medicine*, ed 15, New York, 2001, McGraw-Hill.
13. Suki WN: Phosphorus deficiency and hypophosphatemia. In Goldman L, Bennett JC, editors: *Cecil textbook of medicine*, ed 21, Philadelphia, 2000, Saunders.
14. Mashrani U, Karam JH: Pancreatic hormones and diabetes mellitus. In Greenspan FS, Gardner DG, editors: *Basic and clinical endocrinology*, ed 7, Stamford, Conn, 2003, McGraw-Hill.
15. Magee MF, Bhatt BA: Management of decompensated diabetes: diabetic ketoacidosis and hyperglycemic hyperosmolar syndrome, *Crit Care Clin* 17(1):75-106, 2001.
16. Davidson JK: Diabetic ketoacidosis and the hyperglycemic hyperosmolar state. In Davidson JK, editor: *Clinical diabetes mellitus: a problem-oriented approach*, ed 3, New York, 2000, Thieme.
17. Tonnessen TI: Intracellular pH and electrolyte regulation. In Grenvik A et al, editors: *Textbook of critical care*, ed 4, Philadelphia, 2000, Saunders.
18. Umpierrez GE, Ziegler TR: Diabetic emergencies. In Grenvik A et al, editors: *Textbook of critical care*, ed 4, Philadelphia, 2000, Saunders.
19. Tierney LM et al, editors: *Current medical diagnosis and treatment 2003*, New York, 2003, McGraw-Hill.
20. Eisenbarth GS, Polonsky KS, Buse JB: Type 1 diabetes mellitus. In Larsen PR et al editors: *Williams textbook of endocrinology*, ed 10, Philadelphia, 2003, Saunders.
21. Sherwin RS: Diabetes mellitus. In Goldman L, Bennett JC, editors: *Cecil textbook of medicine*, ed 21, Philadelphia, 2000, Saunders.
22. Rudy DR et al:, Endocrinology. In Rakel RE editor: *Textbook of family practice*, ed 6, Philadelphia, 2002, Saunders.
23. Holcomb SS: Diabetes insipidus, *Dimens Crit Care Nurs* 21(3):94-97, 2002.
24. Jacobs DS et al: Chemistry. In Jacobs DS, Oxley DK, DeMott WR editors, *Jacobs and DeMott laboratory test handbook*, ed 5, Hudson, Ohio, 2001, LexiComp.
25. Wallach J: *Interpretation of diagnostic tests*, ed 7, Philadelphia, 2000, Lippincott Williams & Wilkins.
26. Robinson AG: Posterior pituitary. In Goldman L, Bennett JC, editors: *Cecil textbook of medicine*, ed 21, Philadelphia, 2000, Saunders.
27. Robinson AG, Verbalis JG: Posterior pituitary gland. In Larsen PR et al, editors: *Williams textbook of endocrinology*, ed 10, Philadelphia, 2003, Saunders.
28. Fischbach F: *A manual of laboratory and diagnostic tests*, ed 6, Philadelphia, 2000, Lippincott Williams & Wilkins.
29. Corbett JV: *Laboratory tests and diagnostic procedures with nursing diagnoses*, ed 5, Upper Saddle River, NJ, 2000, Prentice Hall.
30. Ayus JC, Caramelo C: Sodium and potassium disorders. In Grenvik A et al, editors: *Textbook of critical care*, ed 4, Philadelphia, 2000, Saunders.

UNIT NINE

MULTISYSTEM ALTERATIONS

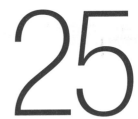

KAREN L. JOHNSON

Trauma

Objectives

- Compare and contrast injuries associated with blunt and penetrating trauma.
- Discuss mechanism of injury, pathophysiology, assessment findings, medical management, and nursing management of traumatic injuries to the head, spinal cord, heart, lungs, and abdomen.
- Use assessment findings to identify potential complications and sequelae of traumatic injuries.

Trauma is the leading cause of death for all age groups under 44 years and costs hundreds of billions of dollars annually. Injury as a result of trauma is no longer viewed as an "accident" in the critical care arena. To reflect this change, "motor vehicle accident" (MVA) has been replaced with *motor vehicle crash* (MVC), and "accident" has been replaced with *unintentional injury*. It is estimated that 30% to 50% of injuries are preventable.[1] Domestic violence and alcohol-related issues are the priority areas for injury prevention and are recommended as routine components of trauma care.[2,3]

MECHANISMS OF INJURY

Trauma occurs when an external force of energy impacts the body and causes structural or physiologic alterations, or "injuries." External forces can be radiation, electrical, thermal, chemical, or mechanical forms of energy. This chapter focuses on trauma from mechanical energy, either blunt or penetrating. Knowledge of the mechanism of injury helps health care providers anticipate and predict potential internal injuries.

Blunt Trauma

Blunt trauma is seen most often with a MVC, contact sports, blunt force injuries, or falls. Injuries occur because of the forces sustained during a rapid change in velocity (deceleration). To estimate the amount of force a person would sustain in an MVC, the person's weight is multiplied by miles per hour of speed the vehicle was traveling. A 130-pound woman in a vehicle traveling 60 mph that hits a brick wall would sustain 7800 pounds of force within milliseconds. As the body stops suddenly, tissues and organs continue to move forward, resulting in lacerations and crush injuries of internal body structures.

Penetrating Trauma

Penetrating trauma occurs with knife, firearm, or impalement injuries that penetrate the skin and damage internal structures. Damage is created along the path of penetration. Penetrating injuries can be misleading because the outside of the wound does not determine the extent of internal injury. Bullets can create internal cavities 5 to 30 times larger than the diameter of the bullet.[4] Once inside the body, the bullet can ricochet off bone and create further damage along its pathway. With penetrating stab wounds, factors that determine the extent of injury include type and length of the object used, as well as the angle of insertion.

PHASES OF TRAUMA CARE
Prehospital Resuscitation

The goal of prehospital care is immediate stabilization and transportation. Stabilization is achieved through airway maintenance, control of external bleeding and shock, immobilization of the patient, and immediate transport by ground or air to the closest appropriate medical facility.[4]

Emergency Department Resuscitation
Primary Survey

On arrival of the trauma patient in the emergency department (ED), the primary survey is initiated. During this assessment, life-threatening injuries are discovered and treated. The five steps in the primary survey comprise the ABCDEs[4] (Table 25-1):

Airway maintenance with cervical spine protection
Breathing and ventilation
Circulation with hemorrhage control
Disability: neurologic status
Exposure/environmental control

The cervical spine must be immobilized in all trauma patients until a cervical spinal cord injury has been definitively ruled out. If the airway is obstructed, foreign bodies are removed. In the presence of ineffective airway clearance, the airway is secured through intubation or cricothyrotomy. Cardiac monitoring is initiated to assess for rhythm disturbances. Life-threatening dysrhythmias are treated according to advanced cardiac life support (ACLS) protocols. External bleeding is identified and controlled. A rapid assessment of circulatory status includes assessment of level of consciousness, skin color, and pulse.

Resuscitation Phase

After the primary survey the resuscitation phase begins. Hypovolemic shock is the most common type of shock that occurs in trauma patients.[4] Hemorrhage must be identified and treated rapidly. Two large-bore peripheral intravenous (IV) catheters (14 to 16 gauge) or a central venous catheter is inserted. During the initiation of IV lines, blood samples are drawn. IV therapy with lactated Ringer's (LR) solution should be administered rapidly. High-flow fluid warmers may be used to deliver warmed IV solutions at rates greater than 1000 milliliters per minute (ml/min). If the patient remains unresponsive to bolus IV therapy, type-specific blood or O-negative blood may be administered.[4] Transfusion of autologous salvaged blood (autotransfusion) can also be used to replace intravascular volume and provide oxygen-carrying capacity. Urinary and gastric catheters are placed, unless contraindicated. Adequate resuscitation is assessed by monitoring for improvement in clinical condition, vital signs, and laboratory values such as arterial blood gases (ABGs), lactic acid level, hemoglobin (Hgb), hematocrit (Hct), and urine output.[4]

Secondary Survey

The secondary survey begins when the primary survey is completed, resuscitation is initiated, and the patient's ABCs are reassessed. During the secondary survey, each body region is thoroughly examined. The history is one of the most important aspects of the secondary survey. Often, head injury, shock, or use of drugs or alcohol may preclude a good history, so the history must be pieced together from other sources. The prehospital providers (paramedics, emergency

Table **25-1** Primary Survey of the Trauma Patient

Survey Component	Nursing Diagnosis	Nursing Assessment/Care
Airway	Ineffective Airway Clearance related to obstruction or actual injury	*Look:* • Is there obvious airway trauma, tachypnea, accessory muscle use, or tracheal shift? *Listen:* • Stridor, hyperresonance, or dullness to percussion? *Feel:* • For air exchange over mouth; insert finger and sweep to clear foreign bodies. Secure airway. • Oropharyngeal • Nasopharyngeal • Endotracheal tube • Cricothyrotomy
Breathing	Ineffective Breathing Pattern related to actual injury Impaired Gas Exchange related to actual injury or disrupted tissue perfusion	Assess for: • Spontaneous breathing • Respiratory rate, depth, and symmetry • Chest wall integrity *Absent breathing:* • Intubate for mechanical ventilation. *Breathing but ineffective:* • Assess life-threatening conditions (e.g., tension pneumothorax, flail chest). Administer supplemental oxygen. Initiate pulse oximetry.
Circulation	Decreased Cardiac Output related to actual injury Alteration in Tissue Perfusion related to actual injury or shock Deficient Fluid Volume related to actual loss of circulating volume	Assess pulse quality/rate. Maintain ECG monitoring. *No pulse:* • Initiate ACLS interventions. *Pulse but ineffective:* • Assess and treat life-threatening conditions (uncontrolled bleeding, shock) Initiate two large-bore IVs or central catheter; obtain serum samples for laboratory tests. Initiate fluid replacement.
Disability	Ineffective Cerebral Tissue Perfusion Risk for Injury related to actual injury of brain or spinal cord Immobilize cervical spine	Assess Glasgow Coma Scale. Assess pupil size/reactivity.
Exposure and environmental control	Risk for Imbalanced Body Temperature	Remove all clothing to inspect all body regions. Prevent hypothermia.

ECG, Electrocardiographic; ACLS, advanced cardiac life support.

medical technicians [EMTs]) usually can provide vital information pertaining to the mechanism of injury (Box 25-1).

During the secondary survey the nurse ensures the completion of special procedures, such as an electrocardiogram (ECG), radiographic studies (chest, cervical spine, thorax, pelvis), and if required, diagnostic peritoneal lavage. Throughout this survey the nurse continuously monitors the patient's vital signs and response to medical therapies. Emotional reassurance to the patient and family also is imperative and ongoing. Emotional support is often provided by an experienced social worker while physicians and nurses are fully occupied with the injured patient.

Definitive Care/Operative Phase

Once the secondary survey has been completed, specific injuries usually have been diagnosed. Definitive care related to specific injuries is described throughout this chapter. Trauma is often referred to as a "surgical disease" because the nature and extent of injuries usually requires operative management. After surgery, depending on the patient's status, a transfer to the critical care unit may be indicated.[5]

Critical Care Phase

Critically ill trauma patients are admitted into the critical care unit as direct transfers from the ED or operating room (OR). If surgery is required, the trauma patient is directly admitted to the CCU from the OR. **Nursing priorities during the critical care phase focus on (1) assessing the injured patient's metabolic demand, (2) supplying oxygen to preserve vital organ function, (3) limiting the extent of secondary injury, and (4) monitoring physiologic response to medical and nursing interventions.** One of the most important nursing roles is assessment of the balance between oxygen delivery and tissue oxygen demand. Oxygen delivery

---

---

must be optimized to prevent further system damage or *secondary injury*. Assessment of circulatory status to forestall development of tissue hypoxia includes noninvasive and invasive monitoring techniques. Prevention and treatment depend on accurate assessment of the adequacy of pulmonary gas exchange, oxygen transport, and cellular oxygen utilization.[6,7]

TRAUMATIC BRAIN INJURY

More than 2 million traumatic brain injuries (TBIs) occur each year in the United States, with approximately 500,000 injuries severe enough to require hospitalization.[8] Approximately 50% of all trauma deaths are associated with head injury, and more than 60% of all vehicular trauma deaths result from TBI.[4]

Mechanism of Injury

Mechanisms of injury include penetrating or blunt trauma to the head. Injury occurs when mechanical forces are transmitted to delicate brain tissues. Penetrating trauma can result from the penetration of a foreign object (e.g., bullet) that causes direct damage to cerebral tissue. Blunt trauma can be the result of acceleration, deceleration or rotational forces. *Acceleration injury* is produced when a solid object (e.g., baseball bat) forcefully hits the skull. For example, if an object hits the skull from behind, the brain will move forward inside the skull towards the point of impact. In *deceleration injury* the brain crashes against the skull after it has hit some object (e.g., dashboard of car). In many cases, TBI is caused by a combination of acceleration and deceleration forces.

Pathophysiology

Review of the pathophysiology of a TBI can be divided into two categories: primary injury and secondary injury. It is important that the critical care nurse understands this pathophysiology because goals of critical care include efforts to reduce morbidity and mortality from primary and secondary injuries.

Primary Injury

The primary injury occurs at the moment of impact as a result of mechanical forces to the head. The extent of and recovery from injury are related to whether the primary injury was localized to an area or whether it was diffuse or widespread throughout the brain. Primary injuries include contusion, laceration, shearing injuries, and hemorrhage. The primary injury may be *mild*, with little or no neurologic damage, or *severe*, with major tissue damage.

Secondary Injury

Secondary injury is the biochemical and cellular response to the initial trauma that can exacerbate the primary injury and cause loss of brain tissue not originally damaged.[9] *Ischemia* is the primary cause in secondary brain injury. Tissue ischemia occurs in areas of poor cerebral perfusion as a result of hypotension and hypoxia. The cells in the ischemic areas become edematous. Extreme vasodilation of the cerebral vasculature occurs in an attempt to supply oxygen to the cerebral tissue.[10] This increase in blood volume increases intracranial volume and elevates intracranial pressure (ICP).

Classification

Brain injuries are described according to the functional changes or losses that occur. Some of the major functional abnormalities seen in head injury are described here.

Skull Fracture

Skull fractures are common but do not act alone to cause neurologic deficits. Skull fractures can be classified as *open* (dura is torn) or *closed* (dura is not torn) or as fractures of the *vault* or of the *base*. Basilar skull fractures usually are not visible on conventional skull x-ray films because the base of the skull is not seen in this view. Therefore the nurse is vigilant in assessing for physical signs of a basilar skull fracture. These can include cerebral spinal fluid (CSF) leaking from the ear (otorrhea) or leaking from the nose (rhinorrhea), Battle's sign (ecchymosis behind the ear), or "raccoon eyes," caused by subconjunctival and periorbital ecchymosis.

A skull fracture is significant because it identifies the patient at high risk of developing an intracranial hematoma. Open skull fractures require surgical intervention to remove bony fragments and close the dura. The major complications of basilar skull fractures are cranial nerve injury and leakage of CSF.

Concussion

A concussion is a brain injury accompanied by a brief loss of neurologic function, especially loss of consciousness,[4] which may last for seconds to an hour. The neurologic symptoms include confusion, disorientation, and sometimes a period of posttraumatic amnesia. Other clinical manifestations after concussion are headache, dizziness, nausea, irritability, inability to concentrate, impaired memory, and fatigue. The diagnosis of concussion is based on the loss of consciousness inasmuch as the brain remains structurally intact despite functional impairment. Patients with a history of 5 or more minutes of loss of consciousness usually are admitted to the hospital for a 24-hour observation period.[4]

Contusion

Contusion, or bruising of the brain, usually is related to acceleration-deceleration injuries, which result in hemorrhage into the brain tissue, often the frontal and temporal lobes. Frontal or temporal contusions can be seen in a coup-contrecoup mechanism of injury (Figure 25-1). *Coup injury* affects the cerebral tissue directly under the point of impact. *Contrecoup injury* occurs in a line directly opposite the point of impact.

The clinical manifestations of contusion are related to the location of the contusion, the degree of contusion, and the presence of associated lesions. Contusions can be small, in which localized areas of dysfunction result in a focal neurologic deficit. Larger contusions can evolve over 2 to 3 days after injury as a result of edema and further hemorrhaging. A large contusion can produce a mass effect that can cause a significant increase in ICP.

Contusions of the tips of the temporal lobe are common and of particular concern. Because the inner aspects of the temporal lobe surround the opening in the tentorium where the midbrain enters the cerebrum, edema in this area can cause rapid deterioration of the patient's condition and can

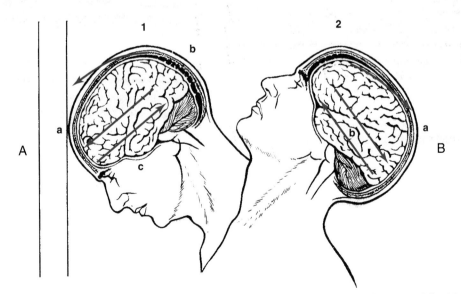

Figure 25-1 Coup and contrecoup head injury after blunt trauma. **A,** Coup injury: impact against object. *a,* Site of impact and direct trauma to brain. *b,* Shearing of subdural veins. *c,* Trauma to base of brain. **B,** Contrecoup injury: impact within skull. *a,* Site of impact from brain hitting opposite side of skull. *b,* Shearing forces throughout brain. These injuries occur in one continuous motion—the head strikes the wall (coup), then rebounds (contrecoup).

lead to *herniation*. Because of the location, this deterioration can occur with little or no warning of a dangerously elevated ICP.

Diagnosis of contusion is made by computed tomography (CT) scan. If the CT scan indicates contusion, especially in the temporal area, the nurse must pay particular attention to neurologic assessments and look for subtle changes in level of consciousness, pupillary signs, and vital signs, regardless of stable ICP.

Medical management of cerebral contusions may consist of medical or surgical therapies. Because a contusion can progress over 3 to 5 days after injury, secondary injury may occur. If contusions are small, focal, or multiple, serial neurologic assessments and possibly ICP monitoring may be indicated. Larger contusions that produce considerable mass effect require surgical intervention to prevent increased ICP as the contusion matures. Outcome of cerebral contusion varies, depending on the location and the degree of contusion.

Hematomas

Extravasation of blood produces a space-occupying lesion on the brain and leads to increased ICP. Three types of hematomas are discussed here (Figure 25-2).

Epidural Hematoma. Epidural hematoma (EDH) is a collection of blood between the inner table of the skull and the outermost layer of the dura, most often associated with skull fractures and middle meningeal artery laceration. A blow to the head that causes a linear skull fracture on the lateral surface of the head may tear the middle meningeal artery. As the artery bleeds, it pulls the dura away from the skull, creating a pouch that expands into the intracranial space. EDH occurs from trauma to the skull and meninges rather than from the acceleration-deceleration forces seen in other types of head trauma.

The classic clinical manifestations of EDH include brief loss of consciousness followed by a period of lucidity. This lucid period is followed by a rapid deterioration in level of consciousness. A dilated and fixed pupil on the same side as the impact area is a hallmark of EDH.[4] The patient may complain of a severe, localized headache and may be sleepy. Diagnosis of EDH is based on clinical symptoms and evidence of a collection of epidural blood identified on CT scan. Treatment of EDH involves surgical intervention to remove the blood and cauterize the bleeding vessels.

Subdural Hematoma. A subdural hematoma (SDH) is the accumulation of blood between the dura and underlying arachnoid membrane. SDH is most often is caused by a rupture in the bridging veins between the brain and the dura.[4] Acceleration-deceleration and rotational forces are the major causes of SDH. There may be associated cerebral contusions with intracerebral hemorrhage.

The three types of SDH are based on the time frame from injury to clinical symptoms: acute, subacute, and chronic. Acute SDHs are hematomas that occur after a severe blow to the head. The clinical presentation of acute SDH is determined by the severity of injury to the underlying brain and the rate of blood accumulation in the subdural space.

Intracerebral Hematoma. Intracerebral hematoma (ICH) results when bleeding occurs within cerebral tissue. Traumatic causes of ICH include depressed skull fractures, penetrating injuries (bullet, knife), or sudden acceleration/ deceleration motion. The ICH can act as a rapidly expanding lesion; however, late ICH into the necrotic center of a contused area also is possible. Sudden clinical deterioration of a patient 6 to 10 days after trauma may be the result of ICH.

Medical management of ICH may include surgical or nonsurgical management. Generally, hemorrhages that do not cause significant elevation of ICP are treated nonsurgically. Over time the hemorrhage may be reabsorbed. If significant problems with elevated ICP occur as a result of the ICH, surgical removal is necessary.

Missile Injuries

Missile injuries are caused by objects that penetrate the skull and produce significant focal damage. The injury may be depressed, penetrating, or perforating (Figure 25-3). *Depressed injuries* are caused by fractures of the skull, with penetration of bone into cerebral tissue. *Penetrating injuries* are caused by objects that enter the cranial cavity but do not exit. *Perforating injuries* are missile injuries that enter and then exit the brain.

Diffuse Axonal Injury

Diffuse axonal injury (DAI) covers a wide range of brain dysfunction caused by acceleration/deceleration and rotational forces. DAI occurs as a result of damage to the axons or disruption of axonal transmission of the neural impulses.

The pathophysiology of DAI is related to the stretching and tearing of axons as a result of movement of the brain

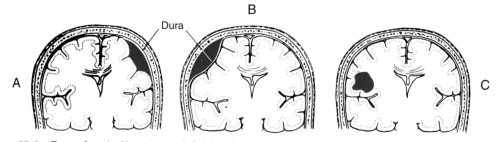

Figure 25-2 Types of cerebral hematomas. **A,** Subdural hematoma. **B,** Epidural hematoma. **C,** Intracerebral hematoma.

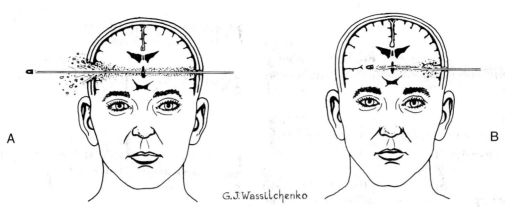

Figure 25-3 Bullet wounds of the head. Bullet wound or other penetrating missile wounds cause an open (compound) skull fracture and damage to brain tissue. Shock wave effects are transmitted throughout the brain. **A**, Perforating injury. **B**, Penetrating injury.

inside the cranium at the time of impact. The stretching and tearing of axons result in microscopic lesions throughout the brain, but especially deep within the cerebral tissue and base of the cerebrum. Disruption of axonal transmission of impulses results in loss of consciousness. Unless surrounding tissue areas are significantly injured, causing small hemorrhages, DAI may not be visible on CT scan but may be visible by magnetic resonance imaging (MRI).

DAI can be classified into three grades based on the extent of the lesions: mild, moderate, or severe. The patient with *mild* DAI may be in a coma for 24 hours and may exhibit periods of decorticate and decerebrate posturing. Patients with *moderate* DAI may be in a coma for longer than 24 hours and exhibit decorticate-decerebrate posturing. *Severe* DAI is usually manifested as a prolonged deep coma with periods of hypertension, hyperthermia, and excessive sweating. Treatment of DAI includes support of vital functions and maintenance of cerebral perfusion pressure (CPP) and ICP within normal limits. The outcome after severe DAI is poor because of the extensive dysfunction of cerebral pathways.

Assessment

Nursing priorities in assessment after traumatic brain injury focus on (1) level of consciousness and (2) motor and sensory function. The neurologic assessment is the most important tool for evaluating the patient with a severe TBI because it can indicate severity of injury, provide prognostic information, and dictate the speed with which further evaluation and treatment must proceed.[10,11] The cornerstone of the neurologic assessment is the Glasgow Coma Scale (GCS). To assist with the initial assessment, TBIs are divided into three descriptive categories on the basis of the patient's GCS score and length of the unconscious state.

Degree of Injury

Mild Injury. Mild TBI is described as a GCS score of 13 to 15, with a loss of consciousness that lasts up to 15 minutes. Patients with mild injury often are seen in the ED and discharged home with a family member who is instructed to evaluate the patient routinely and to bring the patient back to the hospital if any further neurologic symptoms appear.

Moderate Injury. Moderate TBI is described as a GCS score of 9 to 12, with a loss of consciousness for up to 6 hours. Patients with this type of TBI usually are hospitalized. They are at high risk for deterioration from increasing ICP and cerebral edema, and therefore serial clinical assessments are an important function of the nurse. Hemodynamic and ICP monitoring and ventilatory support are not mandatory unless other systemic injuries make them necessary. A CT scan is performed on admission. Repeat CT scans are indicated whenever the patient's neurologic status deteriorates.

Severe Injury. Patients with a GCS score of 8 or less after resuscitation or those who deteriorate to that level within 48 hours of admission have a severe TBI. Patients with severe TBI require intubation and ventilatory support along with ICP and hemodynamic monitoring. A CT scan is performed to rule out any mass lesions that can be surgically removed. Patients are placed in a critical care setting for continual assessment, monitoring, and management.

Diagnostic Procedures

The cornerstone of diagnostic procedures for evaluation of TBI is the CT scan.[11] The CT scan is a rapid, noninvasive procedure that can provide invaluable information about the presence of mass lesions and cerebral edema. Serial CT scans may be used over several days to assess areas of contusion and ischemia and detect delayed hematomas. Electrophysiology studies can aid in ongoing assessments of neurologic function. Evoked-potential studies and electroencephalography (EEG) are becoming widely used in the diagnosis of TBI. MRI is also useful in detecting hematomas and cerebral edema.

Medical Management
Surgical Management

If a lesion, identified by CT scan, is causing a shift of intracranial contents or increasing ICP, surgical intervention is necessary. A craniotomy is performed to remove the EDH, SDH, or large ICH. Occasionally, if an area of contusion is large, hemorrhagic, and associated with an elevated ICP, a craniotomy for removal of the contused area may be performed to relieve pressure and prevent herniation. Patients with previous surgery for penetrating head trauma have an increased incidence of seizures and may be prescribed anticonvulsants.

Nonsurgical Management

Nonsurgical management includes management of ICP, maintenance of adequate CPP and oxygenation, and treatment of any complications. The decision of when to initiate ICP monitoring is critical. ICP monitoring is recommended for patients with a GCS less than 8 and abnormal findings on a head CT scan.[9]

Nursing Management

Nursing priorities in management of traumatic brain injury focus on (1) stabilizing vital signs, (2) preventing further injury, and (3) reducing increased ICP and maintaining adequate CPP. Ongoing nursing assessments are the cornerstone to the care of patients with TBI. Such assessments are the primary mechanism for determining secondary brain injury from cerebral edema and increased ICP.[12,13] In addition to astute neurologic assessments, it is crucial to monitor ventilatory and oxygenation requirements, fluid and electrolyte balance, hemodynamic stability, nutrition, and to provide family support and education.[14]

SPINAL CORD INJURIES

Approximately 10,000 new spinal cord injuries (SCIs) occur annually. The overwhelming majority of injuries occur in young males between ages 16 and 30 years.[15] The diagnosis of SCI begins with a detailed history of events surrounding the incident, precise evaluation of sensory and motor function, and radiographic studies of the spine.

Mechanism of Injury

The type of primary injury sustained depends on the mechanism of injury. Mechanisms of injury can include hyperflexion, hyperextension, rotation, axial loading (vertical compression), and missile or penetrating injuries.

Hyperflexion

Hyperflexion injury most often is seen in the cervical area, especially at the level of the fifth to sixth vertebrae (C5-C6) because this is the most mobile portion of the cervical spine. This type of injury most often is caused by sudden deceleration motion, as in head-on collisions. Injury occurs from compression of the cord as a result of fracture fragments or dislocation of the vertebral bodies. Instability of the spinal column occurs because of the rupture or tearing of the posterior muscles and ligaments.

Hyperextension

Hyperextension injuries involve backward and downward motion of the head. With this injury, often seen in rear-end collisions or diving accidents, the spinal cord itself is stretched and distorted. The resulting neurologic deficits are caused by contusion and ischemia of the spinal cord without significant bony involvement. A mild form of hyperextension is the *whiplash* injury.

Rotation

Rotation injuries often occur in conjunction with a flexion or extension injury. Severe rotation of the neck or body results in tearing of the posterior ligaments and displacement (rotation) of the spinal column.

Axial Loading

Axial loading, or *vertical compression*, injuries occur from vertical force along the spinal cord. This most often occurs with a fall from a height when the person lands on their feet or buttocks. Compression injuries cause burst fractures of the vertebral body that often send bony fragments into the spinal canal or directly into the spinal cord.

Penetrating Injuries

Penetrating injury to the spinal cord can be caused by a bullet, knife, or any object that penetrates the cord. These types of injury cause permanent damage by anatomically transecting the spinal cord.

Pathophysiology

SCIs are the result of a mechanical force that disrupts neurologic tissue or its vascular supply, or both. As with the pathophysiology of TBI, the SCI process includes both primary and secondary injury mechanisms. *Primary* injury is the neurologic damage that occurs at the moment of impact. *Secondary* injury refers to the complex biochemical processes affecting cellular function. Secondary injury can occur within minutes of injury and can last for days to weeks.[16]

Several events after a spinal cord injury lead to spinal cord ischemia and loss of neurologic function. A cascade of events is initiated that includes ischemia, elevated intracellular calcium, and inflammatory changes.[15]

Functional Injury of Spinal Cord

Functional injury of the spinal cord refers to the degree of disruption of normal spinal cord function. This depends on what specific sensory and motor structures within the cord are damaged. SCIs are first classified as complete or incomplete, then further classified according to functional injuries.

Complete Injury

Complete SCI results in a total loss of sensory and motor function below the level of injury. Regardless of the mechanism of injury, the result is a complete dissection of the spinal cord and its neurochemical pathways, resulting in one of two conditions: quadriplegia or paraplegia.

Quadriplegia. With quadriplegia the injury occurs between the C1 to first thoracic (T1) level, and loss of function below the specific level of injury occurs. The potential functional status of differing levels of complete injury is described in Table 25-2.

Paraplegia. A complete injury in the thoracolumbar region (T2 to L1) creates loss of function below this level.[17] Thoracic, L1, or L2 injuries produce paraplegia with variable innervation to intercostal and abdominal muscles.

Incomplete Injury

Incomplete SCI results in a mixed loss of voluntary motor activity and sensation below the level of the lesion. Incomplete SCI exists if any function remains below the level of injury. Incomplete injuries can result in one of a variety of syndromes, which are classified according to the degree of motor and sensory loss below the level of injury.

Spinal Shock

Spinal shock is a condition that can occur shortly after traumatic injury to the spinal cord. Spinal shock is the complete loss of all normal reflex activity below the level of injury and manifests bradycardia and hypotension.[4] The duration of this shock state can persist for up to 1 month after injury.

Blood pressure support is provided by continuous sympathomimetic drug adminstration.

Autonomic Dysreflexia

Autonomic dysreflexia is a life-threatening complication that may occur with SCI. This condition is caused by a massive sympathetic response to a noxious stimulus (full bladder, line insertions, fecal impaction), which results in bradycardia, hypertension, facial flushing, and headache. Immediate intervention is needed to prevent cerebral hemorrhage, seizures, and acute pulmonary edema. Treatment is aimed at alleviating the noxious stimuli[18] (Box 25-2).

Assessment

Upon admission to the ICU, attention to the ABCs is imperative in the patient with known or suspected SCI. **Nursing priorities in assessment after spinal cord injury are directed toward ongoing physical evaluation of (1) airway, (2) breathing pattern, (3) circulation, and (4) neurologic status.**

Spinal Cord Precautions

Stabilization of the spinal cord is mandatory to prevent further injury. Stabilization in the ICU includes bed rest with

---

Table **25-2**	Quadriplegia Functional Status

Vertebra(e)*	Functional Ability
C1-C4	Requires electric wheelchair with breath, head, or shoulder controls.
C5	Needs electric wheelchair with hand control and/or manual wheelchair with rim projections; may require adaptive devices to assist with ADLs.
C6	Independent in manual wheelchair on level surface; may need hand controls; may require adaptive devices for ADLs.
C7	Requires manual wheelchair on most surfaces.
C8-T1	May need adaptive devices.

*Neurologic level of complete injury; C, cervical; T, thoracic.
ADLs, Activities of daily living.

Box **25-2**	Clinical Algorithm for Treatment of Autonomic Dysreflexia

1. If patient is supine, immediately sit patient up.
2. Loosen clothing and constrictive devices.
3. Survey for instigating causes, beginning with urinary system.
4. If indwelling catheter is not present, catheterize patient.
   - Lidocaine jelly may be instilled 5 minutes before catheter insertion.
   - Consider use of a Coudé catheter.
5. If indwelling catheter is present:
   - Check system for kinks and obstructions to flow.
   - Irrigate bladder with small amount of fluid.
   - If not draining, remove catheter and replace.
6. If systolic blood pressure is greater than 150 mm Hg, consider rapid-onset short-duration antihypertensive agent.
7. If acute symptoms persist, suspect fecal impaction.
   - Instill lidocaine jelly into rectum; wait at least 5 minutes.
   - Perform digital examination to check for presence of stool; if present, gently remove.
8. If signs of autonomic dysreflexia persist, stop examination; instill additional lidocaine jelly, and wait 20 minutes to reexamine.

log-rolling maneuvers and a hard cervical collar until definitive stabilization is achieved.

Airway

The primary assessment begins with an evaluation of airway clearance. In an unresponsive person, an oral airway is inserted while the patient's neck is maintained in a neutral position. Endothracheal intubation is used to avoid hypoxemia, which would further damage the spinal cord.

Breathing

Assessment of breathing patterns and gas exchange is made after an airway has been secured. The level of injury dictates the degree of altered breathing patterns and gas exchange.[18] Because complete injuries above the C3 level result in paralysis of the diaphragm, patients with these injuries require intubation and mechanical ventilatory support.

Circulation

The patient with SCI is at high risk for developing alterations in cardiac output and tissue perfusion because the cardiovascular system is subjected to a variety of serious and potential physiologic alterations, including dysrhythmias, cardiac arrest, orthostatic hypotension, emboli, and thrombophlebitis.

Neurologic Status

The initial neurologic assessment may not be an accurate indication of eventual motor and sensory loss. It focuses on the rapid and accurate identification of present, absent, or impaired functioning of the motor, sensory, and reflex systems that coordinate and regulate vital functions. A detailed motor and sensory examination includes the assessment of all 32 spinal nerves for evidence of dysfunction and will occur once the acute stabilization is complete. Ongoing spinal cord assessments must be documented during the critical care phase.

Diagnostic Procedures

Diagnostic radiographic evaluations can identify the severity of damage to the spinal cord. Initial radiographic evaluation includes anteroposterior and lateral views for all areas of the spinal cord. Films of all seven cervical vertebrae and the top of T1 must be obtained to rule out cervicothoracic junction injury. Flexion and extension views can identify subtle ligamentous injuries. CT scan, tomograms, myelography, and MRI also may be used in the diagnostic process.

Medical Management

After assessment and diagnosis of the SCI, medical management begins. The primary treatment goal is to preserve remaining neurologic function. Medical interventions are divided into pharmacologic, surgical, and nonsurgical interventions.

Pharmacologic Management

Methylprednisolone has been shown to improve neurologic outcome after spinal cord injury. Patients with SCI should receive a methylprednisolone bolus followed by a continuous infusion for at least 24 hours and preferably 48 hours (Box 25-3). The treatment must begin within 3 to 8 hours after injury.[19,20] Methylprednisolone decreases posttraumatic spinal cord ischemia, improving energy metabolism, restoring extracellular calcium, and improving nerve impulse conduction.[19]

Surgical Management

Surgical intervention provides spinal column stability in the presence of an unstable injury. Without adequate stabilization, movement and dislocation of the vertebral column could cause a complete neurologic deficit. A variety of surgical procedures may be performed to achieve decompression and stabilization. The question of when surgery should be performed remains controversial.

Laminectomy is the removal of the lamina of the vertebral ring to allow decompression and removal of bony fragments or disk material from the spinal canal. *Spinal fusion* entails the surgical fusion of two to six vertebral elements to provide stability and to prevent motion. Fusion is accomplished through the use of bone parts or bone chips taken from the iliac crest or by use of wire or acrylic glue. The *rodding* procedure stabilizes and realigns larger segments of the spinal column. The rods are attached by screws and glue to the posterior elements of the spinal column, usually to stabilize the thoracolumbar area.

Nonsurgical Management

If the injury to the spinal cord is stable, nonsurgical management is the treatment of choice.

Cervical Injury. Management of cervical injuries involves the immobilization of the fracture site and realignment of any dislocation. This is accomplished through skeletal traction using two-point tongs. Tongs are inserted into the skull through shallow burr holes and are connected to traction weights. Several types of cervical tongs are used, most often the Gardner-Wells and Crutchfield tongs. These tongs can be applied at the bedside with the use of a local anesthetic.

Box **25-3**	Administration of Intravenous Methylprednisolone for Spinal Cord Injury

Based on drug concentration of 62.5 mg/ml:
1. Administer bolus dose 30 mg/kg IV over 15 minutes.
2. Pause for 45 minutes (administer IV fluid to keep vein open).
3. Begin maintenance dose at 5.4 mg/kg/hr IV for 23 hours.
4. Terminate drug administration 24 hours after bolus dose.

After the procedure the patient can be immobilized on a kinetic therapy bed or a regular bed. The *kinetic therapy bed* is the most popular method used for cervical immobilization because it maintains spinal column alignment while providing constant turning motion to reduce pulmonary and skin breakdown. Use of cervical skeletal traction on a regular bed makes it difficult to provide adequate care to the pulmonary system and skin because of the extensive degree of immobility.

After the spinal column has been adequately realigned by means of skeletal traction, a *halo traction brace* often is applied. The halo vest consists of a metal ring secured to the skull with two occipital and two temporal screws. Steel bars anchor the screws to the vest to provide cervical immobilization. The halo traction brace immobilizes the cervical spine, which allows the patient to ambulate and participate in self-care.

Thoracolumbar Injury. Nonsurgical management of the patient with a thoracolumbar injury also involves immobilization. Skeletal traction may be used in high thoracic injury. For the most part, misalignment of the spinal canal does not occur in stable injuries of the thoracolumbar spine. Immobilization to allow fractures to heal is accomplished by bed rest (with bed flat) and the use of a plastic or fiberglass jacket, a body cast, or a brace.

Nursing Management

The goal during the critical care phase is to prevent life-threatening complications while maximizing the functioning of all organ systems. **Nursing priorities in management of spinal cord injury are aimed at (1) preventing secondary damage to the spinal cord, (2) managing cardiovascular and respiratory complications, and (3) coaching the patient to overcome the psychosocial challenges associated with severe neurologic deficit.** Because almost all body systems are affected by SCI, nursing management must also include interventions that optimize nutrition, elimination, skin integrity, and mobility. Prevention of complications that can delay the patient's rehabilitation is one of the goals of critical care.[21,22] In addition, patients with SCI have complex psychosocial needs that require a great deal of emotional support from their family support system and the critical care nurse.[23,24]

THORACIC INJURIES

Thoracic injuries involve trauma to the chest wall, lungs, heart, great vessels, and esophagus. Thoracic trauma most often results from a violent crime or MVC.

Mechanism of Injury
Blunt Trauma

Blunt trauma to the chest is most often caused by MVCs or falls. The underlying mechanism of injury tends to be a combination of acceleration/deceleration injury and direct transfer mechanics, such as a crush injury. Varying mechanisms of blunt trauma are associated with specific injury patterns. After head-on collisions, drivers have a higher frequency of injury than do backseat passengers because the driver comes in contact with the steering assembly. Severe thoracic injuries often are seen in unrestrained vehicle occupants. Falls from greater than 20 feet are associated with thoracic injury.

Penetrating Injury

The penetrating object involved determines the damage sustained. Low-velocity weapons (.22-caliber gun, knife) usually damage only what is in the weapon's direct path. Of particular concern are stab wounds that involve the anterior chest wall close to the heart and great vessels.

Chest Wall Injuries
Rib Fractures

Fractures of certain ribs or multiple rib fractures can cause life-threatening internal injuries. Fractures of the first and second ribs are associated with intrathoracic vascular injuries (brachial plexus, great vessels). Fractures of the seventh through tenth ribs are associated with liver or spleen injuries. The pain associated with rib fractures is aggravated by respiratory excursion. As a result, the patient often splints, takes shallow breaths, and refuses to cough, which results in atelectasis and pneumonia.

Flail Chest

A flail chest occurs when three or more ribs are fractured in two or more places and are no longer attached to the thoracic cage. This results in a free-floating segment of the chest wall. This segment moves independently from the rest of the thorax and results in paradoxical chest wall movement during the respiratory cycle (Figure 25-4). During inspiration the intact portion of the chest wall expands while the injured part is sucked in. During expiration the chest wall moves in and the flail segment moves out. The physiologic impact of impaired chest wall movement includes decreased tidal volume, impaired cough, and hypoventilation, which lead to atelectasis and lung collapse. Often the fractured ribs have punctured the underlying thoracic structures and pneumothorax, hemothorax, or cardiac injury aggravates the chest wall injury to life-threatening proportions.

Ruptured Diaphragm

Diagnosis of a diaphragmatic rupture is often missed in trauma patients because of the subtle and nonspecific symptoms this injury produces. The mechanism of injury appears to be a rapid rise in intraabdominal pressure as a result of compression force applied to the lower part of the chest or upper region of the abdomen. This injury can occur when a person is thrown forward over the tip of the steering wheel in a high-speed deceleration accident. The force can cause the diaphragm, which offers little resistance, to rupture or tear. Abdominal viscera then can enter the thoracic cavity, drawn by the negative pressure in the thorax.

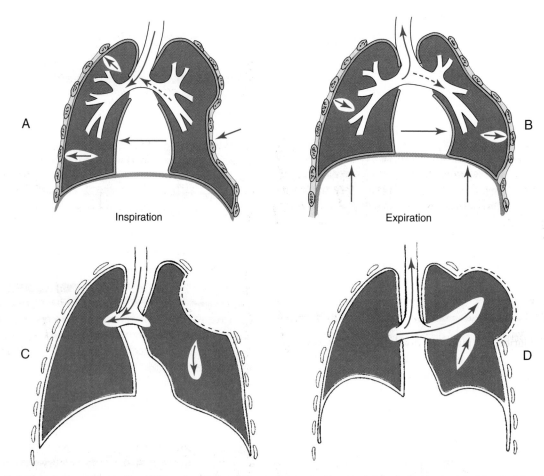

Figure 25-4 Flail chest. **A**, Normal inspiration. **B**, Normal expiration. **C**, Inspiration: area of lung underlying unstable chest wall "sucks in" on inspiration. **D**, Same area "balloons out" on expiration. Note movement of mediastinum toward opposite lung on inspiration. (**A** and **B** redrawn from Rosen P et al: *Emergency medicine: concepts and clinical practice*, vol I, ed 4, St Louis, 1998, Mosby; **C** and **D** from Long BC, Phipps WJ, Cassmeyer VL: *Medical-surgical nursing: a nursing process approach*, ed 3, St Louis, 1993, Mosby.)

Diaphragmatic rupture can be fatal. Massive herniation of abdominal contents into the thoracic cavity can compress the lungs and mediastinum, which then hampers venous return and leads to decreased cardiac output (CO). In addition, herniated bowel can become strangulated and perforate. Treatment of a ruptured diaphragm includes immediate surgical repair.

Pulmonary Injuries
Pulmonary Contusion

A pulmonary contusion is fundamentally a bruise on the lung. Pulmonary contusion often is associated with blunt trauma and other chest injuries, such as rib fractures and flail chest. Pulmonary contusions can occur unilaterally or bilaterally. A contusion manifests initially as a hemorrhage, followed by alveolar and interstitial edema. The edema can remain rather localized in the contused area or can spread to other lung areas. Inflammation affects alveolar-capillary units. As more units are affected by inflammation, further pathophysiologic events may include decreased compliance, increased pulmonary vascular resistance, and decreased pulmonary blood flow. These processes result in a ventilation/perfusion imbalance, causing hypoxemia and poor ventilation. The acute lung injury often progresses over 24 to 48 hours and then slowly resolves unless pulmonary complications occur. The most life-threatening complication is acute respiratory distress syndrome (ARDS).

Tension Pneumothorax

A traumatic tension pneumothorax is caused by an injury that perforates the chest wall and pleural space. Air flows into the pleural space with inspiration and becomes trapped. As pressure in the pleural space increases, the lung on the injured side collapses and the mediastinum is pushed to the opposite side (Figure 25-5). As pressure continues to build, pressure is exerted on the heart and thoracic aorta, which results in decreased venous return and low CO. Oxygenation is hampered because the collapsed lung cannot participate in ventilation.

Clinical manifestations of tension pneumothorax include dyspnea, tachycardia, hypotension, and sudden chest pain.

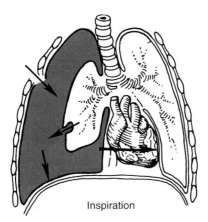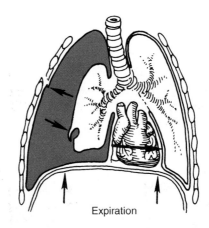

Inspiration   Expiration

Figure 25-5   Tension pneumothorax usually is caused by injury that perforates chest wall or pleural space. Air flows into pleural space with inspiration and becomes trapped. As pressure in pleural space increases, the lung on the injured side collapses and the mediastinum shifts to opposite side. (From Rosen P et al: *Emergency medicine: concepts and clinical practice*, ed 4, St Louis, 1998, Mosby.)

Tracheal deviation is a late sign, noted as the trachea shifts away from the injured side. On the injured side, breath sounds are decreased or absent. Percussion of the chest reveals a hyperresonant sound over the collection of pressurized air. Diagnosis of tension pneumothorax is made by clinical assessment, or with chest radiograph if time and patient condition permit.[4] A large-bore (14-gauge) needle or chest tube is inserted into the affected pleural area. This procedure allows immediate release of air, and a hissing sound is audible as the air escapes and the tension pneumothorax is converted to a simple pneumothorax.

Open Pneumothorax

An open pneumothorax, or "sucking chest wound," is caused by penetrating trauma. Open communication between the atmosphere and intrathoracic pressure results in immediate lung deflation. Air moves in and out of the hole in the chest, producing a sucking sound heard on inspiration. An open pneumothorax produces the same symptoms as a tension pneumothorax. In addition, subcutaneous emphysema may be palpated around the wound.

Initial management of an open pneumothorax involves promptly closing the wound at end expiration with a sterile occlusive dressing (plastic wrap or petroleum gauze) large enough to overlap the wound's edges.[4] This dressing is taped securely on three sides. As the patient breathes in, the dressing is sucked in to occlude the wound and prevent air from entering. A chest tube is inserted as soon as possible.

Hemothorax

Blunt or penetrating thoracic trauma can cause bleeding into the pleural space, resulting in a hemothorax (Figure 25-6). A massive hemothorax results from the accumulation of more than 1500 milliliters (ml) in the chest cavity. The source of bleeding may be the intercostal or internal mam-

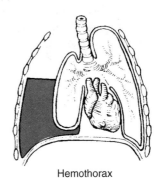

Hemothorax

Figure 25-6   Blunt or penetrating thoracic trauma can cause bleeding into pleural space to form hemothorax.

mary arteries, lungs, heart, or great vessels. Assessment findings include decreased breath sounds and dullness to chest percussion. Massive hemothorax causes hypotension, hypovolemic shock, critically low cardiac output (CO), and tissue ischemia. Urgent resuscitation with IV fluids is initiated, and a chest tube is placed on the affected side to allow drainage of blood.[4]

Nursing Management

Nursing priorities for the patient with traumatic chest or pulmonary injury emphasize delivery of adequate (1) oxygenation, (2) ventilation, and (3) pain management. Assistance with intubation and monitoring of mechanical ventilation may be required to prevent tissue hypoxia and provide adequate ventilatory support. Aggressive removal of airway secretions is important to avoid infection and improve ventilation. Hypoxemia is prevented by continuous pulse oximetry monitoring of arterial oxygen saturation (SpO_2) and ABG analysis. Judicious administration of IV fluids and analgesia is important to improve patient comfort.

Cardiac Injuries
Penetrating Cardiac Injuries

Penetrating cardiac trauma can occur from mechanical injuries as a result of bullets, knives, or impalements. The most common site of injury is the right ventricle because of its anterior position. Mortality is high. Most deaths occur within minutes after injury as a result of exsanguination or cardiac tamponade.

Cardiac Tamponade

Cardiac tamponade is caused by the progressive accumulation of blood in the pericardial sac (Figure 25-7). A progressive accumulation of blood, 120 to 150 ml, increases the intracardiac pressure, compressing the atria and ventricles. The increase in intracardiac pressures leads to diminished venous return, decreased CO, and cardiogenic shock.

Classic assessment findings associated with cardiac tamponade are termed *Beck's triad*: (1) presence of elevated central venous pressure (CVP) with neck vein distention, (2) muffled heart sounds, and (3) hypotension. Pulsus paradoxus may be present. Pulseless electrical activity (PEA) in the absence of hypovolemia and tension pneumothorax strongly suggests cardiac tamponade. If the situation is critical, blood is aspirated from the pericardium using a large-bore needle (pericardiocentesis).[4] Ultrasound may be used to guide needle placement during the pericardiocentesis.[25]

Blunt Cardiac Injuries

The most common causes of blunt cardiac trauma include high-speed MVCs, direct blows to the chest, and falls. The heart is susceptible to blunt traumatic injury. Sudden deceleration (as from contact with a steering wheel) can jolt the heart against the sternum (Figure 25-8). Sudden acceleration can cause the heart to be thrown back against the thoracic vertebrae, such as by a direct blow to the chest from a baseball, a kick from a horse, or a fall. *Blunt cardiac injury* (BCI), formerly called "myocardial contusion," covers the spectrum of myocardial contusion, concussion, and rupture.[26] The chambers injured most often are the right atrium and ventricle because of their anterior position in the chest.

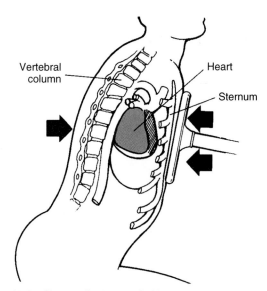

Figure 25-8   Blunt cardiac trauma. Sudden deceleration (as from contact with steering wheel) can cause heart to be thrown against sternum.

Nursing Management

Nursing priorities are directed toward recognizing, preventing, and treating cardiac complications. This includes monitoring the ECG, replacement of essential electrolytes such as magnesium and potassium, and administration of antidysrhythmic medications if required. Chest pain is investigated and treated. Recognition of the potential for heart failure secondary to myocardial damage is important while the critical care nurse utilizes hemodyanmic monitoring to assess the efficacy of CO and tissue perfusion.

ABDOMINAL INJURIES

Abdominal injuries often are associated with multisystem trauma. Injuries to the abdomen are the result of blunt or penetrating trauma. Two conditions that occur with abdominal trauma are hemorrhage and hollow viscera perforation, with peritonitis as a complication.

Mechanism of Injury
Blunt Trauma

Blunt abdominal injuries are common, resulting most often from MVCs, falls, and assaults. In MVCs, abdominal injury is more likely to occur when a vehicle is struck from the side. In the passenger position of the front seat, hepatic injury is increased when the point of impact is on the same side as the passenger. A driver is likely to sustain injury to the spleen when the impact is on the driver's side. Pedestrians hit by motor vehicles are at risk for serious abdominal injuries. Blunt trauma to the thorax can produce injuries to the liver, spleen, and diaphragm. In spinal cord injury, large abdominal arteries and veins can be injured. Deceleration and direct forces can produce retroperitoneal bleeding. Blunt

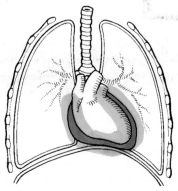

Figure 25-7   Cardiac tamponade is caused by progressive accumulation of blood in the pericardial sac.

abdominal injuries often are hidden and thus are more likely to be fatal than penetrating abdominal injuries.

Penetrating Trauma

Penetrating abdominal trauma is less common and is caused most often by knives or bullets. The danger of penetrating abdominal trauma is that the outside appearance of the wound does not reflect the extent of internal injury. Typically injured organs from knife wounds are the liver, spleen, diaphragm, and colon. Gunshot wounds to the abdomen usually are more serious than stab wounds. A bullet destroys tissue along its path. Once inside the abdomen, a bullet can travel in erratic paths and ricochet off bone. Death from penetrating injuries depends on the injury to major vascular structures and resultant intraabdominal hemorrhage.

Assessment

The initial assessment of the trauma patient, whether in the emergency department or critical care unit, follows the primary and secondary survey techniques as outlined by advanced trauma life support (ATLS) guidelines. Specific assessment findings associated with abdominal trauma are reviewed here.

Physical Assessment

Nursing priorities in assessment of abdominal injury focus on (1) inspecting the abdomen for signs of trauma, (2) auscultating for bowel sounds, (3) percussing to detect intraabdominal fluid or air, and (4) palpating for signs of tenderness or distention.

The location of entry and exit sites associated with penetrating trauma are assessed and documented. Inspection of the patient's abdomen may reveal purplish discoloration of the flanks or umbilicus (Cullen's sign), which is indicative of blood in the abdominal wall. Ecchymosis in the flank area (Turner's sign) may indicate retroperitoneal bleeding or pancreatic injury. A hematoma in the flank area is suggestive of renal injury. A distended abdomen may indicate the accumulation of blood, fluid, or gas secondary to a perforated organ or ruptured blood vessel.

Auscultation of the abdomen may reveal friction rubs over the liver or spleen and may indicate rupture. Bowel sounds are usually absent in severe injury. On percussion, dullness on the lower sides of the abdomen suggests internal bleeding, whereas abdominal distention with a tympanic response to percussion suggests "free air" secondary to a perforated bowel.

The abdomen is palpated for rebound tenderness and rigidity. Presence of these assessment findings indicates peritoneal inflammation. Referred pain to the left shoulder (Kehr's sign) may signal a ruptured spleen or irritation of the diaphragm from bile or other material in the peritoneum. Subcutaneous emphysema palpated on the abdomen suggests free air as a result of a ruptured bowel.

Diagnostic Procedures

Insertion of a nasogastric (NG) tube and urinary catheter are essential for diagnostic and therapeutic reasons. An NG tube will decompress the stomach, and the contents can be checked for blood. The urinary catheter will decompress the bladder and urine can be tested for the presence of blood.

Because of volume depletion and hemoconcentration, Hgb and Hct results may not reflect actual values (artificially high). Serial tests are valuable to diagnose hidden abdominal injuries. Elevated serum amylase and lipase levels can signal pancreatic injuries. Elevated liver enzymes suggest liver trauma. Blood urea nitrogen (BUN) and creatinine will rise if the kidneys are damaged.

A flat-plate radiograph of the abdomen provides a baseline. Abdominal CT scanning can detect hepatic or splenic trauma and retroperitoneal hemorrhage. Ultrasonography may be used to identify hemoperitoneum.[25]

Diagnostic peritoneal lavage (DPL) can exclude or confirm the presence of intraabdominal injury with a high accuracy rate. After the patient's bladder has been emptied, a small incision is made in the abdomen through the skin and into the peritoneum. A small catheter is inserted. If frank blood is encountered, intraabdominal injury is obvious and the patient is taken immediately to the OR. If gross blood is not initially encountered, a liter of fluid (LR solution or 0.9% normal saline) is infused through the catheter into the abdomen. The IV bag is then placed in a dependent position, and abdominal fluid is allowed to drain into the IV bag. The drainage fluid is sent to the laboratory for analysis. If the lavage fluid contains blood, stool, or bile, surgical intervention is often required.

Intraabdominal pressure can be measured through a urinary bladder catheter after the injection of 50 to 100 ml of normal saline.[27,28] The urinary catheter is connected to a hemodynamic transducer system. Serial monitoring of bladder pressures is useful in detecting the onset of intraabdominal hypertension and the progression to abdominal compartment syndrome. Measurements may be classified as mildly elevated (10 to 20 mm Hg), moderately elevated (20 to 40 mm Hg), and severely elevated (greater than 40 mm Hg).[29] Surgical decompression of the abdomen is suggested for abdominal pressures greater than 25 mm Hg that are associated with other assessment findings, such as decreased CO, hypotension, elevated peak inspiratory pressures, and decreased urine output.[30] Bladder pressures should be measured every 2 to 4 hours in all patients in whom intraabdominal hypertension or abdominal compartment syndrome is suspected.[27]

Damage Control Surgery

If the patient is too unstable for definitive operative repair, the trauma surgeon may elect to insert abdominal packing plus any other rapid measures necessary and then take the patient to the ICU for stabilization. This is known as "damage control surgery"[31-35] (Box 25-4).

| Box **25-4** | Damage Control Sequence |

INITIAL OPERATION
1. Control contamination
2. Control hemorrhage
3. Intraabdominal packing
4. Temporary closure

CRITICAL CARE UNIT RESUSCITATION
5. Correct coagulopathy
6. Rewarming
7. Maximize hemodynamics
8. Ventilatory support
9. Injury identification

PLANNED REOPERATION
10. Pack removal
11. Definitive repair

Specific Organ Injuries

Physical assessment findings, CT scan and DPL, aid in making a diagnosis of specific abdominal organ injury. Medical and nursing management vary according to the specific organ injuries. Liver, spleen, and intestinal injuries are seen most often.

Liver Injuries

The liver is the primary organ injured in penetrating trauma and the second most often injured organ in blunt trauma. Detection of liver injury, as with all intraabdominal injuries, is accomplished through physical assessment, CT scan and if needed DPL. Until recently, most liver injuries required operative repair to accomplish hemostasis and healing. Nonoperative interventional radiology procedures are now the standard of care for hemodynamically stable patients with liver injury.[36]

Patients with penetrating or blunt liver trauma who are hemodynamically unstable may require surgical intervention to correct bleeding. Resection of the devitalized tissue is required for massive injuries. Hemorrhage is common with liver injuries, and ligation of the hepatic arteries or veins may be required to control hemorrhage. Drains may be placed intraoperatively to drain areas of blood and to prevent hematomas.

Spleen Injuries

The spleen is the organ most often injured by blunt abdominal trauma and is second to the liver as a source of life-threatening hemorrhage. The treatment of an injured spleen is controversial because of the spleen's importance in preventing infection. Hemodynamically stable patients may be monitored in the critical care unit with serial Hct values and vital signs. Patients who exhibit hemodynamic instability require operative intervention with splenectomy. Patients who have had a splenectomy are at risk for the development

of overwhelming postsplenectomy sepsis with streptococcal pneumonia. These patients require polyvalent pneumococcal vaccine (Pneumovax) to help promote immunity against most pneumococcal bacteria.

Intestinal Injuries

Bowel injuries can result from blunt or penetrating trauma. The diagnosis of small intestinal injuries is difficult. Surgical intervention is usually required in the presence of multiple findings on CT scan (unexplained free air or fluid, pneumoperitoneum, bowel wall thickening, mesenteric fat streaking, mesenteric hematoma, IV contrast extravasation).[1] A DPL may reveal amylase, particulate matter, bacteria, or abnormal cell count ratios.[37] Regardless of the mechanism of injury, intestinal contents (bile, stool, enzymes, bacteria) leak into the peritoneum and cause peritonitis. Surgical resection and repair are required. The patient's postoperative course is dictated by the amount of spillage of intestinal contents. The patient is observed for signs of sepsis and abscess or fistula formation.

GENITOURINARY INJURIES

Trauma to the genitourinary (GU) tract seldom occurs as an isolated injury and is suspected whenever the patient has abdominal or pelvic trauma.[4]

Mechanism of Injury

GU injuries, as with all other traumatic injuries, can result from blunt or penetrating trauma.

Assessment

Nursing priorities in assessment of genitourinary injury are directed toward (1) inspecting the pelvic and perianal area and (2) testing the urine for hematuria.

Evaluation of GU trauma begins after the primary survey has been conducted and immediate life-threatening conditions have been effectively managed. Inspection may reveal blood at the urethral meatus. Bluish discoloration of the flanks suggests retroperitoneal bleeding, whereas perineal discoloration may indicate a pelvic fracture and possible bladder or urethral injury. The conscious patient may complain of flank pain or colic pain. Rebound tenderness can be elicited if intraperitoneal extravasation of urine has occurred. *Hematuria* is the most common assessment finding with GU trauma, although the absence of gross or microscopic hematuria does not exclude a urinary tract injury.[4]

Renal Trauma

Most renal trauma is caused by blunt trauma, resulting in contusions or lacerations without urinary extravasation. Renal injury may be suspected when there is flank ecchymosis and fracture of inferior ribs or spinous processes. Gross or microscopic hematuria may also be present; however, the extent of renal damage is often incongruous with the degree of hematuria.[38] Gross hematuria can be present with minor injuries and usually clears within a few hours. The CT scan is the most accurate modality available for diagnosing renal injuries because it visualizes soft tissue injuries.[4] Contusions (bruises) and minor lacerations can usually be treated with observation, whereas major lacerations and vascular injuries require operative intervention.[4] Postoperative complications can include infection, hemorrhage, infarction, extravasation, calcification, acute tubular necrosis (ATN), and hypertension.

Bladder Trauma

A large percentage of bladder injuries result from pelvic fractures.[38] Physical findings may include lower abdominal bruising, distention, and pain. More definitive findings include difficulty in voiding or incomplete recovery of irrigation fluids from catheterized patients.[38] Definitive diagnosis is made by retrograde urethrogram. Bladder injuries are classified as contusions, extraperitoneal ruptures, intraperitoneal ruptures, or combined injuries. The type of injury depends on the location and strength of the blunt force and volume of urine in the bladder at the time of injury. Extraperitoneal rupture of the bladder usually is managed with catheterization and antibiotics for 7 to 10 days.[38] Unresolved extravasation requires surgical intervention.

Nursing Management

Nursing priorities in interventions for genitourinary injury focus on (1) **monitoring blood volume,** (2) **monitoring electrolyte balance,** and (3) **maintaining the patency of multiple drains and tubes.** Measurement of urine output includes drainage from the urinary catheter and the nephrostomy or suprapubic tubes. Drainage from these areas is recorded separately. Urine output is measured frequently until bloody drainage and clots have cleared. Gentle irrigation of drainage tubes may be required to clear clots and maintain the patency of the tubes.

PELVIC FRACTURES

More patients die from pelvic fractures than from any other skeletal injury, and survivors often suffer prolonged disability.[39] The pelvis is a ring-shaped structure composed of the hip bones, sacrum, and coccyx. Because the pelvis protects the lower urinary tract and major blood vessels and nerves of the lower extremities, pelvic trauma can result in life-threatening hemorrhage as well as urologic and neurologic dysfunction.

Mechanism of Injury

Blunt pelvic trauma is most often caused by MVCs, crushing accidents, and falls from a height greater than 12 feet. Pelvic injuries frequently cause damage to underlying tissues.[4]

Assessment

Nursing priorities in assessment of pelvic fracture focus on (1) **inspecting the pelvic and perianal area,** (2) **assessing neurovascular status of the lower extremities,** and (3) **maintaining surveillance for complications of pelvic trauma.** Signs of pelvic fracture include perianal ecchymosis (scrotum or vulva) indicating extravasation of urine or blood, pain on palpation or "rocking" of the iliac crests, lower limb paresis or hypesthesia, hematuria, and shortening of a lower extremity. Neurovascular assessment of the lower extremities is important in order to recognize potential damage to the many nerves and major vessels that traverse the pelvic area. Knowledge of other potential complications is incorporated into the assessment. The most life-threatening complications include fat embolism syndrome and deep vein thrombosis, which if embolized to the lungs will create a respiratory crisis (see Complications of Trauma).

The diagnosis of pelvic fracture is made by an anteroposterior pelvic radiograph with the patient supine.[39] Further films may be required for definitive treatment, but the timing depends on the patient's hemodynamic stability.

Classification

Pelvic fractures constitute a spectrum of complexity, ranging from a single, closed, nondisplaced fracture of the pelvic ring to a life-threatening condition with multiple fractures and crush injuries associated with significant hemorrhage and internal injuries.[39] *Open* pelvic fractures involve an open wound with direct communication between the site of the fracture and a laceration involving the vagina, rectum, or perineum. Mortality from these injuries is high because of the external exsanguination.[39]

Medical Management

The priority of the medical management of pelvic fractures is to prevent or control life-threatening hemorrhage. Patients with active bleeding are taken directly to the OR for aggressive resuscitation, ligation, and packing to control the exsanguination.[39] Patients who are hemodynamically stable and have stable closed pelvic fractures are usually treated conservatively with bed rest. These patients may receive elective orthopedic stabilization within 2 to 3 days.[39] Definitive management of pelvic fracture may include placement of internal or external fixation devices.

Nursing Management

Nursing priorities in management of pelvic fracture focus on (1) **achieving adequate tissue perfusion,** (2) **preventing further pelvic injury,** and (3) **ensuring adequate pain management.** Massive blood loss creates decreased tissue perfusion. Priority interventions include IV crystalloid, colloid, and blood transfusions. Adequate tissue oxygenation is monitored by means of pulse oximetry, and if needed continuous mixed-venous oxygen saturation (SvO_2). Serial Hct and Hgb evaluation is ongoing.

Pelvic injury is painful. When moving the patient it is important to know whether the physician has classified the closed pelvic fracture as stable or unstable. A *stable* pelvic injury implies that no further pathologic displacement of the pelvis can occur with physical turning or moving. An *unstable* pelvic fracture means that further pathologic displacement of the pelvis can occur with turning or moving.[39] Aggressive pain management strategies should be employed during turning or procedures. Nursing management of external fixation insertion sites is directed at preventing infection. Most institutions have protocols for pin care that require strict compliance.

COMPLICATIONS OF TRAUMA

Ongoing nursing assessments are imperative for early detection of complications often associated with traumatic injuries. A single complication can increase length of hospital stay and decrease survival. The vigilance of critical care nurses is essential.

Nursing Management

Nursing priorities for the patient with a traumatic injury focus on (1) preventing infection, (2) recognizing early signs of respiratory failure, (3) relieving pain, (4) providing nutrition, (5) preventing renal failure, (6) evaluating risk for compartment syndrome, (7) discovering a missed injury, and (8) assessing risk of systemic complications. Various nursing diagnoses are related to care of the trauma patient (Box 25-5). Collaborative management priorities are essential for providing trauma care and ongoing patient support (Box 25-6).

Preventing Infection

Infection remains a major source of mortality and morbidity in critical care units. The trauma patient is at risk for infection because of contaminated wounds, invasive therapeutic and diagnostic catheters, intubation and mechanical ventilation, host susceptibility, and the critical care environment. Nursing management priorities include interventions to decrease and eliminate the trauma patient's risk of infection.

---

nursing diagnosis
priorities   Box **25-5**

Trauma

- Decreased Intracranial Adaptive Capacity related to failure of normal intracranial compensatory mechanisms
- Decreased Cardiac Output related to vasodilation and bradycardia secondary to sympathetic blockage of neurogenic (spinal) shock after spinal cord injury above T6 level
- Ineffective Breathing Pattern related to decreased lung expansion secondary to thoracic trauma (ruptured diaphragm, pneumothorax, hemothorax, rib fractures, pulmonary contusion, flail chest, penetrating and blunt cardiac injuries)
- Risk for Infection risk factor: invasive monitoring devices
- Ineffective Individual Coping related to situational crisis and personal vulnerability

---

Once sepsis is suspected, Gram stain and cultures of blood, urine, sputum, invasive catheters, and wounds are obtained to discover the septic source.

Recognizing Early Signs of Respiratory Failure

Posttraumatic respiratory failure often leads to the development of acute respiratory distress syndrome (ARDS). Trauma patients are especially at risk for the development of ARDS because of sepsis, multiple emergency transfusions, and pulmonary contusions. The presence of more than one of these conditions significantly increases the risk for ARDS for 24 to 72 hours after initial injury.

Fat embolism syndrome (FES) can occur as a complication of major orthopedic trauma. FES appears to develop as a result of fat droplets that leak from fractured bone and embolize to the lungs. Early fixation of long bone fractures has been shown to reduce the incidence of respiratory complications in injured patients.[1]

Deep vein thrombosis (DVT) and the attendant risk of pulmonary embolism are important causes of morbidity and mortality in the multiply injured trauma patient.[1] Trauma patients are at risk for developing DVT because of vascular endothelial injury, coagulopathy, immobility, and bed rest.[42]

Relieving Pain

Relief of pain is a major priority in the care of trauma patients. An issue that often complicates pain management is the high incidence of substance abuse among patients who sustain traumatic injury. *Patient-controlled analgesia* (PCA), when used with adequate safeguards, may be appropriate for trauma patients, including those with a substance abuse history.[41]

Providing Nutrition

Nutritional support is recognized as an essential component in the care of critically ill trauma patients. Within 24 to 48 hours after traumatic injury, predictable stress hypermetabolism occurs, characterized by increased metabolic rate and oxygen consumption.[40] Enteral nutrition should be started within 72 hours. Enteral feeding sites can include the gastric route or any site beyond the pylorus of the stomach, including the duodenum and jejunum. Prompt feeding tube placement by the critical care nurse must be a priority, unless contraindicated by a specific injury or procedure.

Preventing Renal Failure

Assessment and ongoing monitoring of renal function are critical to the survival of the trauma patient. Prevention of renal failure is the best treatment and begins with ensuring adequate renal perfusion. Serial assessments of BUN and serum creatinine levels are used to evaluate renal function. Patients with major crush injuries are susceptible to the development of *myoglobinuria*, with subsequent secondary renal failure. When cells are crushed, intracellular contents are released, particularly potassium and myoglobin (muscu-

Box **25-6** COLLABORATIVE Management

Trauma

1. Triage all trauma patients using the primary trauma survey ABCDE method.
2. Understand the mechanism of injury, and anticipate potential complications associated with that injury.
3. Prevent further harm.
   - Use cervical spine stabilization when appropriate.
   - Support tissue oxygenation by replacing lost blood volume.
   - Assess for adequate tissue oxygen supply (Spo_2 and Svo_2).
   - Perform a thorough secondary survey to detect additional injuries.
   - Anticipate the consequences of secondary injury.
   - Supply nutrition to assist with healing.
   - Provide options for pain management.
   - Maintain a high index of suspicion for missed injury and potential for complications.
4. Provide organ-specific monitoring to detect early changes in compromised organs.
   - ICP and CPP for severe traumatic brain injury (GCS <8).
   - ABGs and Spo_2 for pulmonary contusion, flail chest, hemothorax, and pneumothorax.
   - Intraabdominal (bladder) pressure monitoring for suspected abdominal injury, bleeding, or severe edema.
   - Urine output evaluated for presence of blood, a sign of renal or genitourinary trauma.
   - Support transport to off-unit diagnostic procedures (e.g., CT, MRI) that will yield critical diagnostic information.
5. Surgical repair of damaged tissues.
   - Definitive operative repair.
   - Damage control surgery.
   - External fixation devices (temporary).
6. Anticipate secondary complications, and provide supportive therapy for complications.
   - Acute respiratory distress syndrome (ARDS)
   - Deep vein thrombosis (DVT)
   - Systemic inflammatory response syndrome (SIRS)
   - Multisystem organ dysfunction syndrome (MODS)
   - Infection or sepsis
   - Acute renal failure (ARF)
   - Discovery of a missed injury
7. Provide support for the patient, family, and significant others.
   - Provide information and emotional support.
   - Social workers assist with practical needs and support the patient and those who are in the support network to adjust to the consequences of the unexpected traumatic event.

ABCDE, Airway, breathing, circulation, disability, exposure; *ABGs*, arterial blood gases, *Spo_2*, continuous pulse oximetry oxygen saturation monitoring; *Svo_2*, continuous mixed-venous oxygen saturation monitoring; *ICP*, intracranial pressure monitoring; *CPP*, cerebral perfusion pressure monitoring; *GCS*, Glasgow Coma Scale; *CT*, computed tomography; *MRI*, magnetic resonance imaging.

lar pigment). As myoglobin circulates in the cardiovascular system, this large molecule causes acute renal tubular blockade and subsequent renal failure. Signs of myoglobinuria include dark-red or burgundy urine and decreasing urine output. Definitive diagnosis is made through serial testing of the urine for myoglobin.

Evaluating Risk for Compartment Syndrome

Compartment syndrome is a condition in which increased pressure within a limited space compromises circulation, resulting in ischemia and necrosis of tissues within that space. Among those at high risk for the development of compartment syndrome are patients with lower extremity trauma, penetrating trauma, vascular ruptures, massive tissue injuries, or venous obstruction. Clinical manifestations of compartment syndrome include obvious swelling and tightness of an extremity, paresis, and pain of the affected extremity. The treatment may consist of simple interventions, such as removing an occlusive dressing, to more complex interventions, including a fasciotomy.

Discovering Missed Injury

Nursing assessment of the multiply injured patient in the critical care unit may reveal missed injuries. Missed injuries are often discovered in the first 24 to 48 hours of the hospital stay.[43] Injuries are missed for a variety of reasons. In the critical care unit a missed injury may be suspected if the patient fails to show appropriate response to medical or surgical intervention. Change in the character of drainage from wounds or catheters may represent biliary or duodenal injuries. Hypotension and a falling Hct level despite aggressive fluid administration may indicate an expanding hematoma. The physician must be notified immediately because potential complications of infection and hemorrhage may be fatal. Nurses play a key role in identifying missed injuries, particularly when patients regain consciousness and can communicate.

Assessing Risk for Systemic Complications

Trauma patients are at high risk for systemic complications. *Systemic inflammatory response syndrome* (SIRS) may be triggered by the multiple insults of injury, shock, hypermetabolism, and infection. This can also lead to *multiple organ dysfunction syndrome* (MODS), a clinical syndrome of progressive dysfunction of organ systems.

SUMMARY

Nursing care of the patient with traumatic injuries can be challenging. Vigilant nursing assessments in the critical care unit help to identify life-threatening conditions and enable early and aggressive medical interventions. The critical care nurse must manage multiple organ system interventions in an effort to maintain organ function and prevent further complications. Addressing the nursing priorities may significantly contribute to improving outcomes for traumatically injured patients.

REFERENCES

1. McCarthy MC: Trauma and critical care, *J Am Coll Surg* 190:232, 1999.
2. Sisley A, Jacobs LM, People G: Violence in America: a public health crisis—domestic violence, *J Trauma* 46:1105, 1999.
3. Nilssen O, Ries RK, Rivara FP: The CAGE questionnaire and the Michigan Alcohol Screening Test in trauma patients: comparisons of their correlations with biological markers, *J Trauma* 36:784, 1994.
4. American College of Surgeons: *Advanced trauma life support*, ed 6, Chicago, 1997, The College.
5. Cordonna V: *Trauma reference manual*, Baltimore, 1985, Brady Communications.
6. Mikhail J: Resuscitation endpoints in trauma, *AACN Clin Issues* 10:10, 1999.
7. Porter J, Ivatury R: In search of optimal endpoints of resuscitation in trauma patients: a review, *J Trauma* 44:908, 1998.
8. Geraci EB, Beraci TA: Hyperventilation and head injury: controversies and concerns, *J Neurosci Nurs* 28:381, 1996.
9. Wright MM: Resuscitation of the multiple trauma patient with head injury, *AACN Clin Issues* 10(1):32, 1999.
10. Mansfield RT: Head injury in adults and children, *Crit Care Clin* 13(3):611, 1997.
11. Valadka AB: Evaluating and monitoring head injury: jugular bulb and non-invasive CNS monitoring. In *Proceedings from trauma and critical care 1996*, American College of Surgery Western States Committee on Trauma.
12. Moulton RJ, Pitts LH: Head injury and intracranial hypertension. In Hall JB, Schmidt GA, Wood LD, editors: *Principles of critical care*, New York, 1998, McGraw-Hill.
13. Arbour R: Aggressive management of intracranial dynamics, *Crit Care Nurse* 18(3):30, 1998.
14. Helwick C, Dixon M, Padberg N: Support group for families of trauma patients: a unique approach, *Crit Care Nurse* 15(4):59, 1995.
15. Dubendorf P: Spinal cord injury pathophysiology, *Crit Care Nurs Q* 22(2):31, 1999.
16. Chiles BW, Cooper PR: Acute spinal cord injury, *N Engl J Med* 334:514, 1996.
17. Wirtz KM, La Favor KM, Ang R: Managing chronic spinal cord injury: issues in critical care, *Crit Care Nurse* 16(4):24, 1996.
18. Lisenmeyer T et al: Acute management of autonomic dysreflexia: adults with spinal cord injury presenting to health care facilities, *J Spinal Cord Med* 20:284, 1997.
19. Nayduch D, Lee A, Butler D: High-dose methylprednisolone after acute spinal cord injury, *Crit Care Nurse* 14(4):69, 1994.
20. Bracken MB et al: Administration of methylprednisolone for 24 or 48 hours in the treatment of acute spinal cord injury: results of the Third National Spinal Cord Injury Randomized Controlled Trial, *JAMA* 277:1597, 1997.
21. Lucke KT: Pulmonary management following acute SCI, *J Neurosci Nurs* 30(2):91, 1998.
22. Murphy M: Traumatic spinal cord injury: an acute care rehabilitation perspective, *Crit Care Nurs Q* 22(2):51, 1999.
23. Gill M: Psychosocial implications of spinal cord injury, *Crit Care Nurs Q* 22(2):1, 1999.
24. McIlvoy L, Meyer K, Vitaz T. Use of an acute spinal cord injury clinical pathway, *Crit Care Nurs Clin North Am* 12(4):521, 2000.
25. Rozycki GS et al: The role of ultrasound in patients with penetrating cardiac wounds: a prospective multicenter study, *J Trauma* 46:543, 1999.
26. Eastern Association for the Surgery of Trauma: Practice management guidelines for screening of blunt cardiac trauma, 1998, www.east.org.
27. Lozen Y: Intra-abdominal hypertension and abdominal compartment syndrome in trauma: pathophysiology and interventions, *AACN Clin Issues* 10(1):104, 1999.
28. Gallagher JJ: Procedure for monitoring intra-abdominal pressure via an indwelling urinary catheter, *Crit Care Nurse* 20(1):87, 2000.
29. Nayduch DA, Sullivan K, Reed RL: Abdominal compartment syndrome, *J Trauma Nurs* 4:5, 1997.
30. Cheatham MI: Intra-abdominal hypertension, *New Horizons* 7:96, 1999.
31. Rotundo MR, Zonies DH: The damage control sequence and underlying logic, *Surg Clin North Am* 77:771, 1997.
32. Hirsberg A, Walden R: Physiologic rationale for damage control surgery, *Surg Clin North Am* 77:779, 1997.
33. Zacharias S et al: Damage control surgery, *AACN Clin Issues* 10(1):95, 1999.
34. Mayberry JC: Bedside open abdominal surgery: utility and wound management, *Crit Care Clinics* 16(1):151, 2000.
35. Caruso DM et al: Perihepatic packing of major liver injuries, *Arch Surg* 134:958, 1999.
36. Carrillo EH et al: Interventional techniques are useful adjuncts in nonoperative management of liver injuries, *J Trauma* 46:619, 1999.
37. Fang JF, Chen RJ, Lin BC: Small bowel perforation: is surgery necessary? *J Trauma* 47:515, 1999.
38. Peterson NE: Genitourinary trauma. In Feliciano DV, Moore EE, Mattox KL, editors: *Trauma*, ed 3, Stamford, Conn, 1995, Appleton & Lange.
39. Cryer HG, Johnson E: Pelvic fractures. In Feliciano DV, Moore EE, Mattox KL, editors: *Trauma*, ed 3, Stamford, Conn, 1995, Appleton & Lange.
40. Cheever KJ: Early enteral feeding of patients with multiple trauma, *Crit Care Nurse* 19(6):40, 1999.
41. Acute Pain Management Guidelines Panel: Acute pain management: operative or medical procedures and trauma clinical practice guidelines, AHCPR Pub No 92-0032, Rockville, Md, 1992, Agency for Health Care Policy and Research, Public Health Service, USDHHS.
42. Eastern Association for the Surgery of Trauma: Practice management guidelines for the management of venous thromboembolism in trauma patients, 1998, www.east.org.
43. Sommers MS: Missed injuries: a case of trauma hide and seek, *AACN Clin Issues* 6:187, 1995.

KATHLEEN M. STACY
LORRAINE FITZSIMMONS

26

Shock and Multiple Organ Dysfunction Syndrome

Objectives

- Describe generalized shock response and systemic inflammatory response.
- List the etiologies of hypovolemic, cardiogenic, anaphylactic, neurogenic, and septic shock and multiple organ dysfunction syndrome (MODS).
- Explain the pathophysiology of the five forms of shock and MODS.
- Identify the clinical manifestations of the five forms of shock and MODS.
- Outline the important aspects of the medical management of hypovolemic, cardiogenic, anaphylactic, neurogenic, and septic shock and MODS.
- Summarize nursing priorities for managing a patient with each type of shock or MODS.

evolve Be sure to check out the free exercises on-line at *http://evolve.elsevier.com/Urden/priorities/*

Shock is an acute, widespread process of impaired tissue perfusion that results in cellular, metabolic, and hemodynamic derangements. Impaired tissue perfusion occurs when an imbalance develops between cellular oxygen supply and cellular oxygen demand. This imbalance can occur for a variety of reasons and eventually results in cellular dysfunction, multiple organ dysfunction syndrome (MODS), and death. This chapter presents an overview of the general shock response, or shock syndrome, followed by a discussion of the different shock states and MODS.

SHOCK SYNDROME

Shock is a complex pathophysiologic process that often results in MODS and death. All types of shock eventually result in impaired tissue perfusion and the development of acute circulatory failure or shock syndrome. Shock syndrome is a generalized systemic response to inadequate tissue perfusion[1] with four stages: initial, compensatory, progressive, and refractory. Progression through each stage varies with the patient's prior condition, duration of initiating event, response to therapy, and correction of underlying cause.[2]

Etiology

Shock can be classified as hypovolemic, cardiogenic, or distributive, depending on the pathophysiologic cause. *Hypovolemic* shock results from a loss of circulating or intravascular volume. *Cardiogenic* shock results from the impaired ability of the heart to pump. *Distributive* shock results from maldistribution of circulating blood volume and can be further classified as septic, anaphylactic, or neurogenic. *Septic* shock is the result of microorganisms entering the body. *Anaphylactic* shock results from a severe antibody-antigen reaction. *Neurogenic* shock results from loss of sympathetic tone.[2]

Pathophysiology

During the *initial stage*, cardiac output is decreased and tissue perfusion impaired. As the blood supply to the cells decreases, the cells switch from aerobic to anaerobic metabolism as a source of energy. Anaerobic metabolism produces small amounts of energy but large amounts of lactic acid. Lactic acidemia quickly develops and causes more cellular damage.[2,3]

During the *compensatory stage* the body's homeostatic mechanisms attempt to improve tissue perfusion. The compensatory mechanisms are mediated by the sympathetic nervous system (SNS) and consist of neural, hormonal, and chemical responses. Neural compensation includes an increase in heart rate and contractility, arterial and venous vasoconstriction, and shunting of blood to the vital organs. Hormonal compensation includes activation of the renin response and stimulation of the anterior pituitary and adrenal medulla. Activation of the renin response results in the production of angiotensin II, which causes vasoconstriction

and the release of aldosterone and antidiuretic hormone (ADH), leading to sodium and water retention. Stimulation of the anterior pituitary results in the secretion of adrenocorticotropic hormone (ACTH), which in turn stimulates the adrenal cortex to produce glucocorticoids, causing a rise in blood glucose levels. Stimulation of the adrenal medulla causes the release of epinephrine and norepinephrine, which further enhance the compensatory mechanisms. Chemical compensation includes hyperventilation to neutralize lactic acidosis.[2,3]

During the *progressive stage* the compensatory mechanisms start to fail, and the shock cycle is perpetuated. At the cellular level the small amount of energy created by anaerobic metabolism is not enough to keep the cell functional, and irreversible damage begins to occur. The sodium-potassium pump in the cell membrane fails, causing the cell and its organelles to swell. Cellular energy production comes to a complete halt as the mitochondria swell and rupture. At this point the problem becomes one of oxygen utilization instead of oxygen delivery. Even if the cell were to receive more oxygen, it would be unable to use it because of damage to the mitochondria. The cell's digestive organelles swell, resulting in leakage of destructive enzymes into the cell. Autodigestion occurs with ensuing cell death.[3] Every system in the body is affected by this process (Box 26-1).[4]

During the *refractory stage*, shock becomes unresponsive to therapy and is considered irreversible. As the individual organ systems die, MODS, defined as failure of two or more body systems, occurs. Death is the final outcome.[2]

Box 26-1   Consequences of Shock

CARDIOVASCULAR
Ventricular failure

NEUROLOGIC
Sympathetic nervous system dysfunction
Cardiac and respiratory depression
Thermoregulatory failure
Coma

PULMONARY
Acute respiratory failure
Acute respiratory distress syndrome (ARDS)

RENAL
Acute tubular necrosis (ATN)

HEMATOLOGIC
Disseminated intravascular coagulation (DIC)

GASTROINTESTINAL
Gastrointestinal tract failure
Hepatic failure
Pancreatic failure

Regardless of etiologic factors, death occurs from impaired tissue perfusion because of the failure of the circulation to meet the oxygen needs of the cell.[5]

Assessment and Diagnosis

The patient with a systolic blood pressure (BP) less than 90 mm Hg accompanied by either tachycardia or brady-cardia and altered mental status is considered to be in a shock state.[6] Clinical manifestations will differ according to underlying cause and the stage of the shock and are related to both the cause and the patient's response to shock.[7] (See individual shock sections for a discussion of clinical assessment and diagnosis of the patient in shock.)

Medical Management

The major focus of the treatment of shock is the improvement and preservation of tissue perfusion. Adequate tissue perfusion depends on an adequate supply of oxygen being transported to the tissues and the cell's ability to use it. Oxygen transport is influenced by pulmonary gas exchange, cardiac output (CO), and hemoglobin (Hgb) level. Oxygen utilization is influenced by the internal metabolic environment. Management of the patient in shock focuses on supporting oxygen transport and oxygen utilization.[1,5]

Adequate pulmonary gas exchange is critical to oxygen transport. Establishing and maintaining an adequate airway are the first steps in ensuring adequate oxygenation. Once the airway is patent, emphasis is placed on improving ventilation and oxygenation. Therapies include administration of supplemental oxygen and mechanical ventilatory support.[2,3,6]

Adequate CO and Hgb levels are crucial to oxygen transport. CO depends on heart rate (HR), preload, afterload, and contractility. A variety of fluids and drugs are used to manipulate these parameters. The types of fluids used include both crystalloids and colloids. The categories of drugs used include vasoconstrictors, vasodilators, positive inotropes, and antidysrhythmics.[3,6,8]

Fluid administration is indicated for decreased preload related to intravascular volume depletion and is provided by a crystalloid solution, colloid solution, or both. *Crystalloids* are balanced electrolyte solutions that may be hypotonic, isotonic, or hypertonic. Examples of crystalloid solutions are normal saline (NS), lactated Ringer's (LR) solution, and 5% dextrose in water (D_5W). *Colloids* are protein or starch-containing solutions. Examples of colloid solutions are blood and blood components and pharmaceutic plasma expanders, such as hetastarch, dextran, and mannitol. The choice of fluid depends on the situation. Advantages of colloids include faster restoration of intravascular volume and use of smaller amounts. Colloids stay in the intravascular space as opposed to crystalloids, which readily leak into the extravascular space. Disadvantages of colloids include expense, allergic reactions, and difficulties in typing and crossmatching blood. Colloids also can leak out of damaged capillaries and cause a variety of additional problems, particularly in the lungs.[2,3,8,9] Blood should be used to augment oxygen transport if the patient's Hgb level is low.[8]

Vasoconstrictor agents are used to increase afterload by increasing the *systemic vascular resistance* (SVR) and improving the patient's BP level. Vasodilator agents are used to decrease preload or afterload, or both, by decreasing venous return and SVR. Positive inotropic agents are used to increase contractility. Antidysrhythmic agents are used to influence HR[2,3,8] (Box 26-2).

An optimal metabolic environment is very important to oxygen utilization. Once the oxygen is delivered to the cells, the cells must be able to use it. The major metabolic derangement seen in shock is *lactic acidosis*. Interventions to correct lactic acidosis include correcting the cause, reestablishing perfusion, inducing hyperventilation, and in severe cases, administering sodium bicarbonate. The role of sodium bicarbonate in the treatment of acidosis

---

Box **26-2**	Agents Used in Treatment of Shock

VASOCONSTRICTORS	Dobutamine (Dobutrex)
Epinephrine (Adrenalin)	Epinephrine (Adrenalin)
Norepinephrine (Levophed)	Isoproterenol (Isuprel)
α-Range dopamine (Intropin)	Norepinephrine (Levophed)
Metaraminol (Aramine)	Digoxin (Lanoxin)
Phenylephrine (Neo-Synephrine)	
Ephedrine	**ANTIDYSRHYTHMICS**
	Lidocaine (Xylocaine)
VASODILATORS	Bretylium (Bretylol)
Nitroprusside (Nipride, Nitropress)	Procainamide (Pronestyl)
Nitroglycerin (Nitrol, Tridil)	Labetalol (Normodyne, Trandate)
Hydralazine (Apresoline)	Verapamil (Calan, Isoptin)
Labetalol (Normodyne, Trandate)	Esmolol (Brevibloc)
	Diltiazem (Cardizem)
INOTROPES	
β-Range dopamine (Intropin)	

is controversial because of the associated risks of using it. These include rebound increase in lactic acid production, development of a hyperosmolar state and fluid overload resulting from excessive sodium, shifting of the oxyhemoglobin dissociation curve to the left, and rapid cellular electrolyte shifts. In addition, no overall measurable benefit to the patient has been found.[10]

The patient also should be started on a nutritional support therapy. The type of nutritional supplementation initiated varies according to the cause of shock and should be tailored to the individual patient's need, as indicated by the underlying condition and laboratory data. The enteral route generally is preferred over parenteral feeding.[11]

Nursing Management

The nursing management of a patient in shock is a complex and challenging responsibility. It requires an in-depth understanding of the pathophysiology of the disease and the anticipated effects of each intervention, as well as a solid understanding of the nursing process.[12] (Individual shock sections include discussions of specific interventions for the patient in shock.)

The psychosocial needs of the patient and family dealing with shock are extremely important. These needs, which differ with each patient and family, are based on situational, familial, and patient-centered variables. **Nursing priorities in managing the patient with shock are directed toward (1) providing information on patient status, (2) explaining procedures and routines, (3) supporting the family, (4) encouraging the expression of feelings, (5) facilitating problem solving and decision making, (6) involving the family in the patient's care, and (7) establishing contacts with necessary resources.**[13]

Collaborative management of the patient with shock is outlined in Box 26-3.

Box **26-3** **COLLABORATIVE** Management

Shock

1. Support oxygen transport.
   - Establish a patent airway.
   - Initiate mechanical ventilation.
   - Administer oxygen.
   - Administer fluids (crystalloids, colloids, blood and other blood products).
   - Administer vasoactive medications.
   - Ensure sufficient hemoglobin and hematocrit.
2. Support oxygen utilization.
   - Identify and correct cause of lactic acidosis.
   - Ensure adequate organ and extremity perfusion.
   - Administer sodium bicarbonate for severe acidosis.
   - Initiate nutritional support therapy.
3. Identify underlying cause of shock and treat accordingly.
4. Maintain surveillance for complications.
5. Provide comfort and emotional support.

HYPOVOLEMIC SHOCK
Etiology

Hypovolemic shock occurs from inadequate fluid volume in the intravascular space. The lack of adequate circulating volume leads to decreased tissue perfusion and initiation of the general shock response. Hypovolemic shock is the most common form of shock.[2]

Hypovolemic shock can result from either absolute or relative hypovolemia. *Absolute* hypovolemia occurs when there is an external loss of fluid from the body including whole blood, plasma, or any other body fluid. *Relative* hypovolemia occurs when there is an internal shifting of fluid from the intravascular space to the extravascular space. This can result from a loss in intravascular integrity, increased capillary membrane permeability, or decreased colloidal osmotic pressure[2] (Box 26-4).

Pathophysiology

Hypovolemia results in a loss of circulating fluid volume. A decrease in circulating volume leads to a decrease in venous return, which in turn results in a decrease in end-diastolic volume or preload. Preload is a major determinant of stroke volume (SV) and CO. A decrease in preload results in a decrease in SV and CO. The decrease in CO leads to inadequate cellular oxygen supply and impaired tissue perfusion[2] (Figure 26-1).

Assessment and Diagnosis

The clinical manifestations of hypovolemic shock vary depending on the severity of fluid loss and the patient's ability to compensate. The first, or initial, stage occurs with a fluid volume loss up to 15% or an actual volume loss up to 750 ml. Compensatory mechanisms maintain CO, and the patient appears symptom-free.[14]

The second, or compensatory, stage occurs with a fluid volume loss of 15% to 30% or an actual volume loss of 750 to 1500 ml. CO falls, resulting in the initiation of a variety of compensatory responses. The HR increases in response to increased SNS stimulation. The pulse pressure narrows as the diastolic BP increases because of vasoconstriction. Respiratory rate (RR) and depth increase in an attempt to improve oxygenation. Arterial blood gas (ABG) specimens drawn during this phase reveal respiratory alkalosis and hypoxemia, as evidenced by low arterial carbon dioxide tension ($PaCO_2$) and low arterial oxygen tension (PaO_2), respectively. Urine output starts to decline as renal perfusion decreases. Urine sodium decreases while urine osmolality and specific gravity increase as the kidneys start to conserve sodium and water. The patient's skin becomes pale and cool, with delayed capillary refill because of peripheral vasoconstriction. Jugular veins appear flat as a result of decreased venous return. Decreased cerebral perfusion causes a change in level of consciousness (LOC). The patient may appear disoriented, confused, restless, anxious, or irritable.[7,14]

Box 26-4   Etiologic Factors in Hypovolemic Shock

ABSOLUTE

Loss of Whole Blood

Trauma
Surgery
Gastrointestinal bleeding

Loss of Plasma

Thermal injuries
Large lesions

Loss of Other Body Fluids

Severe vomiting
Severe diarrhea
Massive diuresis

RELATIVE

Loss of Intravascular Integrity

Ruptured spleen

Long bone or pelvic fractures
Hemorrhagic pancreatitis
Hemothorax or hemoperitoneum
Arterial dissection

Increased Capillary Membrane Permeability

Sepsis
Anaphylaxis
Thermal injuries

Decreased Colloidal Osmotic Pressure

Severe sodium depletion
Hypopituitarism
Cirrhosis
Intestinal obstruction

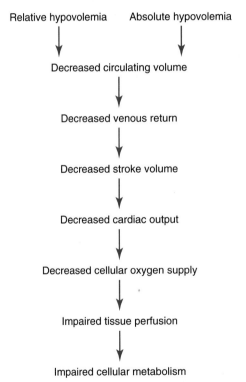

Figure 26-1   Pathophysiology of hypovolemic shock.

The third, or progressive, stage occurs with a fluid volume loss of 30% to 40% or an actual volume loss of 1500 to 2000 ml. The compensatory mechanisms become overwhelmed, and impaired tissue perfusion develops. The HR continues to increase, and dysrhythmias develop as myocardial ischemia ensues. Respiratory distress occurs as the pulmonary system deteriorates. ABG values during this phase reveal respiratory and metabolic acidosis and hypoxemia, as evidenced by a high $PaCO_2$, low bicarbonate (HCO_3^-), and low PaO_2, respectively. Decreased renal perfusion results in the development of oliguria. Blood urea nitrogen (BUN) and serum creatinine levels start to rise as the kidneys begin to fail. The patient's skin becomes ashen, cold, and clammy, with marked delayed capillary refill. The patient appears lethargic as cerebral perfusion decreases and LOC continues to deteriorate.[7,14]

The fourth, or refractory, stage occurs with a fluid volume loss of greater than 40% or an actual volume loss of more than 2000 ml. The compensatory mechanisms completely deteriorate, and organ failure occurs. Severe tachycardia and hypotension ensue. Peripheral pulses are absent, and because of marked peripheral vasoconstriction, capillary refill does not occur. The skin appears cyanotic, mottled, and extremely diaphoretic. The patient becomes unresponsive, and a variety of clinical manifestations associated with failure of the different body systems develop.[14]

Assessment of the hemodynamic parameters of a patient in hypovolemic shock reveals a decreased CO and cardiac index (CI). Loss of circulating volume leads to a decrease in venous return to the heart, which results in a decrease in the preload of the right and left ventricles. This is evidenced by a decline in the right atrial pressure (RAP) and pulmonary artery occlusion pressure (PAOP). Vasoconstriction of the arterial system results in an increase in the afterload of the heart, as evidenced by an increase in SVR.[7]

Medical Management

Treatment of the patient in hypovolemic shock requires an aggressive approach. The major goals of therapy are to correct the cause of the hypovolemia and to restore tissue perfusion. This approach includes identifying and stopping the source of fluid loss and vigorously administering fluid to replace circulating volume.[14,15] Fluid administration can be accomplished with use of either a crystalloid or a colloid solution, or a combination of both. The type of solution used usually depends on the type of fluid lost.[2,8,9,14]

Another therapy available for assisting with resuscitation of the patient in hypovolemic shock is *autotransfusion*, the collection and administration of the patient's own blood. Autotransfusion has been particularly useful in managing the patient with hypovolemic shock caused by chest trauma and hemorrhage.[16]

Nursing Management

Prevention of hypovolemic shock is one of the primary responsibilities of the nurse in the critical care area. Preventive measures include the identification of patients at risk and constant assessment of the patient's fluid balance. Accurate monitoring of intake and output (I&O) and daily weights are essential components of preventive nursing care. Early identification and treatment result in decreased mortality.[2]

The patient in hypovolemic shock may have any number of nursing diagnoses, depending on the progression of the process (Box 26-5). **Nursing priorities are directed toward (1) minimizing fluid loss, (2) enhancing volume replacement, and (3) monitoring the patient's response to care.**

Measures to minimize fluid loss include limiting blood sampling, observing lines for accidental disconnection, and applying direct pressure to bleeding sites. Measures to enhance volume replacement include insertion of large-diameter peripheral intravenous (IV) catheters, rapid administration of prescribed fluids, and positioning the patient with the legs elevated, trunk flat, and head and shoulders above the chest. In addition, monitoring the patient for clinical manifestations of fluid overload is critical to preventing further problems.

CARDIOGENIC SHOCK
Etiology

Cardiogenic shock is the result of failure of the heart to pump blood forward effectively. It can occur with dysfunction of either the right or the left ventricle, or both. The lack of adequate pumping function leads to decreased tissue perfusion and initiation of the general shock response.[2,17] Cardiogenic shock occurs in approximately 6% to 20% of the patients with acute myocardial infarction (MI), and mortality is 72% to 84%.[18]

Cardiogenic shock can result from primary ventricular ischemia, structural problems, and dysrhythmias.[17] The most common cause is acute MI resulting in the loss of 40% or more of the functional myocardium. The damage to the myocardium may occur after one massive MI, or it may be cumulative as a result of several smaller MIs. Structural problems of the cardiopulmonary system and dysrhythmias also may cause cardiogenic shock if they disrupt the forward motion of the blood through the heart[2,17,19] (Box 26-6).

Pathophysiology

Cardiogenic shock results from the impaired ability of the ventricle to pump blood forward, which leads to a decrease in SV and an increase in the blood left in the ventricle at the end of systole. The decrease in SV results in a decrease in CO, which leads to decreased cellular oxygen supply and impaired tissue perfusion. When the underlying problem

---

nursing diagnosis priorities   Box **26-5**

Hypovolemic Shock
- Deficient Fluid Volume related to active blood loss
- Deficient Fluid Volume related to interstitial fluid shift
- Decreased Cardiac Output related to alterations in preload
- Imbalanced Nutrition: Less than Body Requirements related to increased metabolic demands or lack of exogenous nutrients
- Risk for Infection
- Anxiety related to threat to biologic, psychologic, and/or social integrity
- Compromised Family Coping related to critically ill family member

---

Box **26-6**   Etiologic Factors in Cardiogenic Shock

PRIMARY VENTRICULAR ISCHEMIA
Acute myocardial infarction
Cardiopulmonary arrest
Open heart surgery

STRUCTURAL PROBLEMS
Septal rupture
Papillary muscle rupture
Free wall rupture
Ventricular aneurysm
Cardiomyopathies
- Congestive
- Hypertrophic
- Restrictive
Intracardiac tumor
Pulmonary embolus
Atrial thrombus
Valvular dysfunction
Acute myocarditis
Cardiac tamponade
Myocardial contusion

DYSRHYTHMIAS
Bradydysrhythmias
Tachydysrhythmias

involves the left ventricle, the increase in end-systolic volume results in backup of blood into the pulmonary system and subsequent development of pulmonary edema. Pulmonary edema causes impaired gas exchange and decreased oxygenation of the arterial blood, which further impairs tissue perfusion (Figure 26-2). Death may result from cardiopulmonary collapse.[2,17,19]

Assessment and Diagnosis

A variety of clinical manifestations occur in the patient in cardiogenic shock, depending on etiologic factors in pump failure, the patient's underlying medical status, and the severity of the shock state. Some clinical manifestations are caused by failure of the heart as a pump, whereas many relate to the overall shock response (Box 26-7).

Initially the clinical manifestations relate to the decline in CO. These signs and symptoms include systolic BP less than 90 mm Hg; decreased sensorium; cool, pale, moist skin; and urine output less than 30 ml/hr. The patient also may complain of chest pain. Once the compensatory mechanisms are activated, tachycardia develops to compensate for the fall in CO. A weak, thready pulse develops, and heart sounds may reveal a diminished S_1 and S_2 as a result of the decrease in contractility. Respiratory rate increases to improve oxygenation. ABG values at this time indicate res-

piratory alkalosis, as evidenced by a decrease in $PaCO_2$. Urinalysis findings demonstrate a decrease in urine sodium and an increase in urine osmolality and specific gravity as the kidneys start to conserve sodium and water. The patient also may experience a variety of dysrhythmias, depending on the underlying problem.[7,17]

In the patient with left ventricular failure a variety of additional clinical manifestations may be seen. Auscultation of the lungs may disclose crackles and rhonchi, indicating the development of pulmonary edema. Hypoxemia occurs, as evidenced by a fall in PaO_2 using ABG values. Heart sounds may reveal an S_3 and S_4. If right-sided failure occurs, jugular venous distention may become evident.[19]

Once the compensatory mechanisms become overwhelmed and impaired tissue perfusion develops, a variety of other clinical manifestations appear. Myocardial ischemia progresses, as evidenced by continued increases in HR, dysrhythmias, and chest pain. The pulmonary system starts to deteriorate, which leads to respiratory distress. ABG values during this phase reveal respiratory and metabolic acidosis and hypoxemia, as indicated by a high $PaCO_2$, low HCO_3^-, and low PaO_2, respectively. Renal failure is demonstrated by the development of anuria and increases in BUN and serum creatinine levels. Cerebral hypoperfusion manifests as decreasing LOC.[17]

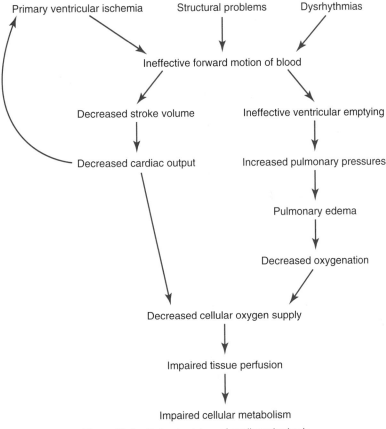

Figure 26-2 Pathophysiology of cardiogenic shock.

Box **26-7** Clinical Manifestations of Cardiogenic Shock

Systolic blood pressure <90 mm Hg
Heart rate >100 beats/min
Weak, thready pulse
Diminished heart sounds
Change in sensorium
Cool, pale, moist skin
Urine output <30 ml/hr
Chest pain
Dysrhythmias
Tachypnea
Crackles
Decreased cardiac output (CO)
Cardiac index (CI) <2.2 L/min/m²
Increased pulmonary artery occlusion pressure (PAOP)
Increased right atrial pressure (RAP)
Increased systemic vascular resistance (SVR)

Assessment of the hemodynamic parameters of a patient in cardiogenic shock reveals a decreased CO and a CI less than 2.2 L/min/m². Inadequate pumping action leads to a decrease in SV, which results in an increase in the left ventricular end-diastolic pressure (LVEDP). This is reflected in an increase in the PAOP. Compensatory vasoconstriction results in an increase in the afterload of the heart, as shown by an increase in the SVR. If right ventricular failure is present, the RAP also will be increased.[7,19]

Medical Management

Treatment of the patient in cardiogenic shock requires an aggressive approach. The major goals of therapy are to treat the underlying cause, enhance the effectiveness of the pump, and improve tissue perfusion. This approach includes identifying the etiologic factors of pump failure and administering pharmacologic agents to enhance CO. Inotropic agents are used to increase contractility, whereas vasodilating agents and diuretics are used for afterload and preload reduction, respectively. Antidysrhythmic agents should be used to suppress or control dysrhythmias that can affect CO.[2,20]

Once the cause of pump failure has been identified, measures should be taken to correct the problem if possible. If the problem is related to an acute MI, measures should be taken to increase myocardial oxygen supply and decrease myocardial oxygen demand. Therapies to increase myocardial oxygen supply include supplemental oxygen, intubation and mechanical ventilation, and coronary artery vasodilator agents such as nitroglycerin. In addition, thrombolytic agents, coronary angioplasty, intracoronary stents, or coronary artery bypass surgery may also be used. Therapies to decrease myocardial demand include activity restrictions, analgesics, and sedatives.[2,18,19]

Two other therapies used to improve the effectiveness of the pumping action of the heart are the *intraaortic balloon pump* (IABP) and *ventricular assist device* (VAD). The IABP is a temporary measure to decrease myocardial workload by improving myocardial supply and decreasing myocardial oxygen demand. The IABP achieves this goal by improving coronary artery perfusion and reducing left ventricular afterload. The VAD is a temporary external pump that takes the place of the patient's ventricle, allowing it to heal.[19]

Nursing Management

Prevention of cardiogenic shock is one of the primary responsibilities of the nurse in the critical care area. Preventive measures include the identification of patients at risk and constant assessment of the patient's cardiopulmonary status.[2] Patients who require IABP therapy need to be observed frequently for complications, including emboli formation, infection, aortic rupture, thrombocytopenia, improper balloon placement, bleeding, improper timing of balloon, balloon rupture, and circulatory compromise of the cannulated extremity.[21]

The patient in cardiogenic shock may have any number of nursing diagnoses depending on the progression of the process (Box 26-8). **Nursing priorities are directed toward (1) limiting myocardial oxygen consumption, (2) enhancing myocardial oxygen supply**, and **(3) monitoring the patient's response to care**.

Measures to limit myocardial oxygen consumption include (1) administering analgesics and sedatives, (2) positioning the patient for comfort, (3) limiting activities, (4) offering support to reduce anxiety, (5) providing a calm and quiet environment, and (6) teaching the patient about their condition. Measures to enhance oxygen myocardial supply include administering supplemental oxygen, monitoring the patient's respiratory status, and administering prescribed medications.

ANAPHYLACTIC SHOCK
Etiology

Anaphylactic shock, a type of distributive shock, is the result of an immediate hypersensitivity reaction. It is a

nursing diagnosis
priorities   Box **26-8**

Cardiogenic Shock

- Ineffective Cardiopulmonary Tissue Perfusion related to acute myocardial ischemia
- Decreased Cardiac Output related to alterations in contractility
- Decreased Cardiac Output related to alterations in heart rate
- Imbalanced Nutrition: Less than Body Requirements related to increased metabolic demands or lack of exogenous nutrients
- Risk for Infection
- Disturbed Body Image related to functional dependence on life-sustaining technology
- Compromised Family Coping related to critically ill family member

life-threatening event that requires prompt intervention. The severe antibody-antigen response leads to decreased tissue perfusion and initiation of the general shock response.[2,22,23]

Anaphylactic shock is caused by an antibody-antigen response. Almost any substance can cause a hypersensitivity reaction (Box 26-9). These substances, known as *antigens*, can be introduced by injection or ingestion or through the skin or respiratory tract. A number of antigens have been identified that can cause a reaction in a hypersensitive person; categories include foods, food additives, diagnostic agents, biologic agents, environmental agents, drugs, and venoms.[2,22-25] Latex allergies are discussed in Box 26-10.

Pathophysiology

The antibody-antigen response (immunologic stimulation) or direct triggering (nonimmunologic activation) of the mast cells results in the release of biochemical mediators. These mediators include histamine, *eosinophilic chemotactic factor of anaphylaxis* (ECF-A), *neutrophilic chemotactic factor of anaphylaxis* (NCF-A), proteinases, heparin, serotonin, leukotrienes (formerly known as slow-reacting substance of anaphylaxis), prostaglandins, and platelet-activating factor (PAF). The activation of the biochemical mediators causes vasodilation, increased capillary permeability, bronchoconstriction, excessive mucus secretion, coronary vasoconstriction, inflammation, cutaneous reactions, and constriction of intestinal wall, bladder, and uterine smooth muscle. Coronary vasoconstriction causes severe myocardial depression. Cutaneous reactions cause stimulation of nerve endings, followed by itching and pain.

ECF-A promotes chemotaxis of eosinophils, thus facilitating the movement of eosinophils into the area. During allergic reactions, eosinophils phagocytose the antibody-antigen complex and other inflammatory debris and release enzymes that inhibit vasoactive mediators such as histamine and leukotrienes. In addition, secondary mediators are produced that either enhance or inhibit the already released biochemical mediators. Bradykinin, a secondary mediator, increases capillary permeability, facilitates vasodilation, and contracts smooth muscles.

Peripheral vasodilation results in decreased venous return. Increased capillary membrane permeability results in the loss of intravascular volume and the development of relative hypovolemia. Decreased venous return results in decreased end-diastolic volume and SV. The decline in SV leads to a fall in CO and impaired tissue perfusion (Figure 26-3). Death may result from airway obstruction or cardiovascular collapse, or both.[2,22,23]

Assessment and Diagnosis

Anaphylactic shock is a severe systemic reaction that can affect any number of organ systems. Clinical manifestations vary in the patient in anaphylactic shock depending on the

---

Box 26-9 Etiologic Factors in Anaphylactic Shock

FOODS
Eggs and milk
Fish and shellfish
Nuts and seeds
Legumes and cereals
Citrus fruits
Chocolate
Strawberries
Tomatoes

FOOD ADDITIVES
Food coloring
Preservatives

DIAGNOSTIC AGENTS
Iodinated contrast dye
Sulfobromophthalein (Bromsulphalein) (BSP)
Dehydrocholic acid (Decholin)
Iopanoic acid (Telepaque)

BIOLOGIC AGENTS
Blood and blood components
Insulin and other hormones
Gamma globulin
Seminal plasma

Enzymes
Vaccines and antitoxins

ENVIRONMENTAL AGENTS
Pollens, molds, and spores
Sunlight
Animal hair

DRUGS
Antibiotics
Aspirin
Narcotics
Dextran
Vitamins
Local anesthetic agents
Muscle relaxants
Barbiturates

VENOMS
Bees and wasps
Snakes
Jellyfish
Spiders
Deer flies
Fire ants

Box 26-10 Latex Allergies

Latex is the milky sap of the rubber tree *Hevea brasiliensis*. It is treated with preservatives, accelerators, stabilizers, and antioxidants to make a more elastic, stable rubber. Reactions to products containing latex can be triggered by either the latex protein or an additive used in the manufacturing process.

Latex reactions can be classified into three different categories: *irritation* (nonallergic inflammation occurring when the skin is abraded), *delayed hypersensitivity* (non-IgE-mediated response to the chemical agents added during the manufacturing process), or *immediate sensitivity* (IgE-mediated response to latex proteins). Although the overall prevalence of latex allergy in the general population is only 1%, it is much higher (28%-67%) in selected groups, such as patients with neural tube defects (spina bifida, myelomeningocele, lipomyelomeningocele) or congenital urologic disorders; those who have undergone multiple surgeries or who have a history of allergy to anesthetic drugs; and health care, rubber industry, or glove manufacturing plant workers.

Five routes of exposure to latex proteins have resulted in systemic reactions: *cutaneous* (contact with moist skin), *mucous membranes* (mouth, vagina, urethra, rectum), *internal tissue* (during surgery and other invasive procedures), *intravascular*, and *inhalation* (exposure to anesthesia equipment or endotracheal tubes or through the aerosolization of glove powder). It has been postulated that the latex allergen adheres to the cornstarch or powder and is released into the air with the manipulation of rubber gloves.

The American Academy of Allergy and Immunology has published guidelines for providing care to persons with latex allergy. All persons at risk for latex allergy should have a careful history and should complete a standardized latex allergy questionnaire. A history suggestive of reactivity to latex includes local swelling or itching after blowing up balloons, dental examinations, contact with rubber gloves, vaginal or rectal examinations, using condoms or diaphragms, and contact with other rubber products. Other historical information that may suggest increased risk of latex allergy includes hand eczema; previous, unexplained anaphylaxis; oral itching after eating bananas, chestnuts, kiwis, and avocados; and multiple surgical procedures in infancy. Patients at high risk should be offered clinical testing for latex allergy.

The patient with a latex allergy should be cared for in a latex-free environment, that is, an environment in which no latex gloves are used and there is no direct patient contact with other latex devices.

Data from Warshaw EM: *J Am Acad Dermatol* 39(1):1, 1998, and Wai DME: *Gastroenterol Nurs* 22:263, 1999.

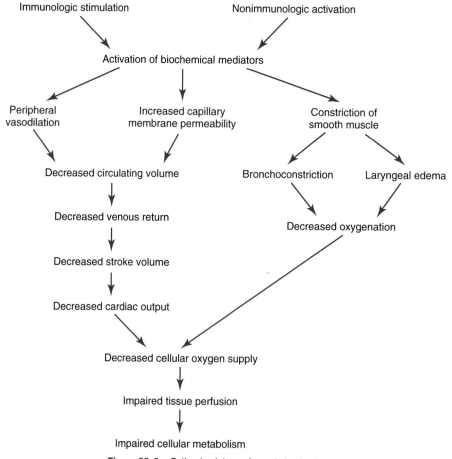

Figure 26-3   Pathophysiology of anaphylactic shock.

extent of multisystem involvement. The symptoms usually start to appear within minutes of exposure to the antigen, peak within 15 to 30 minutes, and resolve over the next several hours[22] (Box 26-11).

The cutaneous effects usually appear first and include pruritus, generalized erythema, urticaria, and angioedema. Usually seen on the face and in the oral cavity and lower pharynx, *angioedema* develops as a result of fluid leaking into the interstitial space. The patient may appear restless, uneasy, apprehensive, anxious and complain of being warm. Respiratory effects include the development of laryngeal edema, bronchoconstriction, and mucus plugs. Clinical manifestations of laryngeal edema include inspiratory stridor, hoarseness, a sensation of fullness or a lump in the throat, and dysphagia. Bronchoconstriction causes dyspnea, wheezing, and chest tightness.[7,22,23] In addition, gastrointestinal (GI) and genitourinary (GU) manifestations may develop as a result of smooth muscle contraction, including diarrhea, vomiting, cramping, abdominal pain, urinary incontinence, and vaginal bleeding.[22,23]

As the anaphylactic reaction progresses, hypotension and reflex tachycardia develop in response to massive vasodilation and loss of circulating volume. Jugular veins appear flat as right ventricular end-diastolic volume is decreased. The eventual outcome is circulatory failure and shock.[7,22,23] The patient's LOC may deteriorate to unresponsiveness.[23]

Assessment of the hemodynamic parameters of a patient in anaphylactic shock reveals a decreased CO and CI. Venous vasodilation and massive volume loss lead to a decrease in preload, which results in a decline in RAP and PAOP. Vasodilation of the arterial system results in a decrease in the afterload of the heart, as evidenced by a decrease in SVR.[7]

Medical Management

Treatment of anaphylactic shock requires an immediate and a direct approach. The goals of therapy are to (1) remove the offending antigen, (2) reverse the effects of the biochemical mediators, and (3) promote adequate tissue perfusion. When the hypersensitivity reaction occurs as a result of administration of medications, dye, blood, or blood products, the infusion should be immediately discontinued. Often it is not possible to remove the antigen because it is unknown or has already entered the patient's system.[22]

Reversal of the effects of the biochemical mediators involves preservation and support of the patient's airway, ventilation, and circulation through oxygen therapy, intubation, mechanical ventilation, and administration of drugs and fluids. Epinephrine is given to promote bronchodilation and vasoconstriction and to inhibit further release of biochemical mediators.[22,26] Usually administered intravenously or via endotracheal tube, the epinephrine dose is 0.1 mg/kg of 1:10,000 dilution IV over at least 3 to 5 minutes

---

Box **26-11** Clinical Manifestations of Anaphylactic Shock

CARDIOVASCULAR
Hypotension
Tachycardia

RESPIRATORY
Lump in throat
Dysphagia
Hoarseness
Stridor
Wheezing
Rales and rhonchi

CUTANEOUS
Pruritus
Erythema
Urticaria
Angioedema

NEUROLOGIC
Restlessness
Uneasiness
Apprehension
Anxiety
Decreased level of consciousness

GASTROINTESTINAL
Nausea
Vomiting
Diarrhea

GENITOURINARY
Incontinence
Vaginal bleeding

SUBJECTIVE COMPLAINTS
Sensation of warmth
Dyspnea
Abdominal cramping and pain
Itching

HEMODYNAMIC PARAMETERS
Decreased cardiac output (CO)
Decreased cardiac index (CI)
Decreased right atrial pressure (RAP)
Decreased pulmonary occlusion pressure (PAOP)
Decreased systemic vascular resistance (SVR)

or 10 ml of 1:10,000 dilution endotracheally. Diphenhydramine (Benadryl), 1 to 2 mg/kg IV every 6 to 8 hours, is used to block the histamine response. Corticosteroids may also be given with the goal of preventing a delayed reaction and stabilizing capillary membranes.[26] Fluid replacement is accomplished by use of a crystalloid or colloid solution. In addition, positive inotropic agents and vasoconstrictor agents may be necessary to reverse the effects of myocardial depression and vasodilation.[2,23,26]

Nursing Management

Prevention of anaphylactic shock is one of the primary responsibilities of the nurse in the critical care area. Preventive measures include the identification of patients at risk and cautious assessment of the patient's response to the administration of drugs, blood, and blood products. A complete and accurate history of the patient's allergies is an essential component of preventive nursing care. In addition to a list of the allergies, a detailed description of the type of response for each one should be obtained.[2]

The patient in anaphylactic shock may have any number of nursing diagnoses, depending on the progression of the process (Box 26-12). **Nursing priorities are directed toward (1) facilitating ventilation, (2) enhancing volume replacement, (3) promoting comfort, and (4) monitoring the patient's response to care.**

Measures to facilitate ventilation include positioning the patient to assist with breathing and instructing the patient to breathe slowly and deeply. Measures to enhance volume replacement include (1) inserting large-diameter peripheral IV catheters, (2) rapidly administering prescribed fluids, and (3) positioning the patient with the legs elevated, trunk flat, and head and shoulders above the chest. Measures to promote comfort include (1) administering medications to

relieve itching, (2) applying warm soaks to skin, and, if necessary, (3) covering the patient's hands to discourage scratching. In addition, observing the patient for clinical manifestations of a delayed reaction is critical to preventing further problems.

NEUROGENIC SHOCK

Neurogenic shock, a type of distributive shock, is the result of the loss or suppression of sympathetic tone. Its onset is within minutes, and it may last for days, weeks, or months depending on the cause. The lack of sympathetic tone leads to decreased tissue perfusion and initiation of the general shock response. Neurogenic shock is the rarest form of shock.[2]

Etiology

Neurogenic shock can be caused by anything that disrupts the SNS. The problem can occur as the result of interrupted impulse transmission or blockage of sympathetic outflow from the vasomotor center in the brain.[2,27] The most common cause is a spinal cord injury above the level of the sixth thoracic vertebra (T6), also known as *spinal shock*.[28] Other causes include spinal anesthesia, drugs, emotional stress, pain, and central nervous system (CNS) dysfunction.[2]

Pathophysiology

Loss of sympathetic tone results in massive peripheral vasodilation, inhibition of the baroreceptor response, and impaired thermoregulation. Arterial vasodilation leads to a decrease in SVR and a fall in BP. Venous vasodilation leads to decreased venous return because of pooling of blood in the venous circuit. A decreased venous return results in a decrease in end-diastolic volume or preload. A decrease in preload results in a decrease in SV and CO, and relative hypovolemia develops. The fall in BP and CO leads to inadequate or impaired tissue perfusion.[28] Inhibition of the baroreceptor response results in loss of compensatory reflex tachycardia. The HR does not increase to compensate for the fall in CO, which further compromises tissue perfusion.[29] Impaired thermoregulation occurs because of loss of vasomotor tone in the cutaneous blood vessels that dilate and constrict to maintain body temperature. The patient becomes *poikilothermic*, or dependent on the environment for temperature regulation[29] (Figure 26-4).

Assessment and Diagnosis

The patient in neurogenic shock usually presents with hypotension, bradycardia, hypothermia, and warm, dry skin. The decreased BP results from massive peripheral vasodilation. The decreased HR is caused by inhibition of the baroreceptor response and unopposed parasympathetic control of the heart. Hypothermia results from uncontrolled heat loss peripherally. The warm, dry skin results from pooling of blood in the extremities and loss of vasomotor control in surface vessels of the skin that control heat loss.[27,29]

---

nursing diagnosis
priorities   Box **26-12**

Anaphylactic Shock

- Deficient Fluid Volume related to relative loss
- Decreased Cardiac Output related to alterations in preload
- Decreased Cardiac Output related to alterations in afterload
- Ineffective Breathing Pattern related to decreased lung expansion
- Impaired Gas Exchange related to ventilation/perfusion mismatching or intrapulmonary shunting
- Imbalanced Nutrition: Less than Body Requirements related to increased metabolic demands or lack of exogenous nutrients
- Risk for Infection
- Ineffective Coping related to situational crisis and personal vulnerability
- Compromised Family Coping related to critically ill family member

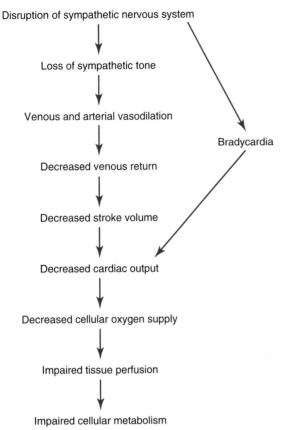

Figure 26-4   Pathophysiology of neurogenic shock.

Assessment of the hemodynamic parameters of a patient in neurogenic shock reveals a decreased CO and CI. Venous vasodilation leads to a decrease in preload, which results in a decline in the RAP and PAOP. Vasodilation of the arterial system causes a decrease in the afterload of the heart, as demonstrated by decreased SVR.[27]

Medical Management

Treatment of neurogenic shock requires a careful approach. The goals of therapy are to treat or remove the cause, prevent cardiovascular instability, and promote optimal tissue perfusion. Cardiovascular instability can occur from hypovolemia, hypothermia, hypoxia, and dysrhythmias. Specific treatments are aimed at preventing or correcting these problems as they occur.

Hypovolemia is treated with careful fluid resuscitation. The minimal amount of fluid is administered to ensure adequate tissue perfusion. Volume replacement is initiated for systolic BP lower than 90 mm Hg, urine output less than 30 ml/hr, or changes in mental status that indicate decreased cerebral tissue perfusion. The patient is carefully observed for evidence of fluid overload.[28] Vasopressors may be used as necessary to maintain BP and organ perfusion.[27]

Hypothermia is treated with warming measures and environmental temperature regulation. The goal is to maintain normothermia and avoid large swings in the patient's body temperature.[29]

The treatment of hypoxia varies with the underlying cause. Chest wall paralysis, retained secretions, pulmonary edema, and suctioning contribute to the development of hypoxia. Management of this problem may include ventilatory support, vigorous pulmonary hygiene, and supplemental oxygen. Continuous pulse oximetry monitoring also may be helpful in recognizing hypoxia early, before complications arise. The major dysrhythmia seen in neurogenic shock is *bradycardia*, which should be treated with atropine.[29]

Nursing Management

Prevention of neurogenic shock is one of the primary responsibilities of the nurse in the critical care area. This includes the identification of patients at risk and constant assessment of the neurologic status. Vigilant immobilization of spinal cord injuries and minimal elevation of the head of bed of the patient after spinal anesthesia are essential components of preventive nursing care. Early identification allows for early treatment and decreased mortality.[2]

The patient in neurogenic shock may have any number of nursing diagnoses, depending on the progression of the process (Box 26-13). **Nursing priorities are directed toward (1) treating hypovolemia, (2) maintaining normothermia, (3) preventing hypoxia, and (4) monitoring for dysrhythmias.**

Venous pooling in the lower extremities promotes the formation of deep vein thrombosis (DVT), which can result in a pulmonary embolism. All patients at risk for DVT should be started on prophylaxis therapy. DVT prophylactic measures include monitoring of calf and thigh measurements, passive range of motion, application of antiembolic/sequential pneumatic stockings, and administration of prescribed anticoagulation therapy.

SEPTIC SHOCK

Septic shock, another form of distributive shock, occurs when microorganisms invade the body. The primary mechanism of

---

nursing diagnosis *priorities*   Box **26-13**

Neurogenic Shock

- Deficient Fluid Volume related to relative loss
- Decreased Cardiac Output related to sympathetic blockade
- Hypothermia related to exposure to cold environment, trauma, or damage to the hypothalamus
- Imbalanced Nutrition: Less than Body Requirements related to increased metabolic demands or lack of exogenous nutrients
- Risk for Infection
- Anxiety related to threat to biologic, psychologic, and/or social integrity
- Compromised Family Coping related to critically ill family member

this type of shock is the maldistribution of blood flow to the tissues, with some areas overperfused and others underperfused.[30] Sepsis is estimated to occur in 300,000 to 500,000 patients annually in the United States, with estimated mortality for septic shock of 45%.[31] A variety of terms may be used to describe the condition experienced by the patient with an infection. In 1991, at the American College of Chest Physicians/Society of Critical Care Medicine Consensus Conference, definitions were developed to describe these conditions (Box 26-14).[32]

Etiology

Septic shock is caused by a wide variety of microorganisms, including gram-negative and gram-positive aerobes, anaerobes, fungi, and viruses. The source of these microorganisms is varied. Exogenous sources include the hospital environment and members of the health care team. Endogenous sources include the patient's skin, GI tract, respiratory tract, and GU tract. Gram-negative bacteria are responsible for more than half of the cases of septic shock.[3,33] Toxic shock syndrome is an example of gram-positive shock caused by *Staphylococcus aureus* (Box 26-15).[34]

Sepsis and septic shock are associated with a wide variety of intrinsic and extrinsic precipitating factors (Box 26-16). All these factors interfere directly or indirectly with the body's anatomic and physiologic defense mechanisms. Several of the intrinsic factors are not modifiable or are very difficult to control. Several of the extrinsic factors may be required for diagnosis and management. All critically ill patients are therefore at risk for the development of septic shock.[31,33]

Pathophysiology

Septic shock is a complex systemic response that is initiated when a microorganism enters the body and stimulates the inflammatory/immune system. Shed protein fragments and the release of toxins and other substances from the microorganism activate the plasma enzyme cascades (complement, kallikrein/kinin, coagulation and fibrinolytic factors) as well as platelets, neutrophils, and macrophages. In addition, the toxins damage the endothelial cells. Once activated, these systems and cells release a variety of mediators that target various organs throughout the body.[35,36]

These mediators initiate a chain of complex interactions that are controlled by numerous feedback mechanisms. Eventually the immune system is overwhelmed, the feedback mechanisms fail, and a process that was designed to protect the body actually harms the body.[3,35] Once the mediators are activated, a variety of physiologic and pathophysiologic events occur that affect capillary membrane permeability, clotting, distribution of blood flow to the tissues and organs, and the metabolic state of the body. Subsequently a systemic imbalance between cellular oxygen supply and demand develops, resulting in cellular hypoxia, damage, and death[3,36] (Figure 26-5).

Damage to the endothelial cells results in continued activation of the mediators, increased capillary membrane permeability, and formation of microemboli. This leads to disruption of blood flow to tissues, more endothelial cell damage, and further propagation of the septic process.[35,36]

Activation of the CNS and endocrine system also occurs as part of the primary response to invading microorganisms. This activation leads to stimulation of the SNS and the

---

Box **26-14** Definitions for Sepsis and Organ Failure

Infection Microbial phenomenon characterized by inflammatory response to presence of microorganisms or invasion of normally sterile host tissue by those organisms.

Bacteremia Presence of viable bacteria in the blood.

Systemic inflammatory response syndrome (SIRS) Systemic inflammatory response to a variety of severe clinical insults. The response is manifested by two or more of the following conditions: (1) temperature >38° C or <36° C; (2) HR >90 beats/min; (3) RR >20 breaths/min or $Paco_2$ <32 mm Hg; and (4) WBC count >12,000/mm³, <4000/mm³, or >10% immature (band) forms.

Sepsis Systemic response to infection, manifested by two or more of the following conditions as a result of infection: (1) temperature >38° C or <36° C; (2) HR >90 beats/min; (3) RR >20 breaths/min or $Paco_2$ <32 mm Hg; and (4) WBC count >12,000/mm³, <4000/mm³, or >10% immature (band) forms.

Severe sepsis Sepsis associated with organ dysfunction, hypoperfusion, or hypotension. Hypoperfusion and perfusion abnormalities may include, but are not limited to, lactic acidosis, oliguria, and acute alteration in mental status.

Septic shock Sepsis-induced shock with hypotension despite adequate fluid resuscitation, along with perfusion abnormalities that may include, but are not limited to, lactic acidosis, oliguria, and acute alteration in mental status. Patients receiving inotropic or vasopressor agents may not be hypotensive when perfusion abnormalities are measured.

Sepsis-induced hypotension Systolic blood pressure <90 mm Hg or reduction of ≥40 mm Hg from baseline in the absence of other causes for hypotension

Multiple organ dysfunction syndrome (MODS) Presence of altered organ function in acutely ill patient such that homeostasis cannot be maintained without intervention.

From American College of Chest Physicians/Society of Critical Care Medicine Consensus Conference Committee: *Crit Care Med* 20:864, 1992.
HR, Heart rate; *RR*, respiratory rate; $Paco_2$, arterial carbon dioxide partial pressure (tension); *WBC*, white blood cell.

Box 26-15 Toxic Shock Syndrome

Toxic shock syndrome (TSS) is a form of septic shock that was first identified in 1978. TSS is a potentially lethal syndrome that is caused by a toxin-producing strain of gram-positive *Staphylococcus aureus*. Although often associated with menstruating women who use tampons, TSS has been reported in men, children, and nonmenstruating women.

The syndrome starts with bacterial colonization or infection of a site. The bacteria release a toxin that is absorbed into the bloodstream and circulated to the rest of the body. Once the toxin is in the bloodstream, the septic cascade is initiated, and septic shock develops.

A few features distinguish TSS. Initially the patient may have flulike symptoms, such as high fever, headache, vomiting, diarrhea, hyperactive bowel sounds, abdominal pain, arthralgia, myalgia, and malaise. The mucous membranes become hyperemic, and pharyngitis, conjunctivitis, vaginitis, and strawberry tongue may develop. In addition, a diffuse erythematous macular rash develops, which progresses to desquamation of the skin in 7 to 10 days. Blood cultures may be negative for bacteremia.

The circulating toxins can also affect the renal, hepatic, hemopoietic, and neurologic systems. Dysfunction of these systems may manifest as elevated levels of blood urea nitrogen (BUN), creatinine, lactic dehydrogenase (LDH), aspartate transferase (AST), bilirubin, and alkaline phosphatase, as well as a decline in platelets. The patient may appear disoriented, confused, and agitated.

Treatment of TSS is essentially the same as the treatment of septic shock. Definitive measures are aimed at identifying the cause of the infection. Supportive measures include administering fluid, antibiotics, and vasoactive agents; treating the fever; and protecting the patient. Generally the acute phase lasts 2 to 5 days.

Data from Manders SM: *J Am Acad Dermatol* 39:383, 1998.

Box 26-16 Precipitating Factors Associated with Septic Shock

INTRINSIC FACTORS
Extremes of age
Coexisting disease
- Malignancy
- Burns
- Acquired immunodeficiency syndrome (AIDS)
- Diabetes
- Substance abuse
- Dysfunction of one or more of major body systems
Malnutrition

EXTRINSIC FACTORS
Invasive devices
Drug therapy
Fluid therapy
Surgical and traumatic wounds
Surgical and invasive diagnostic procedures
Immunosuppressive therapy

release of ACTH. These events trigger the release of epinephrine, norepinephrine, glucocorticoids, aldosterone, glucagon, and renin, which results in the development of a hypermetabolic state and further contributes to the vasoconstriction of the renal, pulmonary, and splanchnic beds. Activation of the CNS also causes the release of endogenous opiates thought to cause vasodilation and decrease myocardial contractility.[37]

Once the initial sequence of events is triggered, a series of pathophysiologic responses occur and eventually culminate in the maldistribution of circulating blood volume. These responses include massive peripheral vasodilation, microemboli formation, selective vasoconstriction, and increased capillary membrane permeability.[3,36] The maldistribution of circulating blood volume eventually results in decreased cellular oxygen supply.[30,31]

Massive peripheral vasodilation results in the development of relative hypovolemia and decreased tissue perfusion. Microemboli formation leads to decreased tissue perfusion and further endothelial cell damage. Selective vasoconstriction results in decreased tissue perfusion of the kidneys, lungs, and GI organs, with eventual system dysfunction. Increased capillary membrane permeability promotes fluid loss from the intravascular space and potentiates the relative hypovolemic effect induced by the massive peripheral vasodilation. The formation of microemboli also is exacerbated because of the increased viscosity of the blood left in the intravascular space.[3,31,36]

The maldistribution of circulating blood volume decreases the amount of oxygen delivered to the cells. This situation leads to a number of cellular derangements that ultimately result in cellular death. The hypermetabolic state created by CNS and endocrine system activation further enhances the situation by increasing the oxygen demands of the cells. A number of metabolic derangements result from CNS and endocrine system activation. A hypermetabolic state increases cellular oxygen demand and contributes to cellular hypoxia. Lactic acid is produced as a result of anaerobic metabolism. Glucocorticoids, ACTH, epinephrine, and glucagon are all catabolic hormones released as part of this response. These hormones favor the use of fats and proteins over glucose for energy production.[37]

The hypermetabolic state also increases the cellular metabolic needs. Increased glucose requirements in conjunction with the high level of catabolic hormones result in the limited ability of the cells to use glucose as a substrate for energy production. This causes glucose intolerance,

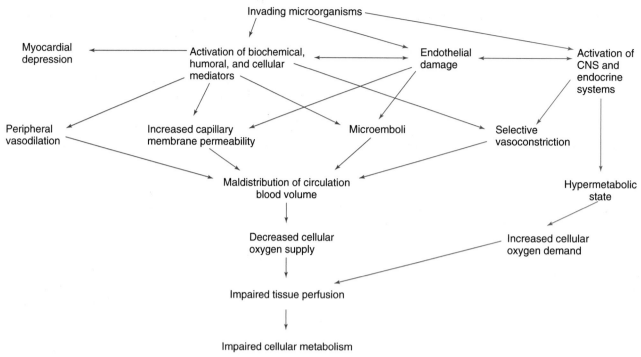

Figure 26-5 Pathophysiology of septic shock.

hyperglycemia, relative insulin resistance, and the use of fat for energy (lipolysis). The relative insulin resistance causes the body to produce more insulin, which inhibits the use of fat as an energy substrate. This promotes the use of protein as an energy substrate and catabolism of protein stores in the visceral organs and skeletal muscles.[37]

Assessment and Diagnosis

The patient in septic shock may present with a variety of clinical manifestations (Box 26-17). During the initial stage, massive vasodilation occurs in both the venous and arterial beds. Dilation of the venous system leads to a decrease in venous return to the heart, which results in a decrease in the preload of the right and left ventricles. This is demonstrated by a decline in RAP and PAOP. Dilation of the arterial system results in a decrease in the afterload of the heart, as shown by a decrease in SVR. The patient's BP falls in response to the reduction in preload and afterload. The patient's skin becomes pink, warm, and flushed as a result of the massive vasodilation.[7,31,36]

HR rises to compensate for the hypotension and in response to increased metabolic, SNS, and adrenal gland stimulation. This results in a normal to high CO and CI. The pulse pressure widens as the diastolic blood pressure decreases because of the vasodilation, and the systolic BP increases because of the elevated CO. A full, bounding pulse develops. Myocardial contractility is decreased, as evidenced by a decline in the left ventricular stroke work index (LVSWI), an effect of myocardial depressant factor, a substance secreted by the pancreas.[7,31,38]

In the lungs ventilation/perfusion mismatching develops as a result of pulmonary vasoconstriction and the formation of pulmonary microemboli. Hypoxemia occurs, and RR increases to compensate for the lack of oxygen. Crackles develop as increased pulmonary capillary membrane permeability leads to pulmonary interstitial edema.[31]

Box 26-17 Clinical Manifestations of Septic Shock
Increased heart rate
Decreased blood pressure
Wide pulse pressure
Full, bounding pulse
Pink, warm, flushed skin
Increased respiratory rate (RR) (early)/decreased RR (late)
Crackles
Change in sensorium
Decreased urine output
Increased temperature
Increased cardiac output (CO) and cardiac index (CI)
Decreased systemic vascular resistance (SVR)
Decreased right atrial pressure (RAP)
Decreased pulmonary artery occlusion pressure (PAOP)
Decreased left ventricular stroke work index
Decreased arterial oxygen tension (Pao_2)
Decreased arterial carbon dioxide tension ($Paco_2$) (early)/increased $Paco_2$ (late)
Decreased bicarbonate (HCO_3^-)
Increased mixed-venous oxygen saturation (Svo_2)

Changes start in LOC as a result of decreased cerebral perfusion, immune mediator activation, hyperthermia, and lactic acidosis. The patient may appear disoriented, confused, combative, or lethargic. Urine output declines because of decreased perfusion of the kidneys. The patient's temperature is elevated in response to pyrogens released from the invading microorganisms, immune mediator activation, and increased metabolic activity.[7,31]

ABG values during this phase reveal respiratory alkalosis, hypoxemia, and metabolic acidosis, as demonstrated by low $PaCO_2$, low PaO_2, and low HCO_3^-, respectively. The respiratory alkalosis is caused by the patient's increased RR. As the patient becomes fatigued, RR decreases and $PaCO_2$ increases, resulting in respiratory acidosis. The metabolic acidosis is the result of lack of oxygen to the cells and the development of lactic acidemia. The mixed-venous oxygen saturation (SvO_2) is increased because of maldistribution of the circulating blood volume and impaired cellular metabolism.[31]

The white blood cell (WBC) count is elevated as part of the immune response to the invading microorganisms. In addition, the WBC differential reveals an increase in immature neutrophils (shift to the left) because the body needs to mobilize increasing numbers of WBCs to fight the infection. Increased serum glucose also occurs as part of the hypermetabolic response and the development of insulin resistance.[37] As impaired tissue perfusion develops, a variety of other clinical manifestations appear, indicating the development of MODS.[31]

Medical Management

Treatment of the patient in septic shock requires a multifaceted approach. The goals of treatment are to control the infection, reverse the pathophysiologic responses, and promote metabolic support. This approach includes (1) identifying and treating the infection, (2) supporting the cardiovascular system and enhancing tissue perfusion, and (3) initiating nutritional therapy. In addition, dysfunction of the individual organ systems must be prevented.

One of the first measures that must be taken in the treatment of septic shock is finding and eradicating the cause of the infection. Blood, urine, sputum, and wound cultures should be obtained to find the location of the infection. Antibiotic therapy should be initiated as soon as possible. If the microorganism is unknown, a broad-spectrum antibiotic should be administered. Once the microorganism is identified, an antibiotic more specific to the microorganism should be started. Administration of antibiotics can be particularly hazardous in gram-negative shock because more endotoxin is released from the cell walls when the microorganisms die, further aggravating the septic process. Surgical intervention to debride infected or necrotic tissue or to drain abscesses also may be necessary to facilitate removal of the septic source.[33,38,39]

In supporting the cardiovascular system and enhancing tissue perfusion, specific interventions are aimed at increasing cellular oxygen supply and decreasing cellular oxygen demand. These treatments include administration of fluids, vasoconstrictor and positive inotropic agents, as well as ventilatory support, temperature control, and reversal of acidosis.[38-40]

Aggressive fluid administration to augment intravascular volume and increase preload is crucial during the initial phase. Crystalloids or colloids may be used depending on the patient's condition. The amount of fluid administered may vary, but generally the goal is to restore PAOP to the range of 15 to 18 mm Hg. The administration of vasoconstrictor agents is indicated to reverse the massive peripheral vasodilation. These agents help increase the SVR and augment the patient's BP. Positive inotropic agents are used to increase contractility and treat myocardial depression. All these medications are titrated to the patient's response.[38-40]

To optimize oxygenation and ventilation, intubation and mechanical ventilation are required. Ventilator settings should be adjusted to provide the patient with PaO_2 greater than 70 mm Hg and pH within normal range. Temperature control also is necessary to decrease the metabolic demands created by hyperthermia. Antipyretic agents and cooling measures often are used.[38,39]

The initiation of nutritional therapy is critical in the management of the patient in septic shock. The goal is to improve the patient's overall nutritional status, enhance the immune system, and promote wound healing. The ideal nutritional supplement for the patient in septic shock should be high in protein because of the metabolic derangements that develop in the hypermetabolic state. The amount of protein calories given depends on the patient's nitrogen balance. In early sepsis the mix of nonprotein calories may be divided evenly between carbohydrates and fats. In the later stages, significant alterations in fat metabolism occur, and the lipid content should be limited to 10% to 15% of the total nonprotein calories. The lipid emulsion should contain long-chain fatty acid triglycerides for their protein-sparing effects.[37,38]

One drug that has recently been approved to treat the patient with severe sepsis is *drotrecogin alfa* (Xigris). A form of activated protein C, it has been shown to reduce the mortality of patients with severe sepsis by helping modulate the inflammatory process. Drotrecogin alfa limits the abnormal coagulation and fibrinolytic processes that are part of the septic cascade. It is administered intravenously at an infusion rate of 24 mcg/kg/hr for a total duration of infusion of 96 hours. It is contraindicated in patients with active internal bleeding, recent hemorrhagic stroke (within 3 months), or recent intracranial/intraspinal surgery(within 2 months); severe head trauma, trauma with an increased risk of life-threatening bleeding, or presence of an epidural catheter; and intracranial neoplasm/mass lesion or evidence of cerebral herniation. The most common serious side effect of drotrecogin alfa is bleeding.[41]

Nursing Management

Prevention of septic shock is one of the primary responsibilities of the nurse in the critical care area. These measures include the identification of patients at risk and reduction of their exposure to invading microorganisms. Handwashing, aseptic technique, and an understanding of how microorganisms can invade the body are essential components of preventive nursing care. Early identification allows for early treatment and decreased mortality.[2,42]

The patient in septic shock may have any number of nursing diagnoses depending on the progression of the process (Box 26-18). **Nursing priorities are directed toward (1) administering prescribed antibiotics, fluids, and vasoactive agents; (2) preventing the development of concomitant infections; (3) observing for complications of nutritional therapy; and (4) monitoring the patient's response to care.** Continual observation to detect subtle changes indicating the progression of the septic process is also important.[42]

MULTIPLE ORGAN DYSFUNCTION SYNDROME
Etiology

The result of progressive physiologic failure of several interdependent organ systems, MODS is defined as the "presence of altered organ function in an acutely ill patient such that homeostasis cannot be maintained without intervention."[32] Dysfunction of one organ may amplify dysfunction in another. Organ dysfunction may be absolute or relative and occurs over varying periods. MODS is the major cause of morbidity in the critically ill patient and may account for up to 80% of all mortality in the critical care unit. MODS is a leading cause of late mortality after trauma.

Lack of consensus regarding acceptable definitions for organ dysfunction, the number of organs involved, and the duration of organ dysfunction has hampered an accurate account of organ dysfunction in critically ill patients. About 7% to 15% of critically ill patients experience dysfunction in at least two organ systems. Patient outcome is directly related to the number of organs that fail. Failure of three or more organs is associated with 90% to 95% mortality.[43]

Although various patient populations are at risk for organ dysfunction, trauma patients are particularly vulnerable because they frequently experience prolonged episodes of circulatory shock, with tissue hypoxemia, tissue injury, and infection.[44] Other high-risk patients include those who have experienced a shock episode associated with a ruptured aneurysm, acute pancreatitis, sepsis, burns, or surgical complications.[44-46] Patients age 65 years and older are at increased risk secondary to their decreased organ reserve.[44]

Pathophysiology

Organ dysfunction may be a direct result of the insult (primary MODS) or may manifest latently and involve organs not directly affected in the initial insult (secondary MODS) (Figure 26-6). Patients can experience both primary and secondary MODS.

Primary MODS

Primary MODS "directly results from a well-defined insult in which organ dysfunction occurs early and is directly attributed to the insult itself."[32] Direct insults initially cause localized inflammatory responses. Examples of primary MODS include the immediate consequences of trauma, such as pulmonary contusion, pulmonary dysfunction after aspiration or inhalation injury, and renal dysfunction as a result of rhabdomyolysis or emergency aortic surgery.[32,47]

---

nursing diagnosis priorities Box **26-18**

Septic Shock

- Deficient Fluid Volume related to relative loss
- Decreased Cardiac Output related to alterations in preload
- Decreased Cardiac Output related to alterations in afterload
- Decreased Cardiac Output related to alterations in contractility
- Impaired Gas Exchange related to ventilation/perfusion mismatching or intrapulmonary shunting
- Imbalanced Nutrition: Less than Body Requirements related to increased metabolic demands or lack of exogenous nutrients
- Risk for Infection
- Anxiety related to threat to biologic, psychologic, and/or social integrity
- Compromised Family Coping related to critically ill family member

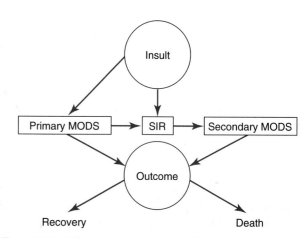

Figure 26-6 Different causes and results of primary and secondary multiple organ dysfunction syndrome (*MODS*). *SIR*, Systemic inflammatory response. (From American College of Chest Physicians/Society of Critical Care Medicine Consensus Conference Committee: *Crit Care Med* 20:868, 1992.)

Primary MODS generally results in one of three patient outcomes: recovery, a stable hypermetabolic state, or death.[43]

Secondary MODS

Secondary MODS is a consequence of widespread systemic inflammation that results in dysfunction of organs not involved in the initial insult.[32] Secondary MODS develops latently after a variety of insults. The early impairment of organs normally involved in immunoregulatory function, such as the liver and GI tract, intensifies the host response to an insult.[48-50]

Systemic Inflammatory Response Syndrome. SIRS is a common initiating event in the development of secondary MODS. The systemic inflammatory response, a continuous process, is an abnormal host response characterized by generalized inflammation in organs remote from the initial insult.[51] SIRS pertains to the widespread inflammation or clinical response to inflammation occurring in patients with a variety of insults (Box 26-19). These insults produce similar or identical systemic inflammatory responses, even in the absence of infection. SIRS is present when two or more of four clinical manifestations are present in the high-risk patient (see Box 26-14). Manifestations of SIRS must represent an acute alteration from the patient's normal baseline and must not be related to other causes (e.g., neutropenia from chemotherapy, leukopenia). When SIRS is a result of infection, the term *sepsis* is used. Organ dysfunction or failure (e.g., acute lung injury, acute renal failure, MODS) is a complication of SIRS.[32,47]

When SIRS is not contained, several consequences may lead to organ dysfunction, including intense uncontrolled activation of inflammatory cells (neutrophils, macrophages, lymphocytes), direct damage of vascular endothelium, disruption of immune cell function, persistent hypermetabolism, and maldistribution of circulatory volume to organ systems.[45] Inflammation becomes a systemic, self-perpetuating, inadequately controlled process that results in organ dysfunction.[48-53]

However, not all patients develop MODS from SIRS. The development of MODS appears to be associated with failure to control the source of inflammation or infection, a persistent perfusion-deficit supply-dependent oxygen consumption (VO_2), or continued presence of necrotic tissue.[54] Normally, under steady-state conditions, VO_2 is relatively constant and independent of oxygen delivery (DO_2) unless delivery becomes severely impaired. The relationship is known as *supply-independent* oxygen consumption. VO_2 is about 25% of DO_2. Consequently, a percentage of oxygen is not used (physiologic reserve). SIRS/MODS patients often develop *supply-dependent* oxygen consumption, in which VO_2 becomes dependent on DO_2 rather than on demand, at a normal or high DO_2. When VO_2 does not equal demand, a tissue oxygen debt develops, subjecting organs to failure.

Clinical Course

The definitive clinical course of secondary MODS has not been completely identified. Clinical observations suggest that organ dysfunction may occur in a progressive pattern; however, organs may fail simultaneously.[44,45,50,55,56] Renal dysfunction, for example, may occur concurrently with hepatic dysfunction. The lungs generally are the first major organs affected. After the initial insult and resuscitation, patients develop a persistent hypermetabolism, a metabolic consequence of sustained systemic inflammation and physiologic stress, followed closely by pulmonary dysfunction, manifested as acute respiratory distress syndrome (ARDS).

Hypermetabolism accompanies SIRS but may not occur immediately after insult. Hypermetabolism generally lasts for 14 to 21 days. During hypermetabolism, changes occur in cellular anabolic and catabolic function, resulting in autocatabolism. *Autocatabolism* manifests as a severe decrease in lean body mass, severe weight loss, anergy, and increased CO and VO_2. The patient experiences profound alterations in carbohydrate, protein, and fat metabolism.[57] Concurrently, GI, hepatic, and immunologic dysfunction may occur, intensifying SIRS. Clinical manifestations of cardiovascular instability and CNS dysfunction may be present. Ongoing perfusion deficits and septic foci continue to perpetuate SIRS. About 25% to 40% of patients die during hypermetabolism.[46] The

---

Box **26-19**	Clinical Manifestations and Conditions Associated with Systemic Inflammatory Response Syndrome

CLINICAL MANIFESTATIONS	Pancreatitis
Temperature >38° C or <36° C	Ischemia
Heart rate >90 beats/min	Multiple trauma with massive tissue injury
Respiratory rate >20 breaths/min or $PaCO_2$ <32 mm Hg	Hemorrhagic shock
WBC count >12,000 cells/mm^3 or <4000 cells/mm^3 or >10% immature (band) forms	Immune-mediated organ injury
	Exogenous administration of tumor necrosis factor or other cytokines
CLINICAL CONDITIONS	Aspiration of gastric contents
Infection	Massive transfusion
Infection of vascular structures (heart and lungs)	Host defense abnormalities

$PaCO_2$, Arterial carbon dioxide tension; *WBC*, white blood cell.

development of renal and hepatic failure is a preterminal event in MODS.[46] Patients with decreased physiologic organ reserve may manifest signs and symptoms of organ dysfunction earlier than previously healthy patients.[58] Survivors may develop generalized polyneuropathy and a chronic form of pulmonary disease from ARDS, complicating recovery.[59] These patients often require prolonged, extensive rehabilitation.

Secondary MODS results from altered regulation of the patient's acute immune and inflammatory responses. Dysregulation, or failure to control the host inflammatory response, leads to the excessive production of inflammatory cells and biochemical mediators that cause widespread damage to vascular endothelium and organ damage.[60] The critically ill patient's compromised immune state also fosters an environment conducive to organ failure.

The inflammatory and immune responses implicated in SIRS and MODS are mediated by certain cells and biochemicals that in turn affect cellular activity. Mediators associated with SIRS and MODS can be classified as inflammatory cells, plasma protein systems, or inflammatory biochemicals (Box 26-20). Activation of one mediator often leads to activation of another. Plasma levels are not always indicative of cellular levels. The biologic activity of inflammatory cells, biochemical mediators, and plasma protein systems and how they work in concert to cause SIRS and MODS are not yet totally defined.

Assessment and Diagnosis

Secondary MODS is a systemic disease with organ-specific manifestations. Organ dysfunction is influenced by numerous factors, including organ host defense function, response time to the injury, metabolic requirements, organ vasculature response to vasoactive drugs, and organ sensitivity to damage and physiologic reserve. The responses of GI, hepatobiliary, cardiovascular, pulmonary, renal, and coagulation systems are discussed here (Box 26-21).

Gastrointestinal Dysfunction

The GI tract plays an important role in MODS. GI organs normally have immunoregulatory functions. Consequently, GI dysfunction amplifies SIRS and gut damage, which may lead to bacterial translocation and endogenous endotoxemia.[48-50,52,53]

Three specific mechanisms link the GI tract and latent organ dysfunction. First, hypoperfusion and shocklike states damage the normal GI mucosal barrier. The GI tract is extremely vulnerable to oxygen metabolite–induced reperfusion injury. Endothelial injury and GI lesions occur in response to mediator-induced tissue damage. In addition, ischemic events and the absence of feedings can disrupt the normal metabolism of the gastric/intestinal lumen and the normal protective function of the gut barrier.[50,60]

Second, the translocation of normal GI bacteria through a "leaky gut" into the systemic circulation initiates and perpetuates an inflammatory focus in the critically ill patient. The GI tract harbors organisms that present an inflammatory focus when translocated from the gut into the portal circulation and are inadequately cleared by the liver. Hepatic macrophages respond to the presence of enteric organisms by producing tissue-damaging amounts of tumor necrosis factor (TNF). Bacterial translocation has been associated with paralytic ileus and drugs typically used in the critically ill patient, including antibiotics, antacids, and histamine blockers.[50]

The third mechanism linking the GI tract and organ dysfunction is *colonization*. The oropharynx of the critically ill patient becomes colonized with potentially pathogenic organisms from the GI tract. Pulmonary aspiration of colonized sputum presents an inflammatory focus. Antacids, histamine antagonists, and antibiotics also increase colonization of the upper GI tract.[50,61]

Hepatobiliary Dysfunction

The liver plays a vital role in host homeostasis related to the acute inflammatory response. In addition, the liver responds

---

Box 26-20 Inflammatory Mediators Associated with SIRS and MODS

INFLAMMATORY CELLS

Neutrophils
Macrophages/monocytes
Mast cells
Endothelial cells

BIOCHEMICAL MEDIATORS

Interleukins
Tumor necrosis factor (TNF)
Platelet-activating factor (PAF)
Arachidonic acid metabolites
• Prostaglandins

• Leukotrienes
• Thromboxanes
Oxygen radicals
• Superoxide radical
• Hydroxyl radical
• Hydrogen peroxide
Proteases

PLASMA PROTEIN SYSTEMS

Complement
Kinin
Coagulation

SIRS, Systemic inflammatory response syndrome.
MODS, Multiple organ dysfunction syndrome.

Box 26-21   Clinical Manifestations of Organ Dysfunction

GASTROINTESTINAL

Abdominal distention
Intolerance to enteral feedings
Paralytic ileus
Upper/lower gastrointestinal bleeding
Diarrhea
Ischemic colitis
Mucosal ulceration
Decreased bowel sounds
Bacterial overgrowth in stool

LIVER

Jaundice
Increased serum bilirubin (hyperbilirubinemia)
Increased liver enzymes (AST, ALT, LDH, alkaline
  phosphatase)
Increased serum ammonia
Decreased serum albumin
Decreased serum transferrin

GALLBLADDER

Right upper quadrant tenderness/pain
Abdominal distention
Unexplained fever
Decreased bowel sounds

METABOLIC/NUTRITIONAL

Decreased lean body mass
Muscle wasting
Severe weight loss
Negative nitrogen balance
Hyperglycemia
Hypertriglyceridemia
Increased serum lactate
Decreased serum albumin, serum transferrin, and
  prealbumin
Decreased retinol-binding protein

IMMUNE

Infection
Decreased lymphocyte count
Anergy

PULMONARY

Tachypnea
ARDS pattern of respiratory failure
• Dyspnea
• Patchy infiltrates
• Refractory hypoxemia
• Respiratory acidosis
• Abnormal oxygen (O_2) indices
Pulmonary hypertension

RENAL

Increased serum creatinine/BUN levels
Oliguria, anuria, or polyuria consistent with prerenal azotemia
  or ATN
Urinary indices consistent with prerenal azotemia or ATN

CARDIOVASCULAR

Hyperdynamic

Decreased pulmonary capillary occlusion pressure (PAOP)
Decreased systemic vascular resistance (SVR)
Decreased right atrial pressure (RAP)
Decreased left ventricular stroke work index (LVSWI)
Increased O_2 consumption
Increased cardiac output (CO)/cardiac index (CI)/heart rate

Hypodynamic

Increased SVR
Increased RAP
Increased LVSWI
Decreased O_2 delivery/consumption
Decreased CO/CI

CENTRAL NERVOUS SYSTEM

Lethargy
Altered level of consciousness
Fever
Hepatic encephalopathy

COAGULATION/HEMATOLOGIC

Thrombocytopenia
DIC pattern

AST, Aspartate transaminase (SGOT); *ALT*, alanine transaminase (SGPT); *LDH*, lactate dehydrogenase; *ARDS*, acute respiratory distress syndrome;
BUN, blood urea nitrogen; *ATN*, acute tubular necrosis; *DIC*, disseminated intravascular coagulation

to SIRS by selectively changing carbohydrate (CHO), fat, and protein metabolism. Consequently, hepatic dysfunction after a critical insult threatens the patient's survival.

The liver normally controls the inflammatory response by several mechanisms. Kupffer cells, which are hepatic macrophages, detoxify substances that might normally induce systemic inflammation, as well as vasoactive substances that cause hemodynamic instability. Failure to detoxify gram-negative bacteria translocated from the GI tract causes endotoxemia, perpetuates SIRS, and may lead to MODS. Additionally, the liver produces proteins and

antiproteases to control the inflammatory response; however, hepatic dysfunction limits this response.[48,49]

The liver and gallbladder are extremely vulnerable to ischemic injury. *Ischemic hepatitis* occurs after prolonged physiologic shock and is associated with centrilobular hepatocellular necrosis. The degree of hepatic damage is related directly to the severity and duration of the shock episode. Terms such as *shock liver* and *posttraumatic hepatic insufficiency* have been used to describe ischemic hepatitis. Both anoxic and reperfusion injury damage hepatocytes and the vascular endothelium.[62] Patients at high risk for ischemic hepatitis after a hypotensive event include those with a history of cardiac failure or cardiac dysrhythmias. Clinical manifestations of hepatic insufficiency are evident 1 to 2 days after the insult. Jaundice and transient elevations in serum transaminase and bilirubin levels occur. Hyperbilirubinemia results from hepatocyte anoxic injury and an increased production of bilirubin from Hgb catabolism. Ischemic hepatitis may either resolve spontaneously or progress to fulminant hepatic failure. Although not a life-threatening complication, ischemic hepatitis can contribute to patient morbidity and mortality as a component of MODS.[62] Researchers have recently proposed that serum bilirubin is a valid indicator of hepatic dysfunction in MODS because it significantly differentiates MODS survivors from nonsurvivors.[63]

Acalculous cholecystitis manifests 3 to 4 weeks after an insult. Its pathogenesis is unclear but may be related to ischemic reperfusion injury, narcotics, and cystic duct obstruction as a result of hyperviscous bile. Mediator-induced gallbladder dysfunction associated with acalculous cholecystitis may be related to the release of thromboxane A_2 and leukotrienes (vasoactive substances) into the microcirculation in response to a damaged endothelium, aggregated platelets, and neutrophils. Clinical manifestations of acalculous cholecystitis may mimic acute cholecystitis with gallstones. Patients may demonstrate vague symptoms, including right upper quadrant pain and tenderness. Critical to the detection of acalculous cholecystitis is the recognition of abdominal distention, unexplained fever, loss of bowel sounds, and a sudden deterioration in the patient's condition. About 50% of patients with acalculous cholecystitis have gallbladder gangrene, and 10% have gallbladder perforation. Consequently, a cholecystectomy may be performed.[64]

Hypermetabolism accompanies SIRS and is often referred to as the "metabolic response to injury." During hypermetabolism and SIRS, the liver perpetuates select changes in metabolism, including increased gluconeogenesis, glucogenesis, lipogenesis, and increased production of acute-phase reactant proteins. Concurrently, the liver decreases synthesis of proteins, particularly albumin and transferrin. This metabolic response is partially mediated by interleukin-1 (IL-1), TNF, select arachidonic acid (AA) metabolites, and the stress hormones.[56]

Pulmonary Dysfunction

The lungs, a frequent and early target organ for mediator-induced injury, are usually the first organs affected in secondary MODS. Acute pulmonary dysfunction in secondary MODS manifests as ARDS. Patients who develop MODS generally develop ARDS; however, not all patients with ARDS develop secondary MODS. ARDS patients who develop SIRS/sepsis concurrently with acute respiratory failure are at the greatest risk for MODS.[45]

ARDS generally occurs 24 to 72 hours after the initial insult. Patients initially exhibit a low-grade fever, tachycardia, dyspnea, and mental confusion. As dyspnea, hypoxemia, and work of breathing increase, intubation and mechanical ventilation are required. Pulmonary function is acutely disrupted, resulting in refractory hypoxemia secondary to intrapulmonary shunting, decreased pulmonary compliance, altered airway mechanics, and radiographic evidence of noncardiogenic pulmonary edema. ARDS is also associated with severe hypermetabolism, equated with running an 8-minute mile, 24 hours a day, 7 days a week.[54]

Mediators associated with ARDS include AA metabolites, toxic oxygen metabolites, proteases, TNF, PAF, and interleukins.[51,59] Intense mediator activity damages the pulmonary vascular endothelium and the alveolar epithelium, resulting in surfactant deficiency, mild pulmonary hypertension, and increased lung water (noncardiogenic pulmonary edema) resulting from increased pulmonary capillary permeability. Pulmonary hypertension and hypoxic pulmonary vasoconstriction result from loss of the vascular bed.

Attempts to quantify the severity of pulmonary dysfunction in ARDS have led to the development of an acute lung injury scoring system. Variables included in the score are chest x-ray findings, magnitude of hypoxemia using PaO_2/FIO_2 (fraction of inspired oxygen) ratio, pulmonary compliance during mechanical ventilation, and use of positive end-expiratory pressure (PEEP) with mechanical ventilation. The total score is intended to provide an index of pulmonary dysfunction.[65] Attempts to predict outcome in MODS patients and quantify the magnitude of pulmonary dysfunction using scoring systems are ongoing.

Renal Dysfunction

Acute renal failure (ARF) is a common manifestation of MODS. The kidney is highly vulnerable to reperfusion injury. Consequently, renal ischemic-reperfusion injury may be a major cause of renal dysfunction in MODS. The patient may demonstrate oliguria or anuria secondary to decreased renal perfusion and relative hypovolemia. The condition may become refractory to diuretics, fluid challenges, and dopamine. Additional signs and symptoms of ARF include azotemia, decreased creatinine clearance, abnormal renal indices, and fluid and electrolyte imbalances. Prerenal oliguria may progress to acute tubular necrosis, necessitating hemodialysis or other renal therapies. The frequent use of nephrotoxic drugs during critical illness also intensifies the risk of ARF.[66] Researchers have proposed that the serum creatinine is a valid indicator of renal function because it significantly differentiates MODS survivors from nonsurvivors.[63]

Cardiovascular Dysfunction

The initial cardiovascular response in SIRS/sepsis is myocardial depression, decreased RAP and SVR, and increased venous capacitance, Vo_2, CO, and HR. Despite an increased CO, myocardial depression occurs and is accompanied by decreased SVR, increased HR, and ventricular dilation. These compensatory mechanisms help maintain CO during the early phase of SIRS/sepsis. An inability to increase CO in response to a low SVR may indicate myocardial failure or inadequate fluid resuscitation and is associated with increased mortality. VO_2 may be twice normal and may be flow dependent. Mediators implicated in the hyperdynamic response include bradykinin, select AA metabolites, PAF, endogenous opioids, and β-adrenergic stimulators.[44,67-69]

As MODS progresses, cardiac failure develops. Cardiac dysfunction is characterized by ventricular dilation, decreased diastolic compliance, and decreased systolic contractile function. Cardiovascular function becomes vasopressor dependent. Cardiac failure may be caused by immune mediators, TNF, acidosis, or myocardial depressant factor (MDF). TNF has a myocardial-depressant effect and is associated with myocardial depression during septic shock.[70] Myocardial depression is exacerbated by myocardial hypoperfusion from a low CO state and persistent lactic acidosis. Cardiogenic shock and biventricular failure occur and lead to death.

Coagulation System Dysfunction

Failure of the coagulation system manifests as *disseminated intravascular coagulation* (DIC). DIC results in simultaneous microvascular clotting and hemorrhage in organ systems because of the depletion of clotting factors and excessive fibrinolysis. Cell injury and damage to the endothelium initiate the intrinsic or extrinsic coagulation pathways (Figure 26-7). The endothelium is closely involved in DIC. Endotoxins may roughen and expose the endothelial lining of blood vessels and consequently stimulate clotting. Low-flow states during hypotensive episodes may damage vessel endothelium and release tissue thromboplastin, with subsequent activation of the extrinsic pathway. A variety of clinical conditions, such as trauma, burns, and radiographic procedures, can also cause damage to the local endothelium and activation of the intrinsic coagulation pathway.[55,71]

DIC is a complex, consumptive coagulopathy that occurs in patients with various disorders (e.g., sepsis, tissue injury, shock) and is an overstimulation of the normal coagulation process. Thrombosis and fibrinolysis are magnified to life-threatening proportions. The initial alteration in DIC is a generalized state of systemic *hypercoagulation* that produces organ ischemia. All organs, particularly the skin, lungs, and kidneys, are involved[55,71] (Box 26-22).

Hemorrhage is the second pathophysiologic alteration in DIC. The lysis of clots (fibrinolysis) normally is initiated by the coagulation cascade. The intensity of the thrombosis enhances an equally intense lysis; however, clot lysis cannot effectively maintain blood vessel patency. Production of fibrin split products exerts further anticoagulant effects, and hemorrhage ensues (Figure 26-7). Clotting factors, platelets, fibrinogen, and thrombin are consumed in large quantities during thrombosis, depleting coagulation substances (Box 26-22).

The abnormal clotting studies in patients with DIC may indicate thrombocytopenia; prolonged clotting times; depressed levels of clotting factors, particularly factor VII; and fibrinogen/fibrin and high levels of breakdown products of fibrinogen and fibrin (fibrin degradation products, D-dimer). Medical management of DIC includes immediate treatment of the underlying cause, transfusion of blood products (e.g., red blood cells, platelets, fresh-frozen plasma) to correct the clotting factor deficiencies, and cryoprecipitate to treat hypofibrinogenemia. The use of heparin therapy in DIC remains controversial. Heparin must be used with caution; however, it is contraindicated in patients with bleeding in critical areas such as the cranium. Antifibrinolytic agents may be used concurrently with heparin therapy but generally are contraindicated because of the risk of thrombotic complications. Strict adherence to bleeding precautions is essential to minimize tissue and vascular trauma.[55,71]

Medical Management

The goals of therapy are prevention and treatment of infection, maintenance of tissue oxygenation, nutritional/metabolic support, and support for individual organs.[44,45,66,72] The use of investigational therapies may be part of the patient's clinical management.

Elimination of the source of inflammation or infection can reduce mortality.[46] Therefore surgical procedures such as early fracture stabilization, removal of infected organs or tissue, and burn excision may be helpful in limiting the inflammatory response. Appropriate antibiotics are needed if the focus cannot be removed surgically.

Despite compliance with meticulous infection control practices, critically ill patients may "infect" themselves. As previously noted, bacterial contamination of the highly vulnerable respiratory tract and pneumonia can result from the colonization by GI tract bacteria. New approaches to infection control have been proposed, including (1) selective decontamination of the GI tract with enteral antibiotics to prevent nosocomial infections, (2) topical antibiotics in the oropharynx to prevent colonization, (3) monoclonal antibodies against endotoxin, and (4) passive antibody protection.[35,65] Gut decontamination and prevention of oropharyngeal colonization reduce the incidence of infection, although morbidity from MODS is not significantly affected.[61]

New approaches to infection and inflammation control currently are being investigated, including immunotherapy. Immunotherapy is antibody therapy that lessens the SIRS to microbes (antiinflammatory immunotherapy) and is based on the principle that antibodies directed against endotoxin can prevent the endotoxin from stimulating SIRS.[73]

Hypoperfusion and resultant organ hypoxemia frequently occur in patients at high risk for MODS, subjecting essential organs to failure. Therefore effective fluid resuscitation and early recognition of supply-dependent VO_2 is essential. Patients at risk for MODS require pulmonary artery

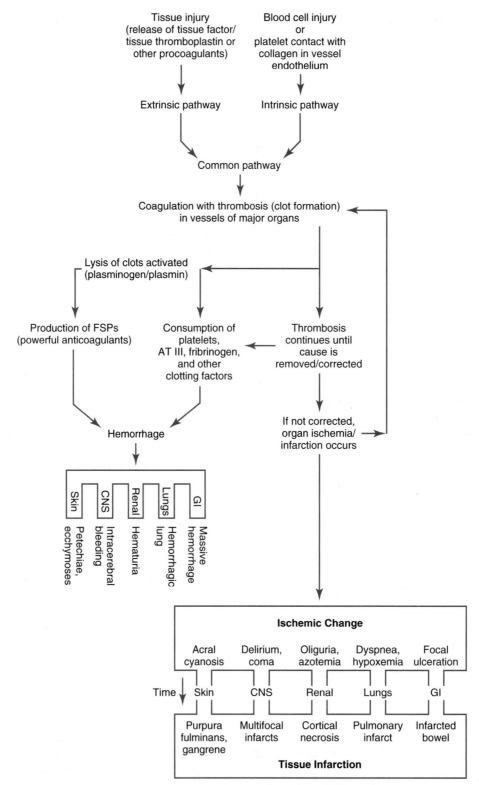

Figure 26-7 Pathophysiology of disseminated intravascular coagulation (DIC). Lysis of clots (fibrinolysis) is a natural consequence of and is activated by coagulation. It is intensified in patients with DIC. DIC is known as a consumptive coagulopathy. During thrombosis, clotting factors are used to form clots. During fibrinolysis, clotting factors are destroyed inside the clot. The end result is a depletion of coagulation substances. *FSPs*, Fibrin split products or fibrin degradation products; *AT III*, antithrombin III ; *CNS*, central nervous system; *GI*, gastrointestinal. (Modified from Carr M: *J Emerg Med* 5:316, 1987.)

Box 26-22   Thrombotic and Hemorrhagic Manifestations of Disseminated Intravascular Coagulation (DIC)

THROMBOTIC

Skin involvement
- Red, indurated areas along vessel wall
- Purpura fulminans (diffuse skin infarction)
- Acral cyanosis
- Necrosis of fingers, toes, nose, and genitalia

Cool, pale extremities with mottling, cyanosis, or edema

Renal involvement

Renal failure

Cerebral infarcts or hemorrhage

Focal neurologic deficits
- Hemiplegia
- Loss of vision

Nonspecific changes
- Altered level of consciousness
- Confusion
- Headache
- Seizures

Bowel infarction

Melena, hematemesis

Abdominal distention

Absent or hyperactive bowel sounds

Thrombophlebitis

Pulmonary embolism

HEMORRHAGIC

Spontaneous hemorrhage into body cavities and skin surfaces

Classic symptom of oozing or bleeding
- Invasive line insertion sites
- Body orifices

Bleeding
- Rectum, vagina, urethra, nose, ears
- Lung, gastrointestinal tract

Petechiae, purpura, or ecchymosis

Gingival, nasal, or scleral hemorrhage on physical examination

Hemorrhaging into all body cavities
- Abdomen
- Retroperitoneal space
- Cranium
- Thorax

---

catheterization, frequent measurements of Do_2 and Vo_2, and arterial lactate levels to guide therapy. Arterial lactate levels provide information regarding the severity of impaired perfusion and the presence of lactic acidosis and differ significantly in MODS survivors and nonsurvivors. Failure to maintain adequate oxygenation to vital organs results in organ dysfunction. Despite adequate Do_2, Vo_2 may not meet the needs of the body during MODS. Patients with ARDS and sepsis frequently manifest supply-dependent oxygen consumption and are unable to use oxygen appropriately despite normal delivery.[67,68,74,75] Possible causes of this flow-dependent Vo_2 include abnormal mitochondrial function, redistribution of blood flow to organs, decreased SVR (secondary to prostaglandins), maldistribution of blood flow, microembolization, and capillary obstruction.[72,74]

Interventions that decrease oxygen demand and increase oxygen delivery are essential. Decreasing oxygen demand may be accomplished through sedation, mechanical ventilation, temperature/pain control, and rest. Do_2 may be increased by (1) maintaining normal Hct and Pao_2 levels, (2) using PEEP, (3) increasing preload or myocardial contractility to enhance CO, and (4) reducing afterload to increase CO. Many critical care clinicians advocate the maintenance of a supranormal Do_2 to increase Vo_2; however, this therapeutic measure has not significantly improved survival, except in select groups of trauma patients.[54]

Hypermetabolism in SIRS/MODS results in profound weight loss, cachexia, and loss of organ function. The goal of nutritional support is the preservation of organ structure and function. Although nutritional support may not alter the course of organ dysfunction, it prevents generalized nutritional deficiencies and preserves gut integrity. The enteral route is preferable to parenteral support.[43,76] Enteral feedings are given distal to the pylorus to prevent pulmonary aspiration. Enteral feedings may limit bacterial translocation. In addition to early nutritional support, the pharmacologic properties of enteral feeding formulas may limit SIRS for select critical care populations. Supplementation of enteral feedings with glutamine and arginine may be beneficial. Enteral feedings with omega-3 fatty acids may lessen SIRS.[76-79]

Recent guidelines have been proposed regarding nutritional support during SIRS for trauma patients. Patients are to receive 25 to 30 kcal/kg/day, with 3 to 5 g/kg/day as glucose. The respiratory quotient is monitored and maintained under 0.9. Long-chain polyunsaturated fatty acids (less than 1.5 g/kg/day) and amino acids (1.5 mg/kg/day) are given. Fat emulsions are limited to 0.5 to 1 g/kg/day to prevent iatrogenic immunosuppression associated with lipids and fat overload syndromes. Plasma transferrin and prealbumin levels are used to monitor hepatic protein synthesis.[56] Efficient protein use must be assessed using nitrogen balance studies.

Organ-specific interventions have not been highly effective in improving survival in MODS. Although organ-specific therapies such as mechanical ventilation and hemodialysis are needed for immediate survival, future medical management must target and control the effects of mediators that cause SIRS and MODS. Animal model studies continue to provide information regarding the efficacy of drugs that prevent organ dysfunction. Several experimental drugs and agents are currently being tested in human clinical trials. However, the initial enthusiasm about inflammatory therapies has been dampened, with many clinical trials reporting negative findings.

Nursing Management

Preventive measures include a multitude of assessment strategies to detect early organ manifestations of this syndrome. Patients who continue to experience sites of inflammation, septic foci, and inadequate tissue perfusion may be at higher risk. Hand hygiene, aseptic technique, and an understanding of how microorganisms can invade the body are essential components of preventive nursing care (Box 26-23).[80]

Nursing management of the patient with acute MODS incorporates a variety of nursing diagnoses (Box 26-24). **Nursing priorities are directed toward** (1) **preventing development of infections**, (2) **facilitating tissue oxygen delivery and limiting tissue oxygen demand**, (3) **facilitating nutritional support**, (4) **providing comfort and emotional support**, and (5) **maintaining surveillance for complications**.

Patients are assessed closely for inflammation and infection. Subtle expressions of infection warrant investigation. Nursing measures include strict adherence to standards of practice to prevent infection. Practices related to infection control with invasive hemodynamic monitoring, urinary catheters, endotracheal tubes, intracranial pressure monitoring devices, total parenteral nutrition (TPN), and wound care must be stringent to prevent further infection.

---

patient safety Box **26-23**

Hand Hygiene

1. Wash hands with soap and water when visibly dirty or contaminated with blood and other body fluids.
   - Wet hands first with water; apply an amount of product recommended by the manufacturer to hands; and rub hands together vigorously for at least 15 seconds, covering all surfaces of the hands and fingers.
   - Rinse hands with water and dry thoroughly with a disposable towel. Use towel to turn off the faucet.
   - Avoid using hot water because repeated exposure may increase risk of dermatitis.
2. If hands are not visibly soiled, use alcohol-based hand rub for routinely decontaminating hands.
   - Apply product to palm of one hand and rub hands together, covering all surfaces of hands and fingers, until hands are dry.
   - Follow manufacturer's recommendations regarding volume of product to use.
3. Decontaminate hands before and after direct contact with patients.

4. Decontaminate hands before and after donning gloves.
   - Wear gloves when contact with blood or other potentially infectious materials, mucous membranes, and nonintact skin could occur.
   - Change gloves during patient care if moving from a contaminated to a clean body site.
   - Remove gloves after caring for a patient.
   - Do not wear the same pair of gloves for the care of more than one patient.
   - Do not wash gloves between uses with different patients.
5. Decontaminate hands after contact with inanimate objects, including medical equipment.
6. Do not wear artificial fingernails or extenders during direct contact with patients at high risk (e.g., in intensive care unit, operating room).
7. Keep natural nail tips less than ¼-inch long.

---

nursing diagnosis priorities Box **26-24**

Multiple Organ Dysfunction Syndrome

- Decreased Cardiac Output related to alterations in preload
- Decreased Cardiac Output related to alterations in afterload
- Decreased Cardiac Output related to alterations in contractility
- Impaired Gas Exchange related to ventilation/perfusion mismatching or intrapulmonary shunting
- Ineffective Renal Tissue Perfusion related to decreased renal blood flow
- Ineffective Cardiopulmonary Tissue Perfusion related to decreased myocardial oxygen supply and/or increased myocardial oxygen demand

- Imbalanced Nutrition: Less than Body Requirements related to increased metabolic demands or lack of exogenous nutrients
- Risk for Infection
- Acute Pain related to transmission and perception of cutaneous, visceral, muscular, or ischemic impulses
- Acute Confusion related to sensory overload, sensory deprivation, and sleep pattern disturbance
- Anxiety related to threat to biologic, psychologic, and/or social integrity
- Compromised Family Coping related to critically ill family member

Measures to limit tissue oxygen consumption include (1) administering analgesics and sedatives, (2) positioning the patient for comfort, (3) limiting activities, (4) offering support to reduce anxiety, (5) providing a calm and quiet environment, and (6) teaching the patient about the condition. Measures to enhance tissue oxygen supply include administering supplemental oxygen, monitoring the patient's respiratory status, and administering prescribed fluids and medications.

REFERENCES

1. Shoemaker WC: Oxygen transport and oxygen metabolism in shock and critical illness: invasive and noninvasive monitoring of circulatory dysfunction and shock, *Crit Care Clin* 12:939, 1996.
2. Rice V: *Shock: a clinical syndrome*, ed 2, Aliso Viejo, Calif, 1997, American Association of Critical-Care Nurses.
3. Jindal N, Hollenberg SM, Dellinger RP: Pharmacologic issues in the management of septic shock, *Crit Care Clin* 16:233, 2000.
4. McMahon K: Multiple organ failure: the final complication of critical illness, *Crit Care Nurse* 15(6):20, 1995.
5. Shoemaker WC: Pathophysiology, monitoring and therapy of circulatory problems, *Crit Care Nurs Clin North Am* 6:295, 1994.
6. Nawas YN, Balk RA: General approach to shock, *Clin Geriatr Med* 10:185, 1994.
7. Summers G: The clinical and hemodynamic presentation of the shock patient, *Crit Care Nurs Clin North Am* 2:161, 1990.
8. Rady MY: Triage of critically ill patients: an overview of interventions, *Emerg Med Clin North Am* 14:13, 1996.
9. Waikar SS, Chertow GM: Crystalloids versus colloids for resuscitation in shock, *Curr Opin Nephrol Hypertens* 9:501, 2000.
10. Forsythe SM, Schmidt GA: Sodium bicarbonate for the treatment of lactic acidosis, *Chest* 117:260, 2000.
11. Heys SD, Walker LG, Smith I, Eremin O: Enteral nutritional supplementation with key nutrients in patients with critical illness and cancer: a meta-analysis of randomized controlled clinical trials, *Ann Surg* 222:467, 1999.
12. Lancaster LE, Rice V: Nursing care planning: overview and application to the patient in shock, *Crit Care Nurs Clin North Am* 2:279, 1990.
13. Jillings CR: Shock: psychosocial needs of the patient and family, *Crit Care Nurs Clin North Am* 2:325, 1990.
14. Baron BJ, Scalea TM: Acute blood loss, *Emerg Med Clin North Am* 14:35, 1996.
15. Britt LD et al: Priorities in the management of profound shock, *Surg Clin North Am* 76:645, 1996.
16. Blansfield J: Emergency autotransfusion in hypovolemia, *Crit Care Nurs Clin North Am* 2:195, 1990.
17. Hollenberg SM: Cardiogenic shock, *Ann Intern Med* 131:47, 1999.
18. Santoro GM, Buonamici P: Reperfusion therapy in cardiogenic shock complicating acute myocardial infarction, *Am Heart J* 138:126, 1999.
19. Alpert JS, Becker RC: Mechanisms and management of cardiogenic shock, *Crit Care Clin* 9:205, 1993.
20. Zaloga GP et al: Pharmacologic cardiovascular support, *Crit Care Clin* 9:335, 1993.
21. Francis GS: Cardiac complications in the intensive care unit, *Clin Chest Med* 20:269, 1999.
22. Freeman TM: Anaphylaxis: diagnosis and treatment, *Prim Care* 25:809, 1998.
23. Mackan MD: Managing the patient with anaphylaxis. Part 1. Mechanisms and manifestations, *Emerg Med* 27(2):68, 1995.
24. Warshaw EM: Latex allergy, *J Am Acad Dermatol* 39(1):1, 1998.
25. Wai DME: A guide to caring for your latex-allergic patient, *Gastroenterol Nurs* 22:262, 1999.
26. Mackan MD: Managing the patient with anaphylaxis. Part 2. Therapeutic strategies, *Emerg Med* 27(3):20, 1995.
27. Frohna WJ: Emergency department evaluation and treatment of the neck and cervical spine injuries, *Emerg Med Clin North Am* 17:739, 1999.
28. Atkinson PP, Atkinson JLD: Spinal shock, *Mayo Clin Proc* 71:384, 1996.
29. Wagner R, Jagoda A: Spinal cord syndromes, *Emerg Med Clin North Am* 15:699, 1997.
30. Balk RA: Pathogenesis and management of multiple organ dysfunction or failure in severe sepsis and septic shock, *Crit Care Clin* 16:337, 2000.
31. Balk RA: Severe sepsis and septic shock: definitions, epidemiology, and clinical manifestations, *Crit Care Clin* 16:179, 2000.
32. American College of Chest Physicians/Society of Critical Care Medicine Consensus Conference Committee: Definitions for sepsis and organ failure and guidelines for the use of innovative therapies in sepsis, *Crit Care Med* 20:864, 1992.
33. Simon D, Trenholme G: Antibiotic selection for patients with septic shock, *Crit Care Clin* 16:215, 2000.
34. Manders SM: Toxin-mediated streptococcal and staphylococcal disease, *J Am Acad Dermatol* 39:383, 1998.
35. Secor VH: The inflammatory/immune response in critical illness: role of the systemic inflammatory response syndrome, *Crit Care Nurs Clin North Am* 6:251, 1994.
36. Crowley SR: The pathogenesis of septic shock, *Heart Lung* 25:124, 1996.
37. Mizock BA: Metabolic derangements in sepsis and septic shock, *Crit Care Clin* 16:319, 2000.
38. Wiessner WH, Casey LC, Zbilut JP: Treatment of sepsis and septic shock: a review, *Heart Lung* 24:380, 1995.
39. Dellinger RP: Current therapy for sepsis, *Infect Dis Clin North Am* 13:495, 1999.
40. Practice parameters for hemodynamic support of sepsis in adult patients in sepsis, *Crit Care Med* 27:639, 1999.
41. Joyce DE, Grinnell BW: Recombinant human activated protein C attenuates the inflammatory response in endothelium and monocytes by modulating nuclear factor-κB, *Crit Care Clin* 30:S228, 2002.
42. Tasota, FJ, Fisher EM, Coulson CF, Hoffman LA: Protecting ICU patients from nosocomial infections: practical measures for favorable outcomes, *Crit Care Nurse* 18(1):54, 1998.
43. Deitch EA, Goodman ER: Prevention of multiple organ failure, *Surg Clin North Am* 79:1471, 1999.
44. Matuschak GM: Multiple systems organ failure: clinical expression, pathogenesis, and therapy. In Hall JB, Schmidt GA, Wood LD, editors: *Principles of critical care*, ed 2, New York, 1998, McGraw-Hill.
45. Cerra FB: The multiple organ failure syndrome, *Hosp Pract* 25(15):169, 1990.
46. Cerra FB: The syndrome of hypermetabolism and multiple systems organ failure. In Hall JB, Schmidt GA, Wood LD, editors: *Principles of critical care*, ed 2, New York, 1998, McGraw-Hill.
47. Lee et al: A current concept of trauma-induced multiorgan failure, *Ann Emerg Med* 38:170, 2001.
48. Hack CE, Zeerleder S: The endothelium in sepsis: source of and target for inflammation, *Crit Care Med* 29:S21, 2001.
49. Kim PK, Deutschman CS: Inflammatory responses and mediators, *Surg Clin North Am* 80:885, 2000.
50. Ayala A: An immune perspective on selective decontamination of the digestive tract, *Crit Care Med* 30:1397, 2002.
51. Bone RC: Toward a theory regarding the pathogenesis of the systemic inflammatory response syndrome: what we do and do not know about cytokine regulation, *Crit Care Med* 24:163, 1996.

52. Rote NS: Inflammation. In McCance KL, Huether SE, editors: *Pathophysiology: the biologic basis for disease in adults and children,* ed 4, St Louis, 2002, Mosby.

53. Marshall JC: Inflammation, coagulapathy, and the pathogenesis of multiple organ dysfunction syndrome, *Crit Care Med* 29:S99, 2001.

54. Bishop M et al: Prospective trial of supranormal values in severely traumatized patients, *Crit Care Med* 20:S93, 1992 (abstract).

55. Levi M, de Jonge E, van der Poll T: Rationale for restoration of physiological anticoagulant pathways in patients with sepsis and disseminated intravascular coagulation, *Crit Care Med* 29:S90, 2001.

56. Cerra FB: Hypermetabolism–organ failure syndrome: a metabolic response to injury, *Crit Care Clin* 5:289, 1989.

57. Cerra FB: Nutritional pharmacology: its role in the hypermetabolism–organ failure syndrome, *Crit Care Med* 18:S154, 1990.

58. Koch T, Geiger S, Ragaller MJR: Monitoring of organ dysfunction in sepsis/systemic inflammatory response syndrome: novel strategies, *J Am Soc Nephrol* 12(suppl 17):53, 2001.

59. Khadaroo RG: ARDS and the multiple organ dysfunction syndrome: common mechanisms of a common systemic process, *Crit Care Clin* 18:127, 2002.

60. Zimmerman JJ, Ringer TV: Inflammatory host responses in sepsis, *Crit Care Clin* 8:163, 1992.

61. Ratschko M, Fenner T, Lankisch PG: The role of antibiotic prophylaxis in the treatment of acute pancreatitis, *Gastroenterol Clin North Am* 28: 641, 1999.

62. Szabo G: Liver in sepsis and systemic inflammatory response syndrome, *Clin Liver Dis* 6:1045, 2002.

63. Meier-Hellmann A: Therapeutic options for the treatment of impaired gut function, *J Am Soc Nephrol* 12(suppl 17):65, 2001.

64. Haglund UH, Arvidsson D: Acute acalculous cholecystitis. In Marston A et al, editors: *Splanchnic ischemia and multiple organ failure,* St Louis, 1989, Mosby.

65. Murray JF et al: An expanded definition of the adult respiratory distress syndrome, *Am Rev Respir Dis* 138:720, 1988.

66. Abernethy VE, Lieberthal W: Acute renal failure in the critically ill patient, *Crit Care Med* 18:203, 2002.

67. Berstern A, Sibbald WJ: Circulatory disturbances in multiple systems organ failure, *Crit Care Clin* 5:233, 1989.

68. Shoemaker WC, Kram HB, Appel PL: Therapy of shock based on pathophysiology, monitoring, and outcome prediction, *Crit Care Med* 18:S19, 1990.

69. Vincent JL, De Backer D: Initial management of circulatory shock as prevention of MSOF, *Crit Care Clin* 5:369, 1989.

70. Kumar A et al: Tumor necrosis factor produces depression of myocardial cell contraction in vitro, *Crit Care Med* 20:S52, 1992 (abstract).

71. Guyton AC, Hall JE: *Textbook of medical physiology,* ed 10, Philadelphia, 2000, Saunders.

72. Macho JR, Luce JM: Rational approach to the management of multiple systems organ failure, *Crit Care Clin* 5:379, 1989.

73. Sheagren JN: Mechanism-oriented therapy for multiple systems organ failure, *Crit Care Clin* 5:393, 1989.

74. Kern JW, Shoemaker WC: Meta-analysis of hemodynamic optimization in high-risk patients, *Crit Care Med* 30:1686, 2002.

75. Edwards JD: Use of survivors' cardiopulmonary values as therapeutic goals in septic shock, *Crit Care Med* 17:1098, 1989.

76. Fitzsimmons L, Hadley SA: Nutritional management of the metabolically stressed patient, *Crit Care Nurs Q* 17:1, 1994.

77. Daly JM, Lieberman MD, Goldfine L: Enteral nutrition with supplemental arginine, RNA, and omega-3 fatty acids in patients after operation: immunologic, metabolic and clinical outcome, *Surgery* 112:56, 1992.

78. Keithley J, Eisenberg P: The significance of enteral nutrition in the intensive care unit patient, *Crit Care Nurs Clin North Am* 5:23, 1993.

79. Cheever KH: Early enteral feeding of patients with multiple trauma, *Crit Care Nurse* 19:40, 1999.

80. Advisory Committee and HICPAC/SHEA/APIC/IDSA Hand Hygiene Task Force: Recommendations of the Healthcare Infection Control Practices, *MMWR* 51:RR-16, 2002.

UNIT TEN

NURSING MANAGEMENT PLANS OF CARE

evolve Be sure to check out the free exercises on-line at *http://evolve.elsevier.com/Urden/priorities/*

NURSING MANAGEMENT PLAN

Activity Intolerance

Definition: Insufficient physiologic or psychologic energy to endure or complete required or desired daily activities.

Activity Intolerance Related to Cardiopulmonary Dysfunction

Defining Characteristics

- Chest pain with activity
- Electrocardiographic changes with activity
- Heart rate elevations 15 beats/min above baseline with activity for patients receiving β or calcium channel blockers
- Heart rate elevations above baseline 5 minutes after activity
- Breathlessness with activity
- Oxygen saturation (SpO_2) <92% with activity
- Postural hypotension when moving from supine to upright position
- Patient report of fatigue with activity

Outcome Criteria

- Heart rate elevations are less than 20 beats/min above baseline with activity and less than 10 beats/min above baseline with activity for patients receiving β or calcium channel blockers.

- Heart rate returns to baseline 5 minutes after activity.
- Chest pain with activity is absent.
- Patient reports tolerance to activity.

Nursing Interventions and *Rationale*

1. Encourage active or passive range of motion exercises while patient is in bed *to keep joints flexible and muscles stretched*.
2. Teach patient to refrain from holding breath while performing exercises and *to avoid Valsalva maneuver*.
3. Encourage performance of muscle-toning exercises at least 3 times daily, *because a toned muscle uses less oxygen when performing work than an untoned muscle*.
4. Progress ambulation *to increase tolerance to activity*.
5. Teach patient to take pulse *to determine activity tolerance*.
   - Take pulse for full minute *before exercise*, and then for 10 seconds and multiply by 6 *at exercise peak*.

Activity Intolerance Related to Prolonged Immobility or Deconditioning

Defining Characteristics

- Decrease in systolic blood pressure (SBP) greater than 20 mm Hg; heart rate increase greater than 20 beats/min with postural change
- Syncope with postural change
- Patient report of lightheadedness with postural change

Outcome Criteria

- SBP decrease is less than 10 mm Hg; heart rate increase is less than 10 beats/min with postural change.
- Syncope or lightheadedness is absent with postural change.

Nursing Interventions and *Rationale*

1. Instruct patient how to perform straight-leg raises, dorsiflexion/plantar flexion, and quadriceps-/gluteal-setting exercises *to increase muscular and vascular tone*.
2. Consult with physician regarding administration of fluids to ensure that patient is hydrated to 24-hour fluid requirements per body surface area (BSA) *to increase preload and thus stroke volume and cardiac output*.
3. Reposition patient incrementally *to avoid syncope*:
   - Head of bed to 45 degrees, and hold until symptom-free.
   - Head of bed to 90 degrees, and hold until symptom-free.
   - Dangle until symptom-free.
   - Stand until symptom-free, and ambulate.

NURSING MANAGEMENT PLAN

Acute Confusion

Definition: Abrupt onset of a cluster of global, transient changes and disturbances in attention, cognition, psychomotor activity, level of consciousness, and/or sleep/wake cycle.

Acute Confusion Related to Sensory Overload, Sensory Deprivation, and Sleep Pattern Disturbance

Defining Characteristics

Early Symptoms

- Sudden onset of global cognitive function impairment (from hours to days)
- Restlessness, agitation, combative behavior
- Drowsiness (can lead to loss of consciousness)
- Slurred speech, inappropriate statements or "word salad," mumbling, inappropriate gestures

- Short attention span (needs questions repeated); inability to learn new material
- Disordered sleep/wake cycle
- Disorientation to person, time, place, and situation
- Difficulty in separating dreams from reality (may experience bizarre dreams or nightmares)
- Anger at staff for continued questions about patient's orientation

Continued

NURSING MANAGEMENT PLAN

Acute Confusion—cont'd

Later Symptoms

- Symptoms that tend to fluctuate throughout the day and night
- Continuation of early symptoms, which may be more frequent or of longer duration
- Illusions
- Hallucinations
- Extreme agitation (e.g., attempts to climb out of bed, pull out catheters, rip off dressings)
- Calling out in loud voice, swearing, attempting to bite/hit people who approach patient

Nursing Interventions and *Rationale*

1. Determine and document patient's dominant spoken language, literacy, and language(s) in which patient is literate. *People may not be literate in their spoken language, or less often, they are literate only in their second language.*
2. Determine and document patient's premorbid degree of orientation, cognitive capabilities, and sensory-perceptual deficits. *Assuming that patient was or was not fully oriented before critical care admission bases nurse's assessment on possibly erroneous assumptions.*

Sensory Overload

1. Initiate each nurse/patient encounter by calling the patient by name and identifying yourself by name, *to foster reality orientation and assist patient in filtering irrelevant or impersonal conversation.*
2. Assess patient's immediate physical environment from patient's viewpoint; explain equipment, sounds, and therapeutic purpose; demonstrate audible and visual alarms; and explain possible alarm conditions. *This decreases alienation of patient from the technologic environment and to reduce inherent sense of fear and urgency accompanying alarm conditions.*
3. For each procedure performed, provide *preparatory sensory information*, that is, explain procedures in relation to the sensations patient will experience, including duration of sensations, *to enhance learning and to lessen anticipatory anxiety.*
4. Limit noise levels. Audible alarms cannot and must not be silenced, and many critical but noisy activities occur in critical care area. However, noise levels produced by clinical personnel exceed those levels designated as "acceptable" and are often greater than those generated by technologic devices. Staff conversations must be kept soft enough that they are inaudible to patient whenever possible. Critical care personnel should assume that everything said at or around a patient's bedside is intended for that patient's awareness and that it will be interpreted as pertaining to the patient. *Conversations "about" but not "to" the patient foster depersonalization and delusions of reference.*
5. Enforce nighttime noise limits.
6. Readjust alarm limits on physiologic monitoring devices as patient's condition changes (improves or deteriorates) *to lessen unnecessary alarm states.*

7. Consider use of headphones and cassette/CD player with patient's favorite and subliminal/classical music, *to effectively filter out assaultive noise of critical care environment and supplant it with familiar, soothing sounds and rhythms.*
8. Modify lighting. Day/night cycles need to by simulated with environmental lighting. Overhead fluorescent lights should never be turned on abruptly without warning the patient, assisting patient from supine position, or shielding patient's eyes with gauze or face cloth. *Continuous bright lighting sustains anxiety and promotes circadian rhythm desynchronization.*
9. To the extent possible, shield patients from viewing urgent and emergent events in critical care unit. *Resuscitation efforts, although difficult to conceal, engender fear in the patient and a sense of instability and vulnerability (e.g., "I'm next").* When such an event occurs, the nurse needs to elicit the patient's cognitive and emotional reaction. Thoughts, impressions, and feelings need to be shared and misconceptions clarified. A useful approach is to emphasize differences between the patient and the person resuscitated (e.g., "He was considerably older," "She was more unstable," "He had serious lung disease").
10. Ensure patients' privacy, modesty, and (at least) dignity. Physical exposure and nudity, although seemingly less important than such priorities as physiologic assessment and stabilization, are primal indignities in all individuals. Patients must be kept minimally exposed. When it becomes necessary in assessment and intervention to expose patient, the nurse should first verbally apologize for this necessity. *To be naked is to feel vulnerable; to be vulnerable is to feel fearful. In this regard, fear is an emotion concomitant to critical care that is preventable through nursing intervention.*

Sensory Deprivation

1. Provide reality orientation in four spheres (personal, place, time, and situation) at more frequent intervals than when testing. Convey this information in the context of routine conversation. For example, "Mr. Clark, this is Tuesday morning and you're in University Hospital. Your heart surgery was yesterday morning, and you're doing well. My name is Joe, and I'm your nurse today." *The patient is made to feel patronized by repetitions such as, "Do you know where you are?"* Given the effects of general anesthesia, narcotic analgesics, sedatives, and sleep, it is expected that some degree of disorientation will exist normally.
2. Ensure patient's visual access to a calendar. The design of most state-of-the-art critical care units now reflects many principles of sensory stimulation. In one coronary care unit designed with a large wall clock, a patient later reflected that one of the most "distressing, frustrating" aspects of his CCU stay unit was the monotonous, inescapable attention to the clock and its painfully slow documentation of time passing.

NURSING MANAGEMENT PLAN

Acute Confusion—cont'd

3. Apprise patient of daily news events and the weather.
4. Touch patient for the express purpose of communicating caring (hold patient's hand, stroke brow, rub skin on aspect of arm). *Touch is the universal language of caring. In the setting of critical care, in which there is considerable physical body manipulation, it is useful and important to contrast assaultive touch with comforting touch.* Touch can be used as a technique for distraction from painful stimuli when used in conjunction with uncomfortable procedures. (See Hallucinations.)
5. Foster liberal visitation by family and significant others. Encourage significant others to touch patient as consistent with their individual comfort level and cultural norms.
6. Structure and identify opportunities for patient to exercise decision-making skills, however small. *Although not so designated, patients with sensory alterations experience a type of "cognitive deprivation" as well.*
7. Assist patients to find meaning in their experiences. Explain the therapeutic purpose of self-care actions they are asked to perform and interventions by staff. *Statements such as, "Will you turn to that side for me?" or "I need you to swallow this medication," implicitly convey that the maneuver has some value for the nurse versus the patient and should be avoided.*
   - Use "thank you" judiciously. *This simple salutation, when used indiscriminately, suggests something was done to benefit the nurse and not the patient.*
   - Patients need to find meaning and to identify their roles in the experience of critical illness and critical care. The sensations that constitute this experience and those that do not are made bearable and intelligible when attached to a larger picture of their condition, treatment, and progress.

Hallucinations

1. Approach patient with calm, matter-of-fact demeanor. The goal of this interaction is for the nurse to demonstrate external control, *to help decrease the anxiety and fear that generally accompany hallucinations and to allow the patient to feel safe. Anxiety is transferable.*
2. Address patient by name, *to provide a useful presentation of reality because self-identity is the last sphere of orientation to vanish.*
3. In responding to patient's description of the hallucination, do not deny, argue, or attempt to disprove the existence of the perceived event. *Statements such as, "There are no voices coming from that air vent" or "Look, I'm brushing my hand across the wall, and there are no bugs," confuse the patient further because the hallucination, although frightening, is his or her perceived reality.*
4. Express to patient that your experiences are dissimilar, and acknowledge how frightening the patient's must be. For example, "I don't hear (see, etc.) what you do, but I know how frightening such an experience must be to you. I'm Joe, your nurse, and I'm going to stay with you until the voices (etc.) go away." Remain with any patient who is experiencing a hallucination. *Feelings of fear and anxiety often accelerate*

when a patient is left alone. The patient needs someone to represent a nonthreatening reality. In addition, validating the patient's feelings demonstrates acceptance and sensitivity to the experience and promotes trust.

5. Do not explore content of the hallucination with patient by asking about its nature or character. *The nurse is the patient's link with reality. Pursuit of a detailed description of a hallucination may signify to the patient that the nurse accepts the patient's sensory distortion as factual. This may further confuse the patient and distance him or her more from reality.*
   - An exception is the patient suspected of experiencing auditory hallucinations (e.g., hearing "voice commands"). To ascertain that the voices are not urging the patient to self-harm, it is appropriate for the nurse to ask simply and concretely, "What are the voices saying?"
   - The nurse can help bridge the gap between the patient's misperception and reality by addressing the feelings (e.g., fear, anxiety) and meanings (e.g., danger, death) engendered by the hallucination. Determining how the misperception affects the patient emotionally, acknowledging those feelings, and using a calm matter-of-fact approach will provide the trust and comfort the patient needs to tolerate this frightening experience. In other words, deal with the *intent* more than the content of the hallucination. *The resultant decrease in anxiety will enable patient to focus more accurately on the immediate environment.*
6. Talk concretely with patient about actual events. For example, "How does your chest incision feel this afternoon, Mr. Clark?" or "Your sister Kate was here to see you, but you were sleeping. She went down to the cafeteria and will be back." or "Your secretions are a little easier for you to cough up today." *Interpretation of reality-based stimuli by nurse encourages patient to focus on actual circumstances and discourages a preoccupation with sensory misperceptions.*
7. In certain circumstances it is appropriate for the nurse simply to distract the patient by changing the topic. This tactic is useful in situations of escalating anxiety and confusion or "when all else fails." Topics must consist of basic themes that are universally understood and culturally congruent (e.g., music, food, weather). Topics may also be of special interest to the patient (e.g., hobbies, crafts, sports). Topics that evoke strong emotions (e.g., politics, religion, or sexuality) should be avoided with most patients, especially for those with reality distortions. *Hallucinations and delusions can be expressions of repressed conflicts associated with religious, sexual, or aggressive issues. Pursuit of such subjects could increase confusion and anxiety.*
8. Consider the following regarding the use of touch. Touch presents a nonthreatening external reality and can therefore be useful in the management of patients with sensory alterations. However, for the patient experiencing hallucinations (as well as delusions and illusions), touch can be readily misinterpreted as, for instance, aggression or pain, or it can actually provide the basis for a tactile illusion.

Continued

NURSING MANAGEMENT PLAN

Acute Confusion—cont'd

Therefore avoid the use of touch as an intervention strategy for any patient who demonstrates escalating anxiety or paranoid, suspicious, or mistrustful thoughts.

9. **Auditory hallucinations**
   - *Patient behaviors*: Head cocked as if listening to an unseen presence; lips moving.
   - *Therapeutic nurse responses*
     — Mr. Clark, you appear to be listening to something.
     — *If patient acknowledges voices*: I don't hear any voices, but I know this is troubling you. The voices will go away. Nothing is going to harm you. I'm Joe, your nurse, and I'll be here with you.
   - *Nontherapeutic nurse responses*
     — Tell me about your conversations with these voices.
     — To whom do these voices belong—anyone you know?
10. **Visual hallucinations**
    - *Patient behaviors*: Staring into space as if focused on an unseen object; startled movements and anxious facial expression.
    - *Therapeutic nurse responses*
      — Mr. Clark, something seems to be troubling you. Tell me what it is.
      — *If patient states he visualizes people, images, or the devil in his environment and implies a sense of danger*: There are only nurses and doctors here, Mr. Clark. I know this must be upsetting, but these images will go away. We're here with you in the hospital. Nothing will happen to you.
    - *Nontherapeutic nurse responses*
      — Describe the people you see. What are they wearing?
      — What does the devil mean in your life? What about God?

Delusions

1. Explain all unseen noises, voices, and activity simply and clearly, **because they readily feed a delusional system**. For example, "That is Dr. Smith; he's come to see you and other patients here in the hospital;" or "The voices and activity you hear are from the bedside of the patient behind this curtain. He's being helped by one of the nurses."
2. Avoid the *negative challenge* (e.g., "Nobody here stole your belongings," "Doctors and nurses do not harm people") of patient's delusions. Similarly, avoid defending the referents of patient's belief (e.g., "Nurses are good," "Doctors mean well"). **Remember, a delusion is a belief, although false, that cannot be changed with logic. To attempt this change is to challenge the patient's belief system and thereby escalate his or her anxiety, further blurring the boundaries between reality and the patient's internally based "logic."**
3. For the patient with persecutory delusions who refuses food, fluids, or medications because of a belief that they have been poisoned or are tainted, permit the refusal unless it is a life-threatening event. Try again in 20 minutes; allow patient to choose an alternative selection of food or to read the label on the unit's medication. Coercion, show of force, or engagement in complicated, logical justifications will only heighten the patient's suspiciousness and possibly reinforce the delusional belief. **When the patient feels more in control, he or she need not rely on the "paradoxical" quality of the delusion to equip him or her with a false sense of power. The patient's power instead is derived from making reality-based decisions**.
4. Staff members should be particularly careful not to engage in unnecessary laughter or whispering within view of the delusional patient. **The delusional patient is hypervigilant, scanning the environment for evidence to corroborate or confirm the belief that staff members are colluding against the patient; laughter and whispers readily suggest this belief, this** *delusion of reference*. **This rationale pertains to patients experiencing hallucinations and illusions as well**.
5. See Hallucinations; refer to principles detailed in third intervention.

Illusions

1. As in the management of delusions, the nurse simply and briefly interprets a reality-based stimulus for the patient in a calm matter-of-fact manner. **Seen and unseen noises, voices, activity, and people can provide the stimulus for a sensory misinterpretation, an** *illusion*.
2. Minimal stimulation should occur in patient's immediate environment. (See Sensory Overload.)
3. Theme of nurse's verbal approach to patient experiencing illusions is similar to that outlined for hallucinations and delusions: address the feeling and *meaning* associated with the experience, not the content of the sensory misinterpretation.
   - *Patient behaviors/response*: Eyes darting, startled movements, frightened facial expression.
     — I know who you are. You're the devil come to take me to hell.
   - *Therapeutic nurse response*
     — I'm Joe, your nurse. I know this experience is troubling for you. You're in the hospital, and no one here will harm you.
   - *Nontherapeutic nurse responses*
     — There are no such things as devils and angels. **Has "parental" tone ("You know better than that"), thus infantilizing the patient and adding to feelings of powerlessness over the environment**.
     — Do you think the devil would be dressed in white? **Reflects obvious logic, which is not in the patient's sensory domain; therefore it cannot be processed and only adds to patient's confused state**.
4. See Hallucinations; refer to principles detailed in fifth intervention.

NURSING MANAGEMENT PLAN

Acute Pain

Definition: Unpleasant sensory and emotional experience arising from actual or potential tissue damage or described in terms of such damage (International Association for the Study of Pain); sudden or slow onset of any intensity from mild to severe with an anticipated or predictable end and a duration of less than 6 months.

Acute Pain Related to Transmission of Perception of Cutaneous, Visceral, Muscular, or Ischemic Impulses

Defining Characteristics

Subjective

- Patient verbalizes presence of pain.
- Patient rates pain on scale of 1 to 10 using visual analog scale.

Objective

- Increase in blood pressure (BP), heart rate (HR), and respiratory rate (RR)
- Pupillary dilation
- Diaphoresis, pallor
- Skeletal muscle reactions (grimacing, clenching fists, writhing, pacing, guarding or splinting of affected part)
- Apprehension, fearful appearance
- May not exhibit any physiologic change

Outcome Criteria

Outcome is highly variable, depending on individual patient and pain circumstance factors.

- Patient verbalizes that pain is reduced to a tolerable level or is totally relieved.
- Patient's pain rating is lower on scale of 1 to 10.
- BP, HR, and RR return to baseline 5 minutes after administration of intravenous (IV) narcotic or 20 minutes after administration of intramuscular (IM) narcotic.

Nursing Interventions and *Rationale*

Modification of Variables that Exacerbate Pain Experience

1. Explain to patient that frequent, detailed, and seemingly repetitive assessments will be conducted *to allow nurse to better understand patient's pain experience, not because existence of pain is in question.*
2. Explain factors responsible for pain. Estimate expected duration of pain if possible.
3. Explain diagnostic and therapeutic procedures to patient in relation to sensations that patient should expect to feel.
4. Reduce patient's fear of addiction by explaining difference between drug tolerance and drug addiction. *Drug tolerance* is a physiologic phenomenon in which a drug does begins to lose effectiveness after repeated doses; *drug dependence* is a psychologic phenomenon in which narcotics are used regularly for emotional, not medical, reasons.
5. Instruct patient to ask for pain medication when pain is beginning and not to wait until pain is intolerable.
6. Explain that physician will be consulted if pain relief is inadequate with the present medication.
7. Instruct patient in the importance of adequate rest, especially when rest reduces pain, *to maintain strength and coping abilities and to reduce stress.*

Pharmacologic Interventions (in Collaboration with Physician)

Postsurgical/Posttraumatic Cutaneous/Muscular/Visceral Pain

1. Medicate with narcotic maximally to break the pain cycles as long as level of consciousness and vital signs are stable. Check patient's previous response to similar dosage and narcotic. First dose received postoperatively is usually reduced by one-half *to evaluate patient's individual response to medication*.
2. Provide continuous analgesia, as required by continuous pain.
   - Establish optimal analgesic dose that brings optimal pain relief.
   - Offer pain medication at prescribed, regular intervals rather than making patient ask, *to maintain more steady blood levels*.
   - Consider waking patient to avoid loss of opiate blood levels during sleep.
3. If administering medication on as-needed (prn) basis, give drug when patient's pain is beginning rather than at its peak. Advise patient to intercept pain, not endure it, or several hours and higher doses of narcotics may be necessary to relieve pain, leading to a cycle of undermedication and pain alternating with overmedication and drug toxicity.
4. Perform rehabilitation exercises (turning, deep breathing, leg exercises, ambulating) shortly before peak of drug effect *because this is optimal time for patient to increase activity with least risk of increasing pain*.
5. When making the transition from one drug to another or from IM or IV to PO medication, use of an equianalgesic chart is helpful. *Equianalgesic* means *approximately* the same pain relief. Many consider the IM and IV dose of medications equianalgesic; however, others recommend using one-half the IM dose for the IV dose. To use analgesics effectively, each patient requires an individual choice of drug, dose, time interval, and route. The patient's response should be closely monitored to determine if the right analgesic choice was made.
6. Assess effectiveness of pain medication.
   - Reevaluate pain 5 minutes after IV and 20 minutes after IM administration; observe patient's behavior; and ask patient to rate pain on scale of 1 to 10.
   - Collaborate with physician to add or delete other medications that potentiate the action of analgesics (e.g., antiemetics, hypnotics, sedatives, muscle relaxants).
   - Observe for indicators of undertreatment (report of pain not relieved; observed restlessness, sleeplessness, irritability, or anorexia; decreased activity level).
   - Observe for indicators of overtreatment (hypotension or bradycardia; RR <10/min; excessive sedation).

Continued

NURSING MANAGEMENT PLAN

Acute Pain—cont'd

Patient-Controlled Analgesia (PCA)

NOTE: PCA allows patients to administer small doses of prescribed medication when they feel the need. Constant levels of the drug in bloodstream mean lower doses can be used to obtain analgesia. Pain control is improved because patient is in control and experiences less fear of unrelieved pain, resulting in reduced net narcotic use and less sedation. Appropriate critical care candidates for PCA are patients who are alert (e.g., burns, trauma without head injury) and some postoperative patients.

1. Instruct patient on what the drug is, the dose, and how often it can be self-administered by pushing button to activate PCA machine.

THERAPEUTIC EXAMPLE: "When you have pain, instead of asking the nurse to bring medication, push the button that activates the machine, and a small dose of the pain medicine will be injected into your IV line. You can keep your pain under control by administering additional medicine as soon as your pain begins to return or increases. Also, push the button before undertaking a painful activity, such as walking. Try to balance your pain relief against sleepiness, and don't activate the machine if you start to feel sleepy. If your pain medicine seems to stop working even when you push the button several times, call the nurse to check your IV. If you're not receiving adequate pain relief, the nurse will call your doctor."

2. Monitor vital signs, especially BP and RR, every hour for the first 4 hours, and assess postural HR and BP before initial ambulation.
3. Monitor respirations every 2 hours while patient is receiving PCA.
4. If patient's respirations decrease to less than 10 per minute or if patient is oversedated, anticipate IV administration of naloxone.

Epidural Narcotic Analgesia

NOTE: Delivery of narcotics, such as morphine or fentanyl, by epidural route to specific receptors in spinal cord selectively blocks pain impulses to brain for up to 24 hours. Effective analgesia can be obtained without many of the negative side effects or serum narcotic concentrations.

1. Keep patient's head elevated 30 to 45 degrees after injection *to prevent respiratory depressant effects*.
2. Observe closely for respiratory depression up to 24 hours after injection. Monitor RR every 15 minutes for 1 hour, every 30 minutes for 7 hours, and every hour for the remaining 16 hours.
3. Assess for adequate cough reflex.
4. Avoid used of other central nervous system (CNS) depressants, such as sedatives.
5. Observe for reports of pruritus, nausea, or vomiting.
6. Anticipate administration of naloxone for respiratory depression (and smaller doses of naloxone for pruritus).
7. Assess for and treat urinary retention.

8. Assess epidural catheter site for local infection. Keep catheter taped securely *to prevent catheter migration*.

Peripheral Vascular Ischemic Pain (Hypothetic Vascular Occlusion of Leg)

1. Correctly identify and differentiate ischemic pain from other types of pain.

NOTE: Ischemic pain is usually a burning, aching pain made worse by exercise and lessened or relieved by rest. Eventually the pain occurs at rest. Coldness and pallor of extremity may be noted, especially if the limb is elevated above the heart level. Rubor and mottling of the skin may be evident from prolonged tissue anoxia and inability of damaged vessels to constrict. Eventually, cyanosis and gangrenous tissue are evident. Chronic ischemia leads to visible changes in the limb, such as flaking skin, brittle nails and hair, leg ulcers, and cellulitis.

2. Administer pain medications, and evaluate their effectiveness as previously described. Remember that the pain of ischemia is chronic and continuous and can make the patient irritable and depressed.
3. Treat the cause of the ischemic pain, and institute measures to increase circulation to the affected part.

Nonpharmacologic Interventions

1. Treat contributing factors.
2. Provide explanation for interventions (see Pharmacologic Interventions).
3. Apply comfort measures.
   - Use relaxation techniques, such as back rubs, massage, warm baths, music and aroma therapy. Use blankets and pillows *to support the painful part and reduce muscle tension*. Encourage slow, rhythmic breathing.
   - Encourage progressive muscle relaxation techniques.
     — Instruct patient to inhale and tense (tighten) specific muscle groups and then relax the muscles as exhalation occurs.
     — Suggest an order for performing tension/relaxation cycle (e.g., start with facial muscles and move down body, ending with toes).
   - Encourage guided imagery.
     (1) Ask patient to recall an experienced image that is very pleasurable and relaxing and involves at least two senses.
     (2) Have patient begin with rhythmic breathing and progressive relaxation and then travel mentally to the scene.
     (3) Have patient slowly experience the scene (how it looks, sounds, smells, feels).
     (4) Ask patient to practice this imagery in private.
     (5) Instruct patient to end the imagery by counting to 3 and saying, "Now I'm relaxed." If patient does not end imagery and falls asleep, purpose of technique is defeated.

NURSING MANAGEMENT PLAN

Anxiety

Definition: Vague uneasy feeling of discomfort or dread accompanied by an autonomic response (the source often nonspecific or unknown to the individual); a feeling of apprehension caused by anticipation of danger. It is an alerting signal that warns of impending danger and enables the individual to take measures to deal with threat.

Anxiety Related to Threat to Biologic, Psychologic, and/or Social Integrity

Defining Characteristics

Subjective

- Verbalizes increased muscle tension
- Expresses frequent sensation of tingling in hands and feet
- Relates continuous feeling of apprehension
- Expresses preoccupation with sense of "impending doom"
- States has difficulty falling asleep
- Repeatedly expresses concerns about changes in health status and outcome of illness

Objective

- Psychomotor agitation (fidgeting, jitteriness, restlessness)
- Tightened, wrinkled brow
- Strained (worried) facial expression
- Hypervigilance (scans environment)
- Startles easily
- Distractibility
- Sweaty palms
- Fragmented sleep patterns
- Tachycardia
- Tachypnea

Outcome Criteria

- Patient effectively uses learned relaxation strategies.
- Patient demonstrates significant decrease in psychomotor agitation.
- Patient verbalizes reduction in tingling sensations in hands and feet.
- Patient is able to focus on the tasks at hand.
- Patient expresses positive, futuristic plans to family and staff.
- Patient's heart rate and rhythm remain within limits commensurate with physiologic status.

Nursing Interventions and *Rationale*

1. Instruct patient in simple, effective relaxation strategies.
   - If not contraindicated for cardiovascular reasons, tense and relax all muscles progressively from toes to head. *Releases muscular tension that may be a stress-related effect resulting from threat or change in patient's health status and outcome of illness.*
   - Perform slow deep-breathing exercises. *Provides slow, rhythmic, controlled breathing patterns that relax patient and distract patient from effects of illness and hospitalization.*
   - Focus on a single object or person in environment. *Helps patient dismiss disorienting stimuli from visual-perceptual field, which can have dizzying, distorted effect. A clear sensorium allows patient to feel more in control of environment.*
   - Listen to soothing music or relaxation tapes (in soft, low tones) with eyes closed. *Produces soothing, relaxing effects that counteract or inhibit escalating anxiety, and provides respites from patient's situational crisis. Closed eyes eliminate distracting visual stimuli and promote more restful environment.*
2. Actively listen to and accept patient's concerns regarding threats from illness, outcome, and hospitalization. *Validates patient as worthwhile individual and assures patient that concerns, no matter how great, will be addressed. Knowledge that patient has avenue for ventilation assuages anxiety.*
3. Help patient distinguish between realistic concerns and exaggerated fears through clear, simple explanations. For example, "Your lab results show that you're doing OK right now," or "The shortness of breath you're experiencing is not unusual," or "The pain you described is expected, and this medication will relieve it." *A patient who is informed about his or her progress and is reassured about expected symptoms and management of care will be better equipped to maintain a more realistic perspective of the illness and its outcome. Thus anxiety emanating from imagined or exaggerated fears will likely be assuaged or averted.*
4. Provide simple clarification of environmental events and stimuli that are not related to the patient's illness and care. For example, "That loud noise is coming from a machine that is helping another patient," or "The visitor behind the curtain is crying because she's had an upsetting day," or "That gurney is here to take another patient to x-ray." *Clarification of events and stimuli that are unrelated to patient helps to disengage patient from anxiety-provoking situations, thus avoiding further anxiety and apprehension.*
5. Assist patient in focusing on building on prior coping strategies to deal with the effects of the illness and care. For example, "What methods have helped you get through difficult times in the past?" or "How can we help you use those methods now?" (See Nursing Management Plan for Ineffective Coping.) *Use of previously successful coping strategies in conjunction with newly learned techniques fortifies patient against anxiety, providing patient with greater control over the situational crisis and decreased feelings of doom and despair.*
6. Give patient permission to deny or suppress effects of the illness and hospitalization that patient cannot cope with or control. For example, "It's perfectly okay to ignore things you can't handle right now," or "How can we help ease your mind during this time?" or "What are some things or tasks that may help distract you?" *Adaptive denial can be helpful in reducing feelings of anxiety in patients with life-threatening illness.*

NURSING MANAGEMENT PLAN

Autonomic Dysreflexia

Definition: Life-threatening, uninhibited sympathetic response of nervous system to noxious stimulus after spinal cord injury at seventh thoracic vertebra (T7) or above.

Autonomic Dysreflexia Related to Excessive Autonomic Response to Noxious Stimuli (e.g., Distended Bladder, Distended Bowel, Skin Irritation)

Defining Characteristics

Major

- Paroxysmal hypertension (sudden periodic elevated blood pressure [BP] greater than 20 mm Hg above patient's normal BP; for many spinal cord injury patients, a normal BP may be only 90/60 mm Hg)
- Bradycardia (most common; pulse <60 beats/min) or tachycardia (>100 beats/min)
- Diaphoresis (above the injury)
- Facial flushing
- Pallor (below the injury)
- Pounding headache (diffuse pain in different portions of head and not confined to any nerve distribution area)

Minor

- Nasal congestion
- Engorgement of temporal and neck vessels
- Conjunctival congestion
- Chills without fever
- Pilomotor erection (goose bumps) below the injury
- Blurred vision
- Chest pain
- Metallic taste in mouth
- Horner syndrome (constriction of pupil, partial ptosis of eyelid, enophthalmos, and sometimes loss of sweating over affected side of face)

Outcome Criteria

- BP has returned to patient's norm.
- Pulse rate is greater than 60 or less than 100 beats/min (or within patient's norm).
- Headache is absent.
- Nasal stuffiness, sweating, and flushing above level of injury are absent.
- Chills, goose bumps, and pallor below level of injury are absent.
- Patient verbalizes causes, prevention, symptoms, and treatment of condition.

Nursing Interventions and *Rationale*

1. Place the patient on cardiac monitor, and assess for bradycardia, tachycardia, or other dysrhythmias. Disturbances of cardiac rate and rhythm can occur because of autonomic dysfunction associated with dysreflexia.
2. Do not leave the patient alone. One nurse monitors BP and patient status every 3 to 5 minutes while another provides treatment.
3. Place head of bed to upright position to decrease BP and promote cerebral venous return.
4. Remove any support stockings or abdominal binder to reduce venous return.
5. Investigate for and remove offending cause of dysreflexia:
   Bladder
   - If indwelling cather not in place, catheterize patient immediately.
     (1) Lubricate catheter with lidocaine jelly before insertion.
     (2) Drain 500 ml of urine, and recheck BP.
     (3) If BP still elevated, drain another 500 ml of urine.
     (4) If BP declines after the bladder is empty, serial BP must be monitored closely *because the bladder can go into severe contractions, causing hypertension to recur*.
     (5) Collaborate with physician regarding the instillation of 30 ml tetracaine through the catheter *to decrease the flow of impulses from the bladder*.
   - If indwelling catheter is in place, check for kinks or granular sediment, which may indicate occlusion.
     — If plugged, irrigate catheter gently with no more than 30 ml of sterile normal saline. If bladder is in tetany, fluid will go in but will not drain out. Atropine may be administered *to relieve bladder tetany*.
     — If unable to irrigate catheter, remove it and prepare to reinsert a new catheter; proceed with its lubrication, drainage, and observation as outlined above.
   Bowel
   - Using glove lubricated with anesthetic ointment, check rectum for fecal impaction.
   - If impaction is felt, *to decrease flow of impulses from bowel*, insert anesthetic ointment into rectum 10 minutes before manual removal of impaction.
   - A low hypertonic enema or a suppository may be given to assist bowel evacuation.
   Skin
   - Loosen clothing or bed linens as indicated.
   - Inspect skin for pimples, boils, pressure sores, and ingrown toenails, and treat as indicated.
6. If symptoms of dysreflexia do not subside, have available the intravenous (IV) solutions and antihypertensive drugs of physician's choosing (e.g., hydralazine, nifedipine, phentolamine, diazoxide, sodium nitroprusside). Administer medications, and monitor their effectiveness. Assess BP and pulse.
7. Instruct patient about causes, symptoms, treatment, and prevention of dysreflexia.
8. Encourage patient to carry medical bracelet or informational card to present to medical personnel in the event dysreflexia may be developing.

NURSING MANAGEMENT PLAN

Compromised Family Coping

Definition: Usually supportive primary person (family member or close friend) provides insufficient, ineffective, or compromised support, comfort, assistance, or encouragement that may be needed by the client to manage or master adaptive tasks related to his/her health challenge.

Compromised Family Coping Related to Critically Ill Family Member

Defining Characteristics

- Disruption of usual family functions and roles
- Inability to accept or deal with crisis situation; use of defense mechanisms (e.g., denial, anger); unrealistic expectations of patient's outcome and care provided; judgmental toward health care providers
- Nonrecognition that family is in state of crisis
- Inappropriate emotional outbursts; arguments among family and with others; inability to respond to each other's feelings or support each other
- Misinterpretation of information; short attention span with repeated questions about information already provided; members not sharing information with each other
- Inability to make decisions regarding changes in family structure or about course of care for ill member; noncooperation among family members
- Expressions of grief, hopelessness, powerlessness, and isolation; do not seek or respond to support services
- Hesitancy to spend time with ill person in the critical care unit, or inappropriate behavior when visiting (may upset patient)
- Neglect of own personal health; fatigue, apathy; refusal of offers for respite time

Outcome Criteria

- The family will express an understanding of course/prognosis of illness, therapies, and alternative measures.
- The family will diminish or resolve conflicts and cooperate in decision making.
- The family will develop trust and mutual support for each member and form a cohesive unit.
- The family will support ill person in making decisions (if capable) or respect prior wishes regarding provision of health care.
- Family efforts will be directed toward a purpose and readjust to changes in life patterns and role function. Members will accept responsibility for changes.
- The family will identify and use effective coping strategies.
- The family will identify and use available resources as needed to facilitate resolution of the crisis.
- The family will have a sense of control and confidence in meeting personal and collective needs.

Nursing Interventions and *Rationale*

1. Identify family's perception of crisis situation. Determine family structure, role developmental phase, and ethnic, cultural, and belief factors that may affect communication with family and the plan of care. Identify strengths of family. *All initial nursing interventions should be directed toward resolving the crisis situation. Understanding and using family theory principles will facilitate this process and individualize care.*

2. Provide honest and accurate information in language persons can understand. Give updated information as appropriate. Listen! *Facilitates open communication among family and health care providers, projects a caring attitude and concern for them and patient, and assists family in making decision and being involved with the plan and goals of care.*

3. Encourage liberal visitation with patient. Before the visit, prepare family for what they will observe in a technical environment. Inform them about patient's appearance and behaviors that may be distressing to them. Explain etiology of patient responses to stimuli (pain, trauma, surgery, medication), and explain that these behaviors are being monitored and are usually temporary. Encourage them to touch the patient and let the patient know of their presence. *Prevents a strong emotional reaction to an unfamiliar and frightening situation, involves family as support to each other and to the patient, demonstrates the nurse's concern for them as persons, and facilitates satisfaction with care being provided for their loved one.*

4. Identify and support effective coping behaviors, *to aid in the family's sense of control and resolution of helplessness/powerlessness.*

5. Observe for signs of fatigue and need for emotional/spiritual support and respite from hospital waiting routine. Encourage family to verbalize feelings. Provide information on available resources. Alert interdisciplinary team members (social, psychologic, spiritual) to family needs. Provide pager device (if available), or obtain phone numbers when family leaves the hospital premises. *Provides support and comfort, facilitates hope, resolves sense of isolation, provides a sense of security, and diminishes guilt feelings for attending to personal needs.*

6. Instruct family in simple care-giving techniques, and encourage participation in patient's care, *to facilitate a sense of "normalcy" to experience, self-confidence, and assurance that good care is being provided.*

7. Serve as advocate for patient and family. Teach family how to negotiate with the health care delivery system, and include them in health care team conferences when appropriate, *to facilitate informed decision making, promote control and satisfaction, and encourage mutual goal setting.*

8. Consider nonbiologic or nonlegal family relationships. Encourage contact with patient and participation in care, *to facilitate holistic care and support of emotional ties and to demonstrate respect for the family unit and relationships.*

9. Provide emotional support and compassion when patient's condition worsens or deteriorates. *Use of touch and expression of concern for the patient and family convey comfort and trust in the health care provider, respect, and assurance that the family's loved one will receive appropriate care and attention.*

NURSING MANAGEMENT PLAN

Decreased Cardiac Output

Definition: Inadequate blood pumped by heart to meet metabolic demands of the body.

Decreased Cardiac Output Related to Alterations in Preload

Defining Characteristics

- Cardiac output (CO) <4.0 L/min
- Cardiac index (CI) <2.5 L/min/m^2
- Heart rate (HR) >100 beats/min
- Urine output <30 ml/hr or 0.5 ml/kg/hr
- Decreased mentation, restlessness, agitation, confusion
- Diminished peripheral pulses
- Blue, gray, or dark-purple tint to tongue and sublingual area
- Systolic blood pressure (BP) <90 mm Hg
- Subjective complaints of fatigue

Reduced Preload

- Right atrial pressure (RAP) <2 mm Hg
- Pulmonary artery occlusion pressure (PAOP) <5 mm Hg

Excessive Preload

- RAP >6 mm Hg
- PAOP >12 mm Hg

Outcome Criteria

- CO 4.0-8.0 L/min
- CI 2.5-4.0 L/min/m^2
- RAP 2-8 mm Hg
- PAOP 5-12 mm Hg

Nursing Interventions and *Rationale*

1. Collaborate with physician regarding administration of oxygen to maintain oxygen saturation (SpO$_2$) greater than 92% *to prevent tissue hypoxia*.
2. Maintain surveillance for signs of decreased tissue perfusion and acidosis *to facilitate early identification and treatment of complications*.
3. Monitor fluid balance and daily weights *to facilitate regulation of patient's fluid balance*.

Reduced Preload Secondary to Volume Loss

1. Collaborate with physician regarding the administration of crystalloids, colloids, blood, and blood products *to increase circulating volume*.
2. Limit blood sampling, observe intravenous (IV) lines for accidental disconnection, apply direct pressure to bleeding sites, and maintain normal body temperature *to minimize fluid loss*.

3. Position patient with legs elevated, trunk flat, and head and shoulders above the chest *to enhance venous return*.
4. Encourage oral fluids (as appropriate), administer free water with tube feedings, and replace fluids that are lost through wound or tube drainage *to promote adequate fluid intake*.
5. Maintain surveillance for signs of fluid volume excess and adverse effects of blood and blood product administration *to facilitate the early identification and treatment of complications*.

Reduced Preload Secondary to Venous Dilation

1. Collaborate with physician regarding administration of vasocontrictors *to increase venous return*.
2. Maintain surveillance for adverse effects of vasoconstrictor therapy *to facilitate early identification and treatment of complications*.
3. If patient is hyperthermic, administer tepid bath, hypothermia blanket, and/or ice bags to axilla and groin *to decrease temperature and promote vasoconstriction*.

Excessive Preload Secondary to Volume Overload

1. Collaborate with physician regarding the administration of drugs.
   - Diuretics *to remove excessive fluid*.
   - Vasodilators *to decrease venous return*.
   - Inotropes *to increase myocardial contractility*.
2. Restrict fluid intake and double concentrate IV drips *to minimize fluid intake*.
3. Position patient in semi-Fowler's or high-Fowler's position *to reduce venous return*.
4. Maintain surveillance for signs of fluid volume deficit and adverse effects of diuretic, vasodilator, and inotropic therapies *to facilitate early identification and treatment of complications*.

Excessive Preload Secondary to Venous Constriction

1. Collaborate with physician regarding the administration of vasodilators *to promote venous dilation*.
2. Maintain surveillance for adverse effects of vasodilator therapy *to facilitate early identification and treatment of complications*.
3. If patient is hypothermic, wrap in warm blankets or administer hyperthermia blanket *to increase temperature and promote vasodilation*.

Decreased Cardiac Output Related to Alterations in Afterload

Definining Characteristics

- CO <4.0 L/min
- CI <2.5 L/min/m^2
- HR >100 beats/min
- Urine output <30 ml/hr

- Decreased mentation, restlessness, agitation, confusion
- Diminished peripheral pulses
- Blue, gray, or dark-purple tint to tongue and sublingual area
- Systolic BP <90 mm Hg
- Subjective complaints of fatigue

NURSING MANAGEMENT PLAN

Decreased Cardiac Output—cont'd

Reduced Afterload

- Pulmonary vascular resistance (PVR) <100 dynes/sec/cm^{-5}
- Systemic vascular resistance (SVR) <800 dynes/sec/cm^{-5}

Excessive Afterload

- PVR >250 dynes/sec/cm^{-5}
- SVR >1200 dynes/sec/cm^{-5}

Outcome Criteria

- CO 4.0-8.0 L/min
- CI 2.5-4.0 L/min/m^2
- PVR 80-250 dynes/sec/cm^{-5}
- SVR 800-1200 dynes/sec/cm^{-5}

Nursing Interventions and _Rationale_

1. Collaborate with physician regarding administration of oxygen to maintain SpO$_2$ greater than 92% _to prevent tissue hypoxia_.
2. Maintain surveillance for signs of decreased tissue perfusion and acidosis _to facilitate early identification and treatment of complications_.

For Reduced Afterload

1. Collaborate with physician regarding administration of vasocontrictors _to promote arterial vasoconstriction and prevent relative hypovolemia_. If decreased preload is present, implement plan for Decreased Cardiac Output Related to Alterations in Preload.
2. Maintain surveillance for adverse effects of vasoconstrictor therapy _to facilitate early identification and treatment of complications_.
3. If patient is hyperthermic, administer tepid bath, hypothermia blanket, and/or ice bags to axilla and groin _to decrease temperature and promote vasoconstriction_.

For Excessive Afterload

1. Collaborate with physician regarding administration of vasodilators _to promote arterial vasodilation_.
2. Collaborate with physician regarding initiation of intraaortic balloon pump (IABP) _to facilitate afterload reduction_.
3. Promote rest and relaxation and decrease environmental stimulation _to minimize sympathetic stimulation_.
4. Maintain surveillance for adverse effects of vasodilator therapy _to facilitate early identification and treatment of complications_.
5. If patient is hypothermic, wrap in warm blankets or administer hyperthermia blanket _to increase temperature and promote vasodilation_.
6. If patient is in pain, treat pain _to reduce sympathetic stimulation_. Implement plan for Acute Pain Related to Transmission and Perception of Cutaneous, Visceral, Muscular, or Ischemic Impulses.

Decreased Cardiac Output Related to Alterations in Contractility

Defining Characteristics

- CO <4.0 L/min
- CI <2.5 L/min/m^2
- HR >100 beats/min
- Urine output <30 ml/hr
- Decreased mentation, restlessness, agitation, confusion
- Diminished peripheral pulses
- Blue, gray, or dark-purple tint to tongue and sublingual area
- Systolic BP <90 mm Hg
- Subjective complaints of fatigue
- Right ventricular stroke work index (RVSWI) <7 g/m^2/beat
- Left ventricular stroke work index (LVSWI) <35 g/m^2/beat

Outcome Criteria

- CO 4.0-8.0 L/min
- CI 2.5-4.0 L/min/m^2
- RVSWI 7-12 g/m^2/beat
- LVSWI 35-85 g/m^2/beat

Nursing Interventions and _Rationale_

1. Collaborate with physician regarding administration of oxygen to maintain SpO$_2$ greater than 92% _to prevent tissue hypoxia_.
2. Maintain surveillance for signs of decreased tissue perfusion and acidosis _to facilitate early identification and treatment of complications_.
3. Ensure preload is optimized. If preload is reduced or excessive, implement plan for Decreased Cardiac Output Related to Alterations in Preload.
4. Ensure afterload is optimized. If afterload is reduced or excessive, implement plan for Decreased Cardiac Output Related to Alterations in Afterload.
5. Ensure electrolytes are optimized. Collaborate with physician regarding administration of electrolyte replacement therapy _to enhance cellular ionic environment_.
6. Collaborate with physician regarding the administration of inotropes _to enhance myocardial contractility_.
7. If myocardial ischemia present, implement plan for Altered Cardiopulmonary Tissue Perfusion.

Decreased Cardiac Output Related to Alterations in Heart Rate or Rhythm

Defining Characteristics

- CO <4.0 L/min
- CI <2.5 L/min/m^2
- HR >100 beats/min

- Urine output <30 ml/hr or 0.5 ml/kg/hr
- Decreased mentation, restlessness, agitation, confusion
- Diminished peripheral pulses
- Blue, gray, or dark-purple tint to tongue and sublingual area

Continued

NURSING MANAGEMENT PLAN

Decreased Cardiac Output—cont'd

- Systolic BP <90 mm Hg
- Subjective complaints of fatigue; HR <60 beats/min
- Dysrhythmias

Outcome Criteria

- CO 4.0-8.0 L/min
- CI 2.5-4.0 L/min/m²
- Absence of dysrhythmias or return to baseline
- HR >60 beats/min

Nursing Interventions and *Rationale*

1. Collaborate with physician regarding administration of oxygen to maintain SpO₂ greater than 92% *to prevent tissue hypoxia*.
2. Ensure electrolytes are optimized. Collaborate with physician regarding administration of electrolyte therapy *to enhance cellular ionic environment and avoid precipitation of dysrhythmias*.
3. Collaborate with physician and pharmacist regarding patient's current medications and effect on heart rate and rhythm *to identify any prodysrhythmic or bradycardiac side effects*.
4. Maintain surveillance for signs of decreased tissue perfusion and acidosis *to facilitate early identification and treatment of complications*.

5. Monitor ST segment continuously *to determine changes in myocardial tissue perfusion*. If myocardial ischemia is present, implement plan for Altered Cardiopulmonary Tissue Perfusion.

For Lethal Dysrhythmias or Asystole

1. Initiate advanced cardiac life support (ACLS) interventions.
2. Notify physician immediately.

For Nonlethal Dysrhythmias

1. Collaborate with physician regarding administration of antidysrhythmic therapy, synchronized cardioversion, and overdrive pacing *to control dysrhythmias*.
2. Maintain surveillance for adverse effects of antidysrhythmic therapy *to facilitate early identification and treatment of complications*.

For Heart Rate less than 60 beats/min

Collaborate with physician on initiation of temporary pacing *to increase heart rate*.

Decreased Cardiac Output Related to Sympathetic Blockade

Defining Characteristics

- Decreased CO and CI
- Systolic BP <90 mm Hg or below patient's baseline
- Decreased RAP and PAOP
- Decreased SVR
- Bradycardia
- Cardiac dysrhythmias
- Postural hypotension

Outcome Criteria

- CO and CI are within normal limits.
- Systolic BP is greater than 90 mm Hg or returns to baseline.
- RAP and PAOP are within normal limits.
- SVR is within normal limits.
- Sinus rhythm is present.
- Dysrhythmias are absent.
- Fainting or dizziness with position change is absent.

Nursing Interventions and *Rationale*

1. Implement measures to prevent episodes of postural hypertension.

- Change patient's position slowly *to allow cardiovascular system to compensate*.
- Apply antiembolic stockings *to promote venous return*.
- Perform range of motion exercises every 2 hours *to prevent venous pooling*.
- Collaborate with physician and physical therapist regarding use of tilt table *to progress the patient from supine to upright position*.
2. Collaborate with physician regarding drug administration.
   - Crystalloids and/or colloids *to increase the patient's circulating volume, which increases stroke volume and subsequently cardiac output*.
   - Vasopressors, if fluids are ineffective, *to constrict the patient's vascular system, which increases resistance and subsequently blood pressure*.
3. Monitor cardiac rhythm for bradycardia and dysrhythmias, *which can further decrease cardiac output*.
4. Avoid any activity that can stimulate the vagal response *because bradycardia can result*.
5. Treat symptomatic bradycardia and symptomatic dysrhythmias according to unit's emergency protocol or ACLS guidelines.

NURSING MANAGEMENT PLAN

Decreased Intracranial Adaptive Capacity

Definition: Intracranial fluid dynamic mechanisms that normally compensate for increases in intracranial volumes are compromised, resulting in repeated disproportionate increases in intracranial pressure (ICP) in response to a variety of noxious and non-noxious stimuli.

Decreased Intracranial Adaptive Capacity Related to Failure of Normal Intracranial Compensatory Mechanisms

Defining Characteristics

- ICP >15 mm Hg, sustained for 15-30 minutes
- Headache
- Vomiting, with or without nausea
- Seizures
- Decrease in Glasgow Coma Scale score of 2 or more points from baseline
- Alteration in level of consciousness, ranging from restlessness to coma
- Change in orientation: disoriented to time and/or place and/or person
- Difficulty or inability to follow simple commands
- Increasing systolic blood pressure (BP) of more than 20 mm Hg with widening pulse pressure
- Bradycardia
- Irregular respiratory pattern (e.g., Cheyne-Stokes, central neurogenic hyperventilation, ataxic, apneustic)
- Change in response to painful stimuli (e.g., purposeful to inappropriate or absent response)
- Signs of impending brain herniation
  - Hemiparesis or hemiplegia
  - Hemisensory changes
  - Unequal pupil size (1 mm or more difference)
  - Failure of pupil to react to light
  - Dysconjugate gaze and inability to move one eye beyond midline if third, fourth, or sixth cranial nerve involved
  - Loss of oculocephalic or oculovestibular reflexes
  - Possible decorticate or decerebrate posturing

Outcome Criteria

- ICP is 15 mm Hg or less.
- Cerebral perfusion pressure (CPP) is greater than 60 mm Hg.
- Clinical signs of increased ICP as previously described are absent.

Nursing Interventions and *Rationale*

1. Maintain adequate CPP.
   - Collaborate with physician regarding administration of volume expanders, vasopressors, or antihypertensives *to maintain the patient's blood pressure within normal range.*
   - Implement measures to reduce ICP.
     - Elevate head of bed 30 to 45 degrees *to facilitate venous return.*
     - Maintain head and neck in neutral plane (avoid flexion, extension, or lateral rotation) *to enhance venous drainage from the head.*
     - Avoid extreme hip flexion.

   - Collaborate with physician regarding administration of steroids, osmotic agents, and diuretics and need for drainage of cerebrospinal fluid (CSF) if a ventriculostomy is in place.
   - Assist patient to turn and move self in bed (instruct patient to exhale while turning or pushing up in bed) *to avoid isometric contractions and Valsalva maneuver.*
2. Maintain patent airway and adequate ventilation and supply oxygen *to prevent hypoxemia and hypercarbia.*
3. Monitor arterial blood gas (ABG) values, and maintain arterial oxygen tension (PaO_2) greater than 80 mm Hg, arterial carbon dioxide tension ($PaCO_2$) at 25 to 35 mm Hg, and pH at 7.35 to 7.45 *to prevent cerebral vasodilation.*
4. Avoid suctioning beyond 10 seconds at a time; hyperoxygenate and hyperventilate before and after suctioning.
5. Plan patient care activities and nursing interventions around patient's ICP response. Avoid unnecessary additional disturbances, and allow patient up to 1 hour of rest between activities as frequently as possible. *Studies have shown the direct correlation between nursing care activities and increases in ICP.*
6. Maintain normothermia with external cooling or heating measures as necessary. Wrap hands, feet, and male genitalia in soft towels before cooling measures *to prevent shivering and frostbite.*
7. With physician's collaboration, control seizures with prophylactic and as-necessary (prn) anticonvulsants. *Seizures can greatly increase the cerebral metabolic rate.*
8. Collaborate with physician regarding administration of sedatives, barbiturates, or paralyzing agents *to reduce cerebral metabolic rate.*
9. Counsel family members to maintain calm atmosphere and avoid disturbing topics of conversation (e.g., patient's condition, pain, prognosis, family crisis, financial difficulties).

Signs of Impending Brain Herniation

1. Notify physician at once.
2. Be sure head of bed is elevated 45 degrees and patient's head is in neutral plane.
3. Administer mainline intravenous (IV) infusion slowly to keep-open rate.
4. Drain CSF as ordered if ventriculostomy in place.
5. Prepare to administer osmotic agents and/or diuretics.
6. Prepare patient for emergency computed tomography (CT) head scan and/or emergency surgery.

Deficient Fluid Volume

Definition: Decreased intravascular, interstitial, and/or intracellular fluid. This refers to dehydration, water loss alone without change in sodium.

Deficient Fluid Volume Related to Absolute Loss

Defining Characteristics

- Cardiac output (CO) <4 L/min
- Cardiac index (CI) <2.2 L/min
- Pulmonary artery occlusion pressure (PAOP), pulmonary artery diastolic pressure (PADP) less than normal or less than baseline, central venous pressure (CVP) less than normal or less than baseline (PAOP <6 mm Hg)
- Tachycardia
- Narrowed pulse pressure
- Systolic blood pressure (BP) <100 mm Hg
- Urine output <30 ml/hr
- Pale, cool, moist skin
- Apprehensiveness

Outcome Criteria

- CO is greater than 4 L/min.
- CI is greater than 2.2 L/min.
- PAOP, PADP, and CVP are normal or back to baseline level.
- Pulse is normal or back to baseline.
- Systolic BP is greater than 90 mm Hg.
- Urine output is greater than 30 ml/hr.

Nursing Interventions and *Rationale*

1. Secure airway and administer high-flow oxygen.
2. Place patient in supine position with legs elevated *to increase preload.* For patient with head injury, consider using low-Fowler's position with legs elevated.
3. For fluid repletion, use the 3:1 rule, replacing three parts of fluid for every unit of blood lost.
4. Administer crystalloid solutions using the fluid challenge technique.
   - Infuse precise aliquots of fluid (usually 5 to 20 ml/min) over 10-minute periods; monitor cardiac loading pressure serially *to determine successful challenging.*
   - If PAOP or PADP elevates more than 7 mm Hg above beginning level, infusion should be stopped.
   - If PAOP or PADP rises only to 3 mm Hg above baseline or falls, another fluid challenge should be administered.
5. Replete fluids first before considering use of vasopressors, *since vasopressors increase myocardial oxygen consumption out of proportion to reestablishment of coronary perfusion in early phases of treatment.*
6. When blood replacement is indicated, replace it with fresh packed red blood cells and fresh-frozen plasma *to keep clotting factors intact.*
7. Move or reposition patient minimally *to decrease or limit tissue oxygen demands.*
8. Evaluate patient's anxiety level, and intervene through patient education or sedation to decrease tissue oxygen demands.
9. Maintain surveillance for signs and symptoms of fluid overload.

Deficient Fluid Volume Related to Decreased Secretion of Antidiuretic Hormone (ADH)

Defining Characteristics

- Confusion and lethargy
- Decreased skin turgor
- Thirst
- Weight loss over short period
- Decreased PAOP
- Decreased CVP
- Urine output >6 L/day
- Serum sodium >148 mEq/L
- Serum osmolality >295 mOsm/kg
- Urine osmolality <100 mOsm/kg
- Urine specific gravity <1.005

Outcome Criteria

- Weight returns to baseline.
- Urine output is greater than 30 ml/hr and less than 200 ml/hr.
- Serum osmolality is 280 to 295 mOsm/kg.
- Urine specific gravity is 1.010 to 1.030.

Nursing Interventions and *Rationale*

1. Record intake and output every hour, noting color and clarity of urine *because color and clarity are an indication of urine concentration.*
2. Monitor electrocardiogram (ECG) rhythm continuously for dysrhythmias caused by electrolyte imbalance.
3. Collaborate with physician regarding administration of vasopressin or desmopressin *to replace ADH.*
   - Monitor patient for adverse effects of medications (i.e., headache, chest pain, abdominal pain) caused by vasoconstriction.
   - Report adverse effects to physician immediately.
4. Collaborate with physician regarding intravenous fluid and electrolyte replacement therapy *to restore fluid balance, correct dehydration, and maintain electrolyte balance.*
   - Administer hypotonic saline *to replace free water deficit.*
5. Provide oral fluids low in sodium such as water, coffee, tea, or orange juice *to decrease sodium intake.*
6. Weigh patient daily (at same time, in same amount of clothing, and preferably with same scale) *to ensure accuracy of readings.*
7. Reposition patient every 2 hours *to prevent skin integrity issues caused by dehydration.*
8. Provide mouth care every 4 hours *to prevent breakdown of oral mucous membranes.*
9. Collaborate with physician regarding administration of medications to prevent constipation *caused by dehydration.*
10. Maintain surveillance for symptoms of hypernatremia (muscle twitching, irritability, seizures), hypovolemic shock (hypotension, tachycardia, decreased CVP/PAOP), and deep vein thrombosis (calf pain, tenderness, swelling).

NURSING MANAGEMENT PLAN

Deficient Fluid Volume—cont'd

Deficient Fluid Volume Related to Relative Loss

Defining Characteristics

- PAOP, PAD pressure, CVP less than normal or less than baseline
- Tachycardia
- Narrowed pulse pressure
- Systolic BP <100 mm Hg
- Urine output <30 ml/hr
- Increased hematocrit level

Outcome Criteria

- PAOP, PADP, and CVP are normal or back to baseline.
- Systolic BP is greater than 90 mm Hg.

- Urine output is greater than 30 ml/hr.
- Hematocrit level is normal.

Nursing Interventions and *Rationale*

Collaborate with physician regarding administration of intravenous (IV) fluid replacements, usually normal saline or lactated Ringer's solution, at a rate sufficient to maintain urine output greater than 30 ml/hr. Colloid solutions are avoided in initial phases (but can be used later) because of risk of increased edema formation *as a result of the increased capillary permeability*.

NURSING MANAGEMENT PLAN

Deficient Knowledge

Definition: Absence or deficiency of cognitive information related to a specific topic.

Deficient Knowledge Related to Cognitive/Perceptual Learning Limitations
(e.g., sensory overload, sleep deprivation, medications, anxiety, sensory deficits, language barrier)

Defining Characteristics

- Verbalized statement of inadequate knowledge of skills
- Verbalization of inadequate recall of information
- Verbalization of inadequate understanding of information
- Evidence of inaccurate follow-through of instructions
- Inadequate demonstration of a skill
- Lack of compliance with prescribed behavior

Outcome Criteria

- Patient participates actively in necessary and prescribed health behaviors.
- Patient verbalizes adequate knowledge or demonstrates adequate skills.

Nursing Interventions and *Rationale*

1. Determine specific cause of patient's cognitive or perceptual limitation.
2. Provide uninterrupted rest period before teaching session *to decrease fatigue and encourage optimal state for learning and retention.*
3. Manipulate environment as much as possible *to provide quiet and uninterrupted learning sessions.*
   - Ensure lights are bright enough to see teaching aids but not too bright.
   - Schedule care and medications *to allow uninterrupted teaching periods.*
   - Move patient to quiet, private room for teaching *if possible.*
4. Adapt teaching sessions and materials to patient's and family's levels of education and ability to understand.

- Provide printed material appropriate to reading level.
- Use terminology understood by patient.
- Provide printed materials in patient's primary language *if possible*.
- Use interpreters during teaching sessions *when necessary*.
5. Teach only present-tense focus during periods of sensory overload.
6. Determine potential effects of medications on ability to retain or recall information.
   - Avoid teaching critical content while patient is taking sedatives, analgesics, or other medications that affect memory.
7. Reinforce new skills and information in several teaching sessions. Use several senses when possible in teaching session (e.g., see a film, hear a discussion, read printed information, demonstrate skills related to self-injection of insulin).
8. Reduce patient's anxiety.
   - Listen attentively, and encourage verbalization of feelings.
   - Answer questions as they arise in a clear and succinct manner.
   - Elicit patient's concerns, and address those issues first.
   - Give only correct and relevant information.
   - Continually assess response to teaching session, and discontinue if anxiety increases or physical condition becomes unstable.
   - Provide nonthreatening information before more anxiety-producing information is presented.
   - Plan for several teaching sessions so information can be divided into small, manageable packages.

Continued

NURSING MANAGEMENT PLAN

Deficient Knowledge—cont'd

Deficient Knowledge Related to Lack of Previous Exposure to Information

Defining Characteristics

- Verbalized statement of inadequate knowledge or skills
- New diagnosis or health problem requiring self-management or care
- Lack of prior formal or informal education about the specific health problem
- Demonstration of inappropriate behaviors related to management of health problem

Outcome Criteria

- Patient verbalizes adequate knowledge about or performs skills related to disease process, its causes, factors related to onset of symptoms, and self-management of disease or health problem.
- Patient actively participates in health behaviors required for performance of a procedure or in those behaviors enhancing recovery from illness and preventing recurrence or complications.

Nursing Interventions and *Rationale*

1. Determine existing level of knowledge or skill.
2. Assess factors that affect the knowledge deficit.
   - Learning needs, including patient's priorities and the necessary knowledge and skills for safety
   - Learning ability, including language skills, level of education, ability to read, preferred learning style
   - Physical ability to perform prescribed skills or procedures; consider effect of limitations imposed by treatment, such as bed rest, restriction of movement by intravenous or other equipment, or effect of sedatives or analgesics.
   - Psychologic effect of stage of adaptation to disease
   - Activity tolerance and ability to concentrate
   - Motivation to learn new skills or gain new knowledge
3. Reduce or limit barriers to learning.
   - Provide consistent nurse/patient contact *to encourage development of trusting and therapeutic relationship*.

- Structure environment *to enhance learning*; control unnecessary noise and interruptions.
- Individualize teaching plan *to fit patient's current physical and psychologic status*.
- Delay teaching until patient is ready to learn.
- Conduct teaching sessions during period of day when patient is most alert and receptive.
- Meet patient's immediate learning needs as they arise (e.g., give brief explanation of procedures when they are performed).
4. Promote active participation in the teaching plan by the patient and family.
   - Solicit input during development of plan.
   - Develop mutually acceptable goals and outcomes.
   - Solicit expression of feelings and emotions related to new responsibilities.
   - Encourage questions.
5. Conduct teaching sessions, using the most appropriate teaching methods.
6. Repeat key principles, and provide them in printed form *for reference at a later time*.
7. Give frequent feedback to patient when practicing new skills.
8. Use several teaching sessions when appropriate. *New information and skills should be reinforced several times after initial learning*.
9. Initiate referrals for follow-up if necessary.
   - Health educators
   - Home health care
   - Rehabilitation programs
   - Social services
10. Evaluate effectiveness of teaching plan, based on patient's ability to meet preset goals and objectives *to determine need for further teaching*.

NURSING MANAGEMENT PLAN

Disturbed Body Image

Definition: Confusion in mental picture of one's physical self.

Disturbed Body Image Related to Actual Change in Body Structure, Function, or Appearance

Defining Characteristics

- Actual change in appearance, structure, or function
- Avoidance of looking at body part
- Avoidance of touching body part
- Hiding or overexposing body part (intentional or unintentional)
- Trauma to nonfunctioning part
- Change in ability to estimate spatial relationship of body to environment

- Verbalization of the following:
  — Fear of rejection or reaction by others
  — Negative feeling about body
  — Preoccupation with change or loss
  — Refusal to participate in or to accept responsibility for self-care of altered body part
- Personalization of part or loss with a name
- Depersonalization of part or loss by use of impersonal pronouns
- Refusal to verify actual change

NURSING MANAGEMENT PLAN

Disturbed Body Image—cont'd

Outcome Criteria

- Patient verbalizes the specific meaning of the change to him or her.
- Patient requests appropriate information about self-care.
- Patient completes personal hygiene and grooming daily with or without help.
- Patient interacts freely with family or other visitors.
- Patient participates in the discussions and conferences related to planning his or her medical and nursing management in the critical care unit and transfer from the unit.
- Patient talks with trained visitors (support-group representatives) at least twice about his or her loss.

Nursing Interventions and *Rationale*

1. Evaluate patient's mental, physical, and emotional state. Recognize assets, strengths, response to illness, coping mechanisms, past experience with stress, and support system.
2. Appraise response of family and significant others. *Body image is derived from the "reflected appraisals" of family and significant others.*
3. Determine patient's goals and readiness for learning.
4. Provide the necessary information to help patient/family adapt to the change. Clarify misconceptions about future limitations.
5. Permit and encourage patient to express significance of the loss or change; note nonverbal behavior responses.
6. Allow and encourage patient's expression of anxiety. *Anxiety is the most predominant emotional response to a body image disturbance.*
7. Recognize and accept use of denial as adaptive defense mechanism when used early and temporarily.
8. Recognize maladaptive denial as interfering with patient's progress and/or alienating support systems. Use confrontation.

9. Provide opportunity for patient to discuss sexual concerns.
10. Touch affected body part *to provide patient with sensory information about altered body structure and function.*
11. Encourage and provide movement of altered body part *to establish kinesthetic feedback. Enables a person to know his or her body as it now exists.*
12. Prepare patient to look at body part. Call the body part by its anatomic name (e.g., stump, stoma, limb) as opposed to "it" or "she." *Use of impersonal pronouns increases a sense of fantasy and depersonalization of the body part.*
13. Allow patient to experience excellence in some aspect of physical functioning—walking, turning, deep breathing, healing, self-care—and point out progress and accomplishment. *Helps to balance patient's sense of dysfunction with function.*
14. Avoid false reassurance. Acknowledge the difficulty of incorporating the altered body part or function into one's body image. *Demonstrates the nurse's sensitivity and promotes trust.*
15. Talk with patient about his or her life, generativity, and accomplishments. *Patients with disturbances in body image frequently see themselves in a distortedly "narrow" sense. Encouraging a wider focus of themselves and their life reduces this distortion.*
16. Help patient explore realistic alternatives.
17. Recognize that incorporating a body change into one's body image takes time. Avoid setting unrealistic expectations and *thereby inadvertently reinforcing a low self-esteem.*
18. Suggest use of additional resources, such as trained visitors who have mastered situations similar to those of patient. Refer patient to a psychiatric liaison nurse or psychiatrist if needed.

Disturbed Body Image Related to Functional Dependence on Life-Sustaining Technology (e.g., ventilator, dialysis, IABP, halo traction)

Defining Characteristics

- Actual change in function requiring permanent or temporary replacement
- Refusal to verify actual loss
- Verbalization of feelings of helplessness, hopelessness, powerlessness, and fear of failure to wean from technology

Outcome Criteria

- Patient verifies actual change in function.
- Patient does not refuse or fight technologic intervention.
- Patient verbalizes acceptance of expected change in lifestyle.

Nursing Interventions and *Rationale*

1. Evaluate patient's response to the technologic intervention.
2. Assess responses of family and significant others. *Body image is derived from the "reflected appraisals" of family and significant others.*
3. Provide information needed by patient and family.
4. Promote trust, security, comfort, and privacy.

5. Recognize anxiety. Allow and encourage its expression. *Anxiety is the most predominant emotion accompanying body image alterations.* Implement plan for Anxiety.
6. Assist patient to recognize his or her own functioning and performance in the face of technology. For example, assist patient to distinguish spontaneous breaths from mechanically delivered breaths. *Will assist in weaning patient from the ventilator when feasible. To establish realistic, accurate body boundaries, a patient needs help to separate self from the technology that is supporting functioning. Any participation or function by patient during periods of dependency is helpful in preventing or resolving an alteration in body image.*
7. Plan for discontinuation of the treatment (e.g., weaning from ventilator). Explain procedure that will be followed, and be present during its initiation.
8. Plan for transfer from the critical care environment.
9. Document care, ensuring an up-to-date management plan is available to all involved caregivers.

NURSING MANAGEMENT PLAN

Disturbed Sleep Pattern

Definition: Time-limited disruption of sleep (natural, periodic suspension of consciousness) amount and quality.

Disturbed Sleep Pattern Related to Fragmented Sleep

Defining Characteristics

- Decreased sleep during one block of sleep time
- Daytime sleepiness
- Decreased sleep
  — Less than one half of normal total sleep time
  — Decreased slow-wave, or rapid eye movement (REM), sleep
- Anxiety
- Fatigue
- Restlessness
- Disorientation and hallucinations
- Combativeness
- Frequent awakenings

Outcome Criteria

- Patient's total sleep time approximates patient's norm.
- Patient can complete sleep cycles of 90 minutes without interruption.
- Patient has no delusions or hallucinations.
- Patient has reality-based thought content.

Nursing Interventions and *Rationale*

1. Assess normal sleep pattern on admission and any history of sleep disturbance or chronic illness that may affect sleep or sedative/hypnotic use. Promote normal sleep activity while patient is in critical care unit. Assess sleep effectiveness by asking patient how his or her sleep in the hospital compares with sleep at home.
2. Promote comfort, relaxation, and a sense of well-being. Treat pain; change, smooth, or refresh bed linens at bedtime; and provide oral hygiene. Eliminate stressful situations before bedtime. Use relaxation techniques, imagery, music, massage, or warm blankets. Other interventions may include having a close family member sit beside the bed and providing the patient with own garments or coverings. Individual patients may prefer quiet or may prefer the background noise of the television or music to best promote sleep. Provide a comfortable room temperature.
3. Minimize noise, particularly that of the staff and noisy equipment. Reduce the level of environmental stimuli. Dim lights at night.
4. Foods containing tryptophan (e.g., milk, turkey) may be appropriate *because these promote sleep.*
5. Plan nap times to assist in approximating the patient's normal 24-hour sleep time.
6. Minimize awakenings *to allow for at least 90-minute sleep cycles.* Continually assess the need to awaken patient, particularly at night. Distinguish between essential and nonessential nursing tasks. Organize nursing management to allow for maximal amount of uninterrupted sleep while ensuring close monitoring of patient's condition. Whenever possible, monitor physiologic parameters without waking patient. Coordinate awakenings with other departments, such as respiratory therapy, laboratory, and x-ray, *to minimize sleep interruptions.*
7. Be aware of the effects of common medications on sleep. *Many sedative and hypnotic medications decrease REM sleep.* Sedative and analgesic medications should not be withheld; rather, drugs that minimally disrupt sleep should be used to complement comfort measures, with dosages reduced gradually as the medication becomes no longer necessary. Do not abruptly withdraw REM-suppressing medications *because this can result in "REM rebound."*
8. Document amount of uninterrupted sleep per shift, especially sleep episodes lasting longer than 2 hours. This can be effectively documented as part of the 24-hour flow sheet and reported routinely, shift to shift. *Sleep pattern disturbance is diagnosed, treated, and resolved more efficiently when formally documented in this manner.*
9. Be aware that the best treatment for sleep pattern disturbance is prevention.
10. Facilitate staff awareness that sleep is essential and health promoting. Assess the critical care unit for sleep-reducing stimuli and work to minimize them.

NURSING MANAGEMENT PLAN

Dysfunctional Ventilatory Weaning Response

Definition: Inability to adjust to lowered levels of mechanical ventilator support that interrupts and prolongs the weaning process.

Dysfunctional Ventilatory Weaning Response (DVWR) Related to Physical, Psychologic, or Situational Factors

Defining Characteristics

Mild DVWR

- Responds to lowered levels of mechanical ventilator support with:
  — Restlessness

  — Slightly increased respiratory rate from baseline
  — Expressed feelings of increased need for oxygen, breathing discomfort, fatigue, and warmth
  — Queries about possible machine malfunction
  — Increased concentration on breathing

NURSING MANAGEMENT PLAN

Dysfunctional Ventilatory Weaning Response—cont'd

Moderate DVWR

- Responds to lowered levels of mechanical ventilator support with:
  — Slight baseline increase in blood pressure <20 mm Hg
  — Slight baseline increase in heart rate <20 beats/min
  — Baseline increase in respiratory rate <5 breaths/min
  — Hypervigilance to activities
  — Inability to respond to coaching
  — Inability to cooperate
  — Apprehension
  — Diaphoresis
  — Eye-widening ("wide-eyed look")
  — Decreased air entry on auscultation
  — Color changes: pale, slight cyanosis
  — Slight respiratory accessory muscle use

Severe DVWR

- Responds to lowered levels of mechanical ventilator support with:
  — Agitation
  — Deterioration in arterial blood gases from current baseline
  — Baseline increase in blood pressure >20 mm Hg
  — Baseline increase in heart rate >20 beats/min
  — Respiratory rate increases significantly from baseline
  — Profuse diaphoresis
  — Full respiratory accessory muscle use
  — Shallow, gasping breaths
  — Paradoxical abdominal breathing
  — Discoordinated breathing with the ventilator
  — Decreased level of consciousness
  — Adventitious breath sounds, audible airway secretions
  — Cyanosis

Outcome Criteria

- Airway is clear.
- Underlying disorder is resolving.
- Patient is rested, and pain is controlled.
- Nutritional status is adequate.
- Patient has feelings of perceived control, situational security, and trust in nurses.
- Patient is able to adapt to selected levels of ventilator support without undue fatigue.

Nursing Interventions and *Rationale*

1. Communicate interest and concern for the patient's well-being, and demonstrate confidence in ability to manage weaning process *to instill trust in patient.*
2. Use normalizing strategies (e.g., grooming, dressing, mobilizing, social conversation) *to reinforce patient's self-esteem and feeling of identity.*
3. Identify parameters of patient's usual functioning before the weaning process begins *to facilitate early identification of problems.*

4. Identify patient's strengths and resources that can be mobilized *to enhance patient's coping and to maximize weaning effort.*
5. Note concerns that adversely affect patient's comfort and confidence, and manage them discretely *to facilitate patient's ease.*
6. Praise successful activities, encourage a positive outlook, and review the patient's positive progress to date, *to increase the patient's perceived self-efficacy.*
7. Inform patient of his or her situation and weaning progress *to permit patient as much control as possible.*
8. Teach patient about weaning process and how patient can participate in the process.
9. Negotiate daily weaning goals with patient *to gain cooperation.*
10. Position patient with head of the bed elevated *to optimize respiratory efforts.*
11. Coach patient in breath control by regular demonstrations of slow, deep, rhythmic patterns of breathing *to assist with dyspnea.*
12. Remain visible in room and reassure patient that help is immediately available if needed, *to reduce patient's anxiety and fearfulness.*
13. Encourage patient to view weaning trials as a form of training, regardless of whether weaning goal is achieved, *to avoid discouragement.*
14. Encourage patient to maintain emotional calmness by reassuring, being present, comforting, talking down if emotionally aroused, and reinforcing idea that patient can and will succeed.
15. Monitor patient's status frequently, *to avoid undue fatigue and anxiety.*
16. Provide regular periods of rest by reducing activities, maintaining or increasing ventilator support, and providing oxygen as needed before fatigue advances.
17. Provide distraction (e.g., visitors, radio, television, conversation) when patient's concentration starts to create tension and increases anxiety.
18. Ensure adequate nutritional support, sufficient rest and sleep time, and sedation or pain control *to promote patient's optimal physical and emotional comfort.*
19. Start weaning early in the day *when patient is most rested.*
20. Restrict unnecessary activities and visitors who do not cooperate with weaning strategies, *to minimize energy demands on the patient during the weaning process.*
21. Coordinate necessary activities *to promote adequate time for rest and relaxation.*
22. Monitor patient's underlying disease process *to ensure it is stabilized and under control.*
23. Advocate for additional resources (e.g., sedation, analgesia, rest) needed by patient *to maximize comfort status.*
24. Develop and adhere to an individualized plan of care *to promote patient's feelings of control.*

NURSING MANAGEMENT PLAN

Excess Fluid Volume

Definition: Increased isotonic fluid retention.

Excess Fluid Volume Related to Increased Secretion of Antidiuretic Hormone (ADH)

Defining Characteristics

- Headache
- Decreased sensorium
- Weight gain over short period
- Intake greater than output
- Increased pulmonary artery occlusion pressure (PAOP)
- Increased central venous pressure (CVP)
- Urine output <30 ml/hr
- Serum sodium <120 mEq/L
- Serum osmolality <275 mOsm/kg
- Urine osmolality greater than serum osmolality
- Urine sodium >200 mEq/L
- Urine specific gravity >1.03

Outcome Criteria

- Weight returns to baseline.
- Urine output is greater than 30 ml/hr.
- Serum sodium is 135 to 145 mEq/L.
- Urine specific gravity is 1.005 to 1030.

Nursing Interventions and *Rationale*

1. Monitor electrocardiogram (ECG) rhythm continuously for dysrhythmias *caused by electrolyte imbalance*.
2. Restrict patient's fluids to 500 ml less than output per day *to decrease fluid retention*.
3. Provide patient chilled beverages high in sodium content such as tomato juice or broth *to increase sodium intake*.
4. Collaborate with physician regarding administration of demeclocycline, lithium, and narcotic agonists *to inhibit renal response to ADH.*
5. Collaborate with physician regarding administration of hypertonic saline and furosemide *for rapid correction of severe sodium deficit and diuresis of free water*.
   - Administer hypertonic saline at rate of 1 to 2 ml/kg/hr until patient's serum sodium is increased no greater than 1 to 2 mEq/L/hr.
6. Weigh patient daily (at same time, in same amount of clothing, and preferably with same scale) *to ensure accuracy of readings*.
7. Provide frequent mouth care *to prevent breakdown of oral mucous membranes*.
8. Initiate seizure precautions *because patient is at high risk as a result of hyponatremia*.
   - Pad side rails of bed to protect patient from injury.
   - Remove any objects from immediate environment that could injure patient in the event of a seizure.
   - Keep appropriate-size oral airway at bedside to assist with postseizure airway management.
9. Collaborate with physician regarding administration of medications to prevent constipation *caused by decreased fluid intake and immobility*.
10. Maintain surveillance for symptoms of hyponatremia (headache, abdominal cramps, weakness) and congestive heart failure (dyspnea, rales, increased CVP/PAOP).

Excess Fluid Volume Related to Renal Dysfunction

Defining Characteristics

- Weight gain that occurs during 24- to 48-hour period
- Dependent pitting edema
- Ascites in severe cases
- Fluid crackles on lung auscultation
- Exertional dyspnea
- Oliguria or anuria
- Hypertension
- Engorged neck veins
- Decrease in urinary osmolality as renal failure progresses
- CVP >15 cm of H_2O
- PAOP 20-25 mm Hg

Outcome Criteria

- Weight returns to baseline.
- Edema or ascites is absent or reduced to baseline.
- Lungs are clear to auscultation.
- Exertional dyspnea is absent.
- Blood pressure returns to baseline.
- Heart rate returns to baseline.
- Neck veins are flat.
- Mucous membranes are moist.

Nursing Interventions and *Rationale*

1. Promote skin integrity of edematous areas by frequent repositioning and elevation of areas where possible. Avoid massaging pressure points or reddened areas of skin *because this results in further tissue trauma.*
2. Plan patient care to provide rest periods *so as not to increase exertional dyspnea.*
3. Weigh patient daily (at same time, in same amount of clothing, and preferably with same scale).
4. Instruct patient about correlation between fluid intake and weight gain, using commonly understood fluid measurements. For example, ingesting 4 cups (1000 ml) of fluid results in an approximate 2-pound weight gain in the anuric patient.

NURSING MANAGEMENT PLAN

Hyperthermia

Definition: Body temperature elevated above normal range.

Hyperthermia Related to Increased Metabolic Rate

Defining Characteristics

- Increased body temperature above normal range
- Seizures
- Flushed skin
- Increased respiratory rate
- Tachycardia
- Skin warm to touch
- Diaphoresis

Outcome Criteria

- Temperature is within normal range.
- Respiratory rate and heart rate are within patient's baseline range.
- Skin is warm and dry.

Nursing Interventions and *Rationale*

1. Monitor temperature every 15 minutes to 1 hour until within normal range and stable, then every 4 hours, *to maintain close surveillance for temperature fluctuations and evaluate effectiveness of interventions.*
   - Use temperature taken from pulmonary artery catheter or bladder catheter if available *because these methods closely reflect core body temperature.*
   - Use tympanic membrane temperature *if core body temperature devices are unavailable.*
   - Use rectal temperature if none of above methods is available.
2. Collaborate with physician regarding administration of antithyroid medications *to block synthesis and release of thyroid hormone.*

3. Collaborate with physician regarding use of cooling blanket *to facilitate heat loss through conduction.*
   - Wrap hands, feet, and genitalia *to protect them from maceration during cooling and decrease chance of shivering.*
   - Avoid rapidly cooling patient and overcooling patient *because this initiates the heat-conserving response (i.e., shivering).*
4. Place ice packs in patient's groin and axilla *to facilitate heat loss through conduction.*
5. Maintain patient on bed rest *to decrease effects of activity on patient's metabolic rate.*
6. Provide tepid sponge baths *to facilitate heat loss through evaporation.*
7. Decrease patient's room temperature *to facilitate radiant heat loss.*
8. Place fan near patient to circulate cool air *to facilitate heat loss through convection.*
9. Provide patient with nonrestrictive gown and lightweight bed coverings *to allow heat to escape from patient's trunk.*
10. Collaborate with physician and respiratory therapist on the administration of oxygen to maintain oxygen satruation (SpO_2) greater than 90% *because patient has increased oxygen consumption secondary to increased metabolic rate.*
11. Collaborate with physician regarding use of antipyretic medications *to facilitate patient comfort.*
12. Collaborate with physician regarding use of intravenous and oral fluids *to maintain adequate hydration of patient.*

NURSING MANAGEMENT PLAN

Hypothermia

Definition: Body temperature below normal range.

Hypothermia Related to Decreased Metabolic Rate

Defining Characteristics

- Reduction in body temperature below normal range
- Shivering
- Pallor
- Piloerection
- Hypertension
- Skin cool to touch
- Tachycardia
- Decreased capillary refill

Outcome Criteria

- Temperature is within normal range.
- Heart rate is within patient's baseline range.

- Skin is warm and dry.
- Capillary refill is normal.

Nursing Interventions and *Rationale*

1. Monitor temperature every 15 minutes to 1 hour until within normal range and stable and then every 4 hours *to maintain close surveillance for temperature fluctuations and evaluate effectiveness of interventions.*
   - Use temperature taken from pulmonary artery catheter or bladder catheter if available *because these methods closely reflect core body temperature.*
   - Use tympanic membrane temperature *if core body temperature devices are unavailable.*

Continued

NURSING MANAGEMENT PLAN

Hypothermia—cont'd

- Use rectal temperature if none of above methods is available.
2. Collaborate with physician regarding administration of thyroid medications *to replace lacking thyroid hormone.*
3. Collaborate with physician regarding the use of fluid-filled heating blanket *to facilitate rewarming through conduction.*
4. Initiate forced air-warming therapy *to facilitate convective heat gain.*

5. Provide patient with warm blankets *to facilitate heat transfer to the patient.*
6. Increase patient's room temperature *to decrease radiant heat loss.*
7. Replace wet patient gown and bed linen promptly *to decrease evaporative heat loss.*
8. Warm intravenous fluids/blood products *to facilitate rewarming through conduction.*

NURSING MANAGEMENT PLAN

Imbalanced Nutrition: Less than Body Requirements

Definition: Intake of nutrients insufficient to meet metabolic needs.

Imbalanced Nutrition: Less than Body Requirements Related to Lack of Exogenous Nutrients and Increased Metabolic Demand

Defining Characteristics

- Unplanned weight loss of 20% of body weight in past 6 months
- Serum albumin <3.5 g/dl
- Total lymphocytes <1500/mm^3
- Anergy
- Negative nitrogen balance
- Fatigue; lack of energy and endurance
- Nonhealing wounds
- Daily caloric intake less than estimated nutritional requirements
- Presence of factors known to increase nutritional requirements (e.g., sepsis, trauma, multiple organ dysfunction syndrome [MODS])
- Maintenance of nothing-by-mouth (NPO) status >7-10 days
- Long-term use of 5% dextrose intravenously
- Documentation of suboptimal calorie counts
- Drug or nutrient interaction that might decrease oral intake (e.g. chronic use of bronchodilators, laxatives, anticonvulsants, diuretics, antacids, or narcotics)
- Physical problems with chewing, swallowing, choking, and salivation and presence of altered taste, anorexia, nausea, vomiting, diarrhea, or constipation

Outcome Criteria

- Patient exhibits stabilization of weight loss or weight gain of ½ pound daily.

- Serum albumin is >3.5 g/dl.
- Total lymphocyte count is >1500/mm^3.
- Patient has positive response to cutaneous skin antigen testing.
- Patient is in positive nitrogen balance.
- Wound healing is evident.
- Daily caloric intake equals estimated nutritional requirements.
- Increased ambulation and endurance are evident.

Nursing Interventions and *Rationale*

1. Inquire if patient has any food allergies and food preferences *to ensure the food provided to patient is not contraindicated.*
2. Monitor patient's caloric intake and weight daily *to ensure adequacy of nutritional interventions.*
3. Collaborate with dietitian regarding patient's nutritional and caloric needs *to determine the appropriateness of patient's diet to meet those needs.*
4. Monitor patient for signs of nutritional deficiencies *to facilitate evaluation of extent of nutritional deficit.*
5. Provide patient with oral care before eating *to ensure optimal consumption of diet.*
6. Assist patient to eat as appropriate *to ensure optimal consumption of diet.*
7. Collaborate with physician regarding the administration of parenteral and enteral nutrition as needed.

NURSING MANAGEMENT PLAN

Impaired Gas Exchange

Definition: Excess or deficit in oxygenation and/or carbon dioxide elimination at alveolar-capillary membrane.

Impaired Gas Exchange Related to Alveolar Hypoventilation

Defining Characteristics

- Abnormal arterial blood gas (ABG) values: decreased arterial oxygen tension (PaO_2), increased arterial carbon dioxide tension ($PaCO_2$), decreased pH, decreased oxygen saturation (SpO_2)
- Somnolence
- Neurobehavioral changes (restlessness, irritability, confusion)
- Tachycardia or dysrhythmias
- Central cyanosis

Outcome Criteria

- ABG values are within patient's baseline.
- Central cyanosis is absent.

Nursing Interventions and *Rationale*

1. Initiate continuous pulse oximetry or monitor SpO_2 every hour.
2. Collaborate with physician regarding administration of oxygen to maintain SpO_2 greater than 90%.
    - Administer supplemental oxygen via appropriate oxygen-delivery device *to increase driving pressure of oxygen in alveoli.*
    - If supplemental oxygen alone is not effective, administer continuous positive airway pressure (CPAP) or mechanical ventilation with positive end-expiratory pressure (PEEP) *to open collapsed alveoli and increase surface area for gas exchange.*
3. Prevent hypoventilation.
    - Position patient in high-Fowler's position or semi-Fowler's position *to promote diaphragmatic descent and maximal inhalation.*
    - Assist with deep-breathing exercises and incentive spirometry with sustained maximal inspiration 5 to 10 times/hr *to help reinflate collapsed portions of lung.* (See plan for Ineffective Breathing Pattern Related to Decreased Lung Expansion.)
    - Treat pain, if present, *to prevent hypoventilation and atelectasis.* Implement plan for Acute Pain Related to Transmission and Perception of Cutaneous, Visceral, Muscular, or Ischemic Impulses.
4. Assist physician with intubation and initiation of mechanical ventilation as indicated.

Impaired Gas Exchange Related to Ventilation/Perfusion Mismatching or Intrapulmonary Shunting

Defining Characteristics

- Abnormal ABG values (decreased PaO_2, decreased SpO_2)
- Somnolence
- Neurobehavioral changes (restlessness, irritability, confusion)
- Central cyanosis

Outcome Criteria

- ABG values are within patient's baseline.
- Central cyanosis is absent.

Nursing Interventions and *Rationale*

1. Initiate continuous pulse oximetry, or monitor SpO_2 every hour.
2. Collaborate with physician regarding administration of oxygen to maintain SpO_2 greater than 90%.
    - Administer supplemental oxygen via appropriate oxygen-delivery device *to increase driving pressure of oxygen in alveoli.*
    - If supplemental oxygen alone is not effective, administer CPAP or mechanical ventilation with PEEP *to open collapsed alveoli and increase surface area for gas exchange.*
3. Position patient to optimize ventilation/perfusion matching.
    - For patient with unilateral lung disease, position with the good lung down *because gravity will improve perfusion to this area, and this will best match ventilation with perfusion.*
    - For patient with bilateral lung disease, position with right lung down *because right lung is larger than left lung and affords a greater area for ventilation and perfusion*, or change position every 2 hours, favoring positions that improve oxygenation.
    - Avoid any position that seriously compromises oxygenation status.
4. Perform procedures only as needed and provide adequate rest and recovery time in between *to prevent desaturation.*
5. Collaborate with physician regarding administration of drugs.
    - Sedatives, *to decrease ventilator asynchrony and facilitate patient's sense of control.*
    - Neuromuscular blocking agents, *to prevent ventilator asynchrony and decrease oxygen demand.*
    - Analgesics, *to treat pain if present.* Implement plan for Acute Pain Related to Transmission and Perception of Cutaneous, Visceral, Muscular, or Ischemic Impulses.
6. If secretions are present, implement plan for Ineffective Airway Clearance Related to Excessive Secretions or Abnormal Viscosity of Mucus.

NURSING MANAGEMENT PLAN

Impaired Spontaneous Ventilation

Definition: Decreased energy reserves results in an individual's inability to maintain breathing adequate to support life.

Impaired Spontaneous Ventilation Related to Respiratory Muscle Fatigue or Metabolic Factors

Defining Characteristics

- Dyspnea and apprehension
- Increased metabolic rate
- Increased restlessness
- Increased use of accessory muscles
- Decreased tidal volume
- Increased heart rate
- Abnormal arterial blood gas (ABG) values: decreased arterial oxygen tension (PaO_2), increased arterial carbon dioxide tension ($PaCO_2$), decreased pH, decreased arterial oxygen saturation (SpO_2)
- Decreased cooperation

Outcome Criteria

- Metabolic rate and heart rate are within patient's baseline.
- Patient experiences eupnea.
- ABG values are within patient's baseline.

Nursing Interventions and *Rationale*

1. Collaborate with physician regarding application of pressure support to ventilator *to assist patient in overcoming the work of breathing imposed by the ventilator and endotracheal tube.*
2. Carefully snip excess length from proximal end of endotracheal tube *to decrease dead space and thereby decrease the work of breathing.*
3. Collaborate with physician and dietitian to ensure that at least 50% of diet's nonprotein caloric source is in form of fat versus carbohydrates *to prevent excess carbon dioxide production.*
4. Collaborate with physician and respiratory therapist regarding best method of weaning for individual patients

because each situation is different and a variety of weaning options are available.
5. Collaborate with physician and physical therapist regarding progressive ambulation and conditioning plan *to promote overall muscle conditioning and respiratory muscle functioning.*
6. Determine most effective means of communication for patient *to promote independence and reduce anxiety.*
7. Develop a daily schedule and post in patient's room *to coordinate care and facilitate patient's involvement in the plan.*
8. Treat pain, if present, *to prevent respiratory splinting and hypoventilation.* Implement plan for Acute Pain Related to Transmission and Perception of Cutaneous, Visceral, Muscular, or Ischemic Impulses.
9. Ensure that patient receives at least 2- to 4-hr intervals of uninterrupted sleep in a quiet, dark room. Collaborate with physician and respiratory therapist regarding use of full ventilatory support at night *to provide respiratory muscle rest.*
10. Place patient in semi-Fowler's position or in a chair at bedside *for best use of ventilatory muscles and to facilitate diaphragmatic descent.*
11. Explain weaning procedure to patient before the trial *so that patient will understand what to expect and how to participate.*
12. Monitor patient during the weaning trial for evidence of respiratory muscle fatigue *to avoid overtiring patient.*
13. Provide diversional activity during the weaning trial *to reduce patient's anxiety.*
14. Collaborate with physician and respiratory therapist regarding removal of ventilator and artificial airway when patient has been successfully weaned.

NURSING MANAGEMENT PLAN

Impaired Swallowing

Definition: Abnormal functioning of swallowing mechanism associated with deficits in oral, pharyngeal, or esophageal structure or function.

Impaired Swallowing Related to Neuromuscular Impairment, Fatigue, and Limited Awareness

Defining Characteristics

Evidence of Difficulty Swallowing

- Drooling
- Difficulty handling oral secretions
- Absence of gag, cough, and swallow reflexes
- Moist, wet, gurgling voice quality
- Decreased tongue and mouth movements
- Presence of dysarthria

- Difficulty handling solid foods
  — Uncoordinated chewing and swallowing
  — Stasis of food in oral cavity
  — Wet-sounding voice or change in voice quality
  — Sneezing, coughing, or choking with eating
  — Delay in swallowing of more than 5 seconds
  — Change in respiratory patterns
- Difficulty handling liquids

NURSING MANAGEMENT PLAN

Impaired Swallowing—cont'd

— Momentary loss of voice or change in voice quality
— Nasal regurgitation of liquids
— Coughing with drinking

Evidence of Aspiration

- Hypoxemia
- Productive cough
- Frothy sputum
- Wheezing, crackles, or rhonchi
- Temperature elevation

Outcome Criteria

- Evidence of swallowing difficulties is absent.
- Evidence of aspiration is absent.

Nursing Interventions and *Rationale*

1. Collaborate with physician and speech therapist regarding swallowing evaluation and rehabilitation program *to decrease the incidence of aspiration.*
2. Collaborate with physician and dietitian regarding nutritional assessment and nutritional plan *to ensure that patient is receiving enough nutrition.*
3. Place patient in upright position with the head midline and the chin slightly down *to keep food in anterior portion of mouth and to prevent food from falling over base of tongue into open airway.*
4. Provide patient with single-textured soft foods (e.g., cream cereals) that maintain their shape *because these foods require minimal oral manipulation.*
5. Avoid particulate foods (e.g., hamburger) and foods containing more than one texture (e.g., stew) *because these foods require more chewing and oral manipulation.*

6. Avoid dry foods (e.g., popcorn, rice, crackers) and sticky foods (e.g., peanut butter, bananas) *because these foods are difficult to manipulate orally.*
7. Provide patient with thick liquids (e.g., fruit nectar, yogurt) *because thick liquids are more easily controlled in the mouth.*
8. Thicken thin liquids (e.g., water, juice) with a thickening preparation or avoid them *because thin liquids are easily aspirated.*
9. Place foods in the uninvolved side of the mouth *because oral sensitivity and function are greatest in this area.*
10. Avoid straws *because straws can deposit the liquid too far back in mouth for patient to handle.*
11. Serve foods and liquids at room temperature *because patient may be overly sensitive to heat or cold.*
12. Offer solids and liquids at different times *to avoid swallowing solids before being properly chewed.*
13. Provide oral hygiene after meals *to clear food particles from the mouth that could be aspirated.*
14. Collaborate with physician and pharmacist regarding oral medication administration *to adjust medication regimen to prevent aspiration and choking and to ensure all prescribed medications are swallowed.*
15. Crush tablets (if appropriate) and mix with food that is easily formed into a bolus, use thickened liquid medications (if available), and/or embed small capsules into food *to facilitate oral medication administration.*
16. Inspect mouth for residue after all medication administration *to ensure medication has been swallowed.*
17. Educate patient and family on the swallowing problem, rehabilitation program, and emergency measures for choking.

NURSING MANAGEMENT PLAN

Impaired Verbal Communication

***Definition*:** Decreased, delayed, or absent ability to receive, process, transmit, and use a system of symbols.

Impaired Verbal Communication Related to Cerebral Speech Center Injury

Defining Characteristics

- Inappropriate or absent speech or responses to questions
- Inability to speak spontaneously
- Inability to understand spoken words
- Inability to follow commands appropriately through gestures
- Difficulty or inability to understand written language
- Difficulty or inability to express ideas in writing
- Difficulty or inability to name objects

Outcome Criterion

- Patient is able to make basic needs known.

Nursing Interventions and *Rationale*

1. Consult with physician and speech pathologist *to determine the extent of patient's communication deficit* (e.g., whether fluent, nonfluent, or global aphasia is involved).
2. Have speech therapist post a list of appropriate ways to communicate with patient in patient's room *so that all nursing personnel can be consistent in their efforts.*
3. Assess patient's ability to comprehend, speak, read, and write.
   - Ask questions that can be answered with a "yes" or a "no." If patient answers "yes" to question, ask the opposite (e.g., "Are you hot?" "Yes." "Are you cold?" "Yes."), *to help determine whether patient really understands what is being said.*

Continued

NURSING MANAGEMENT PLAN

Impaired Verbal Communication—cont'd

- Ask simple, short questions. Use gestures, pantomime, and facial expressions to give patient additional clues.
- Stand in patient's line of vision, giving a good view of your face and hands.
- Have patient try to write with a pad and pencil. Offer pictures and alphabet letters for reference.
- Make flash cards with pictures or words depicting frequently used phrases (e.g., glass of water, bedpan).
4. Maintain an uncluttered environment, and decrease external distractions *that could hinder communication.*
5. Maintain a relaxed and calm manner, and explain all diagnostic, therapeutic, and comfort measures before initiating them.
6. Do not shout or speak in a loud voice. *Hearing loss is not a factor in aphasia, and shouting will not help.*
7. Have only one person talk at a time. *It is more difficult for a patient to follow a multisided conversation.*
8. Use direct eye contact, and speak directly to patient in unhurried, short phrases.
9. Give one-step commands and directions, and provide cues through pictures and gestures.
10. Try to ask questions that can be answered with a "yes" or a "no," and avoid topics that are controversial, emotional, abstract, or lengthy.
11. Listen to patient in unhurried manner, and wait for patient's attempt to communicate.
    - Expect a time lag from when you ask patient something until patient responds.
    - Accept patient's statement of essential words without expecting complete sentences.
    - Avoid finishing sentences for patient, if possible.
    - Wait approximately 30 seconds before providing the word that patient may be attempting to find (except when patient is very frustrated and needs something quickly, such as a bedpan).
    - Rephrase patient's message aloud *to validate it.*
    - Do not pretend to understand patient's message if you do not.
12. Encourage patient to speak slowly in short phrases and to say each word clearly.

13. Ask patient to write the message, if able, or draw pictures if only verbal communication is affected.
14. Observe patient's nonverbal clues for validation (e.g., answers "yes" but shakes head "no").
15. When handing an object to patient, state what it is *because hearing language spoken is necessary to stimulate language development.*
16. Explain what has happened to patient, and offer reassurance about plan of care.
17. Verbally address problem of frustration over inability to communicate, and explain that both nurse and patient need patience.
18. Maintain a calm, positive manner, and offer reassurance (e.g., "I know this is very hard for you, but it will get better if we work on it together").
19. Talk to patient as an adult. Be respectful, and avoid "talking down" to patient.
20. Do not discuss patient's condition or hold conversations in patient's presence without including patient in the discussion. *This may be the reason some aphasic patients develop paranoid thoughts.*
21. Do not exhibit disapproval of emotional utterances or spontaneous use of profanity. Instead, offer calm, quiet reassurance.
22. If patient makes an error in speech, do not reprimand or scold, but try to compliment patient by saying, "That was a good try."
23. Delay conversation if patient is tired. *Symptoms of aphasia worsen if patient is fatigued, anxious, or upset.*
24. Be prepared for emotional outbursts and tears from patients who have more difficulty in expressing themselves than with understanding. Patient may become depressed, refuse treatment and food, ignore relatives, and push objects away. Comfort patient with statements.
    - "I know it's frustrating and you feel sad, but you are not alone. Other people who have had strokes have felt the way you do. We will be here to help you get through this."

NURSING MANAGEMENT PLAN

Ineffective Airway Clearance

Definition: Inability to clear secretions or obstructions from respiratory tract to maintain a clear airway.

Ineffective Airway Clearance Related to Excessive Secretions or Abnormal Viscosity of Mucus

Defining Characteristics

- Abnormal breath sounds (displaced normal sounds, adventitious sounds, diminished or absent sounds)
- Ineffective cough with or without sputum
- Tachypnea, dyspnea
- Verbal reports of inability to clear airway

Outcome Criteria

- Cough produces thin mucus.
- Lungs are clear to auscultation.
- Respiratory rate, depth, and rhythm return to baseline.

Nursing Interventions and *Rationale*

1. Assess sputum for color, consistency, and amount.
2. Assess for clinical manifestations of pneumonia.
3. Provide for maximal thoracic expansion by repositioning, deep breathing, splinting, and pain management *to avoid hypoventilation and atelectasis.* If hypoventilation is present, implement plan for Ineffective Breathing Pattern Related to Decreased Lung Expansion.
4. Maintain adequate hydration by administering oral and intravenous fluids (as ordered) *to thin secretions and facilitate airway clearance.*
5. Provide humidification to airways via oxygen-delivery device or artificial airway *to thin secretions and facilitate airway clearance.*
6. Administer bland aerosol every 4 hours *to facilitate expectoration of sputum.*
7. Collaborate with physician regarding administration of drugs.
   - Bronchodilators, *to treat or prevent bronchospasm and facilitate expectoration of mucus.*
   - Mucolytics and expectorants, *to enhance mobilization and removal of secretions.*
   - Antibiotics, *to treat infection.*
8. Assist with directed coughing exercises *to facilitate expectoration of secretions.* If patient unable to perform cascade cough, consider using huff cough (patients with hyperactive airways), end-expiratory cough (patient with secretions in distal airway), or augmented cough (patient with weakened abdominal muscle), instructing patient as follows.

- *Cascade cough*
  (1) Take deep breath and hold for 1 to 3 seconds.
  (2) Cough out forcefully several times until all air is exhaled.
  (3) Inhale slowly through nose.
  (4) Repeat once.
  (5) Rest, and then repeat as necessary.
- *Huff cough*
  (1) Take deep breath and hold for 1 to 3 seconds.
  (2) Say the word "huff" while coughing out several times until air is exhaled.
  (3) Inhale slowly through nose.
  (4) Repeat as necessary.
- *End-expiratory cough*
  (1) Take deep breath and hold for 1 to 3 seconds.
  (2) Exhale slowly.
  (3) At end of exhalation, cough once.
  (4) Inhale slowly through nose.
  (5) Repeat as necessary, or follow with cascade cough.
- *Augmented cough*
  (1) Take deep breath and hold for 1 to 3 seconds.
  (2) Perform one or more of following maneuvers to increase intraabdominal pressure:
     — Tighten knees and buttocks.
     — Bend forward at the waist.
     — Place a hand flat on upper abdomen just under xiphoid process and press in and up abruptly during coughing.
     — Keep hands on chest wall and press inward with each cough.
  (3) Inhale slowly through nose.
  (4) Rest and repeat as necessary.
9. Suction nasotracheally or endotracheally as necessary *to assist with secretion removal.*
10. Reposition patient at least every 2 hours or use continuous lateral rotation therapy *to mobilize and prevent stasis of secretions.*
11. Consider chest physiotherapy (postural drainage and/or chest percussion) 3 to 4 times per day in a patient with large amounts of sputum *to assist with expulsion of retained secretions.*
12. Allow rest periods between coughing sessions, chest physiotherapy, suctioning, or any other demanding activities *to promote energy conservation.*

NURSING MANAGEMENT PLAN

Ineffective Breathing Pattern

Definition: Inspiration or expiration that does not provide adequate ventilation.

Ineffective Breathing Pattern Related to Decreased Lung Expansion

Defining Characteristics

- Abnormal respiratory patterns (hypoventilation, hyperventilation, tachypnea, bradypnea, obstructive breathing)
- Abnormal arterial blood gas (ABG) values: increased arterial carbon dioxide tension ($PaCO_2$), decreased pH
- Unequal chest movement
- Shortness of breath, dyspnea

Outcome Criteria

- Respiratory rate, rhythm, and depth return to baseline.
- Use of accessory muscles is minimal or absent.
- Chest expands symmetrically.
- ABG values return to baseline.

Nursing Interventions and *Rationale*

1. Treat pain, if present, ***to prevent hypoventilation and atelectasis.*** Implement plan for Acute Pain Related to Transmission and Perception of Cutaneous, Visceral, Muscular, or Ischemic Impulses.
2. Position patient in high-Fowler's or semi-Fowler's position ***to promote diaphragmatic descent and maximal inhalation.***

3. Assist with deep-breathing exercises and incentive spirometry with sustained maximal inspiration 5 to 10 times/hr ***to help reinflate collapsed portions of lung.***
   - *Deep breathing*
     (1) Sit up straight or lean forward slightly while sitting on edge of bed or chair, if possible.
     (2) Take in slow, deep breath.
     (3) Pause slightly, or hold breath for at least 3 seconds.
     (4) Exhale slowly.
     (5) Rest, and repeat.
   - *Incentive spirometry*
     (1) Exhale normally.
     (2) Place lips around mouthpiece, and close mouth tightly around it.
     (3) Inhale slowly and as deeply as possible, noting maximal volume of air inspired.
     (4) Hold maximal inhalation for 3 seconds.
     (5) Take mouthpiece out of mouth, and slowly exhale.
     (6) Rest, and repeat.
4. Assist physician with intubation and initiation of mechanical ventilation as indicated.

Ineffective Breathing Pattern Related to Musculoskeletal Fatigue or Neuromuscular Impairment

Defining Characteristics

- Unequal chest movement
- Shortness of breath, dyspnea
- Use of accessory muscles
- Tachypnea
- Thoracoabdominal asynchrony
- Abnormal ABG values: increased $PaCO_2$, decreased pH
- Nasal flaring
- Assumption of 3-point position

Outcome Criteria

- Respiratory rate, rhythm, and depth return to baseline.
- Use of accessory muscles is minimal or absent.
- Chest expands symmetrically.
- ABG values return to baseline.

Nursing Interventions and *Rationale*

1. Prevent unnecessary exertion ***to limit drain on patient's ventilatory reserve.***

2. Instruct patient in energy-saving techniques ***to conserve patient's ventilatory reserve.***
3. Assist with pursed-lip and diaphragmatic breathing techniques ***to facilitate diaphragmatic descent and improved ventilation.***
   - *Diaphragmatic breathing*
     (1) Sit in upright position.
     (2) Place one hand on abdomen just above waist and other hand on upper chest.
     (3) Breathe in through nose, and feel lower hand push out; upper hand should not move.
     (4) Breathe out through pursed lips, and feel lower hand move in.
4. Position patient in high-Fowler's or semi-Fowler's position ***to promote diaphragmatic descent and maximal inhalation.***
5. Assist physician with intubation and initiation of mechanical ventilation as indicated.

NURSING MANAGEMENT PLAN

Ineffective Cardiopulmonary Tissue Perfusion

Definition: Decrease in oxygen resulting in failure to nourish tissues at capillary level.

Ineffective Cardiopulmonary Tissue Perfusion Related to Acute Myocardial Ischemia

Defining Characteristics

- Angina for more than 30 minutes
- ST-segment elevation on 12-lead electrocardiogram (ECG)
- Elevation of creatine kinase (CK) and CK-MB enzymes
- Apprehension

Outcome Criteria

- Systolic blood pressure (BP) is greater than 90 mm Hg.
- Mean arterial pressure (MAP) is greater than 60 mm Hg.
- Ventricular heart rate is less than 100 beats/min.
- Pulmonary artery (PA) pressures are within normal limits or back to baseline.
- Cardiac index (CI) is greater than 2.2 L /min/m^2.
- Urine output is greater than 0.5 ml/kg/hr or >30 ml/hr.
- 12-lead ECG is normalized without new Q waves.
- Angina is absent.
- CK and CK-MB enzymes are within normal range.
- Patient and family are educated about coronary artery disease (CAD) risk factor modification.

Nursing Interventions and *Rationale*

1. Initiate interventions to control pain.
   - Evaluate 12-lead ECG for signs of myocardial ischemia.
   - Collaborate with physician regarding administration of sublingual nitroglycerin (NTG) and intravenous (IV) NTG infusion *to control pain.*
     — Titrate IV NTG infusion.
     — Maintain systolic BP greater than 90 mm Hg.
   - Collaborate with physician regarding administration of IV morphine.
2. Initiate interventions to decrease myocardial oxygen demand.

- Administer oxygen at 2 L/min to achieve oxygen saturation (SpO$_2$) greater than 92%.
- Promote bed rest, with head of bed elevated 45 degrees.

3. Initiate interventions to lyse clot in coronary artery.
   - Collaborate with physician regarding administration of low-dose aspirin (80 mg to 325 mg) by mouth (PO).
     or
   - Collaborate with physician regarding administration of a thrombolytic agent *to lyse clot in coronary artery.* Maintain systolic BP at greater than 90 mm Hg.
   - Collaborate with physician and pharmacist regarding infusion of IV heparin and monitoring of coagulation studies (activated clotting time, partial thromboplastin time) *to prevent recurrent thrombosis.*
   - Prepare for cardiac catheterization and emergency angioplasty/atherectomy *to remove coronary thrombus.*
4. Monitor patient's hemodynamic and cardiac rhythm status
   - Evaluate cardiac rhythm for presence of dysrhythmias.
     — Collaborate with physician regarding administration of antidysrhythmics.
   - Assess serum electrolytes (potassium, magnesium) and arterial blood gases (ABGs).
     — Collaborate with physician regarding administration of electrolytes *to correct any imbalances.*
   - Monitor ST segment continuously *to determine changes in myocardial tissue perfusion.*
   - Monitor patient's BP at least every hour *because many conditions* (drugs, dysrhythmias, myocardial ischemia) *may cause hypotension* (systolic BP <90 mm Hg).
   - Treat symptomatic dysrhythmias according to unit's emergency protocol or advanced cardiac life support (ACLS) guidelines.

NURSING MANAGEMENT PLAN

Ineffective Cerebral Tissue Perfusion

Definition: Decrease in oxygen resulting in failure to nourish tissues at capillary level.

Ineffective Cerebral Tissue Perfusion Related to Hemorrhage or Vasospasm

Defining Characteristics
Hemorrhage

- Aneurysm grading system according to Hunt and Hess
  — *Grade I*
    - Minimal bleed
    - Asymptomatic or minimal headache
    - Slight nuchal rigidity
  — *Grade II*
    - Mild bleed
    - Moderate to severe headache

- Nuchal rigidity
- Minimal neurologic deficit (e.g., cranial nerve palsies most common: unilateral pupillary dilation, ptosis, dysconjugate gaze)
  — *Grade III*
    - Moderate bleed
    - Drowsiness
    - Confusion
    - Nuchal rigidity
    - Possible mild focal neurologic deficits

Continued

NURSING MANAGEMENT PLAN

Ineffective Cerebral Tissue Perfusion—cont'd

— *Grade IV*
  - Moderate to severe bleed
  - Extremely decreased level of consciousness, stupor
  - Possible moderate to severe hemiparesis
  - Possible early posturing (decorticate or decerebrate)
— *Grade V*
  - Severe bleed
  - Profound coma
  - Posturing
  - Moribund appearance
  - Pathologic reflexes resulting from meningeal irritation
— *Kerning sign*: Resistance to full extension of leg at knee when hip is flexed
— *Brudzinski sign*: Flexion of hip and knee during passive neck flexion
— Photophobia
— Nausea and vomiting

Vasospasm
- Worsening headache
- Confusion and decreasing level of consciousness
- Focal motor deficits such as unilateral weakness of extremities
- Speech deficits such as slurring or receptive or expressive aphasia
- Increasing blood pressure (BP)

Outcome Criteria
- Patient is oriented to time, place, person, and situation.
- Pupils are equal and normoreactive.
- BP is within patient's norm.
- Motor function is bilaterally equal.
- Headache, nausea, and vomiting are absent.
- Patient verbalizes importance of and displays compliance with reduced activity.

Nursing Interventions and *Rationale*
1. Assess for indicators of increased intracranial pressure (ICP) and brain herniation (see plan for Decreased Intracranial Adaptive Capacity Related to Failure of Normal Intracranial Compensatory Mechanism). *ICP will increase during vasospasm only when caused by edema resulting from brain infarction.*
2. Collaborate with physician regarding administration of hypertensive-hypervolemic therapy *to prevent vasospasm.*
   - Administer crystalloid and colloid intravenous (IV) fluids.
   - Monitor pulmonary artery occlusion pressure (PAOP), pulmonary artery diastolic pressure, systemic vascular resistance (SVR), and BP to achieve and maintain prescribed parameters.
3. Monitor lung sounds and chest radiograph reports *because of risk of pulmonary edema associated with fluid overload.*
4. Anticipate administration of nimodipine *to decrease cerebral vasospasm.*
5. Initiate subarachnoid precautions *to prevent rebleeding.*
   - Ensure bed rest in quiet environment *to lessen external stimuli.*
   - Maintain darkened room *to lessen symptoms of photophobia.*
   - Restrict visitors, and instruct them to keep conversation as nonstressful as possible.
   - Administer prescribed sedatives as needed *to reduce anxiety and to promote rest.*
   - Administer analgesics as prescribed *to relieve or lessen headache.*
   - Provide soft, high-fiber diet and stool softeners *to prevent constipation, which can lead to straining and increased risk of rebleeding.*
   - Assist with activities of daily living (ADLs: feeding, bathing, dressing, toileting).
   - Avoid any activity that could lead to increased ICP; ensure that patient does not flex hips beyond 90 degrees and avoids neck hyperflexion, hyperextension, or lateral hyperrotation *that could impede jugular venous return.*

NURSING MANAGEMENT PLAN

Ineffective Coping

Definition: Inability to form a valid appraisal of the stressors, inadequate choices of practiced responses, and/or inability to use available resources.

Ineffective Coping Related to Situational Crisis and Personal Vulnerability

Defining Characteristics
- Verbalization of inability to cope (e.g., "I can't take this anymore," "I don't know how to deal with this.")
- Ineffective problem solving, "problem lumping" (e.g., "I have to eliminate salt from my diet," "They tell me I can no longer mow the lawn," "This hospitalization is costing a mint; what about my kids' future?" "Who's going to change the oil in the car?" "This is an incredible amount of time away from work.")
- Ineffective use of coping mechanisms
  - *Projection*: Blames others for illness or pain.
  - *Displacement*: Directs anger and/or aggression toward family (e.g., "Get out of here," "Leave me alone"); cursing, shouting, or demanding attention; striking out or throwing objects.
  - *Denial*: Denies severity of illness and need for treatment.

NURSING MANAGEMENT PLAN

Ineffective Coping—cont'd

- Noncompliance (e.g., activity restriction, refusal to allow treatment/take medications)
- Suicidal thoughts (verbalizes desire to end life)
- Self-directed aggression (e.g., disconnects or attempts to disconnect life-sustaining equipment; deliberately tries to harm self)
- Failure to progress from dependent to more independent state (refusal or resistance to care for self)

Outcome Criteria

- Patient verbalizes beginning ability to cope with illness, pain, and hospitalization (e.g., "I'm trying to do the best I can," "I want to help myself get better.")
- Patient demonstrates effective problem solving (lists and prioritizes problems from most urgent to least urgent).
- Patient uses effective behavioral strategies to manage stress of illness and care.
- Patient demonstrates interest or involvement in illness or environment.
  — Requests medications when anticipating pain.
  — Questions course of treatment, progress, and prognosis.
  — Asks for clarification of environmental stimuli and events.
  — Seeks out supportive individuals in environment.
  — Uses coping mechanisms and strategies more effectively to manage situational crisis.
  — Demonstrates significant reduction in impulsive, angry, or aggressive outbursts (projection, shouting, cursing) directed toward family.
  — Verbalizes futuristic plans, with cessation of self-directed aggressive acts and suicidal thoughts.
  — Willingly complies with treatment regimen.
  — Begins to participate in self-care.

Nursing Interventions and *Rationale*

1. Actively listen and respond to patient's verbal and behavioral expressions. *Active listening signifies unconditional respect and acceptance for the patient as a worthwhile individual. It builds trust and rapport, guides the nurse toward problem areas, encourages the patient to express concerns, and promotes compliance.*
2. Offer effective coping strategies to help patient better tolerate stressors related to illness and care. Give permission to vent feelings in a safe setting (e.g., "I don't blame you for feeling angry or frustrated," "Others who are ill like you have expressed similar feelings," "I will listen to anything you want to share with me," "We don't have to talk; I'd like to sit here with you," "It's perfectly OK to cry"). *Individuals who are provided with opportunities to express their feelings will be better able to release pent-up emotions and derive a greater sense of relief and comfort. Thus they are less likely to resort to overimpulsive, aggressive acts, which may harm self or others.*
3. Inform family of patient's need to displace anger occasionally but that you will be working to help patient release feelings in more constructive, effective way. *Family members who are*

well informed are better equipped to cope with their loved one's emotional anguish and outbursts. They are less likely to waste energy on feelings of guilt, fear, anger, or despair and can use their strength to help the patient in more constructive ways. The knowledge that their loved one is being cared for emotionally, as well as physically, will offer family members a greater sense of comfort and understanding. They will feel nurtured and respected by the nurse's attempt to include them in the process.

4. With patient, list and number problems from the most to least urgent. Assist patient in finding immediate solutions for most urgent problems; postpone those that can wait; delegate some to family members; and help patient acknowledge problems that are beyond patient's control. *Listing and numbering problems in an organized fashion help to break them down into more manageable "pieces" so that the patient is better able to identify solutions for those that are solvable and to suppress those that are less relevant or not amenable to interventions.*
5. Identify individuals in patient's environment who best help patient to cope, as well as those who do not. Validate your observations with patient (e.g., "I notice you seemed more relaxed during your daughter's visit," "After the clergy left, you were able to sleep a bit longer than usual; would you like to see him more often?" "Your grandson was a bit upset today; I'll be glad to talk to him if you like"). *Supportive persons can invoke a calming effect on the patient's physiologic and psychologic states. Conversely, well-meaning but nonsupportive individuals can have a deleterious effect on the patient's ability to cope and must be carefully screened and counseled by the nurse.*
6. Teach patient effective cognitive strategies to help patient better manage the stress of critical illness and care. Help patient construct pleasant thoughts, situations, or images that can simultaneously inhibit unpleasant realities (e.g., day at beach, walk in park, drinking glass of wine, being with loved one). *Pleasant thoughts and images constructed during critical illness and care tend to inhibit or reduce the intensity of the unpleasant, stressful effects of the experience.*
7. Assist patient in using coping mechanisms more effectively so that patient can better manage situational crisis.
   - Suppression of problems beyond patient's control.
   - Compensation for illness and its effects; focusing on patient's strengths, interests, family, and spiritual beliefs.
   - Adaptive displacement of anger, fear, or frustration through healthy, verbal expressions to staff. *Effective use of coping mechanisms helps to assuage the patient's painful feelings in a safe setting. Thus the patient is strengthened and need not resort to the use of more ineffective defenses to eliminate anxiety.*
8. Initiate suicidal assessment if patient verbalizes desire to die, states that life is not worth living, or exhibits self-directed aggression.

Continued

NURSING MANAGEMENT PLAN

Ineffective Coping—cont'd

- "We know that this is a bad time for you. You're saying repeatedly that you want to die. Are you planning to harm yourself?"
- If the response is "yes," remain with the patient, alert staff members, and provide for psychiatric consultation as soon as possible. Continue to express concern to patient and protect patient from harm.
- *Suicidal thoughts as a result of ineffective coping or exhaustion of coping devices are not uncommon in critically ill patients. If the mood state is distressing enough, a patient may seek relief by attempting a self-destructive act. Although the patient may not imminently have the energy to* succeed *in the attempt, voicing a specific plan signifies a depressed mood state and depletion of coping strategies. Thus immediate intervention is needed, since the attempt may be successful when the patient's energy is restored.*

9. Encourage patient to participate in self-care activities and treatment regimen in accordance with patient's level of progress. Offer praise for patient's efforts toward self-care. *Patients who take an active role in their own treatment and progress are less apt to feel like helpless or powerless victims. This greater sense of control over their illness and environment will guide them more swiftly toward becoming as independent as possible.*

NURSING MANAGEMENT PLAN

Ineffective Peripheral Tissue Perfusion

Definition: Decrease in oxygen resulting in failure to nourish tissues at capillary level.

Ineffective Peripheral Tissue Perfusion Related to Decreased Peripheral Blood Flow

Defining Characteristics

- Weak and unequal peripheral pulses
- Delayed capillary refill
- Ischemic pain from extremity
- Cool skin on extremity
- Pale extremity
- Paresthesias from extremity

Outcome Criteria

- Peripheral pulses are full and equal bilaterally.
- Capillary refill is equal bilaterally.
- Ischemic pain is absent.
- Skin temperature is equal in both extremities.
- Skin is pink and warm in both extremities.
- Paresthesias are absent.

Nursing Interventions and *Rationale*

1. Collaborate with physician regarding the administration of antiplatelet, anticoagulant, and thrombolytic therapy.

2. Collaborate with physician regarding pain management. Implement plan for Acute Pain Related to Transmission and Perception of Cutaneous, Visceral, Muscular, or Ischemic Impulses.
3. Ensure patient is adequately hydrated *to decrease blood viscosity.*
4. Maintain affected extremity in dependent position if possible *to enhance blood flow.*
5. Keep affected extremity warm and protect it from injury. Do not apply heat directly to the affected extremity *because this can result in injury.*
6. Maintain surveillance for pain, pallor, pulselessness, paresthesia, paralysis, and poikilothermia *as indicators of abrupt change in blood flow.*
7. Maintain surveillance for tissue breakdown and arterial ulcers *as indicators of injury.*
8. Prepare patient for possible surgery or interventional procedure to restore blood flow.

NURSING MANAGEMENT PLAN

Ineffective Renal Tissue Perfusion

Definition: Decrease in oxygen resulting in failure to nourish tissues at capillary level.

Ineffective Renal Tissue Perfusion Related to Decreased Renal Blood Flow

Defining Characteristics

- Anuria or oliguria
- Decreased urinary creatinine clearance
- Increased serum creatinine
- Increased blood urea nitrogen (BUN)

- Electrolyte abnormalities ($\uparrow K^+$, $\downarrow Na^+$)
- Increased mean arterial presssure (MAP), pulmonary artery occlusion pressure (PAOP), pulmonary artery diastolic pressure (PADP), and central venous pressure (CVP) secondary to fluid overload

NURSING MANAGEMENT PLAN

Ineffective Renal Tissue Perfusion—cont'd

- Sinus tachycardia
- Metabolic acidosis
- Crackles on lung auscultation
- Engorged neck veins
- Fluid weight gain
- Pitting edema
- Mental status changes
- Anemia

Outcome Criteria

- Cardiac output (CO) is greater than 4.0 L/min.
- Cardiac index (CI) is greater than 2.2 L/min/m^2.
- MAP, PAOP, PADP, and CVP are within normal limits for patient.
- Electrolytes are within normal range.
- Serum creatinine and BUN are within normal range.
- Normal acid-base balance.
- Level of consciousness is normal.
- Lungs are clear on auscultation.
- Urine output is within normal limits, or patient is stable on dialysis.
- Hemoglobin and hematocrit values are stable.

Nursing Interventions and *Rationale*

1. Monitor intake and output, urine output, and patient weight.
2. Collaborate with physician regarding administration of crystalloids, colloids, blood, and blood products *to increase circulating volume and maintain MAP greater than 70 mm Hg.*
3. Collaborate with physician regarding administration of inotropes *to enhance myocardial contractility and increase CI to greater than 2.5 L/min.*
4. Collaborate with physician regarding administration of diuretics to oliguric patient *to flush out cellular debris and increase urine output.*
5. Minimize patient's exposure to nephrotoxic drugs *to decrease damage to kidneys.*
6. Monitor blood levels of drugs cleared by kidneys *to avoid accumulation.*
7. Monitor patient for signs of electrolyte imbalance due to impaired electrolyte regulation.
8. Maintain surveillance for signs and symptoms of fluid overload.
9. Monitor patient's clinical status and response to dialysis *to ensure patient is receiving safe and effective therapy.*

NURSING MANAGEMENT PLAN

Powerlessness

Definition: Perception that one's own action will not significantly affect an outcome; a perceived lack of control over a current situation or immediate happening.

Powerlessness Related to Lack of Control over Current Situation and/or Disease Progression

Defining Characteristics

Severe

- Verbal expressions of having no control or influence over situation
- Verbal expressions of having no control or influence over outcome
- Verbal expressions of having no control over self-care
- Depression over physical deterioration that occurs despite patient's compliance with regimens
- Apathy

Moderate

- Nonparticipation in care or decision making when opportunities are provided
- Expressions of dissatisfaction and frustration about inability to perform previous tasks and/or activities
- Lack of progress monitoring
- Expressions of doubt about role performance
- Reluctance to express true feelings, fearing alienation from caregivers
- Passivity
- Inability to seek information about care

- Dependence on others that may result in irritability, resentment, anger, or guilt
- No defense of self-care practices when challenged

Low

- Passivity

Outcome Criteria

- Patient verbalizes increased control over situation by wanting "to do things my way."
- Patient actively participates in planning care.
- Patient requests needed information.
- Patient chooses to participate in self-care activities.
- Patient monitors progress.

Nursing Interventions and *Rationale*

1. Evaluate patient's feelings and perception of the reasons for lack of power and sense of helplessness.
2. Determine as much as possible the patient's usual response to limited control situations. Determine through ongoing assessment the patient's usual locus of control.

Continued

NURSING MANAGEMENT PLAN

Powerlessness—cont'd

- Believes that influence over life is exerted by luck, fate, and powerful persons (*external locus of control*).
- Believes that influence is exerted through personal choices, self-effort, and self-determination (*internal locus of control*).

3. Support patient's physical control of environment by involving patient in care activities; knock before entering room if appropriate; ask permission before moving personal belongings. Inform patient that, although an activity may not be to patient's liking, it is necessary. *Gives patient permission to express dissatisfaction with environment and regimen.*

4. Personalize patient's care using preferred name *to support patient's psychologic control.*

5. Provide therapeutic rationale for all requested self-care activities and for all staff actions. Reinforce physician's explanations; clarify misconceptions about illness situation and treatment plans. *Supports patient's cognitive control.*

6. Include patient in care planning by encouraging participation and allowing choices wherever possible (e.g., timing of personal care activities; deciding when pain medicines are needed). Point out situations in which no choices exist.

7. Provide opportunities for patient to exert influence over self and body, thereby affecting an outcome. For example, share with the patient the nurse's assessment of patient's breath sounds and explain that sounds can be improved by self-

initiated deep-breathing exercises. *Feedback that the patient has been successful in helping clear lungs reinforces the influence that patient does retain.*

8. Encourage family to permit patient to do as much independently as possible *to foster perception of personal power.*

9. Assist patient to establish realistic short-term and long-term goals. *Setting unrealistic or unattainable goals inadvertently reinforces patient's perception of powerlessness.*

10. Document care to provide for continuity *so that patient can maintain appropriate control over environment.*

11. Assist patient to regain strength and activity tolerance as appropriate, *thus increasing a sense of control and self-reliance.*

12. Increase sensitivity of health care team members and significant others to the patient's sense of powerlessness. Use power over the patient carefully. Use the words "must," "should," and "have to" with caution *because these words communicate coercive powers and imply that the objects of "musts" and "shoulds" are of benefit to the nurse versus the patient.*

13. Plan with patient for transfer from critical care unit to intermediate unit and eventually to home.

NURSING MANAGEMENT PLAN

Risk for Aspiration

Definition: At risk for entry of gastrointestinal secretions, oropharyngeal secretions, solids, or fluids into tracheobronchial passages.

Risk Factors

- Impaired laryngeal sensation or reflex
- Reduced level of consciousness
- Extubation
- Impaired pharyngeal peristalsis or tongue function
  — Neuromuscular dysfunction
  — Central nervous system (CNS) dysfunction
  — Head or neck injury
- Impaired laryngeal closure or elevation
  — Laryngeal nerve dysfunction
  — Artificial airways
  — Gastrointestinal (GI) tubes
- Increased gastric volume
  — Delayed gastric emptying
  — Enteral feedings
  — Medication administration

- Increased intragastric pressure
  — Upper abdominal surgery
  — Obesity
  — Pregnancy
  — Ascites
- Decreased lower esophageal sphincter pressure
  — Increased gastric acidity
  — GI tubes
- Decreased antegrade esophageal propulsion
  — Trendelenburg or supine position
  — Esophageal dysmotility
  — Esophageal structural defects or lesions

Outcome Criteria

- Breath sounds are normal, or there is no change in patient's baseline breath sounds.

NURSING MANAGEMENT PLAN

Risk for Aspiration—cont'd

- Arterial blood gas (ABG) values remain within patient's baseline.
- There is no evidence of gastric contents in lung secretions.

Nursing Interventions and *Rationale*

1. Assess GI function *to rule out hypoactive peristalsis and abdominal distention*.
2. Position patient with head of bed elevated 30 degrees *to prevent gastric reflux through gravity*. If head elevation is contraindicated, position patient in right lateral decubitus position *to facilitate passage of gastric contents across the pylorus*.
3. Maintain patency and functioning of nasogastric suction apparatus *to prevent accumulation of gastric contents*.
4. Provide frequent and scrupulous mouth care *to prevent colonization of oropharynx with bacteria and inoculation of lower airways*.
5. Ensure that endotracheal/tracheostomy cuff is properly inflated *to limit aspiration of oropharyngeal secretions*.
6. Treat nausea promptly; collaborate with physician on an order for antiemetic *to prevent vomiting and resultant aspiration*.

Additional Interventions for Patient Receiving Continuous or Intermittent Enteral Tube Feedings

7. Position patient with head of bed elevated 45 degrees *to prevent gastric reflux*. If a head-down position becomes necessary at any time, interrupt the feeding 30 minutes before the position change.
8. Check placement of feeding tube either by auscultation or radiographically at regular intervals (e.g., before administering intermittent feedings and after position changes, suctioning, coughing episodes, or vomiting) *to ensure proper placement of the tube*.
9. Monitor patient for signs of delayed gastric emptying *to decrease potential for vomiting and aspiration*.
   - For large-bore tubes, check residuals of tube feedings before intermittent feedings and every 4 hours during continuous feedings. Consider withholding feedings for residuals greater than 150% of the hourly rate (continuous feeding) or greater than 50% of the previous feeding (intermittent feeding).
   - For small-bore tubes, observe abdomen for distention, palpate abdomen for hardness or tautness, and auscultate abdomen for bowel sounds.

NURSING MANAGEMENT PLAN

Risk for Infection

Definition: At increased risk for being invaded by pathogenic organisms.

Risk Factors

- Inadequate primary defenses (broken skin, traumatized tissue, decreased ciliary action, stasis of body fluids, change in pH secretions, altered peristalsis)
- Inadequate secondary defenses (decreased hemoglobin, leukopenia, suppressed inflammatory/immune response)
- Immunocompromise
- Inadequate acquired immunity
- Tissue destruction and increased environmental exposure
- Chronic disease
- Invasive procedures
- Malnutrition
- Pharmacologic agents (antibiotics, steroids)

Outcome Criteria

- Total lymphocyte count is greater than $1000/mm^3$.
- White blood cell count is within normal limits.
- Temperature is within normal limits.
- Blood, urine, wound, and sputum cultures are negative.

Nursing Interventions and *Rationale*

1. Wash hands before and after patient care to reduce the transmission of microorganisms.
   - Wet hands.
   - Apply 5 ml of soap and thoroughly distribute over both hands.
   - Vigorously wash hands for 10 to 15 seconds.
   - Rinse and thoroughly dry hands.
2. Use aseptic technique for insertion and manipulation of invasive monitoring devices, intravenous (IV) lines, and urinary drainage catheters *to maintain sterility of environment*.
3. Stabilize all invasive lines and catheters *to avoid unintentional manipulation and contamination*.
4. Use aseptic technique for dressing changes *to prevent contamination of wounds or insertion sites*.
5. Change any line placed under emergent conditions within 24 hours *because aseptic technique is usually breached during an emergency*.
6. Collaborate with physician to change any dressing that is saturated with blood or drainage *because these are media for microorganism growth*.
7. Minimize use of stopcocks and maintain caps on all stopcock ports *to reduce the ports of entry for microorganisms*.
8. Avoid the use of nasogastric tubes, nasoendotracheal tubes, and nasopharyngeal suctioning in patient with suspected cerebrospinal fluid leak *to decrease the incidence of central nervous system infection*.

Continued

NURSING MANAGEMENT PLAN

Risk for Infection—cont'd

9. Change ventilator circuits with humidifiers no more often than every 48 hours *to avoid introducing microorganisms into the system.*
10. Provide the patient with a clean manual resuscitation bag *to avoid cross-contamination between patients.*
11. Provide meticulous mouth care at least every 4 hours and suction oropharyngeal subglottic secretions as needed *to avoid accumulation.*
12. Cleanse in-line suction catheters with sterile saline according to manufacturer's instructions *to avoid accumulation of secretions within the catheter.*
13. Use disposable sterile scissors, forceps, and hemostats *to reduce the transmission of microorganisms.*

14. Maintain a closed urinary drainage system *to decrease incidence of urinary infections.*
15. Keep urinary drainage tubing and bag below level of patient's bladder *to prevent backflow of urine.*
16. Assess urinary drainage tubing for kinks *to prevent stasis of urine.*
17. Protect all access device sites from potential sources of contamination (nasogastric reflux, draining wounds, ostomies, sputum).
18. Refrigerate parenteral nutrition solutions and opened enteral nutrition formulas *to inhibit bacterial growth.*
19. Maintain daily surveillance of invasive devices for signs and symptoms of infection.

NURSING MANAGEMENT PLAN

Situational Low Self-Esteem

Definition: Development of negative perception of self-worth in response to current situation.

Situational Low Self-Esteem Related to Feelings of Guilt about Physical Deterioration

Defining Characteristics
- Inability to accept positive reinforcement
- Lack of follow-through
- Nonparticipation in therapy
- Not taking responsibility for self-care (self-neglect)
- Self-destructive behavior
- Lack of eye contact

Outcome Criteria
- Patient verbalizes feelings of self-worth.
- Patient maintains positive relationships with significant others.
- Patient manifests active interest in appearance by completing personal grooming daily.

Nursing Interventions and *Rationale*
1. Evaluate meaning of health-related situation.
   - How does the patient feel about himself or herself, the diagnosis, and the treatment?
   - How does the present fit into the larger context of his or her life?
2. Assess patient's emotional level, interpersonal relationships, and feelings about self. Recognize patient's uniqueness (how hair is worn, preference for name used).
3. Help patient discover and verbalize feelings and understand the crisis by listening and providing information.

4. Assist patient to identify strengths and positive qualities that increase sense of self-worth. Focus on past experiences of accomplishment and competency. Help patient with positive self-reinforcement. Reinforce the obvious love and affection of family and significant others.
5. Assess coping techniques that have been helpful in the past. Help the patient decide how to handle negative or incongruent feedback about the situation.
6. Encourage visits from family and significant others. Facilitate interactions, and ensure privacy. Help family members entering critical care unit by explaining what they will see. Increase visitors' comfort with equipment; offer chairs and other courtesies.
7. Encourage patient to pursue interest in individual or social activities, even though difficult in critical care unit.
8. Reflect caring, concern, empathy, respect, and unconditional acceptance in nurse-patient relationships.
9. Remember that for the patient, the nurse is a significant other who provides important appraisals of patient and who can facilitate change process.
10. Help family support patient's self-esteem.
11. Provide for continuity of nurse assignment to ensure consistent contacts that can *facilitate support of the patient's self-esteem.*

NURSING MANAGEMENT PLAN

Unilateral Neglect

Definition: Lack of awareness and attention to one side of the body.

Unilateral Neglect Related to Perceptual Disruption

Defining Characteristics

- Neglect of involved body parts and extrapersonal space
- Denial of existence of the affected limb or side of body
- Denial of hemiplegia or other motor and sensory deficits
- Left homonymous hemianopia
- Difficulty with spatial-perceptual tasks
- Left hemiplegia

Outcome Criteria

- Patient is safe and free from injury.
- Patient is able to identify safety hazards in the environment.
- Patient recognizes disability and describes physical deficits present (e.g., paralysis, weakness, numbness).
- Patient demonstrates ability to scan visual field to compensate for loss of function or sensation in affected limb(s).

Nursing Interventions and *Rationale*

1. Adapt environment to patient's deficits *to maintain patient safety*.
   - Position patient's bed with unaffected side facing door.
   - Approach and speak to patient from unaffected side. If patient must be approached from affected side, announce your presence as soon as entering the room *to avoid startling the patient*.
   - Position call light, bedside stand, and personal items on patient's unaffected side.
   - If patient will be assisted out of bed, simplify environment *to eliminate hazards* by removing unnecessary furniture and equipment.
   - Provide frequent reorientation of patient to environment.
   - Observe patient closely, and anticipate patient's needs. Despite repeated explanation, patient may have difficulty retaining information about the deficits.
   - When patient is in bed, elevate affected arm on a pillow *to prevent dependent edema* and support the hand in a position of function.
2. Assist patient to recognize the perceptual defect.
   - Encourage patient to wear any prescriptive corrective glasses or hearing aids *to facilitate communication*.
   - Instruct patient to turn head past midline *to view environment on affected side*.
   - Encourage patient to look at affected side and to stroke limbs with unaffected hand. Encourage handling of affected limbs *to reinforce awareness of affected side*.
   - Instruct patient to look for affected extremity when performing simple tasks *to know location of affected extremity at all times*.
   - After pointing to parts, have patient name the affected parts.

- Encourage patient to use self-exercises (e.g., lifting affected arm with unaffected hand).
- If patient unable to discriminate between concepts of "right" and "left," use descriptive adjectives such as "the weak arm," "the affected leg," or "the good arm" to refer to the body. Use gestures, not just words, to indicate right and left.
3. Collaborate with patient, physician, and rehabilitation team *to design and implement a beginning rehabilitation program for use during the critical care unit stay*.
   - Use adaptive equipment (braces, splints, slings) as appropriate.
   - Teach patient the individual components of any activity separately, then proceed to integrate the component parts into a completed activity.
   - Instruct patient to attend to affected side, if able, and to assist with bath or other tasks.
   - Use tactile stimulation *to reintroduce the arm or leg to the patient*. Rub affected parts with different textured materials *to stimulate sensations* (warm, cold, rough, soft).
   - Encourage activities that require patient to turn head toward affected side, and retrain patient to scan affected side and environment visually.
   - If patient is allowed out of bed, cue patient with reminders to scan visually when ambulating. Assist and remain in constant attendance *because patient may have difficulty maintaining correct posture, balance, and locomotion*. Patient may have vertical-horizontal perceptual problems, with patient leaning to affected side to align with the perceived vertical. Provide sitting, standing, and balancing exercises before assisting patient out of bed.
   - Assist patient with oral feedings.
     (1) Avoid giving patient very hot food items, **which could cause injury**.
     (2) Place patient in upright sitting position, if possible.
     (3) Encourage patient to feed self; if necessary, guide patient's hand to mouth.
     (4) If patient is able to feed self, place one dish at a time in front of patient. When patient is finished with first dish, add another dish. Tell patient what he or she is eating.
     (5) Initially place food in patient's visual field; then gradually move food out of field of vision, and teach patient to scan entire visual field.
     (6) When patient has learned to visually scan environment, offer a tray of food with various dishes.
     (7) Instruct patient to take small bites and to place food in unaffected side of mouth.
     (8) Teach patient to sweep out pockets of food with tongue after every bite *to eliminate retained food in affected side of mouth*.

Continued

NURSING MANAGEMENT PLAN

Unilateral Neglect—cont'd

(9) After meals or oral medications, check patient's oral cavity for pockets of retained material.

4. Initiate patient and family health teaching.
- Assess to ensure that both patient and family understand nature of neurologic deficits and purpose of rehabilitation plan.

- Teach proper application and use of adaptive equipment.
- Teach importance of maintaining a safe environment, and point out potential environmental hazards.
- Instruct family members how to facilitate relearning techniques (e.g., cueing, scanning visual fields).

Appendix

Physiologic Formulas for Critical Care

HEMODYNAMIC FORMULAS

Mean Arterial Pressure (MAP)

$$MAP = \frac{SBP + (2 \times DBP)}{3}$$

SBP = Systolic blood pressure (measured via arterial line or blood pressure cuff)
DBP = Diastolic blood pressure (measured via arterial line or blood pressure cuff)
Normal range: 70 to 100 mm Hg

Cardiac Index (CI)

$$CI = \frac{CO}{BSA}$$

CO = Cardiac output (measured via pulmonary artery catheter)
BSA = Body surface area (calculated value)
Normal range: 2.5 to 4.0 L/min/m^2

Stroke Volume (SV)

$$SV = \frac{CO}{HR} \times 1000$$

CO = Cardiac output (measured via pulmonary artery catheter)
HR = Heart rate (measured via bedside electrocardiogram)
Normal range: 60 to 100 ml/beat

Stroke Volume Index (SVI)

$$SVI = \frac{CI}{HR} \times 1000$$

CI = Cardiac index (calculated value)
HR = Heart rate (measured via bedside electrocardiogram)
Normal range: 33 to 47 ml/m^2/beat

Systemic Vascular Resistance (SVR)

$$SVR = \frac{MAP - RAP}{CO} \times 80$$

MAP = Mean arterial pressure (measured via arterial line or calculated value)

RAP = Right atrial mean pressure (measured via pulmonary artery catheter)
CO = Cardiac output (measured via pulmonary artery catheter)
Normal range: 800 to 1200 dynes/sec/cm^{-5}

Pulmonary Vascular Resistance (PVR)

$$PVR = \frac{PAMP - PAOP}{CO} \times 80$$

PAMP = Pulmonary artery mean pressure (measured via pulmonary artery catheter)
PAOP = Pulmonary artery occlusion pressure or "wedge" pressure (measured via pulmonary artery catheter)
CO = Cardiac output (measured via pulmonary artery catheter)
Normal range: less than 250 dynes/sec/cm^{-5}

Left Ventricular Stroke Work Index (LVSWI)

$$LVSWI = (MAP - PAOP) \times SVI \times 0.0136$$

MAP = Mean arterial pressure (measured via arterial line or calculated value)
PAOP = Pulmonary artery occlusion pressure or "wedge" pressure (measured via pulmonary artery catheter)
SVI = Stroke volume index (calculated value)
Normal range: 50 to 62 g-m/m^2/beat

Right Ventricular Stroke Work Index (RVSWI)

$$RVSWI = (PAMP - RAP) \times SVI \times 0.0136$$

PAMP = Pulmonary artery mean pressure (measured via pulmonary artery catheter)
RAP = Right atrial mean pressure (measured via pulmonary artery catheter)
SVI = Stroke volume (calculated value)
Normal range: 5.0 to 10.0 g-m/m^2/beat

Corrected QT Interval (QTc)

$$QTc = \frac{QT}{\sqrt{RR}}$$

QT = QT interval
RR = R-to-R interval
Upper limit: 0.44 second

Body Mass Index (BMI)

Body Mass Index = Weight(kg) / Height(m)^2

Body Surface Area (BSA)

To calculate (Figure A-1):
1. Obtain patient's height and weight.
2. Mark height on the left scale and weight on the right scale.
3. Draw a straight line between the two points marked on each scale.

The number where the line crosses the middle scale is the BSA value.

PULMONARY FORMULAS
Shunt Equation (Qs/Qt)

$$\text{division rule} = \frac{Qs}{Qt} = \frac{Cc_{O_2} - Ca_{O_2}}{Cc_{O_2} - Cv_{O_2}}$$

Cc_{O_2} = Capillary oxygen content (calculated value)
Ca_{O_2} = Arterial oxygen content (calculated value)
Cv_{O_2} = Venous oxygen content (calculated value)
Normal range: less than 5%

Capillary Oxygen Content (Cco$_2$)

$$Cc_{O_2} = (Hgb \times 1.34 \times Sc_{O_2}) + (Pc_{O_2} \times 0.003)$$

Hgb = Hemoglobin (measured via laboratory sample or arterial blood gas)
Sc_{O_2} = Pulmonary capillary oxygen saturation
Pc_{O_2} = Partial pressure of oxygen in capillary blood

Arterial Oxygen Content (Cao$_2$)

$$Ca_{O_2} = (Hgb \times 1.34 \times Sa_{O_2}) + (0.003 \times Pa_{O_2})$$

Hgb = Hemoglobin (measured via laboratory sample or arterial blood gas)
Sa_{O_2} = Arterial oxygen saturation (measured via arterial blood gas)
Pa_{O_2} = Partial pressure of oxygen in arterial blood (measured via arterial blood gas)
Normal range: 17 to 20 ml/dl

Venous Oxygen Content (Cvo$_2$)

$$Cv_{O_2} = (Hgb \times 1.34 \times Sv_{O_2}) + (0.003 \times Pv_{O_2})$$

Hgb = Hemoglobin (measured via laboratory sample or arterial blood gas)
Sv_{O_2} = Mixed venous oxygen saturation (measured via mixed venous blood gas)

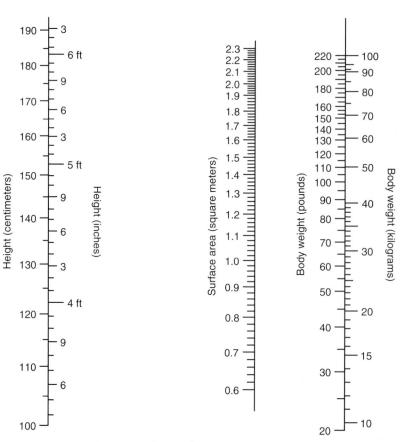

Figure A-1   Body surface area (BSA) nomogram.

Pv_{O_2} = Partial pressure of oxygen in mixed venous blood (measured via mixed venous blood gas)
Normal range: 12 to 15 ml/dl

Alveolar Pressure of Oxygen (PaO$_2$)

$$P_{AO_2} = F_{IO_2} \times (Pb - P_{H_2O}) - Pa_{CO_2}/RQ$$

F_{IO_2} = Fraction of inspired oxygen (obtained from oxygen settings)
Pb = Barometric pressure (assumed to be 760 mm Hg at sea level)
P_{H_2O} = Water pressure in the lungs (assumed to be 47 mm Hg)
Pa_{CO_2} = Partial pressure of carbon dioxide in arterial blood (measured via arterial blood gas)
RQ = Respiratory quotient (assumed to be 0.8)
Normal range: 60 to 100 mm Hg

Arterial/Inspired Oxygen Ratio

$$Pa_{O_2}/F_{IO_2} \text{ ratio} = \frac{Pa_{O_2}}{F_{IO_2}}$$

Pa_{O_2} = Partial pressure of oxygen in arterial blood (measured via arterial blood gas)
F_{IO_2} = Fraction of inspired oxygen (obtained from oxygen settings)
Normal range: greater than 286

Arterial/Alveolar Oxygen Ratio

$$Pa_{O_2}/P_{AO_2} \text{ ratio} = \frac{Pa_{O_2}}{P_{AO_2}}$$

Pa_{O_2} = Partial pressure of oxygen in arterial blood (measured via arterial blood gas)
P_{AO_2} = Partial pressure of oxygen in alveoli (calculated value)
Normal range: greater than 60%

Alveolar-Arterial Gradient

$$P(A\text{-}a)_{O_2} = P_{AO_2} - Pa_{O_2}$$

P_{AO_2} = Partial pressure of oxygen in alveoli (calculated value)
Pa_{O_2} = Partial pressure of oxygen in arterial blood (measured via arterial blood gas)
Normal range: 0 to 20 mm Hg

Dead Space Equation (Vd/Vt)

$$\frac{Vd}{Vt} = \frac{Pa_{CO_2} - Pet_{CO_2}}{Pa_{CO_2}}$$

Pa_{CO_2} = Partial pressure of carbon dioxide in arterial blood (measured via arterial blood gas)
Pet_{CO_2} = Partial pressure of carbon dioxide in exhaled gas (measured via end-tidal CO_2 monitor)
Normal range: 2 to 0.4 (20% to 40%)

Static Compliance (C$_{ST}$)

This value is calculated for mechanically ventilated patients.

$$C_{ST} = \frac{Vt}{PP - PEEP}$$

Vt = Tidal volume (obtained from ventilator)
PP = Plateau pressure (measured via ventilator)
PEEP = Positive end-expiratory pressure (obtained from ventilator)
Normal value: greater than 50 ml/cm H_2O

Dynamic Compliance (C$_{DY}$)

Also called *characteristic*, this value is calculated for mechanically ventilated patients.

$$C_{DY} = \frac{Vt}{PIP - PEEP}$$

Vt = Tidal volume (obtained from ventilator)
PIP = Peak inspiratory pressure (obtained from ventilator)
PEEP = Positive end-expiratory pressure (obtained from ventilator)
Normal value: 40 to 50 ml/cm H_2O

NEUROLOGIC FORMULA
Cerebral Perfusion Pressure (CPP)

$$CCP = MAP - ICP$$

MAP = Mean arterial pressure (measured via arterial line or blood pressure cuff)
ICP = Intracranial pressure (measured via ICP monitoring device)
Normal range: 70 to 150 mm Hg

ENDOCRINE FORMULA
Serum Osmolality

$$\text{Serum Osmolality} = 2\,(Na^+ + K^+) + \frac{Glucose}{18} + \frac{BUN}{2.8}$$

Na^+ = Sodium
K^+ = Potassium
BUN = Blood urea nitrogen
Normal range: 280 to 300 mOsm/kg of water

RENAL FORMULA
Renal Clearance

$$\text{Clearance} = [U] \times \frac{V}{[P]}$$

[U] = Concentration of substance in urine
V = Time
[P] = Concentration of substance in plasma
Normal range: dependent on substance measured

NUTRITIONAL FORMULAS*

Estimate of Caloric Needs

Step 1. Calculate basal energy expenditure (BEE). This is the energy needed for basic life processes, such as respiratory function and maintenance of body temperature.

$$Women: BEE = 795 + 7.18 \times Weight\ (kg)$$

$$Men: BEE = 879 + 10.20 \times Weight\ (kg)$$

Step 2. Multiply by an appropriate stress factor to meet needs of ill or injured patient (see the following table). If patient has more than one stress present (e.g., burn and pneumonia), use only the stress factor for the *highest level* of stress.

Estimate of Protein Needs

Protein needs vary with degree of malnutrition and stress (see the following table).

Example of Calculation of Caloric and Protein Needs

A 28-year-old female patient has a fracture of the left femur and burns of 40% of her BSA after a motor vehicle crash. Her height is 1.65 m (5 ft 5 in) and her weight is 59.1 kg (130 lb).

Energy needs

1. BEE = 795 + 7.18 × 59.1 = 1219 calories/day
2. Energy needs for injury = 1219 calories × 1.75 = 2133 calories/day

Protein needs

Protein needs = 59.1 kg × 1.75 g = 103 g/day

Type of Stress	Multiply Value from Step 2 by:
Fever	1 + 0.13/° C elevation above normal (or 0.07/° F)
Pneumonia	1.2
Major injury	1.3
Severe sepsis	1.5
Burn 15%-30% BSA	
Burn 31%-49% BSA	1.5-2.0
Burn 50% or greater BSA	1.8-2.1

BSA, Body surface area.

Condition	Multiply Desirable Body Weight (kg) by:
Healthy individual	0.8-1.0 g protein
Well-nourished elective surgery patient	
Malnourished or catabolic state	1.2 to 2+ g protein
• Sepsis	
• Major injury	
Burns	
• 15%-30% BSA	1.5 g protein
• 31%-49% BSA	1.5-2.0 g protein
• 50% or greater BSA	2.0-2.5 g protein

BSA, Body surface area.

*Data from Deitch EA: *Crit Care Clin* 11:735, 1995; Owen OE et al: *Am J Clin Nutr* 4:1, 1986; Owen OE et al: *Am J Clin Nutr* 46:875, 1987; Garrel DR, Jobin N, de Jonge LH: *Nutr Clin Pract* 11:99, 1996.

Index